Essential Guide to the Cervical Spine – Volume 2

CLINICAL SYNDROMES AND MANIPULATIVE TREATMENT

RAFAEL TORRES CUECO PHD PT

Professor, Department of Physiotherapy, University of Valencia, Spain
Director of Masters program on Manual Therapy, University of Valencia
President and founder of the Spanish Society of Physiotherapy and Pain (Sociedad Española de Fisioterapia y Dolor SEFID)
Facilitator, WCPT Physical Therapy Pain Network
Instructor, Neuro-Orthopaedic Institute (NOI)
Member of the Spanish Pain Society (Sociedad Española del Dolor SED), Spanish Society of Craneomandibular Dysfunction and Orofacial Pain (Sociedad Española de Disfunción Craneomandibular y Dolor Orofacial SEDCYDO) and the International Association for the Study of Pain (IASP)

FOREWORD BY
LORIMER MOSELEY PhD FACP

Professor of Clinical Neuroscience and Foundation Chair in Physiotherapy, The Sansom Institute for Health Research, University of South Australia, Adelaide, Australia
Senior Principal Research Fellow, Neuroscience Research Australia, Sydney, Australia
NHMRC Principal Research Fellow

ELSEVIER

Edinburgh   London   New York   Oxford   Philadelphia   St Louis   Sydney   Toronto   2017

ELSEVIER

ISBN 978-0-7020-4609-4 (Volume One)
ISBN 978-0-7020-4610-0
ISBN 978-0-7020-4608-7 (2-Volume Set)

British Library Cataloguing in Publication Data
A catalogue record for this book is available from the British Library

Library of Congress Cataloging in Publication Data
A catalog record for this book is available from the Library of Congress

---

Notice

Neither the Publisher nor the Editor assume any responsibility for any loss or injury and/or damage to persons or property arising out of or related to any use of the material contained in this book. It is the responsibility of the treating practitioner, relying on independent expertise and knowledge of the patient, to determine the best treatment and method of application for the patient.

The Publisher

---

your source for books, journals and multimedia in the health sciences

www.elsevierhealth.com

 Working together to grow libraries in developing countries

www.elsevier.com • www.bookaid.org

The publisher's policy is to use **paper manufactured from sustainable forests**

Printed in China

CONTENTS

FOREWORD

■ ■

Neck pain consistently ranks as one of the most burdensome non-fatal health complaints facing humankind. It afflicts about one in 20 people worldwide, keeping them from leading full, productive lives. A significant proportion of those who hurt their neck go on to experience further episodes or ongoing pain that is resistant to treatment. Such situations often lead to a descending spiral of physical, social and economic disadvantage. There is no doubt that effective treatments are badly needed – fixing the problem of neck pain would have a massive positive impact.

Of course, the problem of neck pain is not a simple one, which is probably why it remains so much of a problem. The more we learn about neck pain – indeed the more we learn about pain no matter where it is – the more we realize that it is a multifactorial and multilayered problem. We now know that pain is a complex human experience perhaps best conceptualized as an unpleasant feeling that compels us to take action to protect a body part.

Neck pain is no exception to this rule. In fact, neck pain might be considered particularly complex, in part because the neck is a complex anatomical unit. Think of how many 'nociception-competent' structures there are in the neck – joints, muscles, ligaments and so on; think of the unique requirements of the neck – to offer structural protection to the spinal cord, upon which we depend for our survival, *and* provide for large ranges of movements in multiple planes, *and* support perhaps our biggest asset – our head – all the while catering for all but one of our senses. No other body part has such extraordinary properties.

Let's focus now on the nociceptive competency of the structures of the neck by considering this exchange between Rodeus and Mr Bilby – fictional characters of course – as they describe a metaphor for inbuilt protection of the cervical spinal cord:

Mr Bilby: Rodeus, imagine that you have a very precious piece of jewellery – the most precious item in all the land.

Rodeus: Well, I needn't imagine this, Mr Bilby, for unlike you I am a proud nobleman of the highest class. I am the owner of the Holy Bangle of the Fourth King of the Fourth King – it is surely the most valuable artifact in the land.

Mr Bilby: Excellent, Rodeus, you are right. I am just a small Australian marsupial on the edge of extinction. But tell me this, where might you store this precious bangle?

Rodeus: Of course, I shall not tell you exactly where it is, Mr Bilby, but, for argument's sake and in the spirit of your question, I should choose a place deeply buried behind structures of immense strength, yet in a tomb easily movable should threat approach; I would place sharp-eyed and suspicious guards, focused only on protecting this rare masterpiece; I would place them hand by hand, on every turret, at every corner, in every corridor.

Mr Bilby: I see your bangle must be well protected, Rodeus, but what if the earth shuddered and the whole fortress you have made is itself rocked to and forth?

Rodeus: I would place cushions and padding of the finest silk around the great jewel and I would alert the guards to be especially suspicious and keen-eyed henceforth should such a rocking arrive.

Mr Bilby: And so it is, Rodeus, and so it is. You have protected your bangle well I see – it is housed in a fortress, swathed in soft cushions, and you have installed an alarm system of thousands of guards on every turret and in every corridor – guards who will become more suspicious and vigilant should threat increase.

This exchange captures the extent of protection offered to our cervical spinal cord. It is sensible to be very protective of such a crucial, life-maintaining structure. Couple this with the kinematic and kinetic requirements and we have a truly complex task in deciphering why someone is hurting and how we might go about alleviating it. This is where a book such as this one is so badly needed.

Rafael Torres Cueco has put together a stellar volume that packages all this complexity into a form that is both digestible and sensible. There may be no better person to take on such a gargantuan task – Rafael is both an outstanding clinician and a clever and studious scholar. His grasp of the rich history of musculoskeletal medicine and its most useful role within a wider and fully biopsychosocial model is perhaps unmatched. He has constructed here a resource that matches this rare mix of sage and student, and I fully recommend it to any budding or indeed any established clinician.

I first experienced Rafael's unexampled mix of clinical nous and scientific enquiry when he rose at the end of a lecture I had delivered, strolled to the microphone in the aisle (not that he has ever needed one – his is a voice of remarkable resonance and projection!), and asked me a question that could only have come from a very experienced clinician who was completely on top of scientific developments in a very specific field. There are few who can juggle these two things and Rafael is certainly one of them. The astute reader of this volume will see Rafael's mix of clinical wisdom and scientific rigour in each clarification, in each insightful tip, in each observation.

I was honoured to receive an invitation to write a foreword for Rafael's book. I appreciate the instructive and constructive contributions Rafael has made to my own work and that of my group. I have been most impressed with the service that Rafael has delivered to his community of physiotherapists, doctors and patients. His energy and patience with those of us who are slow on the uptake, his willingness to bring in experts from other fields and his preparedness to share his own expertise with those beyond his immediate group, augur very well indeed for the future of musculoskeletal medicine and physiotherapy.

LORIMER MOSELEY

PREFACE

This book addresses the ever complex and stimulating clinical conditions of the cervical spine and is the companion volume to Essential Guide to the Cervical Spine – Volume One: Clinical Assessment and Therapeutic Approaches. The aim of this book is to offer, firstly, the most up-to-date theoretical information on the pathophysiology and semiology of the different clinical conditions presented by the cervical spine and, secondly, an approach to its treatment in light of scientific evidence and clinical experience. To this aim, an attempt has been made to provide this information supported by best evidence, hence the considerable review of the literature. Another aim has been to show those assessment and therapeutic procedures that have been more effective in the author's clinical practice.

Changes that have taken place in the field of science, as well as in the physiotherapist's professional evolution, have led us towards a new treatment model, which has progressed from a professional practice aiming to apply procedures, towards a clinical model in which the professional must have the ability and responsibility to establish a diagnosis and treatment. To undertake this challenge the professional must become a true clinician and not a mere executor of techniques. For this purpose, key elements in manual therapy are currently: clinical reasoning, an up-to-date knowledge of musculoskeletal pathology, a multimodal approach in the treatment of cervical pain, an understanding of the peripheral and central mechanisms involved in pain and, above all, the need to understand that we are treating a person whose experience of pain is modulated by their beliefs, expectations and behaviours, which are determined by family learning and the social and cultural environment. To do this we must use evidence-based practice, the biopsychosocial model of patient care and an updated view of pain.

The classical care model, namely the biomedical model, considers that the patient's symptoms are the direct result of a disease or dysfunction. The biomedical model has represented an important contribution to health, mainly in the treatment of acute diseases. However, its exclusive interest centred on biological factors which, although necessary, is insufficient in clinical practice.[1] This patho-anatomical model often still applies in the field of manual therapy, which has led to excessive mechanism. In recent decades, the biopsychosocial model has prevailed whereby the patient's clinical presentation, prognosis and treatment outcomes do not depend solely on a particular pathology or physical dysfunction. Beliefs, behaviours and social context are critically important in the manifestations and evolution of the clinical picture. As noted by Waddell,[2] the demand for medical care by a patient depends more on the patient's interpretation of the symptoms and cultural patterns of behaviour associated with the experience of pain. The biopsychosocial paradigm seeks to integrate all biological, psychological, social and cultural factors, and considers that they are all essential in the development, maintenance and exacerbation of pain.

Many of the clinical entities of the cervical spine are subject to considerable controversy as to their pathophysiology and therapeutic possibilities. The first controversy is whether a reliable diagnosis of many of these clinical entities is possible. And it should be noted that the introduction of the biopsychosocial model, although essential to understanding pain, has sometimes entailed misunderstandings regarding the role played by biological and patho-anatomical aspects. It is often mistakenly assumed that patho-anatomical factors are of little importance in clinical decision-making in patients with pain.[3] Many of the current clinical guidelines do not recommend classification or specific treatment based on patho-anatomical aspects except for the exclusion of red flags.[4] It is considered that subgroup identification based on patho-anatomical criteria is not possible except in a very small number of cases. As noted by Hancock when referring to low back pain,[5] almost all consideration of the patho-anatomical diagnosis has disappeared from clinical practice guidelines, which is contrary to the medical approach of most clinical entities or diseases.[6] Without much justification, classifications based on patho-anatomical aspects are said to have a limited clinical utility and that, instead of improving outcomes, they tend to aggravate them.[7,8] It has been assumed that in most patients with neck pain a diagnosis of the causes of pain cannot be reached and therefore the terms 'nonspecific' or 'idiopathic' should be used. But, what does nonspecific actually mean? Basically, that imaging tests are unable to diagnose pain and do not provide relevant information to treat nonspecific pain. This assumption is incorrect because imaging tests are always supplementary tests and never diagnostic in themselves. There is certainly no direct relationship between the patient's pain and the identification of anatomical or degenerative changes in the spine using imaging tests. There is also no evidence that degenerative changes are a risk factor for chronic pain. However, a pathology unrelated to pain in some individuals does not imply that it is not important.

Imaging tests can sometimes be helpful in the diagnosis of the patient's pathology. The belief that they do not provide information relating to the treatment is not entirely correct, since in many cases imaging tests show the state of the tissues as well as changes that determine a different approach to the patient. In fact, imaging tests are sometimes necessary in order to identify serious pathologies or to contraindicate manual therapy and physiotherapy, for example, in cases of severe instability, central canal stenosis, etc.

A frequent misunderstanding, as noted by Hancock et al.,[5] is that until a diagnosis is able to improve the therapeutic outcome, there is no interest in its further research. However, even when there is no evidence that a diagnosis improves the therapeutic results, this does not in any way imply that the diagnosis is incorrect.[5] The diagnosis may be valid before treatment is available. It may also be the first step in designing rational treatment.[5] Besides helping to establish the diagnosis of a clinical condition, it enables the understanding of its natural history and its comparison against the results of an intervention. With the current level of uncertainty as to the causes of pain, a patho-anatomical approach cannot be ruled out either in research or in the clinical context.

Indeed, it is essential to take into account the different psychosocial factors that may be involved in the patient's clinical situation. However, arguments supporting the exclusion of patho-anatomical factors in both clinical and research settings are not compatible with current literature.[6,9,10]

Paradoxically, what happens sometimes after rejecting the identification of a specific pathology, is what we might call tissue-based diagnosis. The therapist endeavours to determine the involvement of the various articular, muscular and neural tissues; and based on the nociceptive response of these tissues or changes in the movement pattern, the therapist generates a diagnostic category. Therapists who use this model often do so based on preferred manual therapy techniques.

Acceptance of the concept of nonspecific pain, as already mentioned, has aroused considerable interest in recent years enabling the subclassification of patients with pain into homogeneous groups with the aim of improving therapeutic outcomes. Classifications that were not based on patho-anatomical criteria were needed. Hence the emergence of recent classifications with respect to common musculoskeletal pain such as low back and neck pain.

Examples of attempted subclassification are those classifications based on clinical aspects considered relevant by a specific physiotherapy model.[11] Other classifications are aimed at identifying patient characteristics that indicate a possible favourable response to a specific treatment. The patient's negative or positive response in the same session or in successive sessions allows the therapist to adjust the treatment to these responses to obtain good therapeutic results.[12-14] However, there is not necessarily a relationship between immediate changes in pain or in physical findings and long-term responses.[15] It seems rather that this model based on patient responses is not necessarily associated with long-term functional improvements. Other classifications are based on the diagnosis of movement dysfunctions. The problem with such classifications is that the movement dysfunctions are very variable, and may be secondary to pain. There is no clear cause–effect relationship between pain and movement control dysfunctions; they can be adaptive or protective behaviours and can be a response to stress, fear, anxiety or misconceptions about the cause of pain. One of the problems that emerge from handling such differing classifications is that the method of evaluation can certainly not be applied to all types of patients with cervical pain. Most research to define patient subgroups is still at the stage of hypothesis generation. No classification system currently relies on sufficient evidence to recommend its use in clinical practice.[16]

Another attempt to subclassify patients is based on the dominant mechanism involved in pain.[17] Although taking into account which mechanisms are dominant (nociceptive, inflammatory, neuropathic, etc.) is relevant to patient management, this approach is not sufficient. Different clinical entities with a very diverse natural history may share the same pain mechanisms.

After reviewing all these classifications, we need to ask: why was the term nonspecific used in the first place? Not because it was impossible to know the causes of pain, as some have stated, but to rationalize and unify the pain patient's care, avoiding unnecessary tests that favour overdiagnosis, etc. The question that then emerges is: should we stop asking ourselves about the causes of neck pain?

In addition, these classification systems raise the following issues. Firstly, do they answer the three main questions asked by patients: What's wrong with me? What can you do for it? What is the prognosis? Secondly, can we establish a discussion with other physiotherapists who are unfamiliar with the classification or with other health professionals? And, finally, do these classification systems improve our understanding of the problem? Therefore, it is necessary to again study tissue pathology and biology, since in the majority of patients with nonspecific neck pain there is a 'specific cause' for their pain. An updated review of the different clinical conditions is necessary and establishing clinical hypotheses is essential for four essential aspects of the therapeutic process: (1) to establish a diagnosis; (2) to know the natural history of the process; (3) to design an appropriate treatment strategy; and (4) to establish a prognosis. We therefore consider that we must continue to investigate the patho-anatomical and neurophysiological mechanisms responsible for neck pain, obviously without forgetting those psychological and social factors that may be involved in its clinical expression.

As pointed out by Jull and Moore,[6] despite social pressure and professional trends, it is critical to possess an up-to-date knowledge of the various clinical conditions that a patient may present with, when evidence also suggests that the use of manual therapy should not be forgotten. As noted, this is not a merely academic issue and the development of appropriate, accurate and reliable strategies to tackle pain depend on an adequate understanding of the causes and mechanisms involved in the clinical syndrome or clinical presentation.[18] Therefore, an up-to-date knowledge of clinical syndromes and their different clinical presentations, their diagnostic criteria, pathophysiology and natural history, specific physical examination and therapeutic possibilities is required. We therefore advocate a bidirectional model. Further research is needed, firstly, with regard to those clinical conditions associated with changes in the structure and function of anatomical elements and, secondly, in connection with the psychosocial aspects involved in the patient's pain. Only then will we have a more balanced view of the 'bio' and 'psychosocial' role in the experience of pain.

This is why the chapters of this book are structured around the different clinical entities that patients can present such as disc pathology and radiculopathy, facet joint pain, cervical and craniocervical instability, cervical myelopathy, the differential diagnosis and treatment of cervicogenic headache, the frequent sensory-motor dysfunctions in patients with neck pain, and those physical and psychological factors that make whiplash a clinically complex entity to manage.

The penultimate chapter is an extensive review of the complications, especially neurovascular accidents, that may occur with manipulative procedures in the cervical spine.

The final chapter is dedicated to what has been a major part of my clinical practice over more than 15 years: the management of patients with complex chronic pain. This chapter reviews aspects of the neurophysiology of pain, describing the evolution in the neurobiological models developed in the last decades and finally an approach from a biopsychosocial integrating perspective is presented.

The model of approach which I have proposed is based on assessing the most relevant factors in different domains: clinical condition and severity and type of associated dysfunction, the relevant physical impairments, pain mechanisms (nociceptive, inflammatory, neuropathic or complex), central sensitization phenomena, patient beliefs (adaptive or maladaptive), patient behaviours (fear-avoidance and illness behaviours) and psychosocial aspects involved. It is crucial to assess social participation and interactions, such as limitations in work or daily activities and social interaction. Our goal as clinicians is not to 'fix' tissue impairment or to improve the patient's physical dysfunction, but to help patients to resume work and social participation and interaction. This book aims to provide theoretical and clinical tools that allow an effective and safe management of the complex pathology of the cervical spine and of patients with complex chronic pain. I hope that this approach will provide the reader with a clear, complete and rigorous reference for clinical, teaching or research work

RAFAEL TORRES CUECO
Valencia 2017

REFERENCES

1. Torres-Cueco R. Aproximación biopsicosocial del dolor crónico y de la fibromialgia. In: Salvat IS, editor. Fisioterapia del Dolor Miofascial y de la Fibromialgia. Sevilla: Universidad Internacional de Andalucía; 2009. p. 78–110.
2. Waddell G. 1987 Volvo award in clinical sciences. A new clinical model for the treatment of low-back pain. Spine 1987;12(7):632–44.
3. Weiner BK. Spine update: the biopsychosocial model and spine care. Spine 2008;33(2):219–23.
4. Childs JD, Cleland JA, Elliott JM, et al. Neck pain: Clinical practice guidelines linked to the International Classification of Functioning, Disability, and Health from the Orthopedic Section of the American Physical Therapy Association. J Orthop Sports Phys Ther 2008;38(9):A1–34.
5. Hancock MJ, Maher CG, Laslett M, et al. Discussion paper: what happened to the 'bio' in the bio-psycho-social model of low back pain? Eur Spine J 2011;20(12):2105–10.
6. Jull G, Moore A. Hands on, hands off? The swings in musculoskeletal physiotherapy practice. Man Ther 2012;17(3):199–200.
7. Deyo RA, Mirza SK, Turner JA, et al. Overtreating chronic back pain: time to back off? J Am Board Fam Med 2009;22(1):62–8.
8. Pransky G, Buchbinder R, Hayden J. Contemporary low back pain research - and implications for practice. Best Pract Res Clin Rheumatol 2010;24(2):291–8.
9. Ford JJ, Hahne AJ. Pathoanatomy and classification of low back disorders. Man Ther 2013;18(2):165–8.
10. Hancock M, Maher C, Macaskill P, et al. MRI findings are more common in selected patients with acute low back pain than controls? Eur Spine J 2012;21(2):240–6.
11. McKenzie R, May S. The lumbar spine, mechanical diagnosis and therapy. 2nd ed. Waikanae: Spinal Publications New Zealand Ltd; 2003.
12. Delitto A, Erhard RE, Bowling RW. A treatment-based classification approach to low back syndrome: identifying and staging patients for conservative treatment. Phys Ther 1995;75(6):470–85, discussion 485-9.
13. Fritz JM, Brennan GP. Preliminary examination of a proposed treatment-based classification system for patients receiving physical therapy interventions for neck pain. Phys Ther 2007;87(5):513–24.
14. Kamper SJ, Maher CG, Hancock MJ, et al. Treatment-based subgroups of low back pain: a guide to appraisal of research studies and a summary of current evidence. Best Pract Res Clin Rheumatol 2010;24(2):181–91.
15. Tuttle N. Is it reasonable to use an individual patient's progress after treatment as a guide to ongoing clinical reasoning? J Manipulative Physiol Ther 2009;32(5):396–403.
16. Fairbank J, Gwilym SE, France JC, et al. The role of classification of chronic low back pain. Spine 2011;36(21 Suppl.):S19–42.
17. Smart KM, Blake C, Staines A, et al. The Discriminative validity of "nociceptive," "peripheral neuropathic," and "central sensitization" as mechanisms-based classifications of musculoskeletal pain. Clin J Pain 2011;27(8):655–63.
18. Carragee EJ, Alamin TF, Miller JL, et al. Discographic, MRI and psychosocial determinants of low back pain disability and remission: a prospective study in subjects with benign persistent back pain. Spine J 2005;5(1):24–35.

ACKNOWLEDGEMENTS

Firstly, I would like to thank all the authors who contributed to this book: Michelle Sterling, Lucy Thomas, Julia Treleaven, Pieter Westerhuis and especially Gwendolen Jull. Most of the knowledge collected in this book is courtesy of Gwendolen Jull and based on her huge contribution (together with her research fellows) to musculoskeletal physiotherapy and manual therapy research. I would also like to thank David Butler, who conveyed his enthusiasm for understanding pain, and Lorimer Moseley, who kindly agreed to write the foreword to this volume.

I would like to thank all those who participated as models: Tamara Gonzálvez, Manuela Gomez and especially Raquel Heredia, and also Yvonne Ribes for the excellent quality of her photographs. Thanks to my colleagues in the Department of Physiotherapy at the University of Valencia. Thanks to my colleagues, Jesus Aguiló-Furio and Mar Machiran-Matallín, who work with me every day treating complex patients. Thanks also to my undergraduate and postgraduate students at the universities where I teach; working with them has forced me to revise my knowledge continuously.

Also, many thanks to the publisher Elsevier and in particular to Rita Demetriou-Swanwick, who showed great interest in this project, and also to Sally Davies and Andrew Riley for their trust and patience.

And, finally, I am grateful to my dear wife and children for their support and encouragement, despite the huge amount of time spent away from home and devoted to my work.

RAFAEL TORRES CUECO
Valencia 2017

PUBLISHER'S ACKNOWLEDGEMENTS

Elsevier wishes to acknowledge the initial Spanish-English translation provided by Rubén Francés García.

Elsevier also wishes to acknowledge the peer review of the English translation which was undertaken by Nicholas Southorn.

CONTRIBUTORS

GWENDOLEN JULL DipPhty GradDipManipTher MPhty PhD FACP
Emeritus Professor, Physiotherapy, School of Health and Rehabilitation Sciences, The University of Queensland, Brisbane, Queensland, Australia

MICHELE STERLING MPhty GradDipManipPhysio BPhty PhD FACP
Director, NHMRC Centre of Research Excellence in Road Traffic Injuries; Associate Director, Centre of National Research on Disability and Rehabilitation Medicine (CONROD); Menzies Health Institute, Griffith University, Parklands, Queensland, Australia

LUCY C. THOMAS MMedSc(Phty) GradDipAppSc(ManipPhty) DipPhys PhD
Lecturer, School of Health and Rehabilitation Sciences, The University of Queensland, Brisbane, Queensland, Australia

RAFAEL TORRES CUECO PhD PT
Professor, Department of Physiotherapy, University of Valencia, Spain; Director of Masters Program on Manual Therapy, University of Valencia; President and founder of the Spanish Society of Physiotherapy and Pain (Sociedad Española de Fisioterapia y Dolor SEFID); Facilitator, WCPT Physical Therapy Pain Network; Instructor, Neuro-Orthopaedic Institute (NOI); Member of the Spanish Pain Society (Sociedad Española del Dolor SED), Spanish Society of Craniomandibular Dysfunction and Orofacial Pain (Sociedad Española de Disfunción Craneomandibular y Dolor Orofacial SEDCYDO) and the International Association for the Study of Pain (IASP)

JULIA TRELEAVEN BPhty PhD
Lecturer, Division of Physiotherapy, School of Health and Rehabilitation Sciences, The University of Queensland, Brisbane, Queensland, Australia

PIETER WESTERHUIS
Physiotherapist, Private Practice, Grenchen, Switzerland; Teacher, Postgraduate Manipulative Therapy, Switzerland, Germany and Austria

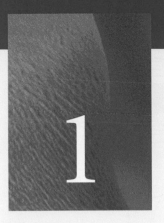

CLINICAL APPROACH TO CERVICAL DISCOGENIC PAIN AND RADICULOPATHY

RAFAEL TORRES CUECO

This chapter describes the syndromes linked to the cervical intervertebral disc, cervical discogenic pain and radicular pain due to disc herniation. It also includes the radicular pain caused by lateral canal stenosis, in whose development participates, besides the disc, the hypertrophic degenerative changes of the structures that make up the intervertebral foramen.

First, we will analyse cervical discogenic pain, before looking at cervical radicular pain, and reviewing the conservative therapeutic options.

As regards cervicobrachial pain, the first thing that should be pointed out is the fact that its differential diagnosis is significantly more complex than that of lumbar radicular syndromes. The clinical signs and symptoms of a cervical radicular complaint are not as evident as those of a lumbar radiculopathy. While in this last case the majority of patients show signs and symptoms typical of a radicular pain syndrome, only one-third of the patients with cervical radiculopathy show an unequivocally radicular cervicobrachial pain.[1]

In daily practice, it is problematic to diagnose, given that different entities can manifest themselves clinically in a similar way to cervical radiculopathy, such as the thoracic outlet syndrome, pain referred to the upper limb of discogenic or facet origin, or the different peripheral nervous compressive syndromes.

DISCOGENIC SYNDROMES

In the cervical spine, two types of clinical syndromes are related to disc pathology: *cervical discogenic pain* and *discogenic radiculopathy*.

This distinction is important since it is commonly thought that disc pathology is exclusively a disc herniation, when the cervical disc, in the same way as the lumbar disc, can be responsible for symptoms without the rupture of the external fibres of the annulus fibrosus and, therefore, without the compression or irritation of the neural elements. Therefore, besides radiculopathy, the cervical disc can be responsible for cervical pain which results from *internal disc disruption* and *painful degenerative changes*.

CERVICAL DISCOGENIC PAIN

Cervical discogenic pain is mainly the consequence of an internal disc disruption. The concept of *internal disc disruption,* described initially by Crock,[2] implies the fissuration of the annulus fibrosus without the external migration of the nuclear material. This entity is produced by a degradation of the nuclear material due to a traumatic injury, an annular injury due to a flexion–rotation mechanism, cervical whiplash or a repetitive shearing of the disc.

The rupture of the innervated portions of the annulus fibrosus determines the appearance of symptoms. Internal disc disruption can be due to a repeated microtrauma or an acute trauma and, in the latter case it can be more frequently symptomatic. Research studies show a high incidence of acute disc injuries after cervical whiplash.[3,4]

There are three types of annulus disruption: concentric or circumferential, radial and marginal or rim lesion (Fig. 1-1). Their development is not related to age, although they are very common from middle-age onwards. *Concentric ruptures* suppose the existence of

1

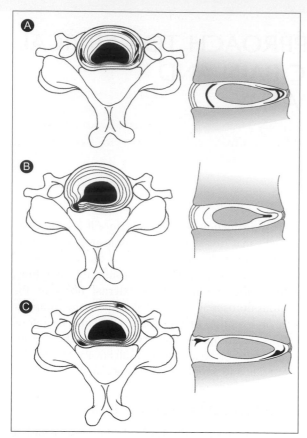

FIGURE 1-1 ■ There are three classifications of annulus fibrosus ruptures: (A) concentric or circumferential, (B) radial and (C) marginal or rim lesions.

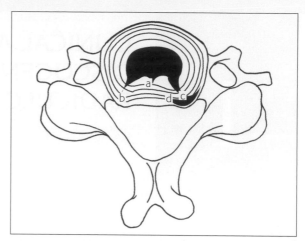

FIGURE 1-2 ■ Internal disc disruption is classified in grades according to the extent of the fissuration: (a) grade 1, when the fissures reach only the internal third of the annulus; (b) grade 2, when the fissures reach the middle third; (c) grade 3, when the fissures reach the external third; (d) grade 4, implies a radial fissure of third degree that expands circumferentially more than 30° in the external third of the annulus fibrosus.

a space between adjoining laminae. *Radial ruptures* imply a transverse disruption of the laminae that progress from the centre to the periphery. These radial ruptures allow for the progressive migration of the nucleus pulposus. *Marginal ruptures* or rim lesions are the consequence of a focal avulsion of the peripheral portion of the annulus that is inserted in the ring apophysis. Their aetiology is frequently traumatic.

The disruption of the annulus is classified according to the extent of the fissuration observed using computed tomography (CT) following a contrast injection[5]:

■ Grade 1: when the fissures only reach the internal third of the annulus.
■ Grade 2: when the fissures reach the middle third.

■ Grade 3: when the fissures reaches the external third.
■ Grade 4: implies a grade 3 radial fissuration that expands circumferentially more than 30° in the external third of the annulus fibrosus (Fig. 1-2).

Three additional grades have been added to this classification:

■ Grade 5: represents the rupture of the disc in all its extension, both focal and circumferential, with the output of contrast outside of the annulus fibrosus.
■ Grade 6: represents a sequestered disc.
■ Grade 7: represents a diffuse annular rupture of a degenerative cause.

The physiopathology of the internal disc disruption is not completely known. It is thought that it is produced as a consequence of a degradation of the nuclear matrix after a fatigue fracture of the cartilaginous endplate.[6]

As a consequence, this situation would lead to a loss of the proteoglycans and the subsequent dehydration of the nucleus, so that a large amount of the load would be transferred to the annulus fibrosus. This excessive stress would cause the radial and concentric fissuration of the annulus fibrosus. Discogenic pain would be the consequence of the inflammation secondary to the disc radial fissuration and the increase in tension suffered by the intact fibres of the annulus.

The *degenerative disc changes* or so-called *degenerative disc disease* implies the existence of annular ruptures, loss of disc height and degeneration of the nucleus pulposus. Degenerative disc disease is, in many cases, the consequence of degenerative changes after an internal disc disruption. The degenerative disease in the cervical spine is difficult to differentiate from involutive changes, and in most cases is not responsible for the symptoms. The disc starts to degenerate from the second decade onwards, as a consequence of a fissuration of the annulus fibrosus. The loss of disc height is the consequence of the radial bulging of the annulus fibrosus, which follows the degradation of the annulus pulposus.[7] Finally, the degenerative changes can lead to an isolated disc resorption.[8] The decrease in disc shock absorption abilities induces vertebral body sclerosis and osteophytes formation.

Discogenic pain patterns

The disc is innervated and can be a source of pain. However, for decades it has been considered that discogenic pain was related to a disc herniation. As previously mentioned in Chapter 5, it was Smith and Nichols[9] and Cloward[10] who showed the capacity of the disc to induce pain and described its referred pain area. The innervation of the cervical disc depends, in its anterior and lateral portion, on the anterior plexus formed by the union of fibres of the lateral sympathetic chain and its corresponding grey ramus communicans, as well as fibres from the primary anterior ramus and, in its posterior portion, on the posterior plexus derived from the recurrent meningeal nerve and the perivascular plexuses associated with the vertebral artery.[11-13] The innervation of the annulus fibrosus is evident in its external third[12] and, according to some authors, it reaches the middle fibres.[11,14]

In light of recent descriptions of the cervical disc, detailed in R. Torres' book *The Cervical Spine: Clinical Evaluation and Therapeutic Approaches*, which show that the posterior and posteroanterior part is practically non-existent, discogenic pain can result from two situations: the stretching or rupture of the annulus in its anterior portion, primarily due to a trauma in hyperextension, or the tension or stretching suffered by the posterior longitudinal ligament (PLL) when being compressed by a disc protrusion.[15]

Discogenic pain can be due to the stretching and rupture of the annulus in its anterior portion, secondary to traumas in hyperextension, or to the tension suffered by the PLL when being compressed by a disc protrusion.

Therefore, internal *disc disruption* can be responsible for pain in the cervical spine and cause referred pain in the thoracic spine and the scapular area. When the disc injury takes places in the C2–C3 and C3–C4 discs, the pain is frequently referred to the craniovertebral region and can determine a cervicogenic headache.[16-25] Also, the protrusion of disc material into the vertebral body can induce pain. In this case, the existence of an inflammatory focus in Schmorl's nodules seems necessary.[26]

Discogenic pain can be expressed as neck pain, but it is especially manifest as referred pain in the scapular and upper thoracic area.[12,21-23,27-31] Occasionally, this pain can be referred to the anterior chest wall simulating an angina.[28,29] Pain can be unilateral and bilateral, which can help to differentiate discogenic referred pain from zygapophyseal joint pain.

Below are detailed the discogenic pain maps described recently by Slipman et al.[31]

- The C2–C3 disc refers neck, suboccipital and facial pain.
- The C3–C4 disc refers posterior and anterior neck pain, suboccipital pain, facial pain, and pain to the area of the trapezius, shoulder, interscapular region and the upper limb.
- The C4–C5 disc refers posterior neck pain, suboccipital, facial pain, and pain to the area of the trapezius and shoulder, the interscapular regions, the upper limb and the anterior chest region.
- The C5–C6 disc refers posterior neck pain, suboccipital, facial pain, and pain to the area of the trapezius, the shoulder, the interscapular area, the anterior thoracic area and the upper limb.
- The C6–C7 disc refers posterior neck pain and suboccipital pain, pain to the area of the

trapezius, the shoulder, the interscapular area and the upper limb.

- The C7–T1 disc refers posterior cervical pain and interscapular pain (Fig. 1-3).

Using the work of Slipman et al.,[31] we can conclude that discogenic pain is very diffuse, and can even refer to the lumbar region. There is significant overlapping between the different discs, and therefore disc pain maps have little clinical use. Although these patterns are much more diffuse, they are topographically similar to those of the zygapophyseal joints that correspond segmentally to the same level, and therefore cannot help to differentiate if pain comes from one articular structure or another. The majority of the discs refer pain to the upper limb, being able to reach the hand, which can simulate a radiculopathy.

Clinical manifestations of cervical discogenic pain

The signs and symptoms of an internal disc disruption in the cervical spine are not clearly defined, contrary to what happens in the lumbar spine, where they are better known clinically.

Clinically, it can be seen as an acute severe pain onset or as an ongoing mild pain that can be episodic. The acute discogenic pain is deep, diffuse and difficult to locate. This pain is usually severe and difficult to bear.

The symptoms are followed by an antalgic posture in flexion or in flexion and side-bending, similar to that of a subject with facet joint synovitis. However, it is not difficult to differentiate secondary wry neck from a discogenic problem from the one of facet origin by their clinical pattern and the history of the onset symptoms. The onset of a discogenic wry neck is usually insidious, so that acute symptoms need a few days to establish themselves, whereas facet joint wry neck appears immediately or a few hours after the movement that triggered it. Discogenic pain is usually much more severe and sickening than facet joint pain, and is frequently accompanied by a malaise and other vegetative signs.

In discogenic wry neck, restriction of mobility is not mechanical, unlike in acute facet joint pain, but the consequence of an antalgic posture resulting from the severity of the symptoms. Discogenic pain does not appear immediately with a posture or movement, but there is a characteristic period of latency between the irritating movement and the onset of pain.

Discogenic pain is diffuse; the patient tends to point to a wide area in the upper trapezius and the thoracic scapular area. Intense discogenic pain is perceived especially in the medial border of the scapula and, in most cases, there is no neck pain. However, if the cervical spine is kept in the position that aggravates the symptoms, a general and diffuse discomfort may appear in the entire cervical region.

Patients with discogenic neck pain have great difficulty finding a posture that alleviates pain. Frequently, postures in which the neck supports the weight of the head aggravate the symptoms, especially in the sitting position. It is common to find a difference in mobility between the positions in which gravity acts and the lying position. Lying down allows for a greater range of mobility without pain, while positions with gravity can provoke an antalgic attitude. Likewise, activities that increase intradiscal pressure, such as Valsalva's manoeuvre, intensify the symptoms, as well as the vibratory stimuli, such as those caused while driving a vehicle.

The symptoms just described, which are characteristic of an internal disc disruption, are also similar to the proximal symptoms of a disc herniation with radicular component. The antalgic posture and the characteristics of the pain are very similar, so that making a distinction between one clinical condition and another will depend on the presence of radicular signs and symptoms.

The diagnosis of cervical discogenic pain is often reached by exclusion, when there are no signs of radiculopathy and the assessment of the zygapophyseal joints is negative. The physical assessment of the disc is characterized by the lack of a painful response to palpation and a negative response to provocation tests of the posterior joints. Discographies can help determine that the pain comes from the intervertebral disc. The reproduction of the patient's pain by injecting a contrast in the disc can help to confirm its discogenic origin (Fig. 1-4).

CLINICAL FEATURES OF CERVICAL ACUTE DISCOGENIC PAIN

- Type of pain: deep, diffuse and difficult to locate.
- Area of pain: medial to the scapula, in most cases with no neck pain.
- Pain intensity: severe and difficult to bear.

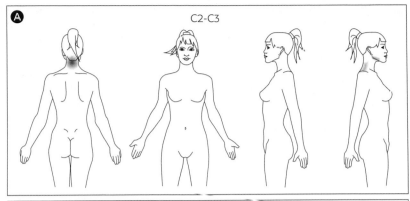

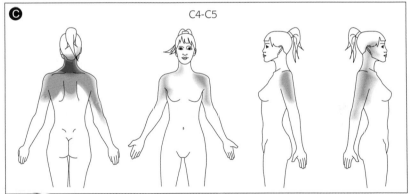

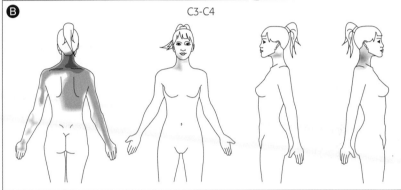

FIGURE 1-3 ■ Discogenic referred pain patterns:(A) C2–C3 discogram; (B) C3–C4 discogram; (C) C4–C5 discogram; (D) C5–C6 discogram; (E) C6–C7 discogram; (F) C7–T1 discogram. *(Modified from Slipman et al.[31])*

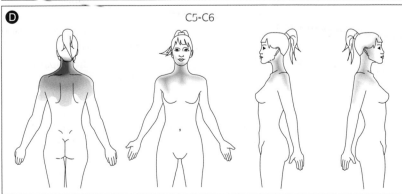

Continued

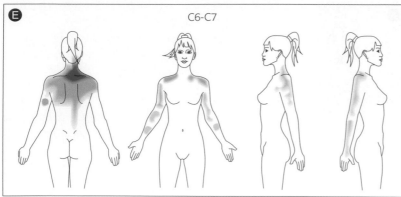

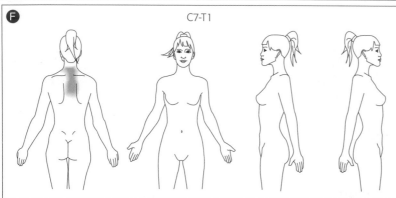

FIGURE 1-3, Cont'd

- Pain latency.
- It is difficult for the patient to find a position that alleviates pain.
- Difference in cervical mobility between positions with gravity and lying positions.
- Antalgic posture in flexion or in flexion and side-bending.
- Progressive clinical onset
- The restriction to mobility is not mechanical.
- The increase in intradiscal pressure and vibratory stimuli intensify the symptoms.
- Discography can help in the diagnosis of discogenic pain

CERVICAL RADICULAR PAIN AND RADICULOPATHY

Radicular pain and radiculopathy can be the consequence of a prolapse of the cervical disc or a degenerative stenosis of the lateral canal, and the latter cause is the most common.

Although in both cases the patient suffers from a radiculopathy, the clinical manifestations and their evolution have several differences. Therefore, the radicular manifestations caused by a disc herniation, and those caused by a degenerative stenosis of the lateral canal, are discussed separately. Before describing the radicular signs secondary to a disc herniation or degenerative origin, it is important to point out that the terms 'radiculopathy' and 'radicular pain' are not synonymous. Although the mechanical compression of the nerve root is an important mechanism of radicular pain, radicular compression can appear with no pain. This difference is obvious in some patients with degenerative stenosis of the lateral canal that show a chronic radiculopathy in which painful symptoms can be absent.

The most frequent cause of cervical radiculopathy is degenerative stenosis of the lateral canal.

There are two types of neuropathic pain: dysaesthetic and somatic neurogenic. Dysaesthetic pain is the

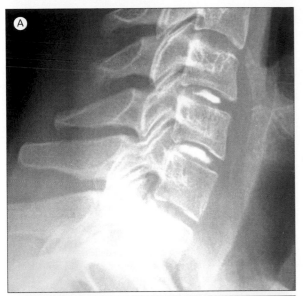

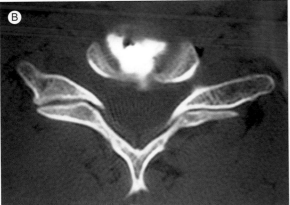

FIGURE 1-4 ■ Cervical discography. Lateral radiographic projection (A) and coronal plane with CT (B).

consequence of pathophysiological changes at the radicular complex, resulting from a mechanical aggression, the alteration of blood perfusion or the diffusion of chemical inflammatory irritants coming from the disc.[32–35]

Somatic neurogenic pain is a consequence of the mechanical or chemical irritation of the connective layers of the radicular complex.[36–38]

These physiopathological changes are manifested by the development of abnormal impulse-generating sites (AIGS) or ectopic pacemaker sites (EPS) in the neural tissue.[39] These EPS especially develop in

structures that lack myelin, such as the dorsal root ganglion (DRG) or those axons that have suffered from a focal demyelization or structural injury. In the radicular complex, the most sensitive element is the DRG.[40,41] Therefore, the direct compression of the nerve root caused by a prolapsed disc is not necessary for this root to suffer pathological changes or changes in sensitization. In fact, inflammation seems to be the main cause of the neural tissue sensitization to mechanical stimuli.[35] Once injured or in a process of regeneration, as a consequence of the development of EPS, they show an increase sensitization to different types of stimuli: mechanical, such as compression or stretching; vascular, like the ischaemia of the radicular complex; and chemical, due to the presence of inflammatory mediators, or to neurotransmitters like noradrenaline (norepinephrine). This increased sensitization explains the behaviour of radicular pain.

Nerve roots can suffer pathological changes in the presence of a disc herniation without necessarily suffering a direct compression.

All these types of sensitizing stimuli have a clinical translation. The clinical manifestation derived from a radicular sensitization has been explained by Gifford.[42]

The sensitization to mechanical stimuli is expressed by pain onset with those movements and postures that imply stretching or compression. This radicular mechanosensitivity to compression or stretching is useful in the clinical assessment of radicular pain. Some examples of sensitivity to stretching are the *arm abduction sign*, and the neurodynamic test of the brachial plexus described by Elvey.[43] These stimuli trigger a sudden discharge of pain that is maintained even when the stimulus is removed. This mechanosensitivity usually has a period of latency, both during the onset as well as the easing off of pain. The roots also suffer a sensitization to ischaemia. The compression of the nerve can compromise the neural blood perfusion. Ischaemia, by decreasing local pH, can increase the discharge of impulses in the abnormal impulse-generating sites. This explains that, often, during the physical assessment, a sustained compression is necessary in order to trigger symptoms.

In a radiculopathy, there is also a sensitization to catecholamines. Ectopic pacemaker sites, as well as nociceptors and dorsal horn neurons, can be sensitized to noradrenaline. One of the structural changes that can be associated is the growth of axonal sympathetic sprouts, both in places were somatic axons have suffered focal demyelization, and around the dorsal root ganglion. It has been speculated that this is the main physiopathological mechanism that underlies the sympathetically maintained pain after a nerve injury. This could explain the potential influence of anxiety in the amplification of radicular pain. It is not infrequent that subjects that have suffered from a radiculopathy, months and years later, refer dysaesthetic symptoms in the upper limb in stressful situations. It is important to highlight that a radiculopathy, especially when it causes changes at the DRG, can lead to neuroplastic changes in the central nervous system (CNS), which will be manifested by a pronounced mechanosensitivity, skin hyperaesthesia and allodynia, and that can induce the transition to chronic pain.[44]

Anatomy of the foramen

It is important to understand the anatomy of the foramen, since the changes that this area of anatomical narrowing undergoes are usually responsible for cervical radiculopathy.

There are differences in the location of the radicular compression between the cervical and the lumbar spine. In the lumbar spine, the roots tend to get trapped at the height of the lateral recess, while in the cervical spine, the root compromise occurs in the foramen. This is because the lateral recesses of the cervical spine are wide, whereas the lateral canal, especially in the lower cervical segments, is occupied by the thick DRG.

The foramina have an oval shape, their sagittal diameter is 10 mm and their anteroposterior diameter is 5 mm. The foramen continue in the channel formed by the union of the anterior and posterior tubercles of the transverse process.

In the lateral canal, three parts can be distinguished: pedicular (between two adjacent pedicles), retrovertebral (behind the vertebral artery) and transversal (in the channel formed by the transverse processes) (Fig. 1-5).

In the first part of the foramen, we find the ventral and dorsal roots, which are separated; in the second, the dorsal root ganglion is found; and in the third, the

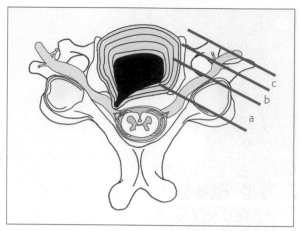

FIGURE 1-5 ■ In the lateral canal three parts can be seen: (a) pedicular (between two adjacent pedicles), (b) retrovertebral (behind the vertebral artery) and (c) transversal (in the canal formed by the transverse processes).

spinal nerve is located, which will immediately be divided between the anterior and posterior primary rami.

The diameter of the intervertebral foramina is amplified or reduced, depending on the position adopted by the cervical spine: flexion and contralateral rotation increase their size, while extension and ipsilateral rotation reduce it[45] (Fig. 1-6).

Neural elements of the foramen

The radicular complex, placed inside the foramen, is relatively well protected against external trauma. Therefore, most likely, its collagen content is lower than in the peripheral nerves. It has no perineurium or endoneurium, and is covered by a thin connective and permeable layer, known as the root sleeve. The lower amount of connective tissue makes it more prone to the compression of neighbouring structures.[46] The DRG, in the cervical spine, is more vulnerable to mechanical irritation than the spinal nerve.

The radicular complex occupies 20–50% of the surface of the foramen,[47,48] and is located in its inferior portion (Fig. 1-7).

The remaining surface is occupied by fat, the venous plexuses in continuity with those of the epidural space, and the recurrent meningeal nerve. The lower cervical roots are the thickest roots in the brachial plexus, and their foramen tends to be narrower,

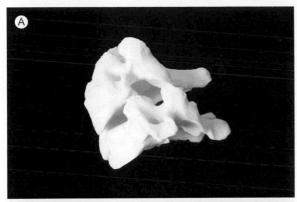

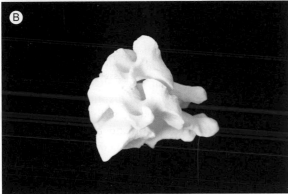

FIGURE 1-6 ■ The diameter of the intervertebral foramen is amplified or reduced, depending on the position adopted by the cervical spine: flexion and contralateral rotation increase its size (A), whereas extension and ipsilateral rotation decrease it (B).

which can explain the high incidence of radiculopathy in these levels.

The higher incidence of radiculopathy on the lower cervical spine can be due to the fact that the lower cervical roots are the thickest of the brachial plexus, and their foramen tend to be narrower.

The spinal nerve is only a few millimetres long, since it is quickly divided in the anterior primary ramus and the posterior primary ramus. The anterior primary rami of C4–T1 determine the formation of the brachial plexus. A third nerve that emerges and is highly significant in pain relating to the intervertebral disc is the sinuvertebral nerve or recurrent meningeal nerve. The recurrent meningeal nerve[11,12,49] originates in the anterior primary ramus of the spinal nerve, as soon as it emerges from the foramen (Fig. 1-8). It receives fibres from the sympathetic system via the grey ramus communicans, and it enters again in the foramen, innervating the anterior structures of the central canal, such as the PLL, the annulus fibrosus, the epidural vessels, the dura mater and the vertebral periosteum. The autonomic components of this nerve would explain the vegetative symptoms that frequently accompany disc injuries.[50]

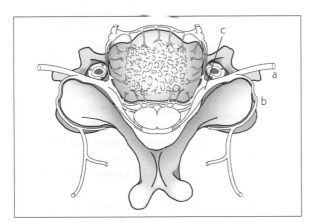

FIGURE 1-7 ■ Three neural elements emerge from the radicular complex and the spinal nerve: the anterior primary ramus (a), the posterior primary ramus (b) and the recurrent meningeal nerve (c).

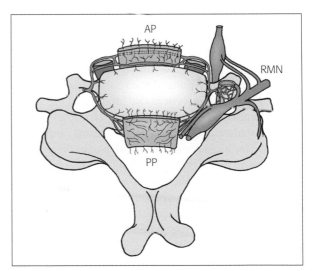

FIGURE 1-8 ■ The recurrent meningeal nerve (RMN) originates in the anterior primary ramus of the spinal nerve, just as it emerges from the foramen, and it configures a posterior plexus (PP) which accompanies the posterior longitudinal ligament. AP, anterior plexus.

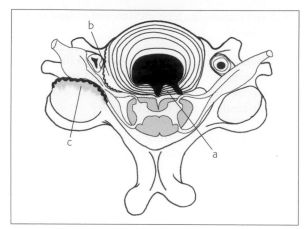

FIGURE 1-9 ■ The compression of the roots of the foramen can occur, in the anterior direction by the disc (a), and by osteophytes of the uncovertebral joint (b), or in the posterior direction by the degenerative hypertrophy of the zygapophyseal joints (c).

Radicular compression

The compression of the roots in the foramen can be caused, in the anterior part, by the disc and the osteophytes of the uncovertebral joint, or in the posterior part by the degenerative hypertrophy of the zygapophyseal joints[51] (Fig. 1-9).

The compression of the nerve roots affects all its components: nerve fibres, connective tissues and blood vessels. If the radicular tissues' ability to adapt to the mechanical deformation is exceeded, they will suffer functional and structural changes.

Functional alterations of the roots are not only the result of the compression in the foramen of the nerve fibres but also the consequence of this compression on their vascularization and their axonal transport systems. The roots are more sensitive than the peripheral nerves to vascular changes. Anything that decreases the space in the foramen tends to alter the gradients of the blood flow pressure along the nerve. The material that occupies the space can be temporary, such as oedema or extruded disc material, or permanent, such as the osteophytes.[52,53]

The compression of the roots of the foramen can determine its functional alteration, not only due to the effect of the direct compression of the roots but also due to the effects of the compression on the vascularization and the axonal transport systems.

The roots, and especially the DRG, do not have a haematoneural diffusing barrier like the wall of the endoneural capillaries of the peripheral nerves. Therefore, the permeability of the microvessels of the ganglion of the dorsal root is higher. These anatomical characteristics predispose the DRG to oedema as a consequence of a mechanical compression.[41] The oedema can lead to intra-articular and periarticular fibrosis, causing structural damage to the nerve fibre.

Maintaining the functional integrity of the root is in part carried out by the axonal transport systems, the anterograde and retrograde systems. Chronic compression is capable of altering these transport systems that play a trophic role in the neuron and may lead to its deterioration. In addition, the axonal transport systems are involved in nociception, as they are related to the synthesis of substances and neuropeptides that induce pain. In particular, the DRG is an important place for the synthesis of neuropeptides, such as substance P and the calcitonin gene-related peptide, as well as other transported substances by the axonal transport systems centrally and peripherally.

The consequences of the compression also depend on the structure on which it is exerted. While an acute compression of a nerve roots only produces a few seconds of repeated discharges, when this is exerted on the DRG, a wider response is triggered with several minutes of axonal activity. If the roots suffer an inflammatory process or a continued irritation, they become sensitized and are capable of triggering prolonged repeated discharges when compressed. These observations can explain why the irritation of the neural structures is a prerequisite for the neurophysiological responses related to pain.

Chronic compression over the roots may induce structural changes, such as demyelination, degeneration and regeneration of the nerve fibres, and atrophy of the DRG.[41]

The effects of compression on the function of the roots depend also on the type of fibres that undergo it. Thus, the function of the motor roots can be more rapidly and completely recovered after the release of the compression than those of the sensitive roots.

Cervical radiculopathy by a disc herniation

The clinical manifestations of cervical radiculopathy caused by disc herniation have marked differences compared to the lumbar spine.

These differences are related to the different anatomy of the cervical disc, both in its external morphology and its internal composition, and its relationships with the neural elements. However, few studies have examined the morphology and biochemistry of the cervical disc, in contrast with the many studies conducted on the lumbar intervertebral disc. This is an interesting situation if we take into account the important development of cervical disc surgery over the last few years.

New contributions to the anatomy of the cervical disc show that there are pronounced morphological differences between the lumbar and cervical discs, in a way that, necessarily, the pathological or degenerative changes that the cervical disc suffers demand a different interpretation. The cervical nucleus pulposus does not have a gelatinous consistency, but is formed by a core of fibrocartilaginous tissue,[54–58] which, due to the development of the uncovertebral joints in adults, is split in two-thirds of its anteroposterior diameter, often leaving an isolated strip of fibrocartilage.[59–61]

The disc nuclear prolapse is therefore less frequent than the lumbar one, except in serious traumatic accidents. When a disc herniation takes place, it is usually posteromedial, in contrast with the lumbar spine, which is usually posterolateral, since the unciform processes behave like true anatomical barriers that make it difficult for the disc to migrate in this direction and, therefore, the radicular pain is less frequent in the cervical spine (Fig. 1-10). In middle-aged individuals it is frequent to observe a bulging of the annulus

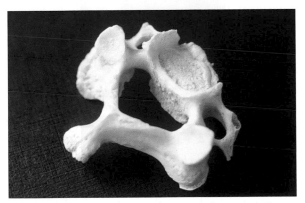

FIGURE 1-10 ■ The unciform processes act as anatomical barriers, making the migration of the disc material in the posterolateral direction difficult.

fibrosus accompanied by osteophytic spurs in the spinal canal.

- The cervical disc nuclear prolapse is less frequent than the lumbar.
- The cervical disc herniation is usually posteromedial, in contrast with the lumbar herniation, which is normally posterolateral.
- In middle-aged individuals it is frequent to observe a bulging of the annulus fibrosus accompanied by osteophytes in the spinal canal.

Cervical disc herniation

The recognition of the relationship between cervicobrachial pain and disc herniation is relatively recent. In 1943, Semmes and Murphey[62] showed that a brachialgia could be derived from a cervical disc herniation, almost a decade after the publication of the classic work by Mixter and Barr[63] on the relationship between sciatica and lumbar disc herniation.

In the 1950s, cervical disc surgery began to develop. In 1955, Robinson and Smith[64] described the anterior disc removal technique. Since then, different modifications of this approach have been developed, associated with arthrodesis, as well as posterior approaches, such as laminectomy and laminoplasty, for the treatment of a cervical disc herniation. Yet, in the last few decades the practice of cervical disc surgery has seen a significant increase. This has been encouraged by the extension of the indications of surgery, a larger number of surgeons who know the technique and, particularly, by advances made in diagnostic imaging techniques.

Cervical disc herniations are not common. The ratio of symptomatic disc herniations in the cervical spine to those in the lumbar spine is 1 to 10.[65] Yet, excessive diagnostic dependence on magnetic resonance imaging (MRI) has currently led to a situation of overdiagnosis of disc herniations.[66] If magnetic resonances are not interpreted with caution, small posterior bulging, without compromising the nerve structures, may lead to the diagnosis of disc hernia susceptible to surgical resection.

In the cervical spine, pathological changes in the disc, such as disc herniation, can often be mistaken for involutive changes that appear in the cervical disc throughout the life of an individual, and that do not have any pathological significance. In fact, one of the

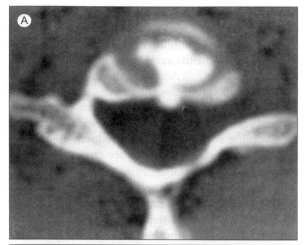

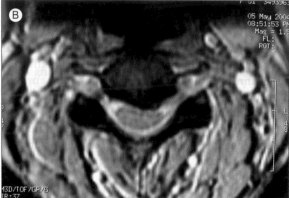

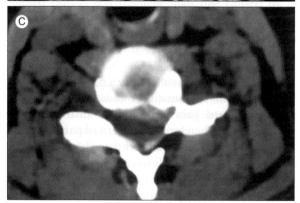

FIGURE 1-13 ■ Posteromedial disc herniation in a discography (A) and posteromedial in MRI (B) and CT (C).

In fact, it is not uncommon to observe in surgery that the extruded material does not cause physical pressure on the spinal nerve. The notion that a disc injury physically compresses the neural tissues does not account for the majority of disc injuries observed in clinical practice.[76]

A small extruded disc herniation is capable of causing as much pain and as significant structural damage to the roots as larger disc herniation, which indicates that mechanical compression, in itself, is not the only mechanism underlying pain. Surgery practiced with local anaesthetics has shown that the roots induce a pain response when subject to mechanical stress only when they show signs of inflammation.[40,77]

Therefore, in radicular pain, secondary tissue changes are necessary involved. Moreover, clinical observation shows that the sequestered discs are frequently associated with radicular pain that is more pronounced than in contained herniations. These observations coincide with experimental studies which show that only the contact of the nucleus pulposus with the nerve root, without a compression mechanism, is capable of altering the conduction velocity and generating histological changes on Schwann's cells, which are identical to those seen in a human disc herniation.[32,78–85] From these studies, it can be concluded that nerve compression, although related to radicular pain, does not constitute the most significant aspect in the changes that the radicular complex undergoes.[32,83,86–88]

Research conducted in the last few years has highlighted that radicular pain and radiculopathy are related to the irritating and neurotoxic properties of nuclear material.[32–34,78,83] The experimental application in the epidural space of autologous nucleus pulposus induces an inflammatory reaction, as well as functional and structural changes in the nerve roots and in the DRG.[32,78,89–94]

The nucleus pulposus has direct neurotoxic effects on the axons by blocking axonal growth.[83] These changes in the nerve roots can be seen 24 hours after the application of nucleus pulposus,[95] and this effect is not observed when applying tissue from the annulus fibrosus.[96]

The alteration of nerve conduction caused by the nucleus can be completely eradicated with the intravenous injection of high doses of methylprednisolone, if applied within the first 24 hours after the application of the nucleus pulposus.[97] This observation justifies the administration of corticoids in an acute radiculopathy in order to minimize the structural deterioration of the root.

The neurotoxic action of the nucleus pulposus can be caused by a minimal fissuration of the outermost annulus, without observing extruded disc material in a magnetic resonance or during surgery.[94,98] This would explain how a radiculopathy and radicular pain are possible without an obvious disc herniation. Both clinical and experimental evidence indicate that the biochemical irritation of the roots caused by the nucleus pulposus plays a crucial role in the production mechanisms of radicular pain.

Over the last few years, there has been significant progress in the study of the chemical and immunological mediators which are responsible for the neurogenic inflammation of the roots. These inflammatory and immune mediators play a crucial role both in the symptoms and the functional changes of the roots. Radicular pain and radiculopathy caused by a disc herniation are the consequence of the neurotoxic action of proinflammatory cytokines and inflammatory substances that are released when the extruded nucleus pulposus has contact with the radicular complex.[32–34,78,99–113] This inflammatory and immunological response leads to the spontaneous regression of the cervical disc herniation. Although it was initially thought that this phenomenon was uncommon,[114] today, we know that it actually corresponds to the natural evolution of the herniated disc.[88] In recent years, many studies have demonstrated that a cervical disc herniation evolves towards its progressive disappearance in the majority of patients.[52,88,115–123]

- Radicular pain and radiculopathy caused by a disc herniation are the consequence of the neurotoxic action of proinflammatory cytokines and inflammatory substances that are released when the extruded nucleus pulposus has contact with the radicular complex
- This inflammatory and immunological response leads to the spontaneous regression of the cervical disc herniation.

The regression of a disc herniation depends on its situation in relation to the PLL, and it is more pronounced in extruded discs that are exposed to the epidural space. In fact, the more extruded the disc, the more important its volume reduction.[52,117,119,124]

The basis for this inflammatory reaction is the contact between the avascular tissues, such as the nucleus, with another tissue that is extremely vascularized, such as the roots. This inflammatory reaction causes the neovascularization of the extruded disc material.[125–127]

This neovascularization involves macrophage activity, which is responsible for the reduction in the size of the disc herniation,[125,126,128–133] The fragments of the cartilaginous endplate, which in some cases accompany the material of the nucleus and the annulus, do not undergo this process of reabsorption and can even hinder the neovascularization process.[117,131,134,135]

The neovascularization process around the herniated nuclear material determines a high-intensity zone in the T2 sequence in MRI with a contrast medium. The contrast medium uptake by the herniated fragments suggests a chemical radiculopathy, secondary to inflammation at the point where there is a solution of continuity in the annulus fibrosus.[136] This unequivocal sign of neovascularization is associated with a positive prognosis. However, it has been primarily observed in lumbar disc herniations.

Saal et al.[86] have highlighted that extruded disc herniations, as they occur in the lumbar spine, have a more positive prognosis than contained herniations. Conceptually, this is consistent with the premise that contained discs are a clinical entity that is physiopathologically different from a nucleus extrusion.

From a therapeutic point of view, it is interesting to understand that the alterations of conduction derived from an experimentally induced disc herniation reach their peak on the seventh day, and then they start to recover until the second month, when a complete recovery can be seen. Therefore, radiculopathy usually tends to be reversed spontaneously in 1 or 2 months.[87,88]

As a conclusion, an essential aspect in the treatment of a disc herniation is knowing its natural history, especially in light of the latest studies, which show that an extruded cervical disc herniation suffers a spontaneous regression. Radicular pain and radiculopathy caused by disc herniation are the consequence of an immune and inflammatory process induced by the contact of the nucleus pulposus with the neural tissue in the epidural space. The neovascularization and subsequent phagocytosis suppress the neurotoxicity of the disc material and lead to its disintegration.

Unlike past interventionist attitudes, which held that disc herniation, in the majority of cases, should be extirpated, today there is evidence to prove that extruded disc herniations undergo a progressive regression. The progressive disappearance of the herniated disc material implies a benign natural evolution of the radiculopathy caused by a disc herniation.

The favourable long-term prognosis of this condition, with up to 75% rate of natural recovery, as well as the demonstration with imaging studies of the decrease in size and the progressive disappearance do not justify surgery, except in exceptional cases.[88,117,137]

Radiculopathy caused by disc herniation frequently shows a positive evolution as long as an adequate control of the symptoms is maintained and neurological deterioration is avoided.

Cervical radiculopathy caused by a disc herniation is, therefore, in the majority of cases, a self-limited condition with a positive natural evolution. A large epidemiological study demonstrated that over a 5-year follow-up period nearly 90% percent of patients were asymptomatic or only mildly incapacitated by the pain.[138]

Usually, radicular pain disappears in a few weeks, as a consequence of the disintegration of the extruded material responsible for the radicular irritation.[139]

However, despite this, a surgical treatment is chosen frequently. Classically, this decision has been made based on the presence of neurological deficit symptoms and severe pain or pain that persists after a non-operative treatment between 2 and 8 weeks. The type of non-operative treatment used is limited to different unspecific measures.[140] In this way, and for unjustified reasons, extruded disc herniations have been frequently considered a clear surgical indication,[141] when repeated MRI explorations have allowed us to understand and confirm that extruded disc fragments have disappeared or decreased significantly in size, so that they stopped compressing neural elements.[52,88,114,116,117,121]

Until very recently, the comparative studies between non-operative and surgical treatment of cervical radiculopathy which have been conducted, have shown that non-surgical treatment has the same level of efficiency without the disadvantages and risks of a surgical intervention,[86,142–146] Currently, most authors recommend a non-surgical treatment for cervical radiculopathy, caused both by disc herniation and lateral canal stenosis,[86,142–144,146–150] even with the presence of amyotrophy.[117]

One example is the work of Saal et al.,[86] who showed that of 24 patients with a prolapsed disc, after a conservative treatment based on specific physical therapy, traction and non-steroidal anti-inflammatory drugs, 20 showed good or excellent results, which equates to 83% of patients receiving conservative treatment According to Saal, the results of the conservative treatment are superior to natural history.

An interesting comparative study between a conservative and surgical treatment was conducted by Heckmann et al.[142] In this study of 60 patients with cervical radiculopathy, 39 were treated with a conservative treatment and 21 with surgery. All of them had brachialgia with sensitive, motor and reflex deficit signs, as well as a disc prolapse confirmed by an MRI. An average follow-up period of 5.5 years was conducted. In the group that received a non-operative treatment, the brachialgia improved in 100%, the sensitive signs improved completely or noticeably in 97%, the reflexes were normalized in 59.2% and the motor weakness improved in 94.1%.

In addition, conservative treatment is preferable to surgery, since this form of therapy does not entail secondary consequences. It is known that 25% of patients that had discectomy and arthrodesis will suffer degenerative changes in the segments adjacent to the fused segment within a period of 10 years.[151] It is speculated that this is related to increased biomechanical stress on the motion segment adjacent to the fused area.[141,152,153] It has been experimentally demonstrated that this surgery increases the intradiscal pressure in the adjacent discs[154,155] and leads to adaptive hypermobility, which would explain the early deterioration of the segments near the fused segment.[155]

It has been stated that although this osteoarthritic degeneration is frequent, it does not necessarily imply a clinical deterioration.[156] However, this has been disproved by recent studies, including one by Goffin et al.[157] These authors studied the frequency with which a degenerative deterioration is caused in the adjacent segments after the anterior interbody fusion and its impact on the clinical situation. In 180 patients that had surgery, a clinical and radiological follow-up was conducted 6 weeks after surgery and then 60 months later. After this period, a progression of degenerative changes was seen radiologically in 92% of patients, with a clinical deterioration associated to most of them. One of the factors responsible for degenerative changes in the adjacent segments after an anterior fusion is a kyphotic change in the cervical spine.[158]

Fouyas et al.[159,160] conducted a Cochrane systematic review in 2002 to determine if a surgical treatment of radiculopathy leads to better outcomes than a non-operative treatment.[159,160] In this meta-analysis, a study of Persson et al.[145] was chosen, as a prospective randomized controlled study. In this study 81 patients were randomly divided into three groups that received three different types of treatment: surgery, physical therapy and immobilization with a hard neck collar. After 3 months, the group that received the surgical treatment had better results in the symptoms and in sensitive and motor deficits; however, after a year there were no significant differences between the three groups. According to the review, the results of surgery are similar to those obtained with conservative treatment. Although the short-term benefits can be superior with a surgical treatment, the fact that they are similar in the long term, in addition to the risks that follow this treatment, does not justify using surgery as a form of treatment.[160]

The Cochrane systematic review was updated in 2010 by the same group.[161] This review concluded that today there is low-quality evidence that surgery may provide pain relief faster than physiotherapy or hard collar immobilization in patients with cervical radiculopathy, but there is little or no difference in the long term.

■ There are no significant differences between the outcomes obtained with a conservative and a surgical treatment of a cervical disc herniation.
■ The treatment of the vast majority of patients with cervical radiculopathy should be conservative.
■ Surgical treatment of cervical radicular pain caused by disc herniation is indicated when a neurological deficit is shown, and when this

worsens despite using an adequate conservative treatment, and when it is manifested with a pyramidal neurological symptomatology.

The treatment of the vast majority of patients with cervical radiculopathy should be conservative. In cervicobrachial pain caused by disc herniation, surgery is indicated when it determines a neurological deficit, and when it worsens despite using an adequate conservative treatment. Also, it is indicated when it is manifested with a pyramidal neurological symptomatology, lateral hemisection syndrome and paraparaesis or tetraparaesis.[66]

A conservative treatment, which requires medical treatment in addition to physical therapy, must be sufficient, and adequate control of the evolution of the clinical signs and pain is crucial, while waiting for the herniation to disappear.[52,88,117]

CERVICOBRACHIAL PAIN CAUSED BY LATERAL CANAL STENOSIS

Lateral canal stenosis is the primary cause relating to the frequency of cervical radiculopathy, reaching between 70% and 75% of all cases.[162] The stenosis is the consequence of degenerative hypertrophy, which, in the majority of cases, is of the interbody, zygapophyseal and uncovertebral joints.[163–166]

As described previously, the articular degenerative changes in the cervical spine are practically universal.[167] Matsumoto et al.[68] showed that, using MRI, degenerative changes can be seen in asymptomatic subjects in 17% of males and 12% of females of 20 years of age, and in 86% and 89% of individuals above the age of 60. The stenosis of the lateral canal is seen radiographically in more than 80% of subjects with cervical spondylosis, especially in the C5–C6 and C6–C7 segments.[168] However, the majority do not present symptoms. Boden et al.,[76] in a study with MRI conducted in 63 asymptomatic subjects, observed that 14% of subjects below the age of 40 had a foraminal stenosis or herniation, and this percentage reached 25% in subjects above the age of 40. Therefore, although the reduction in the diameter of the foramen is a very common phenomenon, it does not necessarily imply the presence of symptoms in the majority of individuals.[76] The scarce correlation between cervical degenerative changes and the symptoms imply that the findings seen in imaging tests should be interpreted with caution.

- In the cervical spine involutive and degenerative changes cannot be differentiated.
- Spondylosis is a practically universal phenomenon and is not necessarily associated symptomatology.

Degenerative foraminal stenosis occurs gradually, as do the symptoms which derive from it. Since stenosis is more pronounced in the middle portion of the foramen, just at the level of the unciform process and the facet joints, the foramen acquires the shape of an eight, and the roots are pushed frequently towards the upper half of the foramen (Fig. 1-14).

Cervical spondylosis is a process that affects all the articular systems of the cervical spine and is accompanied by degenerative changes in the discs, osteophytes in the vertebral bodies and hypertrophy of the zygapophyseal joints and laminae.

Now, we briefly describe the progressive changes that should initially be considered as a natural age-related process, and that can develop into a pathological situation,[169] taking into account that, from a morphological perspective, these changes are indistinguishable.[69]

The degenerative process of the intervertebral disc is seen in the nucleus, the annulus and the cartilaginous endplate, although it is more pronounced in the nucleus. The disc suffers a dehydration mainly in the nucleus pulposus.[170]

The progressive reduction of the volume in the nucleus pulposus[171] is associated with the fissuration of the annulus fibrosus.[3] All of this leads to a decrease in height and to the bulging of the annulus fibrosus, manifesting itself in the form of a hard disc herniation, which tends to reduce the light of the foramen.[172] The disc degeneration determines the growth of osteophytes on the body margins.[67,165,173,174]

The loss of disc height also modifies the anatomical relationship of the articular facets, which will contribute to a greater decrease of the foraminal diameter.

Thus, the inferior facet of the upper vertebra tends to glide downwards and backwards, while the upper facets of the underlying vertebra tend to be more anterior and superior. The degenerative changes that are seen in the articular facets are subchondral sclerosis, the formation of osteophytes and the loss of articular cartilage. The articular capsule suffers a thickening and, occasionally, synovial cysts can significantly reduce the light of the foramen. The decrease in the anteroposterior diameter of the foramen is caused mainly by the hypertrophy of the lower facet.[165] Therefore, facet hypertrophy and the hypertrophy of the laminae and the yellow ligament can contribute to the development of radiculopathy.[175] With the thinning of the disc, the uncovertebral joints bear higher compressive loads and they also suffer degenerative changes. This hyperpressure leads to an osteophytosis of the unciform process towards the lateral canal that can compress the spinal nerves or the vertebral artery.[176] The DRGs of C5–T1 are very thick and laterally are close to the uncovertebral joints. In some subjects, these osteophytes are extremely long and can compress the anterior part of the spinal cord.[177,178] (Fig. 1-15).

The structural changes of the disc and the zygapophyseal joints are responsible for the development of segmental instability.[179] The local instability, if it is associated with retrolisthesis, can further increase the compression.

Foraminal stenosis must be considered to be a dynamic condition, since the flexion and extension movements of the cervical spine modify the size of the foramen, and therefore can increase or decrease the compression. With flexion, the size of the intervertebral foramen increases, and with ipsilateral rotation

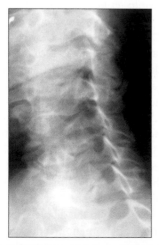

FIGURE 1-14 ■ Oblique projection with degenerative stenosis of the foramen at several levels.

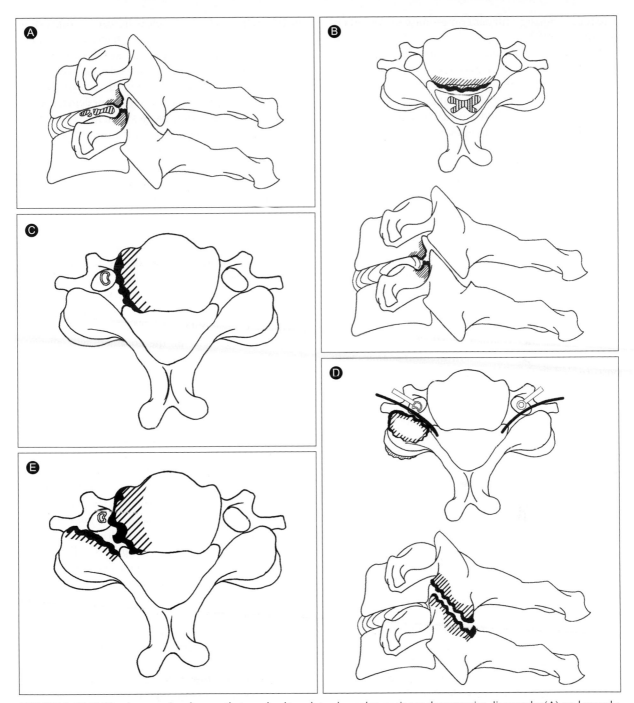

FIGURE 1-15 ■ The degenerative changes that can lead to a lateral canal stenosis are degenerative discopathy (A) and spondylosis (B), uncarthrosis (C), degenerative hypertrophy of the facet joint (D) and the degenerative hypertrophy of the facet and unciform joint (E).

it reduces, causing a higher compromise of the radicular complex.[180,181]

By way of conclusion, degenerative changes in the interbody, zygapophyseal and uncovertebral joints can increase the vulnerability of the nerve roots to mechanical stress. It is therefore clear that the possibility of the roots being compromised during movement increases when the degenerative changes increase.

The *clinical condition* is often the consequence of an overload that alters a fragile balance in subjects with a previously stenosed canal due to degenerative changes. The trigger factor can be a joint synovitis or a direct radicular irritation caused by osteophytes or inflammatory changes in a root that has already been mechanically compromised.

It is very important to highlight that the biomechanics of the radicular compression caused by a spinal stenosis is different from that caused by a disc herniation. The spinal stenosis is generally a slow process that allows for a certain degree of adaptation of the tissues lodged inside the foramen. Furthermore, the compression is dynamic and intermittent. It changes with posture and it occurs in more than one place along the nerve roots. However, in a disc herniation, there is higher focal compression than in degenerative stenosis. As previously described, in a disc herniation, two irritative phenomena can be associated on the root: compression and the neurotoxic effects of the nucleus pulposus. The combination of these two mechanisms, as it occurs in a disc herniation, is the most frequent cause of severe radicular pain.[182] Although the degenerative stenosis can further reduce the lateral canal diameter, it generates less symptoms than a hernia.

- The stenosis of the lateral canal is the first cause of cervical radiculopathy.
- The clinical presentation of radiculopathy due to canal stenosis is different from the disc herniation. Although it may reduce the diameter of the canal significantly, it generally causes less symptoms than a hernia.
- The degenerative stenosis of the lateral canal often manifests with a chronic radiculopathy, in which radicular pain can be moderated and even absent.

The dysfunction of the nerve roots is not only related to the intensity of the compression but also linked to its duration. A rapidly induced compression causes more pronounced tissue changes and higher functional deterioration than when the compression is induced at a slower rate. Therefore, an acute compression induces more pronounced changes than a progressive compression, as a root oedema, axonal transport reduction and changes in nerve conduction. These physiological effects that depend on the velocity of the compression are based probably on the viscoelastic properties of the radicular tissues. Hence the disc herniation causes higher structural and functional deterioration than a lateral stenosis, which evolves slowly throughout the years. The clinical presentation of the radiculopathy caused by canal stenosis is therefore different from a disc herniation.

The degenerative stenosis of the lateral canal is often manifested with a chronic radiculopathy in which radicular pain can be moderate or even absent. However, these patients can suffer somatic referred pain of the zygapophyseal joints. In these cases, the surgical enlargement of the foramen will alleviate the radiculopathy, but it will not have any effects on the somatic referred pain.

Natural history of the degenerative radiculopathy

It is very important to understand the natural history of the degenerative radiculopathy, since the results of its treatment, both conservative and surgical, should be compared to the natural evolution of the disease, before recommending a particular treatment. It is commonly assumed that patients with radiculopathy due to a cervical canal stenosis will continue to be symptomatic and that their symptoms will progress unless they are subject to surgery. However, there is no evidence to validate this claim.

The natural evolution of radiculopathy due to degenerative stenosis was investigated by Lees and Turner,[169] who observed the evolution of 51 patients with cervical radiculopathy over a period of 19 years: 45% of the patients had a single episode of radiculopathy without a relapse; 30% had moderate symptoms; and 25% had persistent symptoms that worsened – i.e. only a quarter of the patients that did not have surgery worsened. Also it is worth mentioning the study of Persson et al.[145] with patients with cervical radicular pain caused by foraminal stenosis dating back to more than 3 months, and in which it was demonstrated that after 12 months there were no clinical or functional differences between those that received a surgical or a non-operative treatment.

Saal et al.[124] have recently shown that the conservative treatment can be a therapeutic option in lateral canal stenosis. In their study, they applied a non-operative treatment in 53 patients, of which 77% had neurological deficits, and they conducted a follow-up for 2 years. After the treatment, 88% of patients recovered the neurological deficit, and in 94% the radicular arm pain disappeared.

Diagnosis of cervicobrachialgias

The differential diagnosis of cervical radicular pain and radiculopathy is significantly more complex than in the lumbar spine. Radicular pain has been defined as pain whose distribution coincides with the innervation of a particular root.[179]

However, pain distribution on the upper limb provides few arguments to infer that pain is radicular, since many times other entities share a similar pain pattern, such as discogenic and zygapophyseal referred pain, thoracic outlet syndromes, referred pain from the shoulder, and even peripheral neuropathies of the upper limb.

An initial differentiation should be made between the clinical presentation of radicular pain due to a disc herniation and pain derived from a stenosis of the lateral canal. The radicular cervicobrachialgia caused by a disc herniation is frequently manifested in an acute or subacute manner, while the stenosis of the cervical canal appears in an insidious and chronic way.

A radiculopathy caused by a disc herniation can be often suspected because of the characteristics and the behaviour of the pain. The classic pattern is characterized by starting with an intense and burning pain in the areas of the upper thoracic region, especially on the medial border of the scapula,[183] and after a few days a severe pain appears on the upper limb, associated to paraesthesia, a very uncomfortable feeling of heaviness of the arm, weakness and progressive weakness of the related muscles. In a recent study, Tanaka et al.[183] showed that the proximal areas of radicular pain can be useful to identify the affected root. According to this study, pain in the suprascapular region frequently indicates a radicular irritation of C5 or C6. Pain in the

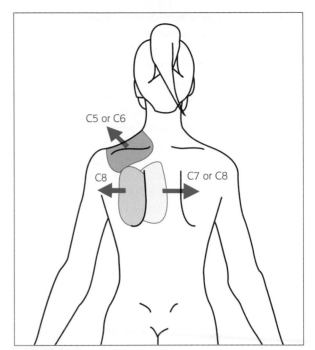

FIGURE 1-16 ■ Proximal radicular pain map. *(Adapted from Tanaka et al.[183])*

interscapular region suggests the affectation of the C7 or C8 root, and pain on the scapula suggests the affectation of the C8 roots (Fig. 1-16).

Pain is usually extremely severe and constant, since it is related to an acute radicular inflammatory condition. The patient has difficulty finding pain-alleviating positions, and pain is accompanied by discomfort and sometimes even nausea. This situation can be linked to the radicular vegetative components or to the fact that the same innervation of the disc, by the sinuvertebral nerve, links these components. It is common for the pain to worsen at night, making it difficult to sleep. Distal pain can be more important than proximal pain, which makes it different from referred pain. A characteristic of radicular pain of disc origin, which is also shared by the discogenic pain, is pain latency. When a movement irritates the neural tissues, pain does not appear immediately, but is delayed for a few seconds. The previous phenomenon is frequently accompanied by another one, known as the *pain wave*, which means that pain severity increases progressively, is maintained at its highest level for a few seconds, and takes a few seconds to subside progressively. Therefore, during the physical assessment, provocation manoeuvres should be performed slowly in order to prevent this unpleasant phenomenon.

Radiculopathy caused by a lateral canal stenosis is characterized primarily by the progressive onset of radicular signs, and pain can be moderate.

Age is an important aspect when differentiating a radiculopathy related to a disc herniation from one caused by a lateral canal stenosis. In general, patients with a disc herniation are usually younger than 40 years old, while patients of ≥ 50 years old show, more often, a degenerative stenosis of the lateral canal.

In order to understand the clinical presentation of a patient with a cervical radiculopathy, we must remember that the compression and irritation can occur in the emergence of the roots, the DRG, or at the level of the spinal nerve and, therefore, always before the division of the spinal nerve in an anterior and posterior primary ramus. The radicular symptomatology does not exclusively include the area of the anterior primary ramus, manifested as a brachialgia, but also the area of the posterior primary ramus. This would explain why pain, especially in the initial phases, is usually more severe proximally, in the area innervated by the posterior ramus, than distally, in the upper limb. This fact could also be linked to an inflammation of the disc and it could be nothing more than discogenic referred pain. Regardless of the cause, it is common to see patients with cervical radiculopathy that has been diagnosed as an acute thoracic pain.

Physical assessment

Observation

The *observation* of the posture of the cervical spine and the upper limb can help to determine if the patient's symptomatology is radicular. The analysis of the relationship between pain and the different postures and movements has diagnostic relevance, since in a cervicobrachialgia the sensitization of the neural tissue to mechanical stimuli is crucial.

Patients with radiculopathy, regardless of their aetiology, show an antalgic posture in flexion or in flexion and contralateral side-bending, and they present reduced range of movement towards the side of the brachialgia. This antalgic posture increases the diameter of the foramen and it decreases the pressure exerted on the inflamed roots. A small percentage of patients with an acute radicular disorder found relief by adopting postures that lean towards the side of pain.[42] Although this antalgic behavior may seem counterproductive, it is able to reduce tension over the root. This antalgic posture would be similar to the direct pattern of the lumbar spine that is seen frequently in L5 disc herniations. The inability to obtain a contralateral side-bending enough to displace the root from the extruded disc material leads to an antalgic pattern in ipsilateral side-bending that allows for an effective decrease in tension over the S1 root.

The symptoms worsen in situations that increase the intrathecal pressure, such as physical activity, coughing, etc.; this is why Valsalva's sign may be positive. Pain is more intense at night, making it difficult to sleep. As the supine position normally tends to increase the lordosis, the patient avoids rest in bed and prefers to remain seated in order to sleep. Some patients can only sleep with two or three pillows in order to maintain sufficient cervical flexion. Progressively, the proximal pain starts to decrease, and the paraesthesia begins to worsen, as do motor and distal sensitive signs.

A cervical radiculopathy can be expressed in other ways.[42] Sometimes, the patient refers a severe pain in the medial border of the scapula that is not accompanied by brachial pain, which would lead one to attribute these symptoms to a joint dysfunction of the thoracic spine. However, provocation tests of the cervical spine aggravate the symptoms, and the decrease of the reflexes and the strength of the related muscles is obvious. On other occasions, the clinical presentation can simulate a peripheral neuropathy, such as a carpal tunnel syndrome, since the patient only refers acute distal paraesthesia with minimum pain on the upper limb. Pain can also be referred to the anterior chest wall, which simulates pain caused by a cardiac ischaemia.[29,184] It is recommended to rule out cervical radiculopathy in every patient with symptoms in the thoracic region or the upper limb.

The radiculopathy of the upper cervical segments, C2–C3, can be manifested as suboccipital pain, headaches and facial paraesthesia.[21,185]

It can also manifest itself, although infrequently, as a bilateral cervicobrachialgia, as a consequence of a massive disc herniation. Symptoms of acute paraplegia,[186] Brown–Séquard syndrome[187–190] and even tetra-paraesthesias[191,192] have been described.

There is a characteristic *clinical sign* of an acute radiculopathy: patients can manage to relieve brachial pain by placing the arm in abduction and supporting the forearm above the head (Fig. 1-17). This manoeuvre significantly decreases radicular pain. This pain relief sign with shoulder abduction[193–193] was described by Davidson et al.[193] and it has been demonstrated experimentally on fresh specimens that it significantly reduces the intraforaminal pressure in the C5, C6 and C7 roots.[180] It can be considered as characteristic of a cervical disc herniation.[194] This posture is often adopted by the patient when sitting down for a long period of time.

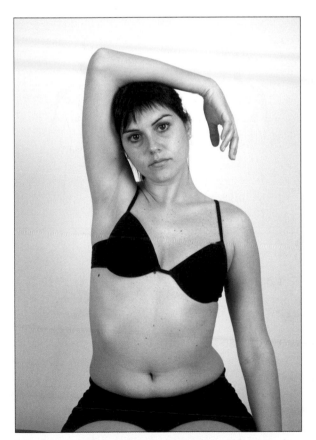

FIGURE 1-17 ■ The shoulder abduction relief sign is characteristic of an acute radiculopathy. The patient can reduce the symptoms of the upper limb by maintaining it in abduction and supporting the forearm over the head.

The mechanism that explains this pain relief is the decrease in tension over the roots. Although the shoulder abduction brings the plexus closer to the coracoid, when accompanied by an elevation of the scapula and it is moving closer to the spine, the tension of the neural elements is reduced, and the neural tension is reduced even more when the elbow is flexed.

Another position of the upper limb that patients also use to decrease pain is supporting the affected arm with the contralateral arm, so that the shoulder stays slightly elevated and the shoulder is separated from the trunk. Its effect on pain is linked to the reduction of the tension on the roots.

- Radicular pain in the upper limb is a highly irritable clinical situation.
- When the signs and symptoms suggest radicular origin, the physical assessment should be brief, without insisting on pain provocation or neurodynamic tests.

A very important aspect that we must consider in patient assessment is that cervicobrachialgia is a syndrome with a high level of irritability. The physical assessment of a patient with radiculopathy should be extremely careful. A small irritation of the inflamed neural tissues can dramatically aggravate the symptoms in the following hours and days. If the signs and symptoms suggest a radicular origin, the physical assessment should be brief, without insisting on pain provocation or neurodynamic tests, or any movement that can reproduce pain.

Radicular pain patterns

As described previously, the neurological level of the radiculopathy cannot be inferred exclusively based on the distribution of pain. The topography of pain does not indicate whether pain is radicular; nor can it be used to determine the neurological level of the radiculopathy, as the case may be. Even so, subjects with zygapophyseal or discogenic show a referred pain area that is more proximal than subjects with radicular pain.[23,196]

Pain in the shoulder girdle and the arm can be somatic referred or radicular, while pain perceived on the forearm and the hand is more likely to be of radicular origin. The proximal area of reference for radicular pain has already been shown in Figure 1-16.

The distribution of radicular pain does not follow a dermatomic pattern as has been commonly affirmed. This concept is erroneous and can lead to unsuitable therapeutic decisions.[1,70,71,197] The study of Slipman et al.[198] has shown that radicular pain is frequently outside the distribution of the dermatome maps and differs from the skin area where the sensitive deficit is manifested. These authors have proposed the term 'dynatome' to refer to the area where the radicular pain is perceived. Therefore, radicular pain, particularly with a dysaesthetic character, is expressed in a topographic area that does not necessarily coincide with the dermatome (Fig. 1-18). *Paraesthesia*, as well as the area of skin hypoaesthesia, the dermatome, are more reliable from a diagnostic point of view.

Even so, we must be careful when attributing the symptoms to a specific root based only on the location of the hypoaesthesia or the paraesthesia. The characteristics of radicular pain allow us to differentiate it from somatic pain which has the same distribution. Radicular pain is usually dysaesthetic, which patients refer to as a burning, sharp shooting or a deep cramp. However, in subjects that show a radiculopathy caused by stenosis of the lateral canal, pain can be somatic, being perceived as deep, diffuse and in ill-defined locations.

Provocation test

Movements that modify the mechanical interface and neurodynamic tests are used as provocation tests.

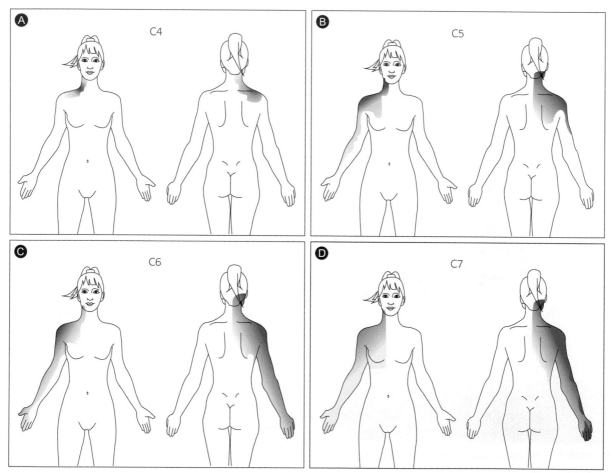

FIGURE 1-18 ■ Dynatome maps: (A) C4 dynatome; (B) C5 dynatome; (C) C6 dynatome; and (D) C7 dynatome. *(Modified from Slipman et al.[198])*

Mechanical interface test. Mechanical interface tests are those that reduce the area of the intervertebral foramen, such as extension, side-bending and rotation towards the side of pain. Initially, and with the purpose of avoiding the excessive irritation of the root, each one of the movements should be performed in isolation. In order to further sensitize these positions, pressure can be applied for 20 to 30 seconds. Subsequently, if the responses are not significant, Spurling's test can be used, which associates an extension, side-bending and rotation with an axial compression component (Fig. 1-19). It has been shown with MRI,[45] as well as in studies with specimens,[199] that this manoeuvre reduces the light of the foramen. This test is clinically useful for confirming a cervical radiculopathy and, although it does not have excessive sensitivity, it has very good specificity.[200]

We must take into account that the test is considered to be positive when the symptoms, such as paraesthesia or pain, are distal. The onset of proximal pain does not mean that the subject is suffering from a radiculopathy. The same movement combination implies an increase in the convergence and pressure over the zygapophyseal joints, which, if irritated, can refer proximal pain in the thoracic pain as the radicular pain does.

Other useful diagnostic tests for cervical radiculopathy are the compression and distraction tests.[201] The reproduction of brachial pain with compression and relief with distraction suggests a radiculopathy. A variant of the compression test, which sometimes amplifies the symptoms, is as follows: compression is applied starting from the flexion of the cervical spine, and maintaining this flexion, the cervical spine is taken to a moderate extension (Fig. 1-20).

Neurodynamic test. Neurodynamic tests are very useful for the assessment and differential diagnosis of radiculopathies.[43,201–209] The aim of this test is to assess the mechanosensitivity of neural tissues. Of the three neurodynamic tests, the upper limb neurodynamic test 1 (ULNT1) or brachial plexus tension test, originally described in 1979 by Elvey[43] is one of the best regarding an assessment of cervical radicular pain[201,203,207]

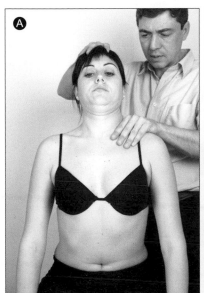
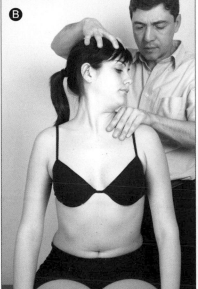
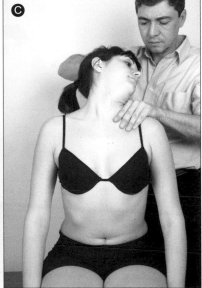

FIGURE 1-19 ■ Mechanical interface tests. The therapist passively directs the patient's cervical spine towards extension, side-bending and rotation towards the side of the pain. Initially, each one of the movements is performed in isolation and the response is observed (A). In order to make the test even more sensitive, a compression can be applied (B). Then, the Spurling's manoeuvre is performed (C).

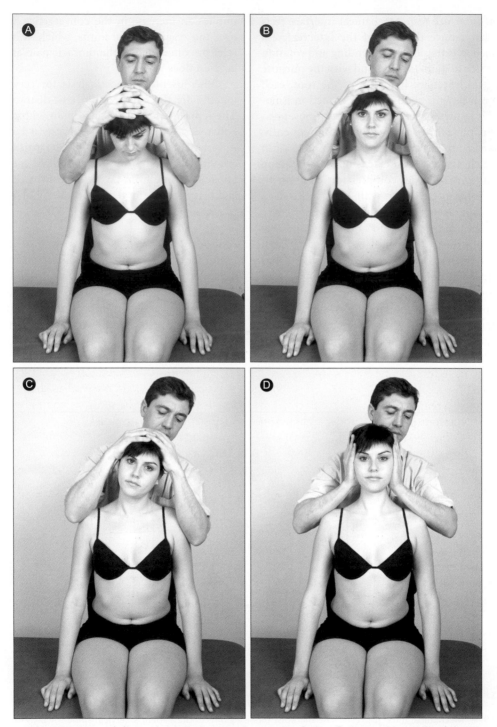

FIGURE 1-20 ■ Compression and distraction test. Compression starting from a flexion position (A) and directing the cervical spine to extension (B). In order to sensitize the test more, a cervical side-bending to the side of pain is added and compression can be applied (C). Relief of the symptoms with distraction (D).

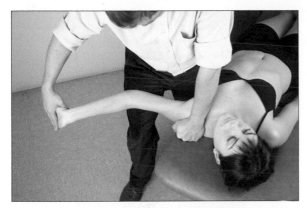

FIGURE 1-21 ■ Neurodynamic test for the upper limb 1 (ULNT1).

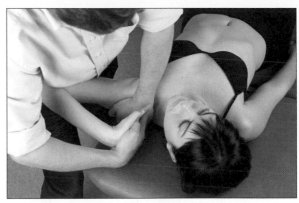

FIGURE 1-22 ■ Neurodynamic test for the upper limb 3 (ULNT3).

(Fig. 1-21). It has been demonstrated in specimens that this test transmits tension efficiently to the cervical roots, at the expense of the tension induced on the median nerve.[207]

Clinically, it has been also demonstrated that it is capable of identifying symptoms in the brachial plexus[210] and its interexaminer reliability has been demonstrated.[205]

It is necessary to remember that it is much easier to aggravate the symptoms with a neurodynamic test in the upper limbs than in the lower ones. Nerves are more fragile and their trajectory is more complex in the upper limb and, therefore, this test must be performed carefully when there is an acute radiculopathy. Neurodynamic tests offer subjective information, such as the tension feeling that is perceived by the patient, as well as the reproduction of the symptoms, and objective information, such as the amplitude of movement and the perception of resistance by the therapist.[211] It is necessary to compare the responses with the contralateral member. There are different variants regarding the order of each of the components of the test. In radiculopathies of C8, the ULNT3 can be used, since it transmits the tension via the cubital nerve (Fig. 1-22).

Another test that can confirm that the patient suffers from a radiculopathy is the palpation of the anterior and medial portion of the transverse processes. If a gentle palpation of this area reproduces intense pain on the scapula or along the upper limb, there is greater reason to suspect a radiculopathy. For a review of the reliability and diagnostic accuracy of different clinical tests in cervical radiculopathy, the study of Wainner et al.[201] is recommended.

Neurological examination

The only way to provide evidence for a radiculopathy during the clinical evaluation is by assessing the neurological deficits. It is essential to locate the implied segment based on the sensitive and motor deficit and the osteotendinous reflexes.

Dermatomal maps can be useful for identifying a particular neurological level based on the area where a particular alteration of sensitivity is observed.[212,213] However, their reliability is not absolute since there is significant variability[214–216] and in a significant number of patients the described classic maps do not match.[217]

This lack of correlation between the sensitive alteration and the dermatomal maps could be linked to the anatomical variants in the division of the roots, spinal nerves, plexuses and intersegmental anastomoses between the spinal roots.[11,218,219] Moriishi et al.[219] dissected the spine cord of 100 adults and found that 61% of them showed anastomosis between the posterior roots of the cervical spine. The sensitive innervation of the same area comes almost always from at least two roots.[220,221]

In addition, both at the plexus and at the peridural level, a redistribution of the fibres occurs. Therefore, we should avoid an overly rigid and simplistic view of the dermatomal maps.

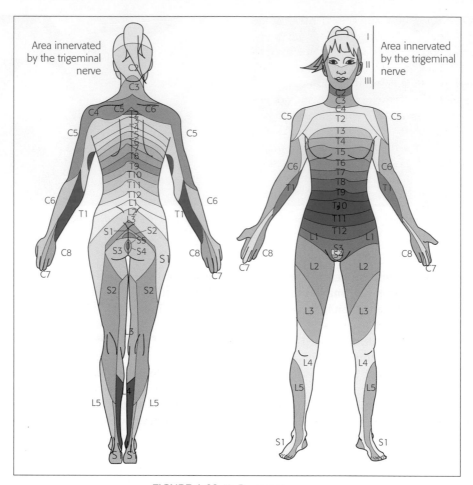

FIGURE 1-23 ■ Dermatome map.

In order to explore the dermatome, the most reliable method is to evaluate the modifications by means of perception of fine touch, using a cotton swab.

The C1 level cannot be explored, as it does not provide skin innervation. The C2 dermatome includes the posterior part of the head behind the ears. The C3 dermatome corresponds to the anterior and posterior region of the neck. The C4 dermatome corresponds to a skin strip above the clavicle, the anterior face of the shoulders and the region of the trapezius. The C5 dermatome corresponds to the regions of the shoulder, including the lateral face of the arm. In the C6 dermatome, sensitive alterations are perceived in the thumb and the index finger. In C7, sensory changes in the middle finger, with a certain degree of overlapping

with the adjacent fingers are seen. The dermatome of C8 corresponds to the cubital hand and cubital fingers. The T1 dermatome encompasses the internal face of the forearm (Fig. 1-23).

The assessment of the myotome, as well as the osteotendinous reflexes, is important, since they provide objective signs of radiculopathy. It must be remembered that the innervation of a muscle does not usually depend on a single root, so that the sign that is being sought is not paralysis, but muscle weakness. Therefore, the tests are based on requesting repeated contractions that could show muscle weakness.

The myotome of C5 is explored with the abduction of the shoulder, since the deltoid is almost entirely innervated by the C5 root. The C6 myotome is explored with the flexion of the elbow, and the extension of the wrist. The myotome of C7 is explored with the extension of the elbow and the fingers. The motor component of the C8 root is explored with the thumb opposition and the flexion of the fingers. The T1 myotome is explored with the abduction and adduction of the fingers. In order to evaluate the myotome, the muscle is placed in an intermediate position and the patient is asked to maintain an isometric contraction for several seconds, against the forces applied by the therapist.

The *alteration of the osteotendinous reflexes*, hyporeflexia or areflexia, indicate a greater or lesser interruption of the reflex arc. The bicipital reflex evaluates primarily the root of C5, the brachioradial reflex or radial style, informs the root of C6 and, finally, the triciptal reflex evaluates the root of C7. It must be highlighted that the isolated decrease of the reflexes that is not accompanied by sensitive motor changes may lack clinical significance, since the reflex response can be modified by non-pathological circumstances, such as stress or anxiety.

Differential diagnosis

There are other entities that demand a differential diagnosis with cervical radiculopathy, such as facet or discogenic referred pain, shoulder pathology, upper limb neuropathies, thoracic outlet syndrome and Parsonage–Turner syndrome.[222,223]

Zygapophyseal and discogenic referred symptoms can be similar to cervicobrachialgia, in addition to possible radiographic signs of spondylosis. However, its reference pattern reaches the hand less frequently, and proximal pain is always more intense than distal pain.

Parsonage–Turner syndrome or acute brachial plexus neuritis can easily be confused with a cervical radiculopathy.[223,224] This syndrome is characterized by an acute onset of severe pain, which disappears after a few days or weeks. As soon as it disappears, a marked weakness or even paralysis develops in the muscles of the upper limb (Fig. 1-24). A marked upper limb weakness coincides with a rapid decrease of the symptoms.[223,225] This behaviour makes it different from radiculopathy, since a radiculopathy needs a few days to be developed. This temporal pain profile preceding weakness is important to establish a prompt diagnosis

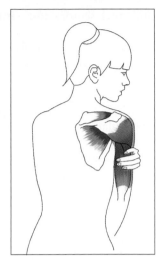

FIGURE 1-24 ■ The Parsonage–Turner syndrome is characterized by a severe pain on the shoulder girdle and the upper limb, followed by a weakness and severe muscle atrophy. *(Modified from Waldman S. Síndromes dolorosos poco frecuentes. Madrid: Elsevier; 2004.)*

and to differentiate this condition from cervical radiculopathy. The symptoms of a radiculopathy can be aggravated by cervical movements, while they have no influence at all on the Parsonage–Turner syndrome. The other difference is that with Parsonage–Turner syndrome two or more nerves are involved but a radiculopathy is restricted to one root. The weakness is commonly seen in the supraspinatus, infraspinatus, deltoid and the biceps muscles as this syndrome primarily affects the upper trunk of the brachial plexus.

Entrapment upper limb neuropathies can also appear in similar ways to a cervicobrachialgia. To distinguish between a radiculopathy and a peripheral nerve lesion, the neurological examination, the location of pain, a Tinel sign and the history play an important role. Relating to motor signs, the weakness in cervical radiculopathy is usually partial or incomplete, because nearly all muscles are innervated by more than one spinal nerve. Therefore severe weakness and atrophy is quite rare. In a radiculopathy, deep tendon reflexes are depressed or absent. Sensory symptoms in a radiculopathy follow a dermatomal pattern. Decreased sensitivity and paraesthesia occur in the distal extent of the dermatome of the involved spinal nerve and total sensory loss virtually never occurs.

The thoracic outlet syndromes can also be responsible for a similar clinical presentation. These syndromes are described in Chapter 3.

Muscle referred pain can, in some cases, simulate a cervicobrachialgia. These muscles, whose pain pattern can simulate a radicular pain are infraspinous, scalenus, serratus anterior, latissimus dorsi, subscapular, rotator teres major muscle, pectoralis major and minor, supraspinous and triceps (Fig. 1-25). It is important to note that the existence of referred pain muscle does not rule out that the pain is radicular. Muscle referred pain is usually an epiphenomenon that is associated with many pain aetiologies.

Pancoast's tumour can simulate a cervical radiculopathy. Radicular pain with a progressive worsening, which is resistant to treatment, in subjects with a history of smoking, should lead to suspicions of this entity. Less frequently, cervical or thoracic spinal tumours and demyelinating diseases show similar signs.

Diagnostic imaging techniques

The diagnosis of a radiculopathy can be performed with the subjective and the physical assessment. However, imaging tests can provide interesting information.

Conventional radiology, although it provides limited information, is usually the initial exploration in the evaluation of the cervical spine. It does not offer information relating to soft tissues and, therefore, it cannot be used to diagnose a disc herniation. It only provides indirect information of disc degeneration, when a decrease in the intersomatic space is seen, as well as an anterior or posterior osteophytosis.[73] Conventional radiology can be useful to observe degenerative changes of the interbody and zygapophyseal joints. Oblique projections show the intervertebral foramen, and can have interest when diagnosing lateral canal stenosis.

Currently, MRI is the most widely used imaging technique for the diagnosis of cervical spine pathology. MRI is the preferred imaging test because it lets us see, as a whole, the relationship between the bony structures and soft tissues, such as the disc and the neural tissues. An MRI provides an excellent vision of the intervertebral disc, information regarding the location and magnitude of the hernia, and also allows the visualization of the neural tissues, such as the roots and the spinal cord (Fig. 1-26). It can also show Modic changes in bone marrow. CT scans offer a better definition of the bony structures and could be indicated in cervical spine trauma.

Cervical *discography* is used, on the one hand, to recognize the internal injuries to the intervertebral disc, and on the other hand, as a test to provoke discogenic pain. While this test is usually painless in normal discs, it is highly provocative in all those subjects with intense discogenic pain.[22,23] However there is still controversy in the use of discography as diagnostic tool because it is an invasive technique and, consequently, it is not free of risks (Fig. 1-27).

Neurophysiological evaluation

Neurophysiological evaluation, electromyography and nerve conduction studies are useful when locating the radicular level. However, in most cases, these diagnostic evaluations are not necessary when the characteristic symptoms of a radiculopathy are present, although they are an efficient means of differentiating this entity from a peripheral neuropathy. Neurophysiological studies are therefore indicated when there is diagnostic doubt between a cervical radiculopathy and other peripheral neurological entities.

MANAGEMENT OF CERVICOBRACHIALGIAS

This section explains the treatment of a radiculopathy caused by a disc herniation and a lateral canal stenosis. The management of these two entities is not significantly different. In most cases, with an adequate initial treatment, there is a decrease in pain in a few weeks. It must be noted that, often a radiculopathy caused by a disc herniation with severe pain requires a shorter treatment period than that which is necessary to treat a cervical facet joint syndrome, whose symptoms are more benign. However, it is essential, in the first case, to have an adequate management of the condition during the acute phase.

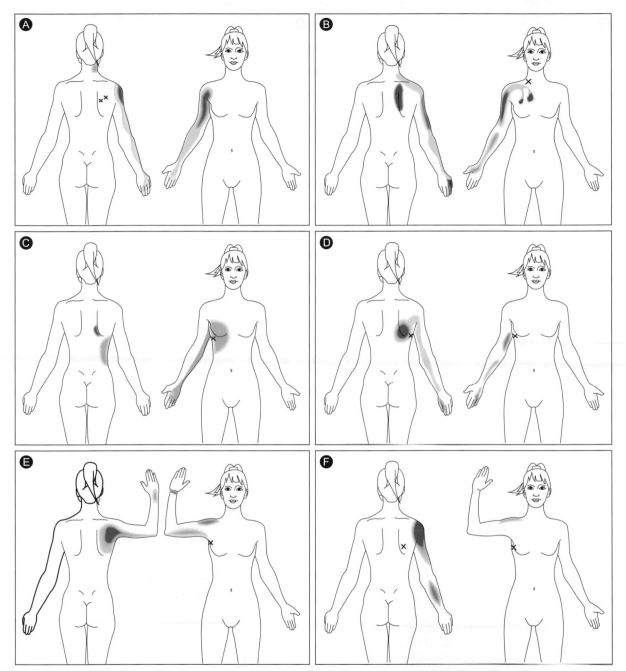

FIGURE 1-25 ■ Myofascial referred pain patterns that can simulate a radiculopathy: (A) infraspinous, (B) scalene muscles, (C) serratus anterior, (D) latissimus dorsi, (E) subscapular, (F) teres major muscle, (G) pectoralis major, (H) pectoralis minor, (I) supraspinous and (J) triceps.   *Continued*

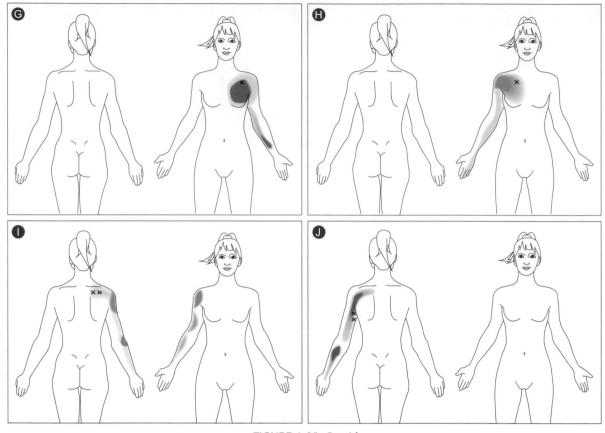

FIGURE 1-25, Cont'd

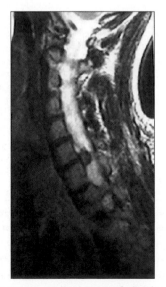

FIGURE 1-26 ■ Voluminous soft disc herniation.

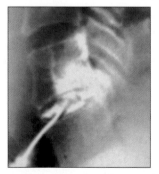

FIGURE 1-27 ■ Discography that shows a posterior migration of the disc material.

148. Schimandle JH, Heller JG. Nonoperative treatment of degenerative cervical disk disease. J South Orthop Assoc 1996;5(3): 207–12.

149. Truumees E, Herkowitz HN. Cervical spondylotic myelopathy and radiculopathy. Instr Course Lect 2000;49:339–60.

150. Eubanks JD. Cervical radiculopathy: nonoperative management of neck pain and radicular symptoms. Am Fam Physician 2010;81(1):33–40.

151. Hilibrand AS, Carlson GD, Palumbo MA, et al. Radiculopathy and myelopathy at segments adjacent to the site of a previous anterior cervical arthrodesis. J Bone Joint Surg Am 1999; 81(4):519–28.

152. Baba H, Furusawa N, Imura S, et al. Late radiographic findings after anterior cervical fusion for spondylotic myeloradiculopathy. Spine 1993;18(15):2167–73.

153. Maiman DJ, Kumaresan S, Yoganandan N, et al. Biomechanical effect of anterior cervical spine fusion on adjacent segments. Biomed Mater Eng 1999;9(1):27–38.

154. Pospiech J, Stolke D, Wilke HJ, et al. Intradiscal pressure recordings in the cervical spine. Neurosurgery 1999;44(2):379– 84, discussion 384–5.

155. Eck JC, Humphreys SC, Lim TH, et al. Biomechanical study on the effect of cervical spine fusion on adjacent-level intradiscal pressure and segmental motion. Spine 2002;27(22): 2431–4.

156. Cherubino P, Benazzo F, Borromeo U, et al. Degenerative arthritis of the adjacent spinal joints following anterior cervical spinal fusion: clinicoradiologic and statistical correlations. Ital J Orthop Traumatol 1990;16(4):533–43.

157. Goffin J, Geusens E, Vantomme N, et al. Long-term follow-up after interbody fusion of the cervical spine. J Spinal Disord 2004;17(2):79–85.

158. Katsuura A, Hukuda S, Saruhashi Y, et al. Kyphotic malalignment after anterior cervical fusion is one of the factors promoting the degenerative process in adjacent intervertebral levels. Eur Spine J 2001;10(4):320–4.

159. Fouyas IP, Statham PF, Sandercock PA, et al. Surgery for cervical radiculomyelopathy. Cochrane Database Syst Rev 2001;(3):CD001466.

160. Fouyas IP, Statham PF, Sandercock PA. Cochrane review on the role of surgery in cervical spondylotic radiculomyelopathy. Spine 2002;27(7):736–47.

161. Nikolaidis I, Fouyas IP, Sandercock PA, et al. Surgery for cervical radiculopathy or myelopathy. Cochrane Database Syst Rev 2010;(1):CD001466.

162. Carette S, Fehlings MG. Clinical practice. Cervical radiculopathy. N Engl J Med 2005;353(4):392–9.

163. Yu YL, Woo E, Huang CY. Cervical spondylotic myelopathy and radiculopathy. Acta Neurol Scand 1987;75(6):367–73.

164. Ebraheim NA, Lu J, Biyani A, et al. Anatomic considerations for uncovertebral involvement in cervical spondylosis. Clin Orthop 1997;(334):200–6.

165. Humphreys SC, Hodges SD, Patwardhan A, et al. The natural history of the cervical foramen in symptomatic and asymptomatic individuals aged 20–60 years as measured by magnetic resonance imaging. A descriptive approach. Spine 1998; 23(20):2180–4.

166. Boyd-Clark LC, Briggs CA, Galea MP. Segmental degeneration in the cervical spine and associated changes in dorsal root ganglia. Clin Anat 2004;17(6):468–77.

167. Fenlin JM Jr. Pathology of degenerative disease of the cervical spine. Orthop Clin North Am 1971;2(2):371–87.

168. Lee C, Woodring JH, Rogers LF, et al. The radiographic distinction of degenerative slippage (spondylolisthesis and retrolisthesis) from traumatic slippage of the cervical spine. Skeletal Radiol 1986;15(6):439–43.

169. Lees F, Turner JW. Natural history and prognosis of cervical spondylosis. Br Med J 1963;5373:1607–10.

170. Resnick D. Degenerative diseases of the vertebral column. Radiology 1985;156(1):3–14.

171. Kumaresan S, Yoganandan N, Pintar FA, et al. Morphology of young and old cervical spine intervertebral disc tissues. Biomed Sci Instrum 2000;36:141–6.

172. Lu J, Ebraheim NA, Huntoon M, et al. Cervical intervertebral disc space narrowing and size of intervertebral foramina. Clin Orthop Relat Res 2000;370:259–64.

173. Kumaresan S, Yoganandan N, Pintar FA, et al. Contribution of disc degeneration to osteophyte formation in the cervical spine: a biomechanical investigation. J Orthop Res 2001;19(5): 977–84.

174. Gore DR, Sepic SB, Gardner GM. Roentgenographic findings of the cervical spine in asymptomatic people. Spine 1986; 11(6):521–4.

175. Epstein JA, Epstein BS, Lavine LS, et al. Cervical myeloradiculopathy caused by arthrotic hypertrophy of the posterior facets and laminae. J Neurosurg 1978;49(3):387–92.

176. Balla JI, Langford KH. Vertebral artery compression in cervical spondylosis. Med J Aust 1967;1(6):284–6.

177. Bohlman HH, Emery SE. The pathophysiology of cervical spondylosis and myelopathy. Spine 1988;13(7):843–6.

178. Clark CR. Cervical spondylotic myelopathy: history and physical findings. Spine 1988;13(7):847–9.

179. Dai L. Disc degeneration and cervical instability. Correlation of magnetic resonance imaging with radiography. Spine 1998;23(16):1734–8.

180. Farmer JC, Wisneski RJ. Cervical spine nerve root compression. An analysis of neuroforaminal pressures with varying head and arm positions. Spine 1994;19(16):1850–5.

181. Yoo JU, Zou D, Edwards WT, et al. Effect of cervical spine motion on the neuroforaminal dimensions of human cervical spine. Spine 1992;17(10):1131–6.

182. Olmarker K, Myers RR. Pathogenesis of sciatic pain: role of herniated nucleus pulposus and deformation of spinal nerve root and dorsal root ganglion. Pain 1998;78(2):99–105.

183. Tanaka Y, Kokubun S, Sato T, et al. Cervical roots as origin of pain in the neck or scapular regions. Spine 2006;31(17): E568–73.

184. Mitchell LC, Schafermeyer RW. Herniated cervical disk presenting as ischemic chest pain. Am J Emerg Med 1991;9(5): 457–60.

185. Chen TY. The clinical presentation of uppermost cervical disc protrusion. Spine 2000;25(4):439–42.
186. Suzuki T, Abe E, Murai H, et al. Nontraumatic acute complete paraplegia resulting from cervical disc herniation: a case report. Spine 2003;28(6):E125–8.
187. Watters MR, Stears JC, Osborn AG, et al. Transdural spinal cord herniation: imaging and clinical spectra. AJNR Am J Neuroradiol 1998;19(7):1337–44.
188. Rumana CS, Baskin DS. Brown–Séquard syndrome produced by cervical disc herniation: case report and literature review. Surg Neurol 1996;45(4):359–61.
189. Kobayashi N, Asamoto S, Doi H, et al. Brown–Séquard syndrome produced by cervical disc herniation: report of two cases and review of the literature. Spine J 2003;3(6):530–3.
190. Mastronardi L, Ruggeri A. Cervical disc herniation producing Brown–Séquard syndrome: case report. Spine 2004;29(2):E28–31.
191. Kotilainen EM, Karki T, Satomaa OK. Traumatic cervical disc herniation –tetraparesis in a patient kicked by a horse. Acta Orthop Scand 1997;68(2):176–7.
192. Sadanand V, Kelly M, Varughese G, et al. Sudden quadriplegia after acute cervical disc herniation. Can J Neurol Sci 2005;32(3):356–8.
193. Davidson RI, Dunn EJ, Metzmaker JN. The shoulder abduction test in the diagnosis of radicular pain in cervical extradural compressive monoradiculopathies. Spine 1981;6(5):441–6.
194. Beatty RM, Fowler FD, Hanson EJ Jr. The abducted arm as a sign of ruptured cervical disc. Neurosurgery 1987;21(5):731–2.
195. Fast A, Parikh S, Marin EL. The shoulder abduction relief sign in cervical radiculopathy [see comment]. Arch Phys Med Rehabil 1989;70(5):402–3.
196. Lord SM, Barnsley L, Wallis BJ, et al. Chronic cervical zygapophysial joint pain after whiplash. A placebo-controlled prevalence study. Spine 1996;21(15):1737–44, discussion 1744–5.
197. Bove GM, Zaheen A, Bajwa ZH. Subjective nature of lower limb radicular pain. J Manipulative Physiol Ther 2005;28(1):12–14.
198. Slipman CW, Plastaras CT, Palmitier RA, et al. Symptom provocation of fluoroscopically guided cervical nerve root stimulation. Are dynatomal maps identical to dermatomal maps? Spine 1998;23(20):2235–42.
199. Nuckley DJ, Konodi MA, Raynak GC, et al. Neural space integrity of the lower cervical spine: effect of normal range of motion. Spine 2002;27(6):587–95.
200. Tong HC, Haig AJ, Yamakawa K. The Spurling test and cervical radiculopathy. Spine 2002;27(2):156–9.
201. Wainner RS, Fritz JM, Irrgang JJ, et al. Reliability and diagnostic accuracy of the clinical examination and patient self-report measures for cervical radiculopathy. Spine 2003;28(1):52–62.
202. Elvey R. Treatment of arm pain associated with abnormal brachial plexus tension. Aust J Physiother 1986;32:225–30.
203. Quintner JL. A study of upper limb pain and paraesthesiae following neck injury in motor vehicle accidents: assessment of the brachial plexus tension test of Elvey. Br J Rheumatol 1989;28(6):528–33.
204. Butler DS. Mobilisation of the nervous system. Melbourne, Australia: Churchill Livingstone; 1991.
205. Yaxley G, Jull G. A modified upper limb tension test: an investigation of responses in normal subjects. Aust J Physiother 1991;37:143–51.
206. Selvaratnam PJ, Matyas TA, Glasgow EF. Noninvasive discrimination of brachial plexus involvement in upper limb pain. Spine 1994;19(1):26–33.
207. Kleinrensink GJ, Stoeckart R, Mulder PG, et al. Upper limb tension tests as tools in the diagnosis of nerve and plexus lesions. Anatomical and biomechanical aspects. Clin Biomech (Bristol, Avon) 2000;15(1):9–14.
208. van der Heide B, Allison GT, Zusman M. Pain and muscular responses to a neural tissue provocation test in the upper limb. Man Ther 2001;6(3):154–62.
209. Shacklock M. Improving application of neurodynamic (neural tension) testing and treatments: a message to researchers and clinicians. Man Ther 2005;10(3):175–9.
210. Selvaratnam PJ, Matyas TA, Glasgow EF. Noninvasive discrimination of brachial plexus involvement in upper limb pain. Spine 1994;19(1):26–33.
211. Balster SM, Jull GA. Upper trapezius muscle activity during the brachial plexus tension test in asymptomatic subjects. Man Ther 1997;2(3):144–9.
212. Foerster O. The dermatomes in man. Brain 1933;102:1–39.
213. Keegan J, Garrett F. The segmental distribution of cutaneous nerves in the limbs of man. Anat Rec 1948;102:409–37.
214. Thomas R, Nanson J. Dermatomal disparity. Anaesthesia 1998;53(6):613.
215. Owen JH, Padberg AM, Spahr-Holland L, et al. Clinical correlation between degenerative spine disease and dermatomal somatosensory-evoked potentials in humans. Spine 1991;16(Suppl. 6):S201–5.
216. Owen JH, Bridwell KH, Lenke LG. Innervation pattern of dorsal roots and their effects on the specificity of dermatomal somatosensory evoked potentials. Spine 1993;18(6):748–54.
217. Nemecek AN, Avellino AM, Goodkin R, et al. Mapping dermatomes during selective dorsal rhizotomy: case report and review of the literature. Surg Neurol 2003;60(4):292–7, discussion 297.
218. Goldstein B. Anatomic issues related to cervical and lumbosacral radiculopathy. Phys Med Rehabil Clin N Am 2002;13(3):423–37.
219. Moriishi J, Otani K, Tanaka K, et al. The intersegmental anastomoses between spinal nerve roots. Anat Rec 1989;224(1):110–16.
220. Dux M, Jancso G. A new technique for the direct demonstration of overlapping cutaneous innervation territories of peptidergic C-fibre afferents of rat hindlimb nerves. J Neurosci Methods 1994;55(1):47–52.
221. Takahashi Y, Nakajima Y, Sakamoto T, et al. Capsaicin applied to rat lumbar intervertebral disc causes extravasation in the groin skin: a possible mechanism of referred pain of the intervertebral disc. Neurosci Lett 1993;161(1):1–3.
222. McGillicuddy JE. Cervical radiculopathy, entrapment neuropathy, and thoracic outlet syndrome: how to differentiate?

Invited submission from the Joint Section Meeting on Disorders of the Spine and Peripheral Nerves, March 2004. J Neurosurg Spine 2004;1(2):179–87.

223. Mamula CJ, Erhard RE, Piva SR. Cervical radiculopathy or Parsonage–Turner syndrome: differential diagnosis of a patient with neck and upper extremity symptoms. J Orthop Sports Phys Ther 2005;35(10):659–64.

224. Saleem F, Mozaffar T. Neuralgic amyotrophy (Parsonage–Turner syndrome): an often misdiagnosed diagnosis. J Pak Med Assoc 1999;49(4):101–3.

225. Misamore GW, Lehman DE. Parsonage–Turner syndrome (acute brachial neuritis). J Bone Joint Surg Am 1996;78(9):1405–8.

226. Hoving JL, Gross AR, Gasner D, et al. A critical appraisal of review articles on the effectiveness of conservative treatment for neck pain. Spine 2001;26(2):196–205.

227. Cornefjord M, Olmarker K, Otani K, et al. Effects of diclofenac and ketoprofen on nerve conduction velocity in experimental nerve root compression. Spine 2001;26(20):2193–7.

228. Strobel K, Pfirrmann CW, Schmid M, et al. Cervical nerve root blocks: indications and role of MR imaging. Radiology 2004;233(1):87–92.

229. Slipman CW, Lipetz JS, Jackson HB, et al. Therapeutic selective nerve root block in the nonsurgical treatment of atraumatic cervical spondylotic radicular pain: a retrospective analysis with independent clinical review. Arch Phys Med Rehabil 2000;81(6):741–6.

230. Naylor JR, Mulley GP. Surgical collars: a survey of their prescription and use. Br J Rheumatol 1991;30(4):282–4.

231. Colachis SC Jr, Strohm BR, Ganter EL. Cervical spine motion in normal women: radiographic study of effect of cervical collars. Arch Phys Med Rehabil 1973;54(4):161–9.

232. Johnson RM, Owen JR, Hart DL, et al. Cervical orthoses: a guide to their selection and use. Clin Orthop Relat Res 1981;154:34–45.

233. Fisher SV, Bowar JF, Awad EA, et al. Cervical orthoses effect on cervical spine motion: roentgenographic and goniometric method of study. Arch Phys Med Rehabil 1977;58(3):109–15.

234. Hall TM, Elvey RL. Nerve trunk pain: physical diagnosis and treatment. Man Ther 1999;4(2):63–73.

235. Hall T, Elvey RL. Management of mechanosensitivity of the nervous system in spinal pain syndromes. In: Boyling J, Jull G, editors. Grieve's modern manual therapy: the vertebral column. 3rd ed. Edinburgh: Churchill Livingstone; 2004. p. 413–31.

236. Allison GT, Nagy BM, Hall T. A randomized clinical trial of manual therapy for cervico-brachial pain syndrome – a pilot study. Man Ther 2002;7(2):95–102.

237. Tan JC, Nordin M. Role of physical therapy in the treatment of cervical disk disease. Orthop Clin North Am 1992;23(3):435–49.

238. Wong AM, Leong CP, Chen CM. The traction angle and cervical intervertebral separation. Spine 1992;17(2):136–8.

239. Humphreys SC, Chase J, Patwardhan A, et al. Flexion and traction effect on C5-C6 foraminal space. Arch Phys Med Rehabil 1998;79(9):1105–9.

240. Constantoyannis C, Konstantinou D, Kourtopoulos H, et al. Intermittent cervical traction for cervical radiculopathy caused by large-volume herniated disks. J Manipulative Physiol Ther 2002;25(3):188–92.

241. Swezey RL, Swezey AM, Warner K. Efficacy of home cervical traction therapy. Am J Phys Med Rehabil 1999;78(1):30–2.

242. Moeti P, Marchetti G. Clinical outcome from mechanical intermittent cervical traction for the treatment of cervical radiculopathy: a case series. J Orthop Sports Phys Ther 2001;31(4):207–13.

243. Zylbergold RS, Piper MC. Cervical spine disorders. A comparison of three types of traction. Spine 1985;10(10):867–71.

244. Joghataei MT, Arab AM, Khaksar H. The effect of cervical traction combined with conventional therapy on grip strength on patients with cervical radiculopathy. Clin Rehabil 2004;18(8):879–87.

245. Graham N, Gross A, Goldsmith CH, et al. Mechanical traction for neck pain with or without radiculopathy. Cochrane Database Syst Rev 2008;(3):CD006408.

246. Elvey R, Hall T. Neural tissue evaluation and treatment. In: Donatelli R, editor. Physical therapy of the shoulder. 3rd ed. New York: Churchill Livingstone; 1997. p. 131–52.

247. Hall T, Elvey R. Evaluation and treatment of neural tissue pain disorders. In: Donatelli R, Wooden M, editors. Orthopaedic physical therapy. 3rd ed. Philadelphia: Churchill Livingstone; 2001.

248. Coppieters MW, Stappaerts KH, Wouters LL, et al. The immediate effects of a cervical lateral glide treatment technique in patients with neurogenic cervicobrachial pain. J Orthop Sports Phys Ther 2003;33(7):369–78.

249. Vicenzino B, Collins D, Wright A. The initial effects of a cervical spine manipulative physiotherapy treatment on the pain and dysfunction of lateral epicondylalgia. Pain 1996;68(1):69–74.

250. Cowell IM, Phillips DR. Effectiveness of manipulative physiotherapy for the treatment of a neurogenic cervicobrachial pain syndrome: a single case study – experimental design. Man Ther 2002;7(1):31–8.

251. Vicenzino B, Neal R, Collins D, et al. The displacement, velocity and frequency profile of the frontal plane motion produced by the cervical lateral glide treatment technique. Clin Biomech (Bristol, Avon) 1999;14(8):515–21.

252. Coppieters MW, Stappaerts KH, Wouters LL, et al. Aberrant protective force generation during neural provocation testing and the effect of treatment in patients with neurogenic cervicobrachial pain. J Manipulative Physiol Ther 2003;26(2):99–106.

253. Sweeney J, Harms A. Persistent mechanical allodynia following injury of the hand. Treatment through mobilization of the nervous system. J Hand Ther 1996;9(4):328–38.

254. Kaye S, Mason E. Clinical implications of upper limb tension test. Physiotherapy 1989;75:750–2.

255. Beneliyahu DJ. Chiropractic management and manipulative therapy for MRI documented cervical disk herniation. J Manipulative Physiol Ther 1994;17(3):177–85.

256. Beneliyahu DJ. Magnetic resonance imaging and clinical follow-up: study of 27 patients receiving chiropractic care for cervical and lumbar disc herniations. J Manipulative Physiol Ther 1996;19(9):597–606.

257. Brouillette DL, Gurske DT. Chiropractic treatment of cervical radiculopathy caused by a herniated cervical disc. J Manipulative Physiol Ther 1994;17(2):119–23.

258. Pollard H, Tuchin P. Cervical radiculopathy: a case for ancillary therapies? J Manipulative Physiol Ther 1995;18(4): 244–9.

259. Eriksen K. Management of cervical disc herniation with upper cervical chiropractic care. J Manipulative Physiol Ther 1998;21(1):51–6.

260. Rathore S. Use of McKenzie cervical protocol in the treatment of radicular neck pain in a machine operator. J Can Chiropr Assoc 2003;47(4):291–7.

261. Abdulwahab SS, Sabbahi M. Neck retractions, cervical root decompression, and radicular pain. J Orthop Sports Phys Ther 2000;30(1):4–9, discussion 10–12.

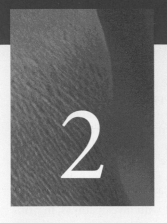

2

CLINICAL APPROACH TO CERVICAL SPONDYLOTIC MYELOPATHY

RAFAEL TORRES CUECO

Cervical spondylotic myelopathy is a common disorder involving chronic progressive compression of the cervical spinal cord due to spondylotic changes or other degenerative pathological conditions.[1,2] Cervical spondylotic myelopathy is the most serious condition that can occur as a result of degenerative changes in the cervical spine. It is important to review this entity, since it is the most frequent cause of spinal cord dysfunction from middle age onwards. The prevalence of degenerative cervical myelopathy has increased in parallel with the increase of the human life span.[3]

Spondylosis is part of the normal involutive process that affects all individuals. More than half of the middle-aged population shows radiological changes that are characteristic of spondylosis. At age 60, these changes are seen in 85% of individuals and in almost all individuals of 80 years of age and above.[4] These changes are accompanied by some degree of observable stenosis, not only in subjects with neck pain but also in more than 25% of asymptomatic subjects.[5] However, only between 10% and 15% of individuals with cervical spondylosis will develop a radiculopathy or a myelopathy.[6]

Cervical spondylotic myelopathy (CSM) was originally described by Stookey[7] in 1928. According to him, the spinal cord compression was caused by cartilaginous nodes deriving from degenerated cervical discs. The consideration of cervical spondylotic myelopathy as its own separate entity began with the works of Brain et al.[8] in 1952. Four years later, Clarke and Robinson[9] published their experiences of treating patients with myelopathy and distinguished it from a radiculopathy caused by a disc herniation.

The most frequent cause of myelopathy is degenerative canal stenosis, which accounts for approximately 55% of all types of cervical myelopathy,[10] although there are other causes, such as compression caused by a voluminous central disc herniation, the ossification of the posterior longitudinal ligament, very common among Asians, traumatic injuries and tumours[11] (Fig. 2-1).

The symptoms of a CSM can be very diverse, according to the location and severity of the spinal cord compression. Spondylotic changes can occur simultaneously in several levels, and they can also affect the intervertebral foramen, leading to a combination of myelopathy and radiculopathy. The myelopathy can be manifested with subtle signs, such as a decrease in balance and manual dexterity, or serious disturbances, such as incontinence or tetraparesis. It is more common in males, and the typical course is usually progressive,[12] with a gradual or episodic symptoms worsening,[3] although in some cases they can trigger sudden neurological signs after a minor injury or a minimal overload.[13]

NATURAL HISTORY

The natural history of a myelopathy is diverse, and some individuals experience improvement, while others get worse. There is also uncertainty, as no good-quality prospective cohort studies of untreated patients have been conducted.[14]

Statements regarding the prognosis of the myelopathy have been controversial ever since the first studies were carried out. In 1956, Clarke and Robinson[9] published their experiences with 120 patients with CSM.

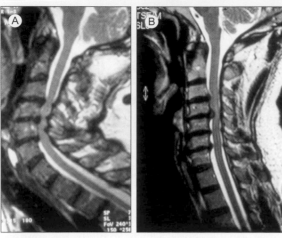

FIGURE 2-1 ■ In the MRI (A) a severe CSM can be seen; in the MRI (B) the stenosis is the result of a voluminous C4–C5 disc herniation.

Although they saw that conservative treatment and immobilization were capable of improving the symptoms, 75% of the patients that did not undergo surgery tended to suffer a progressive neurological deterioration. Contrary to this conclusion, in 1963, Less and Turner[15] researched the natural history of the disease, as well as the efficiency of conservative treatment in 44 patients with symptoms of CSM, of which 57% had an severe form,[16] They observed that patients with symptoms that dated back more than 10 years had a significant disability, and most of them also suffered a significant progression of the disease. However, those who had moderate symptoms had a better prognosis; even among 15 patients that initially had acute symptoms, all but one continued to have moderate or severe symptoms even after a long-term follow-up. Lees and Turner concluded that a degenerative CSM is manifested normally with long periods of non-progressive disability, and only in a few cases is there a progressive deterioration.

The natural history of the CSM was also studied by Nurick[17] in 36 patients treated with a conservative treatment and with a follow-up period of 20 years. Among the 27 patients that initially showed a moderate disability, 18 continued to have the same disability in the final evaluation. Among those that initially had moderate-to-acute symptoms, two-thirds presented the same symptoms at the end of the follow-up.

Fouyas et al.,[18,19] in a Cochrane review in 2002 showed that the belief that patients with CSM will progress to a progressive disability without surgical intervention cannot be supported by reliable evidence. The disease can not only remain unchanged for long periods of time but also, in some patients with a severe disability, can even improve without treatment.[17] Likewise, there is no evidence to support the widespread belief that patients with a radiculopathy will develop a myelopathy over the following years.[19] Therefore, the evolution of a patient with myelopathy is, in principle, unpredictable: while some patients experience a benign clinical evolution, others suffer a worsening of their neurological condition. When a patient starts to show signs of myelopathy, the rule of thirds is often used.[20] According to this rule, one-third of the patients will improve, one-third will remain the same and one-third will worsen. Patients with progressive spinal cord symptoms and signs, such as the alteration of gait, hand impairments and neurogenic bladder, who do not respond to conservative treatment, should be considered candidates for surgery. Surgery can stop the myelopathy from progressing and can bring about a functional improvement in many patients, although the prognosis varies significantly and complete remission is very infrequent.[1] Motor symptoms tend to be more progressive and improve to a lesser extent than the sensory symptoms. In conclusion, CSM is a highly variable condition. Some patients may benefit from surgery, whereas others with mild forms of the condition can be managed with conservative treatment.[14]

PATHOPHYSIOLOGY

The pathophysiology of myelopathy caused by cervical spondylosis is the consequence of a combination of mechanical, degenerative and vascular factors.[21–24]

The cervical central canal is limited, at the front, by the vertebral bodies and the discs covered by the posterior longitudinal ligament; laterally, by the pedicles and articular pillars and, behind, by the laminae and the yellow ligament. When its dimensions are normal, there is enough space to comfortably accommodate the spinal cord, the meningeal layers, the ligaments and the epidural fat. Cervical myelopathy is caused as a result of a decrease in the dimensions of the central canal, and there is direct correlation between the severity of the spinal cord compromise and the decrease in the sagittal diameter of the canal.[25] This central canal, in normal subjects, has a sagittal diameter of 17–18 mm from C3 to C7 levels,[26] with a slight variation between sexes. The dimensions of the cervical canal are smaller among the Japanese and other Asian populations.[27] The thickness of the spinal cord varies slightly from C1 to C7 and it measures between 8.5 and 11.5 mm approximately, with the average being 10 mm.[28] The relationship between the central canal and the neuroaxis varies according to the level: whereas in C1–C3, the spinal cord occupies less than half of the canal, in the C4–C7 segments, it occupies two-thirds. A normal canal is wide enough so that no spinal cord compression occurs even when spondylotic changes develop.

The severity of the CSM is related, although not entirely, to the magnitude of the compression.[29,30] The symptoms of spinal cord compression appear when the spinal cord suffers a 30% reduction of its thickness, or when its transversal area is less than 60 mm².[31]

The transverse area is related to the prognosis of the post-surgical results: in patients with a transversal area of more than 30 mm² it is possible to have a functional recovery after a decompression, but there would be a very poor possibility anywhere below this value; 30 mm² is considered to be a critical thickness, and below this value the spinal cord cannot recover itself.[32,33]

In the development of the canal stenosis, it is necessary to differentiate between *static, dynamic* and *vascular factors*. Static factors are the congenital canal stenosis and the cervical spondylosis as well as other less frequent factors, such as the ossification of the posterior longitudinal ligament. Dynamic factors imply the reduction of the diameter of the canal during the movements of the cervical spine. Finally, vascular factors refer to the alteration of the blood perfusion at the spinal cord level, as a consequence of the static and dynamic factors.

Static factors

Constitutional stenosis

The presence of degenerative changes in the cervical spine has been shown to be age-related and is noted in both symptomatic and asymptomatic subjects.

Therefore, cervical spondylosis itself does not normally lead to a myelopathy. The ample tolerance of the spinal cord to compression means that in order for the degenerative changes to lead to a myelopathy, it is necessary for a narrow central canal to have existed previously. When this situation occurs, a trivial trauma or moderate degenerative changes may lead to a myelopathy.[34]

In 1996, Hinck and Sachdev[35] proposed the concept of *developmental stenosis* of the cervical spinal canal. Subsequently, it has been considered the most important factor in the establishment of a CSM.[29] In order to evaluate the developmental stenosis, the *constitutional sagittal diameter* is measured (Fig. 2-2). This diameter is the distance between the midpoint of the back of vertebral body and the anterior border of the lamina. This distance does not change with degenerative changes.[28] The average values of a normal canal are 20 mm for C2, and 17–18 mm for the C3–C7 segments. It is considered that there is a constitutional stenosis when, in a lateral radiography, the diameter of the cervical canal is less than 13 mm.[36,37]

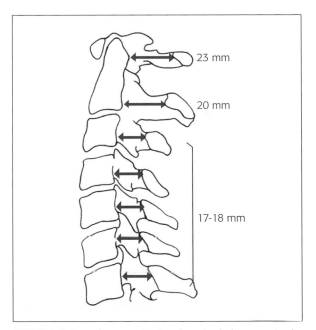

FIGURE 2-2 ■ The constitutional sagittal diameter is the distance between the midpoint of the back of vertebral body and the anterior border of the lamina. The average values of a normal canal are between 20 mm for C2 and 17–18 mm for the C3–C7 segments.

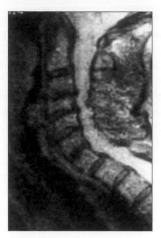

FIGURE 2-3 ■ This MRI shows a severe cervical spondylotic central canal stenosis.

Cervical spondylosis

As previously described, a constitutional stenosis is a pre-existing condition for a myelopathy; however, ultimately, it will be the degenerative changes that will determine a stenosis that is capable of compromising the spinal cord and determining its clinical progression. These changes include the disc degeneration and posterior spur proliferation, the hyperostosis of the uncovertebral joints in the anterolateral direction and the facet hypertrophy, together with the hypertrophy and buckling of the yellow ligament (Fig. 2-3).

The cascade of degenerative phenomena begins with the deterioration of the intervertebral disc.[36] This process is established in an insidious manner and, under normal circumstances, it does not cause symptoms.[38] The decrease in disc height leads to an increase in the sagittal diameter with a variable degree of bulging inside the spinal canal.

The disc degeneration, due to the hypermobility and instability that accompany it, leads to a reactive hyperostosis, with a proliferation of osteophytic bars across the back of the degenerated disc, further reducing the space for the spinal cord. Due to the disc degeneration and the associated instability, zygapophyseal and uncovertebral joints will suffer hypertrophy, projecting osteophytes in the canal and decreasing its diameter. In the same way, a fibrosis of the yellow ligament and a hypertrophy of the laminae in the posterior part of the central canal will be developed. All

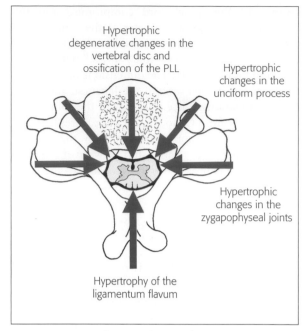

Hypertrophic degenerative changes in the vertebral disc and ossification of the PLL

Hypertrophic changes in the unciform process

Hypertrophic changes in the zygapophyseal joints

Hypertrophy of the ligamentum flavum

FIGURE 2-4 ■ In the CSM, there are hypertrophic degenerative changes in the vertebral body as large osteophytic bars, disc degeneration and bulging, hypertrophic changes in the unciform processes and the zygapophyseal joints and the hypertrophy of the ligamentum flavum lead to a circumferential reduction of the size of the canal. PLL, posterior longitudinal ligament.

these hypertrophic degenerative changes lead to a decrease in the circumferential dimensions of the canal (Fig. 2-4).

Degenerative changes in the cervical spine alter the morphology of the lordosis. The cervical spondylosis and the subsequent decrease in disc height lead to a segmental stiffness and a kyphotic deformity. This deformity often results in the appearance of compensatory hyperextension and hypermobility in the adjacent segments. The mechanical hyperfunction that the latter segments begin to suffer causes them to be unstable and leads to accelerated degenerative changes. Thus, the modifications of the physiological lordotic curve, together with the alteration of the static and dynamic balance of the cervical spine, favour the appearance of instability that accentuates articular deterioration and facilitates the development of stenosis in multiple levels. The most important reduction in the diameter of the canal occurs between the osteophytes of the posteroinferior edge of the vertebral

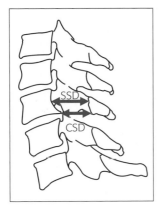

FIGURE 2-5 ■ The *spondylotic sagittal diameter* (SSD) is the distance between the posteroinferior edge of the vertebral body and the lower edge of the lamina. The *constitutional sagittal diameter* (CSD) is the distance between the midpoint of the back of vertebral body and the anterior border of the lamina.

TABLE 2-1	
Cervical developmental sagittal stenosis	
Diameter	
10 mm or less	With cervical spondylosis, likely to develop a myelopathy
10–13 mm	Pre-myelopathy group
13–17 mm	Tendency towards symptomatic spondylosis
> 17 mm	Less prone to develop the disease

body and the inferior portion of the lamina. This distance is the *spondylotic sagittal diameter* (SSD) (Fig. 2-5). The measurement of this diameter is very important, since it represents the most precise sagittal measurement to quantify the degenerative stenosis.[28]

Edwards and LaRocca[39] compared the constitutional sagittal diameter (CSD) and the SSD in patients with spondylosis. The difference between the two diameters, they called the *spondylosis index*, represents the degree of degenerative narrowing for each cervical segment. They found that patients with a cervical canal that was previously narrow were symptomatic, with a spondylotic index of only 2 mm. This value can be compared with the 3.45 mm that is needed in patients with normal canal dimensions. These researchers suggested that there was a group of 'pre-myelopathic' subjects whose sagittal diameter of the canal varied between 10 and 13 mm. In this group, a narrowing of approximately 2 mm would be enough to develop a myelopathy. In contrast, subjects with a sagittal diameter of 17 mm or more had a very low risk of developing a myelopathy (Table 2-1). It can be concluded that, in the development of a myelopathy, a degenerative narrowing is necessary in subjects that previously had a congenital narrow canal.[36]

Ossification of the posterior longitudinal ligament

Cervical myelopathy due to the ossification of posterior longitudinal ligament (PLL) or (OPLL) or poste-

rior longitudinal ligament ossification (PLLO) is a relatively common cause of myelopathy in Japan,[40] where the incidence is higher than 4% of the population.[41] In fact, it was a Japanese researcher, Tsukimoto, who described it for the first time in 1960.[42] Although it is much less prevalent in Europe and the United States, it is more common than originally thought, and it can be identified thanks to imaging techniques such as CT scans or magnetic resonance. Currently, it is thought that approximately one-quarter of North American and Japanese patients with cervical myelopathy have an ossification of the PLL.[43–45] This condition is seen more frequently in the higher cervical segments: 70% in C2–C4, 15% in T1–T4 and 15% in L1–L3.[46] The incidence is twice as common in males as in females.[46,47]

There seems to be a relationship between the ossification of the PLL and the *diffuse idiopathic skeletal hyperostosis*. This name, adopted by Resnick et al.,[48] has replaced the former name of *Forestier and Rotes-Querol disease*. Among patients that suffer from this condition, 60% have an ossification of the PLL, which has led to it being considered as an atypical form of diffuse idiopathic skeletal hyperostosis.[48–51]

There are some studies that relate its high prevalence in Japanese and other Asian population groups to their diet.[52] Other authors suggest that obesity and glucose intolerance are a risk factor for its development.[41]

The ossification of the PLL has been classified into different types[53] (Fig. 2-6):

■ *Continuous type*: the ossification is extended to the adjacent vertebral bodies.
■ *Segmental type*: the ossification is limited to the posterior rim of the vertebral body.

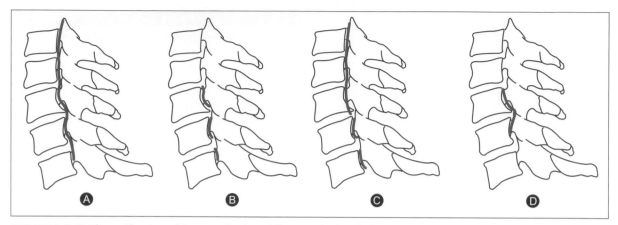

FIGURE 2-6 ■ The ossification of the posterior lateral ligament is classified into four types: (A) continuous type, the ossification is extended to the adjacent vertebral bodies; (B) segmental type, the ossification is limited to the posterior rim of the vertebral body; (C) mixed type, mixture of a continuous and a segmental type; and (D) herniated type, ossification after intervertebral disc herniation.

- *Mixed type*: this is a mixture of the continuous and segmental types.
- *Herniated type*: ossification after intervertebral disc herniation.

In the ossification of the PLL, although the cause of the spinal cord compression is static, the dynamic factors also contribute to the development of neurological deficits.[40,54,55] It seems that a mechanism of hyperextension is responsible for the onset of an acute neurological injury.[40]

The symptoms of myelopathy in this condition begin to appear early, in the early 50s and sometimes even earlier.[46] Although the neurological deterioration usually develops gradually, in 10% of cases it can appear suddenly after a mild trauma.[40,55] The risk of developing symptoms is high when the ligament occupies 40% of the canal.[47]

There is another entity that is similar to the ossification of the PLL, the *hypertrophy of the posterior longitudinal ligament*.[56,57] The hypertrophy of this ligament seems to be related to a disc herniation and degeneration of the cervical disc. The protrusion of the intervertebral disc could favour the development of a hyperplasia of the chondral tissue[56] and the evolution of the ligament hypertrophy would lead to a myelopathy, and on occasions, to the ossification of the PLL.

There is no agreement regarding the possible relationship between the hypertrophy and the ossification of the PLL. Some authors state that hypertrophy is an early stage or an atypical pattern of ossification,[56,57] and consider it to be a 'PLL ossification in evolution'.[47] On the contrary, others believe that the hypertrophy is a degenerative process characterized by a metaplasia of the collagenous fibres of the ligament into chondrocytes, but without ossification. This would distinguish it from the ossification of the PLL, since it would be considered to be an atypical form of diffuse idiopathic skeletal hyperostosis.[48,49]

Dynamic factors

Dynamic factors can have a significant influence on both the vertical dimensions and the cross-sectional area of the spinal canal. The central canal does not have a stable length; rather, it is modified by the spine's flexion and extension movements. From the position of extension to flexion, the total length of the canal increases between 5 and 9 cm, and this lengthening occurs especially in the cervical and lumbar regions.[58,59] This change in length causes a displacement of the spinal cord as a whole in relation to its fibro-osseous case. Neck flexion causes a gliding of the entire spinal cord cephalically, and the straight leg raise in a caudal direction (Fig. 2-7). As regards the cervical spine, the spinal cord is displaced 3 mm during the cervical flexion, and the direction of the movement changes according to the level[60,61]: above C5–C6, its

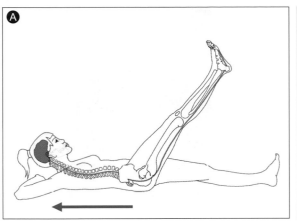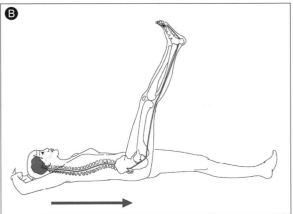

FIGURE 2-7 ■ The direction of the displacement of the cord is in the cranial direction during cervical flexion (A) and in the caudal direction during the straight leg raise (B).

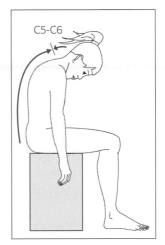

FIGURE 2-8 ■ The cord is displaced 3 mm during the cervical flexion: in the caudal direction above the C5–C6 segments and in the cranial direction below these segments. *(Modified from Shacklock.[60])*

displacement is in the caudal direction, and below this level, it is in the cranial direction[59,61] (Fig. 2-8).

In addition to being displaced, the spinal cord undergoes a lengthening. Yuan et al.,[61] in a study conducted in normal subjects with an MRI, showed that the spinal cord, between the neutral and flexion positions, increases in length 10% and 6% along the posterior and anterior surfaces, respectively. This lengthening implies an increase in the tension of the

spinal cord, the roots and its meningeal layers, as well as changes in the arterial and venous perfusion.

The cord can also suffer transversal movements inside the canal due to the tension generated by the movements of the upper limbs. This is evidenced by the fact that when an upper limb neurodynamic test triggers symptoms in a limb, if this position is maintained, the symptoms can be modified when performing the same test on the other limb.[62]

The cross-sectional area of the central canal suffers variations during the movements of neck flexion and extension. In normal cervical kinematics, the extension between adjacent vertebrae causes a reduction of the diameter of the canal.[63,64] In the presence of degenerative changes, this diameter can be reduced to a critical level.[64,65]

Flexion, by increasing the length of the cervical canal, induces an increase of the tension over the cord and can cause ischaemia. If, in addition, there are osteophytes in the posterior face of the vertebral bodies, the anterior part of the cord can be compressed against them during this movement.[66]

On the other hand, when the cervical spine is extended, the yellow ligament buckles inside the canal, and this causes a decrease in the cross-sectional area of the cervical canal.[36] As the disc and the yellow ligament are at the same height, if both are protruded in the canal and at the same time a cervical extension is performed, and it is highly probable that there will be irritation or spinal cord compression. It has also been shown that ventral osteophytes can reduce upward and downward movements of the spinal cord during sagittal physiological movements.[67]

Another factor that increases the risk of cord compression during extension is an increase in the cord cross-sectional area linked to the shortening of the cord in this movement. The combination of a maximum reduction of the diameter of the canal with an increase in the spinal cord cross-sectional area increases the risk of cord compression. This 'impingement' or compression is limited to the part of the cord located between the posteroinferior margin of the vertebral body, on the front, and the lamina and the yellow ligament of the inferior vertebra, on the back.[65]

This clinical situation can be observed when asymptomatic subjects with advanced cervical spondylosis suffer from a hyperextension injury or a cervical whiplash. There have even been published cases of severe acute neurological deterioration of non-traumatic cause as, for example, when intubating a patient before surgery.[5,68]

In some cases, this acute neurological deterioration can occur after minimal mechanical stress, such as in the case reported by Young et al.[4] involving a 56-year-old individual who, after taking a nap in the supine position for 1 hour on the floor, developed a severe tetraplegia.

Degenerative spondylolisthesis

The phenomenon of degenerative spondylolisthesis and its involvement in CSM has been the subject of studies over the last few years.[69–71] The magnitude of the listhesis, both anterior and posterior, rarely exceeds 2–3 mm, but it has the potential to aggravate the canal stenosis.[72] The onset of degenerative listhesis is a result of the degeneration of the triarticular complex, which, in addition to intervertebral disc degeneration,[73] suffers from osteoarthritis and facet joint instability. It is considered that there is spondylolisthesis when the displacement of the vertebral body in relation to the vertebral body of the lower vertebra is higher than 2 mm (Fig. 2-9).

The most severe cases of dynamic stenosis are the degenerative spondylolisthesis in elderly subjects[69,70] and dynamic stenosis, as a consequence of a previous arthrodesis in the lower cervical spine.[73]

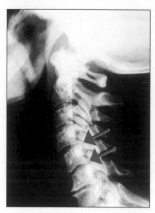

FIGURE 2-9 ■ This radiography shows a severe degeneration of the lower segments and a spondylolisthesis of the C4–C5 segment.

Degenerative spondylolisthesis in elderly subjects

Since the first description by Perlman and Hawes,[74] cervical spondylolisthesis, known often as vertebral subluxation,[63] has been considered a very uncommon phenomenon,[75,76] contrary to what occurs in the lumbar spine. However, this entity in the cervical spine is much more frequent than what was initially thought, especially in elderly patients.[26,71] In patients over 65 years old who show a CSM, a spondylolisthesis is observed in approximately 70% of cases, with an anterior or posterior displacement higher than 3 mm.[69,77] Therefore, the myelopathy of the elderly patient is mainly dynamic.[77]

Myelopathy in elderly patients is distinguished by the fact that it is established in different vertebral levels in comparison with younger patients. Whereas in younger patients the stenosis appears in the lower cervical segments, C5–C6 and C6–C7, in elderly patients it appears more frequently in the C3–C4 segment, followed by the C4–C5 segment.[69–71]

The lower cervical spine tends to show early osteoarthritic degeneration, with a higher amount of degenerative change in the anterior interbody joint. This osteophytic hypertrophy reduces the central canal diameter and, therefore, it is primarily considered to be a static stenosis. The lower cervical spine evolves, as previously described, towards stiffness, which in some cases leads to true spontaneous arthrodesis. Paradoxically, this stiffness protects the lower segments from listhesis. The degenerative changes do

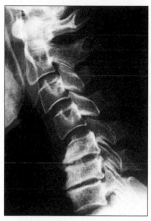

FIGURE 2-10 ■ Compensatory hypermobility of the C4–C5 segment in a spondylosis of the lower cervical spine.

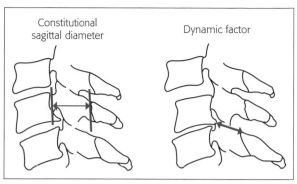

FIGURE 2-11 ■ The dynamic factor (DF) is a better indicator of a dynamic stenosis in extension than the constitutional sagittal diameter (CSD). It corresponds to the distance between the posteroinferior margin of the soma and the anterior margin of the lamina of the underlying vertebra, with the cervical spine in extension. A distance shorter than 12 mm constitutes a positive DF.

not affect the disc of the upper cervical segments so early, since they evolve towards hypermobility with the purpose of maintaining an adequate cervical function (Fig. 2-10). This compensatory hypermobility imposed on the segments C3–C4 or C4–C5[70,71] is one of the factors responsible for the high occurrence of myelopathy due to spondylolisthesis in elderly patients.[70]

The spondylolisthesis of the upper cervical segments in these patients is also related to changes in posture that are age-associated. Ageing is accompanied by an increase of thoracic kyphosis, which affects the rest of the spine. Equally, the lower cervical spine tends to show kyphosis and, in some cases, there is a significant anterior tilt of the vertebral segments. This situation favours the attempt of the C3 vertebra to compensate for this anterior angulation with a retrolisthesis and hypermobility in extension. This retrolisthesis in extension is the dynamic factor, and it is measured from the posteroinferior edge of the vertebral body and the anterior margin of the lamina of the underlying vertebra, with the cervical spine in extension. A distance lower than 12 mm is considered a positive dynamic factor (Fig. 2-11).

In conclusion, in elderly patients, a dynamic stenosis is added to the static stenosis and the upper levels C3–C4 and C4–C5 are usually the most affected levels.[71]

Another factor that should be considered in elderly patients, regarding the dynamic character of the stenosis, is the rapid progression of the myelopathy. Barnes and Saunders[78] showed that the progression of the myelopathy can be stabilized in subjects with a reduced cervical mobility, while in subjects with maintained cervical mobility, the development of the pathology can be dramatic.

> In subjects with reduced cervical mobility, the evolution of myelopathy can be stabilized, while in subjects with maintained cervical mobility, the development can be dramatic.

Also, the study conducted by Tani et al.[69] showed that a significant listhesis, associated with a pronounced angular mobility at the level of the spondylolisthesis, increases the probability of the spinal cord being compromised. Thus, a listhesis of ≥ 3.5 mm, combined with a 20% mobility, is accompanied by a focal conduction block.[79]

Dynamic stenosis after surgery

Despite the fact that cervical arthrodesis is a frequently used surgical procedure in patients with CSM, there are cases where the symptoms worsen after surgery.[80–82] This is attributed to post-surgical degenerative changes.

As a result of the immobility of the segments with arthrodesis, the mobile segments suffer higher functional demands, favouring the development of an instability that can lead to a spinal canal dynamic stenosis. Therefore, before surgery, there should be an evaluation of whether there is an underlying dynamic factor in the neighbouring segments to those who are going to undergo an arthrodesis. The presence of this dynamic factor is a clear risk factor of post-surgical deterioration,[83] especially with a multiple level arthrodesis.

The alterations, both dynamic and static, suffered by the cervical spine can result in a cord compression and an alteration of its vascular perfusion. Ogino et al.[29] described, in necropsy studies, the changes suffered by the cord in patients with CSM and found that the compression of the spinal cord was associated with an extensive destruction of grey and white matter and an extensive demyelination.

Vascular factors

The pathological alterations are not only derived from the direct mechanical compression on the neural elements: the vascular phenomena associated with such compression also play an important role. The concept of ischaemic injury of the cord was presented by Nurick.[84] Experimental studies conducted on animals have confirmed the role ischaemia plays in the myelopathy caused by spinal canal stenosis.[29,85–87] More recently, Yoshizawa[88] has reviewed the role that blood perfusion changes have on the physiopathology of the myelopathy. The anterior spinal artery is responsible for the irrigation of 65–70% of the spinal cord. With the progress of the compressive phenomena at the cord, the blood perfusion of the terminal branches of the anterior spinal artery within the cord is interrupted.[89] If this alteration of the perfusion is prolonged in time, the ischaemia causes demyelination and neural damage, as well as the loss of axoplasmic flow.[90] Therefore, it is evident that the ischaemia further aggravates the pathological effects of compression.[91,92]

The alteration of the cerebrospinal fluid (CSF) flow is also involved in the development of a myelopathy. The cerebrospinal fluid plays an important role in the nutrition and elimination of waste from the spinal cord and roots. The reduction of subarachnoid space as a consequence of the canal stenosis can block the cerebrospinal fluid flow, causing an alteration of the cord trophism (88). Compression can alter the hematoencephalic barrier due to venous congestion (88).

The irritation of the neuroaxis and its connective layers can trigger a neurogenic inflammation phenomenon that increases neural deterioration and favours the development of adherences.

CORD COMPRESSION PATTERNS

A myelopathy can manifest itself clinically in many different ways, depending on the most affected tracts. Among the different classification systems that have been developed, the most widely used is the one put forth by Crandall and Batzdorf,[93] based on the differential susceptibility of the different spinal tracts. It distinguishes five different syndromes:

- *Transverse lesion syndrome*: this is the most common syndrome and it affects the posterior columns and the spinothalamic and corticospinal tracts.
- *Motor system syndrome*: it is characterized by how it exclusively affects the corticospinal tract, and it is manifested by weakness in the upper limb, gait changes and spasticity.
- *Central cord syndrome*: the weakness of the upper limbs is greater than that of the lower limbs, and the hands are severely affected.
- *Brown–Séquard syndrome*: this involves unilateral cord compression. The compression of the corticospinal tract leads to an ipsilateral hemiparesis. The compression of the dorsal column-medial lemniscus tract leads to loss of vibration sense and fine touch, loss of proprioception while the compression of the spinothalamic tract causes loss of pain and temperature sensation.
- *Brachial cord syndrome:* this combines cervical radicular compression with signs of compression of the long tracts caused by cord compression. This syndrome is characterized by radicular pain, paraesthesias, hyperreflexia, long tracts signs, weakness and gait alterations. The best prognosis is after surgical decompression.

The differential diagnosis should rule out other neurological diseases, such as multiple sclerosis and amyotrophic lateral sclerosis. Multiple sclerosis can also lead to sensitive and motor alterations in the upper and lower limbs. However, in contrast with CSM, it has outbreaks, and it usually presents a dysfunction of the cranial nerves, which can be manifest themselves in a physical examination with an abnormal mandibular reflex. Amyotrophic lateral sclerosis affects the motor neuron and therefore there are no alterations in superficial and deep sensitivity. Other pathological entities, such as spinal cord tumours and syringomyelia, can lead to similar symptoms as a myelopathy. However, MRI can establish a definite diagnosis.

The clinical presentation of the CSM is classified, according to Crandall and Batzdorg,[93] into five syndromes:

- Transverse lesion syndrome.
- Motor system syndrome.
- Central cord syndrome.
- Brown–Séquard syndrome.
- Brachial cord syndrome.

Clinical signs and symptoms

Patients with CSM present a wide spectrum of signs and symptoms, depending on the magnitude of the spinal dysfunction, on the level of the compression and the chronicity of the process. While some subjects do not have any symptoms, others can end up being severely disabled.

Myelopathy is characterized by affecting the upper motor neuron on levels located below the compression, and the dysfunction of the lower motor neuron at the level of the spinal compression. The dysfunction of the upper motor neuron manifests itself primarily in the form of spasticity and gait changes, and the dysfunction of the lower motor neuron is translated into sensitive-motor deficit signs, such as hyporeflexia and fasciculations.

Initial clinical manifestations are usually the decrease in manual dexterity and subtle alterations of balance and gait. The difficulty in handling small objects is characteristic, as when trying to fasten buttons. Spasticity is referred to in the beginning by the patient as a stiffness feeling in the legs.

It is not infrequent for the signs of the lower limbs to be asymmetrical, with one limb being more affected than the other. The alterations of sensitivity in the form of hyperaesthesia are very frequent, as shown by allodynia when in contact with clothing. Incontinence and sexual dysfunction are less frequent, but, when

present, they are associated with a severe clinical condition.

Myelopathy can occur alongside a radiculopathy, since the development of a spondylosis leads to a foraminal stenosis.

Physical examination

The diagnosis of CSM can be challenging, particularly in the early stages. Many different signs and symptoms can be present in the upper quadrant, such as neck pain and stiffness, paraesthesia, pain, allodynia, radicular signs in one or two upper limbs and the loss of hand dexterity. In the lower quadrant there may be symptoms like clumsiness in gait and hyperreflexia.

Motor signs

The most frequent sign of myelopathy is weakness of the lower limbs, as a result of the affected corticospinal tracts. If the pathology progresses, the posterior tracts will be affected, with a subsequent alteration of proprioception. This will result in a characteristic gait in which the patient extends his support base in order to maintain balance. Although not as common, it is also possible to see motor signs in the upper limbs. The signs of the dysfunction of the long tracts, such as spasticity and hyperreflexia of the arms, are accompanied by signs of lower motor neurons at the level of the injury, such as muscle atrophy and fasciculations.

The hand of the patient with myelopathy has a characteristic dysfunction that was described by Ono et al.[94] as the *myelopathy hand*. Patients show a loss of power of adduction and extension of the fourth and fifth fingers and an inability to grip and release rapidly with these fingers. This alteration is assessed with the so-called *finger-escape sign* (Fig. 2-12). To assess this sign, the patient is asked to keep the fingers extended. The test is positive if the ring and little fingers are flexed and abducted. The assessment should also check the patient's ability to open and close the hands quickly. Normal adults can perform such rapid grip and release movements more than 20 times in 10 seconds. This is called the *grip-and-release test*.[94] These spastic behaviours of the hand are associated with a sensitive deficit.

Ebara et al.[95] distinguished a different type of dysfunction of the hand in patients with myelopathy, which they named *amyotrophic myelopathic hand*. This

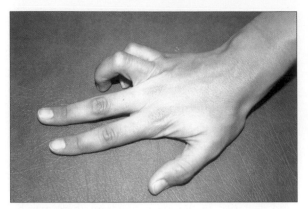

FIGURE 2-12 ■ Finger escape sign. When the patient is asked to keep the fingers in extension, the ring and small fingers are flexed and abducted.

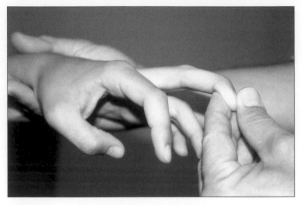

FIGURE 2-13 ■ Hoffman's sign is positive when following the therapist flexing the terminal phalange of the middle finger of the patient rapidly, a flexion of the thumb occurs at the level of the interphalangeal joint.

is characterized by localized wasting and weakness of the intrinsic and extrinsic hand muscles, without spasticity or sensory loss.

Motor function assessment in the lower limbs is performed by asking the patient to do tandem walking, to walk on their tiptoes and heels and single leg stance.

Sensory signs

Sensory changes vary widely, depending on the location and extension of the spinal cord dysfunction. The sensory impairments in the upper limbs are the result of both spinal cord compression and the affected roots in several levels. Pain and paraesthesia in the upper limbs are the most frequent signs.

When the myelopathy is chronic or severe, it is common to lose deep touch sense, vibratory and proprioceptive sensitivity. However, the loss of the vibratory sensitivity can also occur in a diabetic neuropathy, a thyroid disease or an alcoholic or metal intoxication. Romberg's test is used to evaluate if the alteration of the proprioceptive sensitivity is due to the affected posterior columns. Alternatively, as previously described, the patient is asked to walk in a straight line.

Confirmatory test

Deep tendon reflex changes are important when assessing patients with CSM. Generally, the lower limbs show hyperreflexia. Upper limb deep reflexes can be hyperreflexic or hyporeflexic, depending on the

level of cord injury. The reliability and diagnostic accuracy of this test has been studied by Cook et al.[96]

In the diagnosis of the CSM it is very important to explore the presence of some pathological reflexes, such as Hoffmann's sign, the inverted supinator sign, Babinski's sign and *clonus*.

Hoffmann's sign, also known as the finger flexor reflex, is useful when attempting to verify if the corticospinal tract is involved. This sign is triggered when the terminal phalange of the middle finger is flexed rapidly. The test is positive if the thumb is flexed at the level of the interphalangeal joint (Fig. 2-13).

An inverted supinator sign is observed when performing a brachioradialis tendon reflex. When positive, instead of a normal slight wrist extension, radial deviation and supination, the response is a spastic contraction of the finger and wrist flexors (Fig. 2-14).

The compression of the upper cervical spinal cord (C1–C3) can exacerbate the scapulohumeral reflex. In order to obtain this reflex, the tip of spine of the scapula and the acromion are tapped in the caudal direction. A hyperreactive reflex causes the elevation of the scapula and the abduction of the shoulder (Fig. 2-15).

Babinski's sign is explored by stimulating the lateral side of the sole of the foot. A negative response is expressed with the flexion of the fingers, and the positive response is expressed with the extension of the first toe associated with the separation of the rest of the toes (Fig. 2-16).

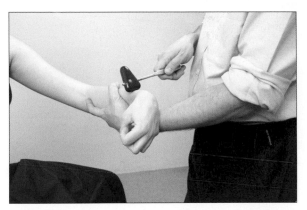

FIGURE 2-14 ■ An inverted supinator sign is observed when performing a brachioradialis tendon reflex. When positive, the response is a spastic finger and wrist flexion.

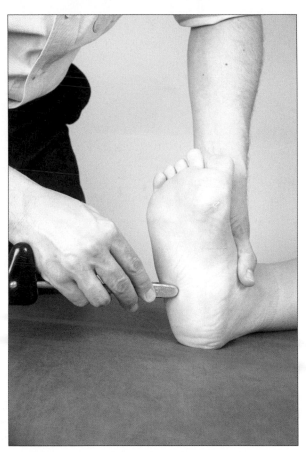

FIGURE 2-16 ■ A positive Babinski sign is the extension of the first toe associated with the separation of the rest of the toes.

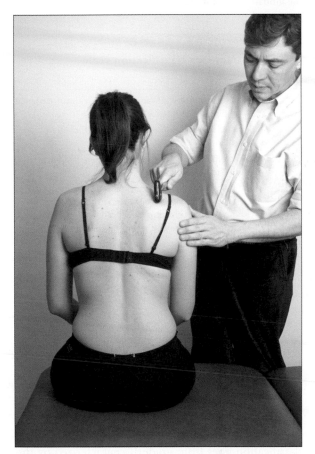

FIGURE 2-15 ■ The compression of the upper cervical spinal cord (C1–C3) can exacerbate the scapulohumeral reflex. A hyperreactive reflex causes the elevation of the scapula and the abduction of the shoulder.

It is very important to remember that the presence of hyperreflexia does not make it possible to differentiate a myelopathy from a supraspinal disease or injury. Therefore, it is interesting to evaluate the *mandibular reflex*. This reflex involves the masseter and temporal muscles, innervated by the fifth cranial nerve. In order to explore this reflex, the patient is asked to keep his mouth slightly open, and then the chin is tapped. The presence of a hyperreactive reflex (excessive contraction in the direction that the mouth closes) indicates an intracranial pathology or a systemic disease, such as hyperthyroidism or hypercalcaemia (Fig. 2-17). Therefore, if the mandibular reflex is positive, the hyperreflexia should not be attributed to a myelopathy, but to a neurological involvement of the structures located above the foramen magnum.

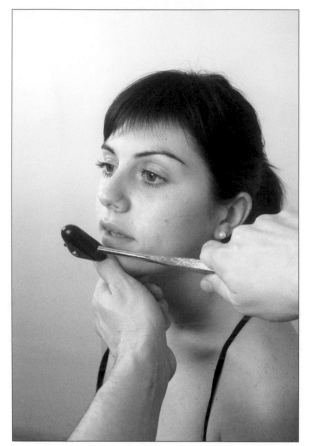

FIGURE 2-17 ■ In order to explore the mandibular reflex, the patient is asked to keep the mouth open slightly, and the therapist taps the chin. The presence of a hyperreactive reflex indicates an intracranial pathology or a systemic disorder.

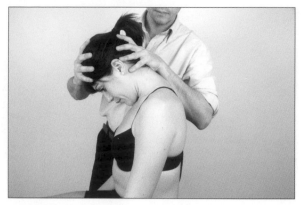

FIGURE 2-18 ■ Lhermitte's sign is positive when the examiner flexes the patient's head and the patient refers a sensation of electric discharge that runs down the back and into the limbs.

TABLE 2-2	
Nurick's classification scale	
Grade	
0	Signs or symptoms of radiculopathy without evidence of spinal cord disease
1	Signs of spinal cord disease but no difficulty in walking
2	Slight difficulty in walking that did not prevent full-time employment
3	Difficulty in walking that prevents full-time employment or the ability to perform all housework but that is not severe enough to require someone else's help to walk
4	Able to walk with someone else's help or the aid of a frame
5	Chairbound or bedridden

Another sign that can indicate cord compression is Lhermitte's sign. While the patient is sitting down, the examiner passively flexes the patient's head. The test is positive if the subject reports an electric sensation that runs down the back and into the limbs (Fig. 2-18).

Neurodynamic tests, such as the passive neck flexion, the passive neck flexion while sitting down (cervical slump) and the slump test in all its variants, can provide information regarding neural mechanosensitivity, as well as the presence of distal symptoms. The changes seen in this type of tests can help to evaluate the progression of the patient throughout treatment (Fig. 2-19). In subjects with myeloradicular symptoms the upper limb neurodynamic tests can also be used to assess neural mechanosensitivity.

Cervical myelopathy assessment scales

It is important to use scales in order to quantify the degree of neurological deterioration in the myelopathy. The first scale to be developed was Nurick's scale,[17] which evaluates the loss of motor function. This classification goes from grade 1, characterized by the presence of signs of myelopathy, but with a normal gait, up to grade 5 or severe myelopathy, whereby the patient is unable to walk (Table 2-2).

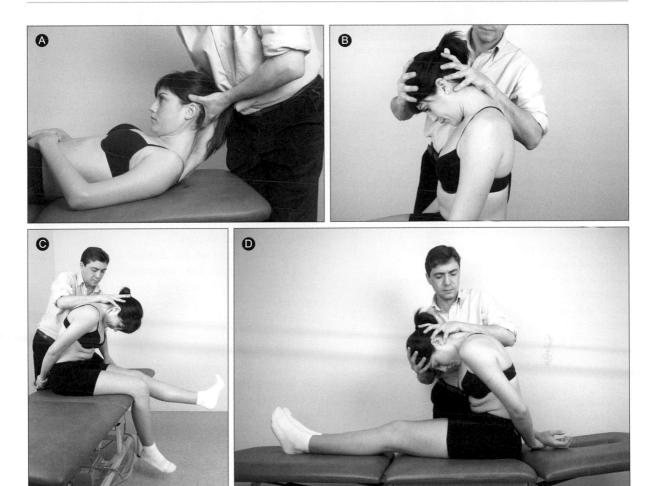

FIGURE 2-19 ■ The neurodynamic tests, such as the passive neck flexion (A), the passive neck flexion in the sitting position (cervical slump) (B), slump test (C) and the slump long sitting test (D) provide very interesting information to evaluate the neural mechanosensitivity. The range of movement applied during these tests should be adapted to the clinical situation of the patient.

Although Nurick's scale is well established and widely used, it is of limited use since it only measures the function of the lower limbs. One of the most commonly used scales is the *Japanese Orthopaedic Association Score* (JOA score).[97] This scale quantifies the severity of a myelopathy based on the motor dysfunction in the lower and upper limbs, the degree of sensory deficits and the sphincter's dysfunction. This scale has been subsequently reviewed and validated.[98,99] The maximum reference value is 17, which corresponds to a normal function (Table 2-3). According to this scale, a myelopathy is considered to be mild when the score is between 17 and 14 points, moderate between 13 and 6, and severe between 5 and 0 points.[100]

Recently, the JOA has developed a new assessment scale for cervical myelopathy, the *Cervical Myelopathy Evaluation Questionnaire* (JOACMEQ), which includes items related to the quality of life,[101] and it has been proven to provide a reliable evaluation.[102] Other myelopathy evaluation scores that have been developed are the Cooper myelopathy scale,[103] the modified Prolo score[104] and the European myelopathy score.[105] Singh et al.[106] have recently published a systematic review of the validity and reliability of assessment tools on cervical spondylotic myelopathy.

TABLE 2-3

The modified Japanese Orthopedic Association score as described by Benzel et al.[98]

	Score
I. Motor dysfunction score of upper extremities	
Inability to move hands	0
Inability to eat with a spoon but able to move hands	1
Inability to button shirt but able to eat with a spoon	2
Able to button shirt with great difficulty	3
Able to button shirt with slight difficulty	4
No dysfunction	5
II. Motor dysfunction score of the lower extremities	
Complete loss of motor and sensory function	0
Sensory preservation without ability to move legs	1
Able to move legs but unable to walk	2
Able to walk on flat floor with a walking aid (i.e. cane or crutch)	3
Able to walk up- and/or downstairs with hand rail	4
Moderate to significant lack of stability but able to walk up- and/or downstairs without hand rail	5
Mild lack of stability but able to walk unaided with smooth reciprocation	6
No dysfunction	7
III. Sensation	
Complete loss of hand sensation	0
Severe sensory loss or pain	1
Mild sensory loss	2
No sensory loss	3
IV. Sphincter dysfunction	
Unable to urinate voluntarily	0
Marked difficulty with micturition	1
Mild to moderate difficulty with micturition	2
Normal micturition	3

COMPLEMENTARY DIAGNOSTIC TESTS

Radiographic evaluation

There are different ways to identify a myelopathy caused by a cervical canal stenosis through imaging tests. The lateral projection of a conventional radiography can show a congenital stenosis, a degenerative stenosis, the ossification of the PLL and the presence of listhesis. Dynamic radiographies in flexion and extension are useful when evaluating the range of motion and the presence of segments with ankylosis or instability.[90]

For the radiographic evaluation of the constitutional stenosis with lateral radiography, the radiographic focus is placed 1.5 m away and is directed towards C5. The constitutional sagittal diameter, as described previously, is the distance between the midpoint of the back of vertebral body and the spinolaminar line. The cervical canal is wider in its superior portion, as can be seen in the C1 and C2 levels, where its mean diameter is 24 mm and 21 mm, respectively. However, in the lower levels, from C3 and C7, the dimensions are between 15 and 25 mm, with an average of 17 and 18 mm.[26,72,107–109]

The lower limit of the normal sagittal diameter is 14 mm,[110] and the constitutional stenosis is shown when the diameter of the cervical canal is ≤ 12 mm.[72,90,111,112]

The degenerative stenosis is evaluated using the spondylotic sagittal diameter, which is the distance from the lower margin of the vertebra, including the osteophytes' neoformations, to the anterior edge of the lamina. This diameter represents the most precise sagittal measurement to quantify the spondylotic stenosis.

The difference between the constitutional diameter and the spondylotic diameter provides us with the spondylotic index, also known as the segmental stenosis index. In subjects with constitutional stenosis, an index of 1.5 to 2 mm is enough for clinical manifestations characteristics of myelopathy to appear.[39,113]

The evaluation of the *dynamic canal stenosis* in a lateral radiography is performed by measuring, with the cervical spine in extension, from the lower edge of the vertebral body to the anterior margin of the lamina of the lower vertebra. A diameter that is 12 mm or less is considered a positive dynamic factor. The magnitude of the posterior listhesis with the cervical spine in extension is the most important diagnostic parameter of the dynamic stenosis (31, 114).

Pavlov's ratio

The absolute values of the cervical canal dimensions can be inaccurate due to the variability of the radiographic magnification. In order to avoid this problem, Pavlov et al.[115] designed a method to determine cervical stenosis after observing that there was a correlation

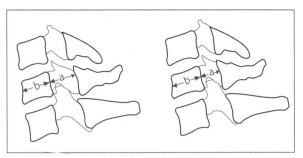

FIGURE 2-20 ■ Pavlov's ratio is the difference between the anteroposterior diameter of the vertebral boy and the sagittal diameter of the canal. Normal Pavlov's ratio (a) and narrow canal (b).

between the sagittal canal diameter and the sagittal vertebral body diameter. This is the Pavlov's ratio, also known as Torg's ratio,[116] and it relates to the difference between the anteroposterior diameter of the vertebral body and the sagittal canal diameter. A value ≥ 1 corresponds to a normal distance (Fig. 2-20). It is considered that there is absolute stenosis, and therefore a high risk of developing a myelopathy, when this ratio is ≤ 0.82.

An aspect that must be considered is the discrepancy in this ratio between males and females. Whereas the diameter of the canal is identical in both sexes, the diameter of the vertebral body is larger in males than in females,[117,118] and this is related to the higher incidence of this condition in males. Hukuda and Kojima[117] compared Pavlov's ratio in healthy males and females, and observed that, while 4.4% of females had a stenotic canal, the percentage rose to 19.4% in males. In a previous study, these authors proved that a large vertebral body is a risk factor for myelopathy.[119] As it is thought that a large vertebral body is associated with osteophytes or a larger disc, males that have a larger vertebral body are more prone to suffer from a myelopathy than women.

Nevertheless, the reliability of this method has been questioned over the last few years due to the possibility of false positives.[28,107,120] Blackley et al.[120] showed that there is poor correlation between Pavlov's ratio and the true sagittal diameter of the canal measured by a CT scan. They concluded that this ratio is of limited use when evaluating the true diameter of the cervical canal.

Prasad et al.[107] have compared Pavlov's ratio using plain radiographies with MRI, measuring the area of section of the cervical spinal cord and the space occupied by the CSF. They concluded that there is weak correlation between Pavlov's diameter and a possible cord compression. On the other hand, the area of the central canal and, therefore, the space available for the spinal cord, not only depends on the sagittal diameter but also on the coronal diameter. As it is known, in a normal cervical canal, the coronal diameter is greater than the sagittal diameter.

Although the pathology of the cervical canal stenosis occurs primarily in the sagittal plane, a narrowing that occurs exclusively at this plane may not indicate a significant reduction in the cross-sectional canal area.[107] Because of wide anatomical variations observed in normal subjects, this ratio is not in itself sufficient to predict the presence of a myelopathy. However, it is a method that is indeed validity provided that it is easy to perform and can alert possible cervical canal stenosis.

Another method used to identify the presence of a constitutional stenosis by using a lateral radiography is known as the safety space. In a lateral radiograph, the cervical canal can be divided into three parts: pedicular, articular and laminar (Fig. 2-21). The safety space corresponds with this last laminar part and should measure an average of 4 mm (Fig. 2-22).

The safety space may be reduced in subjects that have a hypoplasia of the laminae, or as a consequence of the degenerative hypertrophy of the zygapophyseal joints. However, there can be a constitutional stenosis with a normal safety space. For example, this may be the case when there is hypoplasia of the pedicles or when these have excessive coronal plane alignment, or in subjects with an excessive anteroposterior diameter of the vertebral body, as happens frequently in Asian people (Fig. 2-23).

Imaging techniques, such as CT and MRI in particular, can provide more reliable evaluations of cervical stenosis and myelopathy. A CT offers good information regarding the bone architecture in the sagittal plane and, therefore, of the bone elements responsible for the stenosis, such as the osteophytes or the calcification of the PLL, as well as the soft tissues that can reduce the area of the canal. The effectiveness of the technique increases with a contrast medium.

The CT–myelography can show the degree of spinal compression and, when performed in flexion and extension positions, it can help to identify a dynamic stenosis. Yet, it has several disadvantages with regard to an MRI: it is an invasive technique and does not allow for the observation of intramedullary cord changes. MRI allows for an evaluation of the soft tissues and the spinal cord,[121] and helps to visualize the non-osseous causes of stenosis, such as disc protrusions and the hypertrophy of the yellow ligament. The diameter of the canal can be analysed in sagittal and axial projections.

The MRI has shown that there are wide variations in the spinal cord diameter within normal population members. Therefore, the measurement of the diameters of the bone case with plain X-rays is not sufficient to evaluate the severity of the cervical myelopathy.[122] The degree of cord compression can be quantified in MRI with the measurement of the sagittal diameter of the spinal cord, its cross-sectional area and the space occupied by the CSF. The sagittal diameter of the cervical cord varies between 5 and 11.5 mm, and the average is 10 mm.[28] The spinal cord cross-sectional area should be equal or higher to 40 mm^2. The magnitude of this area in the MRI has demonstrated a good correlation with the severity of the myelopathy, the duration of the process and the functional recovery after surgery in patients with canal stenosis myelopathy.[123,124] Furthermore, the MRI has the advantage of allowing us to observe the signs of cord parenchymal damage, such as a high-intensity signal on T2 sequences, and a decrease in signal intensity in T1 (Fig. 2-24).

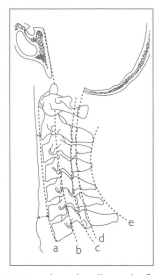

FIGURE 2-21 ■ In a lateral radiograph, five lines can be seen: anterior vertebral line (a), posterior vertebral line (b), posterior pillar line (c), spinolaminar line (d) and posterior spinous line (e). The central canal is located between the posterior vertebral line and the spinolaminar line. The safety space corresponds to the laminar portion of the canal and should measure an average of 4 mm.

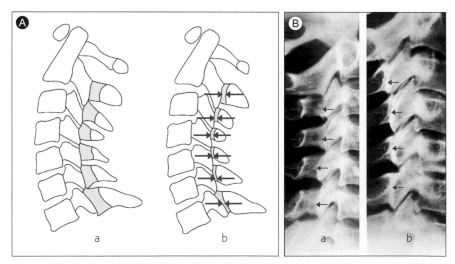

FIGURE 2-22 ■ (A) In this diagram, in grey, can be seen a normal safety space (a) and a reduction of it (b). (B) In the radiograph, a normal canal (a) and a narrow canal due to reduction of the safety space (b) are shown.

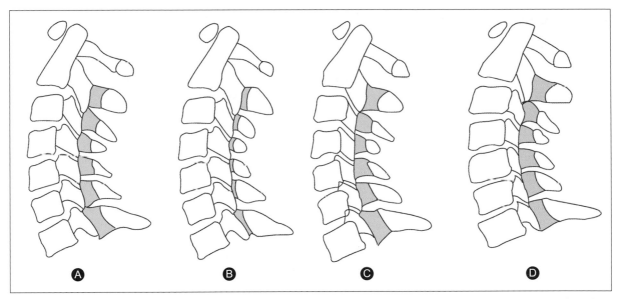

FIGURE 2-23 ■ Normal canal (A). The central canal can be narrow constitutionally, with a normal safety space, when there is hypoplasia of the pedicles (B), or these pedicles have an excessive orientation in the coronal plane (C), or in subjects with an excessive anteroposterior diameter of the vertebral body (D).

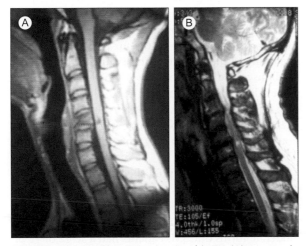

FIGURE 2-24 ■ A low-intensity signal in T1 (A), as seen in the MRI, associated with a high-intensity signal in T2 (B) indicates serious damage with necrosis and myelomalacia and a poor recovery prognosis.

The meaning of the high-intensity signal is not completely clear. Some researchers consider it to be a sign of myelomalacia and of irreversible spinal cord changes[125] and, therefore, a sign of a poor prognosis for the myelopathy. However, others state that, although it reflects pathological changes, it is not correlated with the severity of the myelopathy and cannot be used as a predictive value.[126–128]

At present, it is considered that a high-intensity signal indicates an unspecific and broad spectrum of cord damage, such as inflammation, oedema, ischaemia, gliosis or myelomalacia.[129,130] In patients with a mild myelopathy, a high-intensity signal is not related to bad conservative treatment outcomes or to the severity of the myelopathy.[131] Differences have been established in the high-intensity signal images between irreversible and reversible damage.[132] Irreversible changes, such as a myelomalacia or a cystic necrosis, provide an image with a bright area with well-defined margins, while in a reversible damage, the oedema is less bright and the margins are not as well defined in T2 sequences. However, it is not always possible to differentiate between reversible and irreversible damage. There is a more agreement in relation to the sign of low-intensity signal in T1 sequences. A low-intensity signal in T1[128,129] associated to a high-intensity signal in T2, indicates severe damage with necrosis and myelomalacia and, therefore, a poor prognosis of recovery.[123,125,129,133,134]

CONSERVATIVE TREATMENT

There have been several trials and systematic reviews into the use of a structured physical therapy programme for the treatment of cervical spondylosis, including CSM. The treatment of CSM is still controversial, especially in its mild and moderate forms, in which no rapid progression is observed. The effectiveness of the conservative treatment and its capacity to modify the natural history of the CSM had not been thoroughly studied until recently. Following the publication of the study by Clarke and Robinson in 1956, several studies have found that conservative treatment is not effective in the long term.[9,17,135] However, the initial publication did show that different conservative measures could improve the symptoms in 50% of the subjects. It is generally believed that the results of surgical treatment are better than those obtained by conservative treatment and, therefore, the conservative treatment tends to be rejected, and surgery is considered the first choice for a therapeutic intervention,[123,136,137] However, this belief has been questioned by some researchers,[138–141] who have shown that in some cases surgery does not achieve better outcomes than conservative treatment. The conservative treatment is currently recognized as a therapeutic alternative for a mild CSM, with good outcomes in a high percentage of patients in the long term.[131,135,142–148] There are recent studies that compare the outcomes of the surgical and the conservative treatments.

In 2000, the *Cervical Spine Research Society* conducted a prospective multicentric non-randomized study[149] in order to find out the effectiveness of the conservative and surgical treatments. In this trial, 43 patients were treated, 54% of them receiving a medical treatment and 46% a surgical treatment. The follow-up period was not very long, lasting for a period of between 8 and 13 months. Patients who were treated conservatively noted worsening in their ability to perform everyday activities, and the functional state of those treated with surgery improved significantly. As for the improvement of their neurological symptoms, neither group showed a significant change in the symptoms of the lower limbs. However, the patients that were treated with surgery had an improvement of the symptoms in their upper limbs. This improvement could be due to the fact that upper limb symptoms are related to a radiculopathy that, as previously described, is frequently associated with a myelopathy.

Certainly, surgery is recommended in cases of severe myelopathies and in moderate-to-severe cases, since it stops further neurological deterioration. The clinical outcomes vary according to the severity of the myelopathy, the extent of the condition and other factors related to the patient.[150] The neurological improvement, both after ventral or posterior surgical procedures, is variable,[151] although it seems to be different from the natural history of the CSM, since 50% of patients end up being seriously disabled.

On the other hand, as previously described, there are several studies that advocate the conservative treatment of a mild myelopathy. A factor that must be taken into account when choosing this treatment is the high morbidity, both neurological and non-neurological, of the different surgical treatments employed in the treatment of this pathology.[81,138,148,152–156]

Matsumoto et al.[131] conducted a study regarding the non-operative treatment of CSM. Thirty-four (65%) patients had an area of high-intensity signal (HIS) on MRI examination. Their results showed that the average JOA score began at 14.0 and remained at 14.4 on average after a follow-up period of 3 years. According to their results, conservative therapy stabilized the course of myelopathy. A satisfactory outcome was evident in a 78% and in a 65%, without HIS and with HIS, respectively. A HIS regression was recorded in 18% of patients on follow-up imaging. This regression was associated with a significant improvement in JOA scores.

Kadanka et al.,[144,145] published in 2000 and 2002, respectively, the results of prospective randomized studies, with the purpose of comparing the results of the conservative and surgical treatments in mild and moderate forms of CSM. Patients had a score of 12 or higher in the JOA score. After a follow-up period of 2 or 3 years, the functional improvement of the patients that had surgery was not statistically superior that of the patients treated with a conservative treatment. Therefore, there is no solid evidence to indicate that decompressive surgery improves the clinical outcomes in patients with a mild myelopathy, which does not mean that surgery is contraindicated. The purpose of surgery is to stop the progression and avoid a sudden deterioration as a consequence of a minor trauma. The results of this work show that the conservative treatment can have the same outcomes as surgery in these mild forms, at least during the first 3 years.

In order to clarify this situation, in 2002 a Cochrane systematic review was published by Fouyas et al.[18,19] to determine if surgical treatment of myelopathy is associated with an improved outcome as compared with conservative management. The review was also intended to outline whether the timing of surgery (immediate or delayed) had an impact on outcomes. The trial of Bednarik et al.[157] carried out on 49 patients with cervical myelopathy was chosen as the reference study. In this study different parameters were used to analyse disability following conservative and surgical treatments. The parameters used were upper and lower motor neuron function, proprioception, coordination, paraesthesia in the limbs and sphincter control, using the JOA scale. The study demonstrated that patients that received a conservative treatment improved significantly after 6 months. There were no differences between the two groups at 12 and 24 months after the beginning of the treatment. According to this systematic review, the results of surgery are not always satisfactory and can be similar to those obtained through conservative treatment. It is not clear if the risks of surgery compensate for the long-term benefits.[19] This review concludes that, despite the 4000 interventions performed in the United Kingdom each year for a pathology related to a cervical spondylosis, there is no conclusive evidence to support the surgical treatment of cervical radiculomyelopathy. The Cochrane systematic review was updated in 2010 by the same group.[158] The conclusion of this review was that there is very low-quality evidence to show that patients with mild myelopathy feel subjectively better shortly after surgery, but there is little or no difference in the long term.

Another review was carried out by Hirpara et al.[159] in 2012 regarding the use of non-operative modalities to treat symptomatic cervical spondylosis. The review concludes that CSM patients initially treated with surgery obtain greater improvements in pain, muscle strength and sensory function in the early follow-up period, but at 1 year there is no difference between groups either objectively or in terms of patient satisfaction.

Rhee et al.[160] published a systematic review in 2013 concerning the non-operative management of cervical myelopathy. The authors recommend surgical treatment in patients with moderate-to-severe myelopathy and non-operative treatment as a treatment option for mild myelopathy. However, the authors acknowledge that further comparative studies between these two management strategies are needed. They add that there is also a need to compare specific types of non-operative treatments with the natural history of myelopathy.

As a conclusion, non-operative management may have better results than previously thought, especially when used early in the initial phases of the disease. Conservative therapy can stop the progression of CSM and reverse the symptoms in some patients with a mild myelopathy.[161]

Conservative treatment: criteria and indications

After this review, it is interesting to highlight the criteria used to advocate a conservative treatment, which can be summarized as the duration of the disorder, the severity of the signs and symptoms, the aetiology and severity of the stenosis and the patient's age.

The *duration of the myelopathy* is one of the most significant parameters in the prognosis and the outcomes after surgical or conservative treatment.[162] The conservative treatment is effective primarily in patients with initial signs of myelopathy. It is recommended to begin the treatment when the first signs and symptoms appear, since its effectiveness is very limited in subjects with a myelopathy of more than 5 years.[64,146] The initial symptoms of myelopathy are frequently neck pain and a restricted range of cervical motion.[163] In patients that do not yet show cord compression signs, and when imaging tests point to a pre-myelopathic situation, it is recommended to initiate a conservative treatment to limit the possible progression to a myelopathy.

The selection between conservative or surgical treatment depends on the *severity of the signs and symptoms*.[22,23] Conservative treatment is only recommended for mild or moderate forms of spondylotic myelopathy, particularly in patients that can walk without crutches, with a score of ≥ 2 in the motor dysfunction of the upper extremities JOA score, with a JOA global score of ≥ 12 points, or with a Nurick's grade of ≤ 3.[141,164,165]

Regarding the *stenosis severity*, the conservative treatment should be followed in cases of mild-to-moderate stenosis. It is considered that a myelopathy has a bad prognosis when the central canal diameter/vertebral body diameter ratio is ≤ 0.8.[33] Likewise, the transversal area of the spinal cord, at the level of the maximum compression, is a basic parameter for treatment outcomes.[141,162] All those parameters that in conventional radiography and in MRI indicate a severe canal stenosis contraindicate, initially, the conservative treatment. As previously described, the increase in signal intensity in an MRI in the T2 sequences does not necessarily imply bad outcomes in the conservative treatment in patients with a mild myelopathy.[131,141]

The possibilities of the conservative treatment are also defined by the aetiology of the stenosis. If it is reversible, such as in cases of soft disc herniation or listhesis,[162,164] surgery should be postponed until the effects of the conservative treatment are confirmed.[12,162] Several studies have shown that conservative treatment is an effective management option for mild CSM caused by cervical soft disc herniation.[162,164] In a study by Matsumoto et al.,[164] 27 patients with a mild CSM caused by cervical soft disc herniation were treated conservatively. This treatment was effective in 63% of patients, of which 59% showed a spontaneous regression of the disc herniation with a concomitant resolution of the neurological symptoms. As described in Chapter 1, currently, it is known that the extruded disc material suffers a regression that tends to decrease the herniated mass, which can even disappear.[166] This phenomenon is caused primarily when the disc material is located in the epidural space and when there are clear signs of vascularization.[167] If, on the contrary the aetiological factors that are either unchangeable, such as constitutional, or progressive, such as the ossification of the PLL, then surgical treatment should be considered.[148,162,165]

Age is a controversial factor when it comes to assessing the influence of conservative treatment outcomes. While some studies affirm that advanced age influences the prognosis of the conservative treatment negatively,[150,168] others found no correlation.[141,148]

The effectiveness of the conservative treatment also depends on cervical mobility and the patient's sex.[78] Being a female and having a significant cervical mobility facilitates the worsening of the neurological status.[146] Furthermore, conservative treatment for CSM is considered to be effective if it is performed intensively in selected patients.[146]

TREATMENT TECHNIQUES

The conservative treatment does not attempt to resolve the cervical myelopathy, but to contribute to the improvement of the neurological function, reduce pain and other symptoms, and improve the subject's quality of life.

Manual therapy

Manual therapy, in its various forms, is not contraindicated for CSM. However, the high-velocity manipulation techniques with impulse are indeed contraindicated, not only for myelopathies but also in the presence of significant degenerative changes in the cervical spine. Mobilization, traction and accessory movement techniques, as well as neurodynamic techniques, can improve a patient's clinical condition.[169]

In any case, none of the examples of treatment techniques outlined in this section should be performed indiscriminately. It is essential to only select the techniques that are suitable for the patient's clinical situation, and they should be evaluated at all times to monitor if there is a worsening of the symptoms or neurological function during or after the application of the techniques. In order to improve the symptoms of the patient, it may also be necessary to immobilize the patient with a neck collar that keeps the cervical spine in slight flexion.[15,17,135,142]

Cervical traction

Despite the fact that traction was previously contraindicated,[9,90] it is currently one of the most commonly used methods in the treatment of this type of patient.[131,142,146] Its effectiveness can be derived from its capacity to modify the relationship between the neural tissues and the central canal. It should be applied with caution and progressively, and checks should be

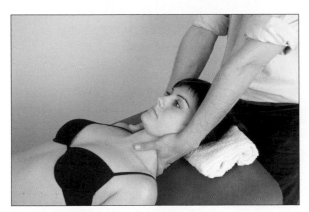

FIGURE 2-25 ■ Intermittent manual traction.

carried out at all times to see if there is an aggravation of symptoms. It is important to know what structure is the most relevant in the spinal stenosis: that is, if the stenosis is caused primarily by anterior structures, such as the disc or the vertebral body osteophytes, the traction in flexion should be avoided, since it would aggravate the compressive forces over the anterior portion of the spinal cord.

On the other hand, when the posterior structures are responsible for that, as in the cases of zygapophyseal, laminae hypertrophy or ligamentum flavum buckling, applying traction in flexion could reduce the compressive forces. Both intermittent and continuous traction can be useful[170,171] (Fig. 2-25). Some authors recommend a protocol of intensive continuous traction in a hospital environment.[146,172,173]

Mobilization techniques

Mobilization techniques can be aimed at the mechanical interface or the neural tissues. The *mechanical interface mobilization techniques* are indicated, except for subjects with significant dynamic stenosis, for whom an increase in mobility could aggravate neurological deterioration. The objective of these techniques is to reduce the compressive forces that act on the neural elements. Therefore, it is necessary, as in the traction technique, to first evaluate which structures are involved in the stenosis. The use of these techniques should be cautious and progressive. High-velocity manipulation techniques, or those that imply end range amplitudes, are contraindicated. The tech-

niques that are best suited this type of patients are low-amplitude physiological and accessory joint mobilization techniques.

The *lateral side-glide technique* should be applied on a position that causes minimum stress for the cervical spinal cord, associating progressively a small traction component. This mobilization can be performed, especially if the patient has a myeloradiculopathy, with a positioning of the upper limbs that could modify tension on the cervical roots.

An example of a side-glide technique is that which involves the therapist holding the patient's cervical spine and head between their hands and introducing a left and right segmental side-glide movement of low-amplitude rhythmically. Initially, with the purpose of not soliciting the neural tissues excessively, the hands of the patient rest on the abdomen, in a position without any neural tension. Then, one or the two upper limbs can be placed in extension, in order to apply more neural tension (Fig. 2-26).

In the *physiological movements*, the isolated mobilization in side-bending and rotation in initial degrees can be incorporated from the first treatment sessions (Fig. 2-27). The procedure can be continued with a combined movement of side bending and ipsilateral rotation to which a small component of traction can be added. The mobilization in flexion should be very moderate in the cases where the structures responsible for the stenosis are ventral.

Several techniques can be applied at distance, especially in cases where the use of a direct approach could initially lead to symptoms worsening. For instance, the mobilization of the thoracic and lumbar spine can be an interesting strategy to help to reduce stress over the neural tissues of the cervical spine. Below, a few examples of manual treatments are outlined.

Neurodynamic techniques

The *nerve tissue mobilization techniques* can be used to treat cervical canal stenosis, except in the cases where there is significant irritability. The objective is to reduce the mechanosensitivity of the neural tissue, improve its blood perfusion and help with the dispersion of the intraneural or extraneural oedema. The type and technique and its intensity depends on the patient's clinical situation. At first, sliders techniques

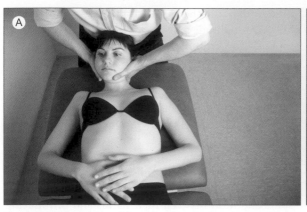
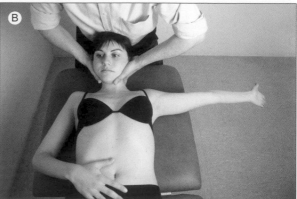

FIGURE 2-26 ■ Side-glide technique. During the translation, the patient keeps the arms on the abdomen (A) and when the translation ceases, the patient extends the upper limb (B).

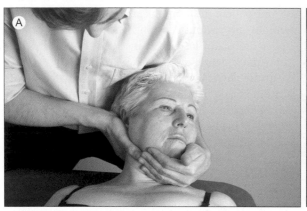
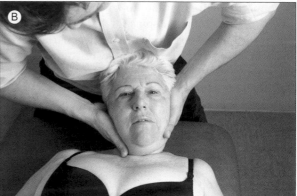

FIGURE 2-27 ■ Mobilization in rotation (A) and side-bending (B) in the initial phases can be added in the first treatment sessions.

seem more appropriate for this entity than tensioner techniques. However, the latter can be introduced as the neural mechanosensitivity decreases. In both types of techniques, the mobilization can start from the periphery, as in the case of a radiculopathy, and then the neuromeningeal tissues can be mobilized more intensely. The recommended neurodynamic techniques are those where the neural tissue is mobilized with the upper and lower limbs, and those aimed at mobilizing the neuroaxis.

Upper limb neurodynamic techniques. The purpose of the neurodynamic techniques is to transversally mobilize the neuroaxis, which can be seen as the shape of an 'H' laying down. Any tension applied on one of

the ends will tend to be dissipated by the others. At first, all the techniques will be performed in grade I and II, until a patient;s response can be observed. If the symptoms are not aggravated, there will be a progression to the III and IV grades of mobilization. Some examples of this technique have been described in Chapter 1 (Fig. 2-28 and 2-29).

CERVICAL SLUMP OR PASSIVE NECK FLEXION. *Patient's position:* supine position, initially with the hands on the abdomen (neural anti-tension position for the upper limbs).

Therapist's position: stood at the head of the table.

Procedure: the therapist applies a cervical flexion movement rhythmically and repeatedly (Fig. 2-30). Subsequently, the upper limbs are placed in different

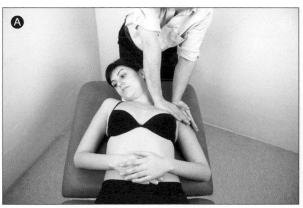
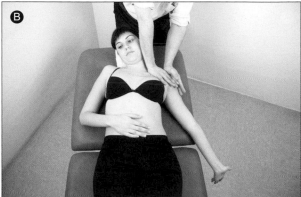

FIGURE 2-28 ■ Neural slider manoeuvre (ULNT2). The patient maintains the cervical spine in slight side-bending and contralateral rotation (A). The therapist applies a depression of the shoulder girdle and, when releasing this depression, the patient extends the elbow (B).

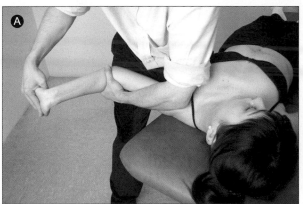
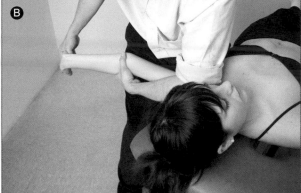

FIGURE 2-29 ■ The neural slider manoeuvre (ULNT1) associates a lateral traction of the upper limb (A) with an elbow flexion (B).

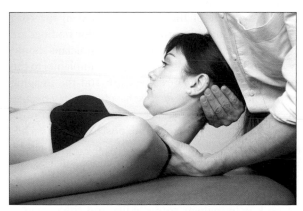

FIGURE 2-30 ■ Passive neck flexion.

degrees of shoulder abduction and elbow extension in order to introduce a greater component of initial tension on the neural tissues. In order for the technique to be a neural gliding technique, the patient can be asked to flex the elbow or raise the shoulder girdle during the neck flexion (Fig. 2-31). This manoeuvre can be performed with an upper limb or with both simultaneously. In the latter case, the excursion of the neural tissue movement is reduced.

CRANIOCERVICAL SPINE FLEXION. This manoeuvre is most commonly used when the patient's symptoms do not allow for a cervical flexion (Fig. 2-32). If the clinical situation of the patient allows it, in order to include a gliding component, the patient can perform

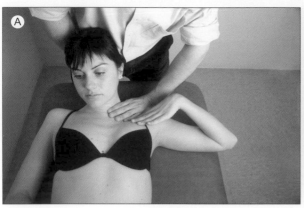
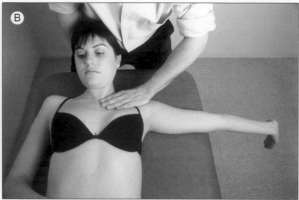

FIGURE 2-31 ■ Passive neck flexion associated with a neural slider (A and B).

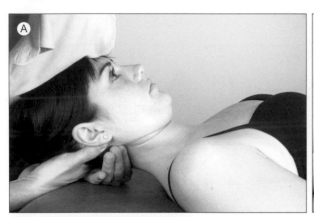
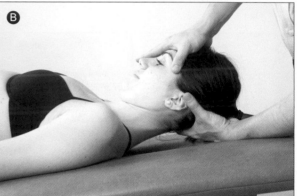

FIGURE 2-32 ■ Flexion of the craniocervical spine stabilizing C2 (A) and with fronto-occipital grip (B).

an active elevation of the straight leg or an abduction of the upper limb by decreasing craniocervical traction (Fig. 2-33).

THORACIC MOBILIZATION IN THE SUPINE POSITION. *Patient's position*: supine position.
Therapist's position: standing at the head of the table.
Procedure: the therapist places a wedge on the upper thoracic region, which acts as a fulcrum, and with one hand performs a flexion of the cervical spine. Using the other hand, on the anterior thoracic region, the therapist applies anteroposterior pressure towards the fulcrum located on the thoracic spine (Fig. 2-34).

Surgical treatment

In patients with a severe or moderate-to-severe myelopathy, and in those with a mild myelopathy with a progression of the neurological signs, it is advisable to opt for surgery. Post-surgical outcomes vary according to the severity of the myelopathy.[150,151,174-177]

The decision to undergo surgery is based on a thorough knowledge of the factors involved in the cord dysfunction. Since abnormal radiographic findings are common in asymptomatic subjects,[38] clinicians should be careful when linking the patient's complaints to the results of the physical examination and the imaging tests. The goal of surgery is to obtain an effective decompression of the spinal cord. In a cervical myelopathy both the anterior and posterior approaches are employed. The decision to use one approach or the other is based on different factors, such as the cause of the spinal compression, the number of segments involved, the vertebral alignment, the severity of neck pain, patient comorbidity and the surgeon's familiarity with the different techniques.

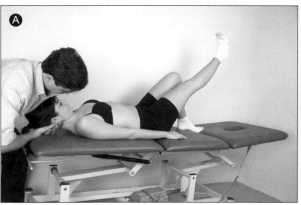 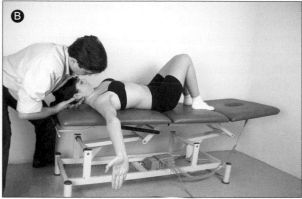

FIGURE 2-33 ▪ Flexion of the craniocervical spine associated with a straight leg raise (A) and an abduction of the upper limb (B).

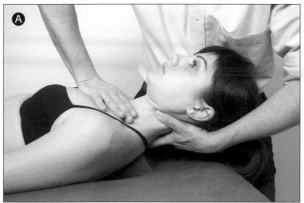 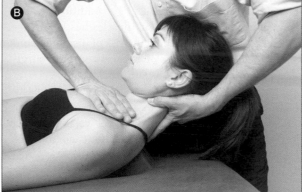

FIGURE 2-34 ▪ (A, B) Anteroposterior thoracic mobilization in the supine position associated with a cervical flexion using a wedge on the thoracic spine.

The aforementioned approach is well suited to cases in which the stenosis is ventral to the spinal cord, as in the case of a disc herniation, an anterior osteophytosis or the ossification of the PLL. Decompression is commonly used when the stenosis is present in one or two levels. This approach allows for a direct visualization and the possibility of removing the elements responsible for the stenosis without manipulating the spinal cord. When a vertebral alignment is neutral or kyphotic, the anterior procedures restore the cervical lordosis. The recovery of the lordosis allows for the spinal cord to be displaced in a posterior direction, diminishing its anterior compression. After the decompression, the vertebral stability is achieved with a segmental arthrodesis. The problem with the aforementioned approach is the high rate of failure of the arthrodesis when performed in more than two or three levels.[178–183]

With regard to posterior approaches, laminectomy and laminoplasty allow for a wide decompression of the spinal cord. This surgical approach is used when there are several levels implicated in the myelopathy and the source of the cord compression is posterior. The problem of a laminectomy is that, by eliminating the posterior elements, it often leads to the development of a deformity in kyphosis or listhesis.[184] In order to expose the lamina, the semispinalis cervicis muscle must be sectioned and this leads to its caudal retraction. Vasavada et al.[185] have demonstrated that this muscle is responsible for more than 37% of cervical extension and plays a crucial role in maintaining the cervical lordosis. Nolan and Sherk[186] also pointed out that the extensor muscles act as dynamic stabilizers and that by eliminating the attachments of the semispinalis muscles, the laminectomy leads to a significant loss of the normal cervical alignment. The level of recovery in patients with a severe loss of cervical lordosis is much lower than in those that maintain a normal curvature.[187] Furthermore, the loss of lordosis can cause a persistence of the stress suffered by the neural structures.[188]

Pain is another challenge derived from a posterior approach, and it can affect 40–60% of individuals following a laminoplasty.[189,190] Therefore, posterior decompression is only recommended when the stenosis is present in several levels.[70,156,176] Additionally, the reattachment of the posterior muscles has been suggested as a means of reducing the risk of instability and kyphotic deformity.[189,191,192] The most common surgical method is an open-door laminoplasty.[187]

The loss of lordosis after a cervical laminoplasty is also related to the loss of muscular stabilization, and this proves the importance of establishing a post-surgical rehabilitation programme as soon as possible.[193]

CONCLUSION

Conservative treatment can be an effective therapeutic option and is especially indicated for patients with a mild myelopathy, and when the aetiology is reversible.[15,17,142] However, prolonging a conservative treatment without seeing any significant functional improvements can eliminate the possibility of obtaining good results after surgery, since a long preoperative period can have adverse effects on the final outcome of surgery.[131,194] More caution should be taken when choosing between conservative and surgical treatment with patients suffering from myelopathy than with radiculopathy patients.[164] With current knowledge of the physiopathology of stenosis in a CSM, there has been a decrease of early surgery for mild forms of the condition.

Currently, it is considered important to carefully select candidates for surgery, in order to obtain the best possible outcomes and ensure that outcomes are better than those of the conservative treatment or the natural history of the disease.

If a conservative treatment is chosen, it is crucial to perform a frequent assessment of the patient's neurological condition in order to monitor progress for at least 3 months after beginning treatment. If a neurological deterioration is observed during this period, then surgical decompression should be considered.[164]

REFERENCES

1. Edwards CC 2nd, Riew KD, Anderson PA, et al. Cervical myelopathy. Current diagnostic and treatment strategies. Spine J 2003;3(1):68–81.
2. Kalsi-Ryan S, Karadimas SK, Fehlings MG. Cervical spondylotic myelopathy: the clinical phenomenon and the current pathobiology of an increasingly prevalent and devastating disorder. Neuroscientist 2013;19(4):409–21.
3. Ito T, Oyanagi K, Takahashi H, et al. Cervical spondylotic myelopathy. Clinicopathologic study on the progression pattern and thin myelinated fibers of the lesions of seven patients examined during complete autopsy. Spine 1996; 21(7):827–33.
4. Young IA, Burns SP, Little JW. Sudden onset of cervical spondylotic myelopathy during sleep: a case report. Arch Phys Med Rehabil 2002;83(3):427–9.
5. Greene KA, Gorman WF, Sonntag VK. Gentle cervical hyperextension causing quadriplegia in an older man with symptomatic cervical spondylosis. J Am Geriatr Soc 1998;46(2): 208–9.
6. Teresi LM, Lufkin RB, Reicher MA, et al. Asymptomatic degenerative disk disease and spondylosis of the cervical spine: MR imaging. Radiology 1987;164(1):83–8.
7. Stookey B. Compresion of the spinal cord due to ventral extradural cervical chondromas. Arch Neurol Psychiatry 1928;20:275–91.
8. Brain WR, Northfield D, Wilkinson M. The neurological manifestations of cervical spondylosis. Brain 1952;75(2):187–225.
9. Clarke E, Robinson PK. Cervical myelopathy: a complication of cervical spondylosis. Brain 1956;79(3):483–510.
10. Bernhardt M, Hynes RA, Blume HW, et al. Cervical spondylotic myelopathy. J Bone Joint Surg Am 1993;75(1):119–28.
11. Fischgrund J, Herkowitz H. Cervical degenerative disease. In: Garfin S, Vaccaro A, editors. Orthopedic knowledge update spine. Illinois: AAOS; 1997. p. 75–86.
12. Heller JG. The syndromes of degenerative cervical disease. Orthop Clin North Am 1992;23(3):381–94.
13. Yu YL, Woo E, Huang CY. Cervical spondylotic myelopathy and radiculopathy. Acta Neurol Scand 1987;75(6):367–73.
14. Fouyas IP, Sandercock PA, Statham PF, et al. How beneficial is surgery for cervical radiculopathy and myelopathy? BMJ 2010;341:c3108.
15. Lees F, Turner JW. Natural history and prognosis of cervical spondylosis. Br Med J 1963;5373:1607–10.

16. Phillips DG. Surgical treatment of myelopathy with cervical spondylosis. J Neurol Neurosurg Psychiatry 1973;36(5):879–84.
17. Nurick S. The natural history and the results of surgical treatment of the spinal cord disorder associated with cervical spondylosis. Brain 1972;95(1):101–8.
18. Fouyas IP, Statham PF, Sandercock PA, et al. Surgery for cervical radiculomyelopathy. Cochrane Database Syst Rev 2001;(3):CD001466.
19. Fouyas IP, Statham PF, Sandercock PA. Cochrane review on the role of surgery in cervical spondylotic radiculomyelopathy. Spine 2002;27(7):736–47.
20. Heller J. Surgical treatment of degenerative cervical disc disease. In: Fardon D, Garfin S, editors. Orthopedic knowledge update spine 2. Illinois: AAOS; 2002. p. 299–309.
21. Taylor AR. Vascular factors in the myelopathy associated with cervical spondylosis. Neurology 1964;14:62–8.
22. Sampath P, Bendebba M, Davis JD, et al. Outcome in patients with cervical radiculopathy. Prospective, multicenter study with independent clinical review. Spine 1999;24(6):591–7.
23. McCormack BM, Weinstein PR. Cervical spondylosis. An update. West J Med 1996;165(1–2):43–51.
24. Bohlman HH. Cervical spondylosis and myelopathy. Instr Course Lect 1995;44:81–97.
25. Fehlings MG, Skaf G. A review of the pathophysiology of cervical spondylotic myelopathy with insights for potential novel mechanisms drawn from traumatic spinal cord injury. Spine 1998;23(24):2730–7.
26. Hayashi H, Okada K, Hamada M, et al. Etiologic factors of myelopathy. A radiographic evaluation of the aging changes in the cervical spine. Clin Orthop 1987;214:200–9.
27. Lee HM, Kim NH, Kim HJ, et al. Mid-sagittal canal diameter and vertebral body/canal ratio of the cervical spine in Koreans. Yonsei Med J 1994;35(4):446–52.
28. Herzog RJ, Wiens JJ, Dillingham MF, et al. Normal cervical spine morphometry and cervical spinal stenosis in asymptomatic professional football players. Plain film radiography, multiplanar computed tomography, and magnetic resonance imaging. Spine 1991;16(6 Suppl.):S178–86.
29. Ogino H, Tada K, Okada K, et al. Canal diameter, anteroposterior compression ratio, and spondylotic myelopathy of the cervical spine. Spine 1983;8(1):1–15.
30. Bucciero A, Vizioli L, Tedeschi G. Cord diameters and their significance in prognostication and decisions about management of cervical spondylotic myelopathy. J Neurosurg Sci 1993;37(4):223–8.
31. Penning L, Wilmink JT, van Woerden HH, et al. CT myelographic findings in degenerative disorders of the cervical spine: clinical significance. AJR Am J Roentgenol 1986;146(4):793–801.
32. Fujiwara K, Yonenobu K, Hiroshima K, et al. Morphometry of the cervical spinal cord and its relation to pathology in cases with compression myelopathy. Spine 1988;13(11):1212–16.
33. Fujiwara K, Yonenobu K, Ebara S, et al. The prognosis of surgery for cervical compression myelopathy. An analysis of the factors involved. J Bone Joint Surg Br 1989;71(3):393–8.
34. Bernhardt M, Hynes RA, Blume HW, et al. Cervical spondylotic myelopathy. J Bone Joint Surg Am 1993;75(1):119–28.
35. Hinck V, Sachdev N. Developmental stenosis of the cervical spinal canal. Brain 1966;89:27–36.
36. Parke WW. Correlative anatomy of cervical spondylotic myelopathy. Spine 1988;13(7):831–7.
37. Martin-Laez R, Pinto-Rafael JI, Carda-Llop JR, et al. [Current controversies in pathophysiology of cervical spondylotic myelopathy.]. Neurologia 2004;19(10):738–60.
38. Boden SD, McCowin PR, Davis DO, et al. Abnormal magnetic-resonance scans of the cervical spine in asymptomatic subjects. A prospective investigation. J Bone Joint Surg Am 1990;72(8):1178–84
39. Edwards WC, LaRocca H. The developmental segmental sagittal diameter of the cervical spinal canal in patients with cervical spondylosis. Spine 1983;8(1):20–7.
40. Koyanagi I, Iwasaki Y, Hida K, et al. Acute cervical cord injury associated with ossification of the posterior longitudinal ligament. Neurosurgery 2003;53(4):887–91, discussion 891-2.
41. Shingyouchi Y, Nagahama A, Niida M. Ligamentous ossification of the cervical spine in the late middle-aged Japanese men. Its relation to body mass index and glucose metabolism. Spine 1996;21(21):2474–8.
42. Kojima T, Waga S, Kubo Y, et al. Surgical treatment of ossification of the posterior longitudinal ligament in the thoracic spine. Neurosurgery 1994;34(5):854–8, discussion 858.
43. Epstein N. The surgical management of ossification of the posterior longitudinal ligament in 51 patients. J Spinal Disord 1993;6(5):432–54, discussion 454-5.
44. Epstein NE. The surgical management of ossification of the posterior longitudinal ligament in 43 North Americans. Spine 1994;19(6):664–72.
45. Matsunaga S, Sakou T, Arishima Y, et al. Quality of life in elderly patients with ossification of the posterior longitudinal ligament. Spine 2001;26(5):494–8.
46. Epstein N. Ossification of the cervical posterior longitudinal ligament: a review. Neurosurg Focus 2002;13(2):ECP1
47. Epstein NE. Ossification of the posterior longitudinal ligament in evolution in 12 patients. Spine 1994;19(6):673–01.
48. Resnick D, Shaul SR, Robins JM. Diffuse idiopathic skeletal hyperostosis (DISH): Forestier's disease with extraspinal manifestations. Radiology 1975;115(3):513–24.
49. Forestier J, Rotes-Querol J. Senile ankylosing hyperostosis of the spine. Ann Rheum Dis 1950;9(4):321–30.
50. Resnick D, Guerra J Jr, Robinson CA, et al. Association of diffuse idiopathic skeletal hyperostosis (DISH) and calcification and ossification of the posterior longitudinal ligament. AJR Am J Roentgenol 1978;131(6):1049–53.
51. Kamizono J, Matsunaga S, Hayashi K, et al. Occupational recovery after open-door type laminoplasty for patients with ossification of the posterior longitudinal ligament. Spine 2003;28(16):1889–92.
52. Wang PN, Chen SS, Liu HC, et al. Ossification of the posterior longitudinal ligament of the spine. A case-control risk factor study. Spine 1999;24(2):142–4, discussion 145.

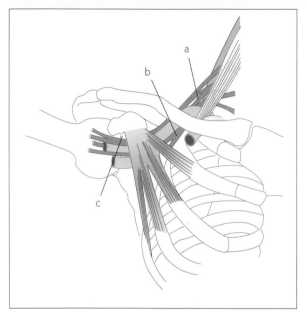

FIGURE 3-1 ■ The thoracic outlet is composed of three anatomical narrowing areas: the interscalene triangle (a), the costoclavicular space (b) and the retropectoral space (c).

after a clavicle or first rib fracture, or functional changes that are secondary effects of a trauma, such as the hypertrophy of the scalene muscles.

In order to understand the physiopathology of the TOS, it is important to consider it as a dynamic entity in which postural alterations or alterations of the activity that the subject performs have a profound effect. Changes in the static and dynamic balance of the shoulder girdle and the cervical and thoracic spine can reduce space that is available to maintain the normal function of the neurovascular structures. At present, it is believed that these postural changes are critical factors in the development of a TOS.[8,24–29]

The TOS is a dynamic entity in which the changes in the static and dynamic balance of the shoulder girdle and the cervical and thoracic spine can favour its development.

CLASSIFICATION

As previously discussed, the structures that can suffer from compression are the brachial plexus and the subclavian artery and vein. Depending on the structure that suffers the compression, the TOS can be classified as a *neurogenic syndrome, arterial syndrome* or *venous syndrome.* Given that it is often difficult to obtain positive objective tests, a fourth category is *non-specific TOS,* also known as symptomatic TOS and, presumably, *neurogenic TOS.*[9–11,30–34] The non-specific TOS category is used when a patient has chronic pain, symptoms that suggest that the brachial plexus is affected, but the objective neurological evaluation is normal.[30]

When a patient has a cervical rib and acute vascular insufficiency it is easy to recognize a vascular TOS.[8,35] Likewise, when a subject has atrophy of the intrinsic muscles of the hand and the electrophysiological studies do not show more distal affectation, a neurogenic TOS is easily recognized. Unfortunately, from a diagnostic perspective, many of the patients do not show these obvious characteristics. The non-specific TOS is the most common type found during clinical practice.[8]

INCIDENCE

The incidence of the TOS diagnosed as such is low.[4,6,10,25,26,31,36–41] The occurrence of the truly neurogenic TOS is estimated to be approximately one in one million cases.[42] By way of example, an electrodiagnosis centre that examines 3500 patients each year will only detect four or five cases.[31] However, there is uncertainty regarding the real incidence of all the types of TOS, especially if the non-specific TOS is included. This is because patients usually suffer the symptoms intermittently; however, they are not acute, and therefore they are not diagnosed.

As far as age is concerned, it is rare to find the condition before puberty and after menopause.[8,43] The most common age period for the onset of symptoms is between 25 and 50 years of age.[10,43] Incidence in children is an exception to the rule, although there have been some cases, and in all of them there was a clear structural anomaly, such as a cervical rib.[44,45]

The TOS can occur in elderly patients; yet, when there are nerve compression symptoms in patients that are older than 60, a radiculopathy caused by a canal stenosis should be suspected and, clearly, if the patients are smokers, a pulmonary tumoural pathology is likely.[41]

The TOS is two to four times more common in women than in men.[6,8,10,27,43,46–49] This difference has been explained by the fact that, during growth, the scapula gradually descends through the posterior part of the thorax, and this descent is greater in women.

ANATOMY OF THE THORACIC OUTLET

The possible places where a compression of the neurovascular structures can occur are the interscalene triangle, the costoclavicular space and the retropectoral space.

Interscalene triangle

The interscalene triangle is limited in its anterior part by the scalenus anterior, in its posterior part by the scalenus medius, and in its base by the first rib (Fig. 3-2).

In the interscalene triangle, the subclavian artery is located above the first rib, describing a curve, passing between the scalenus anterior and the scalenus medius, and it immediately faces downward and outward. The

brachial plexus is found in this space and is behind and above the subclavian artery, and the roots of C8 and T1 are very close to the artery. However, the subclavian vein is located in front of the scalenus anterior and, consequently, it is not usual to suffer compression at this level (Fig. 3-3). This anatomically narrow space can suffer from a greater amount of narrowing due to different anomalies, such as a cervical rib, morphological changes in the first rib and the scalene muscles or the presence of abnormal fibrous bands.[6,10,50–54]

Costoclavicular space

This space is made up, in its upper part, of the costoclavicular ligament, the subclavian muscle and the

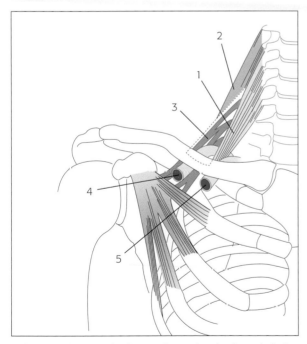

FIGURE 3-2 ■ In the interscalene triangle the subclavian artery is located above the first rib, between the anterior scalenus (1) and the middle scalenus (2). The brachial plexus (3) is behind and above the subclavian artery (4). The subclavian vein (5) is in front of the anterior scalenus, and this level does not usually suffer compression.

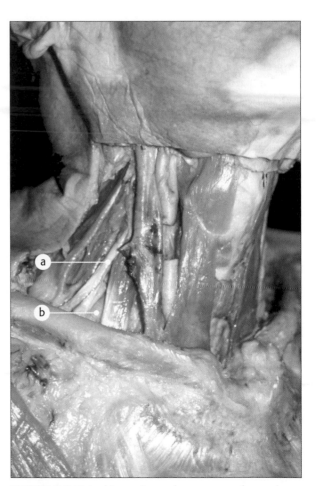

FIGURE 3-3 ■ In this specimen, the structures that make up the interscalene triangle and run through it are shown: brachial plexus (a) and the subclavian artery (b).

medial portion of the clavicle, and in its lower part, of the first rib (Fig. 3-4). It is divided in an anterior and posterior part. The subclavian vein runs through the anterior part of the costoclavicular space, and the brachial plexus and the subclavian artery go through the posterior part (Fig. 3-5).

All of the neurovascular structures that cross the costoclavicular space can suffer compression. This clinical situation is linked to congenital or acquired changes in the subclavian muscles, in the scalenus anterior or the costoclavicular ligament.[2,43,49,55-60] It can also be the consequence of a clavicle or first rib fracture, as well as of postural alterations that modify the relationship between these two bones and the adjacent soft tissues.

Retropectoral space

The retropectoral space or subcoracoid tunnel is limited in its upper part by the coracoid process, in its anterior part by the tendon of the pectoralis minor, and in its posterior part by the first ribs. The space undergoes narrowing during the abduction process, since the neurovascular bundle is propped up against the coracoid process, while compressed by the tendon of the pectoralis minor (Fig. 3-6). The hyperabduction syndrome was described by Wright[61] in 1945. Its name highlights the fact that the compression is produced during this movement.

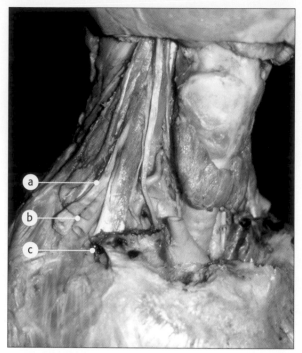

FIGURE 3-5 ■ In this specimen, the first rib has been dissected and the structures that run through the costoclavicular space are shown: brachial plexus (a), subclavian artery (b) and subclavian vein (c).

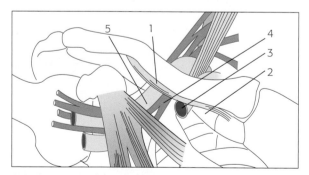

FIGURE 3-4 ■ The costoclavicular space is composed, in its upper portion, of the costoclavicular ligament and the subclavian muscle (1), and the medial portion of the clavicle, and in its lower portion, of the first rib (2). It is divided into two areas, an anterior and a posterior area. The subclavian vein (3) runs through the anterior area, and the brachial plexus (4) and the subclavian artery (5) run through the posterior part.

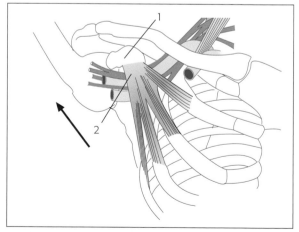

FIGURE 3-6 ■ The retropectoral space is composed of the coracoid process (1) in its upper portion, the tendon of the pectoralis minor (2) in its anterior part and the first ribs in its posterior part.

The compression in this space can be the result of changes in the pectoralis minor muscle, such as hypertrophy or fibrosis, and the existence of fibrous or fibromuscular bands, such as the muscular arch of the armpit, also known as the pectorodorsal muscle or Langer's muscle.[23,62–67] This musculotendinous structure is the most common anatomical variant in the axillary region, present in 2–3% of the population. It is located transversally in the armpit. It usually begins in the wide dorsal muscles, and it is directed towards the pectoralis major in order to be inserted in the bicipital groove or the coracoid process.[62,65,66,68–75]

AETIOLOGY

The aetiology of the TOS can be divided into congenital and acquired. The latter can also be classified as traumatic, due to overload or as a consequence of postural alterations. The most common anatomical causes that lead to the TOS are congenital or acquired anomalies, to which some types of trauma or mechanical overload can be added.[76] Neurovascular compression can occur in any of the three spaces of the thoracic outlet, and they are more frequent in the interscalene triangle.[10]

Alterations in the interscalene triangle

The most common alterations that occur in the interscalene triangle are determined by anatomical, congenital or acquired changes in the scalene muscles. This group of alterations can be responsible for the scalenus anterior or anticus syndrome, also known as the Naffziger syndrome.[77–79] Although this name refers to the anterior component of the group of scalene muscles, these anomalies can be related to the scalenus minimus or the scalenus medius.[2] These anomalies include the complete joining point of the scalenus anterior and medius,[2,80] the joint insertion of both, which causes the narrowing of the base of the interscalene triangle,[37,80] a more anterior insertion of the scalenus medius in the first rib[80] or the *presence* of the supernumerary scalene muscles[43] (Fig. 3-7).

Acquired changes in the scalene muscles can be the consequence of an overload or a trauma. With regards to the latter case, different studies have shown that the scalene muscles develop a hypertrophy or spasm.[43,46,81–83] This explains why the presence of a TOS is not

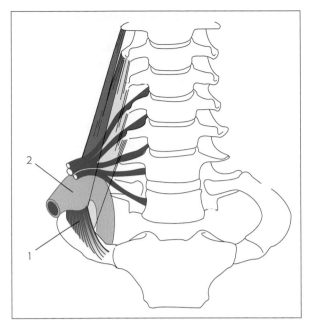

FIGURE 3-7 ▪ The interscalene triangle with an abnormally anterior insertion of the middle scalenus (1), which, together with the anterior scalenus, determines a narrowing of this space, as well as the poststenotic dilatation of the subclavian artery (2).

uncommon following cervical whiplash.[32,81] Machleder et al.[83] studied the histochemical changes that occur in the muscular fibres of the scalene muscles before and after a trauma. They found that the slow-contraction type I fibres were replaced by rapid-contraction type II fibres that can generate tetanic contractions. Sanders et al.[81] observed the same changes, and also noted an increase in the connective tissue in the scalene muscles following a trauma. These changes in composition lead to an increase in the tension and rigidity of the scalene muscles.

Fibrous bands

Another anomaly that occurs in the soft tissues and that can cause compression in the interscalene space is the existence of fibrous bands: numerous types have been described.[50,84,85] These fibrous structures can accompany the scalenus anterior, medius or minimus, or can be free, and are found to originate in the cervical rib or in an abnormal first rib, in the transverse process of C7 or Sibson's fascia.[54] These fibrous bands are, more often than costal anomalies, responsible for a TOS.[6,10,50,53,54,86] In a study conducted with 200 patients that had surgery for a TOS, Makhoul and Machleder[43] found that 66% of them had obvious anomalies in the soft tissues and only 8.5% had a cervical rib or an abnormal first rib.

Cervical rib

The first mention of a cervical rib found in medical literature is attributed to Galeno in the 2nd century BC[15] (Fig. 3-8). The cervical rib is present in approximately 0.2% and 1–5% of the population. It is bilateral in 50–80% of cases[6,46,54,87–90] and is more commonly found in women.[6,46] The symptomatic side corresponds to the dominant arm in more than 72% of patients.[46] The existence of a cervical rib does not necessarily mean that a subject will suffer a TOS. Sanders and Hammond[88] have shown that only 10% of subjects with a cervical rib develop symptoms.

Classification of the cervical rib

Gruber,[91] in 1869, classified the different types of cervical ribs and divided them into four groups (Fig. 3-9):

- Type I corresponds to a hypertrophic transverse process of C7 (Fig. 3-10).

- Type II is a rudimentary rib with a free end and with no connection to the first rib.
- Type III is an incomplete cervical rib that connects to the first rib with fibrous bands.
- Type IV is a complete cervical rib that is connected to the first rib with a cartilaginous pseudo-joint (Fig. 3-11).

Except for situations in which the cervical rib articulates with the sternal manubrium through a costal cartilage, the cervical rib always tends to be linked to the first thoracic rib. In many cases, the first rib does not necessarily cause the compression: rather, it is caused by the fibrous bands that link it to the first rib.

Other classification systems have been developed, such as the one devised by Sargent.[92] This classification divides the cervical rib into five different categories: I, hypertrophy of the transverse process of C7; II, a small rib related to the first rib through a fibrous prolongation; III, a rib that is long enough to accompany the eighth cervical nerve; IV, a rib joined to the first thoracic rib or that articulates with it; and V, a complete cervical rib with a cartilaginous junction with the first costal cartilage or with the sternal manubrium.

The most common type of cervical rib is the type III rib, followed by the type I, according to Gruber's classification.[46]

It is interesting to point out that there is a relationship between the presence of a cervical rib and transitional anomalies in the lumbosacral spine (Fig. 3-12). In a study conducted with 471 subjects that had a cervical rib, more than 73% showed a sacralization of L5.[93] The link between the cervical rib and sacralization can be explained by the embryological development of the vertebral spine.

As previously discussed, the TOS can occur without any type of structural anomalies, as a consequence of postural alterations, such as the descent of the shoulder girdle, which leads to the compression of the neurovascular bundle against the first rib.

Alterations in the costoclavicular space

The compression in the costoclavicular space seems to have been described by Falconer and Weddell[94] in 1943 for the first time. This clinical situation can be due to an enlargement or fibrosis of the subclavian muscle, as well as the costoclavicular ligament[2,43,49,55–59] (Figs 3-13

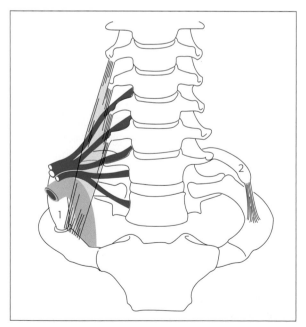

FIGURE 3-8 ■ Cervical rib that is joined to the first rib (1), and cervical rib associated with a fibrous band (2).

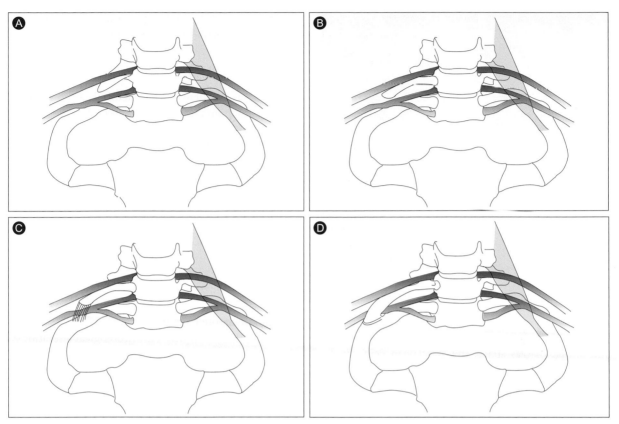

FIGURE 3-9 ■ Gruber's classification. Type I (A) corresponds to a hypertrophic transverse process of C7. Type II (B) is a rudimentary rib with a free end and with no connection to the first rib. Type III (C) is an incomplete cervical rib connected to the first rib by fibrous bands. Type IV (D) is a complete cervical rib joined to the first rib with a cartilaginous pseudo-joint.

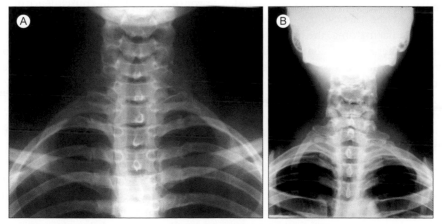

FIGURE 3-10 ■ In the radiographs a transverse megaprocess of C7 is seen on the left side (A) and in the complete cervical rib (B) bilaterally.

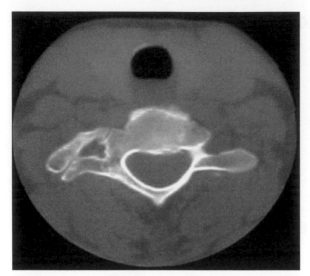

FIGURE 3-11 ■ CT scan in which a cervical rib is seen with its costovertebral and costotransverse joint.

and 3-14). In this space, the subclavian vein can be compressed by the anterior insertion of the scalenus anterior,[60] or the presence of the described supernumerary muscles, such as the subclavius posticus.[95,96] The stenosis in the costoclavicular space can be caused by a hypertrophic transverse process of C7.[97]

The costoclavicular space can be reduced by a clavicle or first rib fracture.[98] In these cases, the situations that are most commonly associated with the development of the TOS are the fractures of the middle third of the clavicle with a significant displacement[98-100] and the pseudo-arthrosis of the clavicle[101,102] or the first rib.[103] The body of the haematoma, the hypertrophic consolidation or the alteration of the surrounding tissues are responsible for the TOS to a greater extent than the fracture.

The compression in this space can be due to postural changes that lead to a horizontalization and descent of the clavicle or to an elevation of the first rib caused by a spasm or a retraction of the scalene muscles.

Alterations in the retropectoral space

As previously described, the compression in this space can be due to hypertrophy of the pectoralis minor muscle and the presence of fibrous or fibromuscular muscles, such as the muscular arch of the armpit.[23,24,62-69,104,105] Also, postural alterations can foster neurovascular compression within this space.

PHYSIOPATHOLOGY

The TOS is frequently multifactorial, although it is evident that anatomical anomalies of bone or soft tissues may also be involved in the compression. Many patients that suffer from TOS do not show any signs of these alterations, in the same way that many individuals that show these anatomical anomalies do not present any type of symptoms. All of this seems to indicate that neurovascular compression in the thoracic outlet is derived from a combination of factors, underlying morphological variations, structural modifications and histological changes in the muscles and the soft tissues, induced by excessive functional requirements or traumas.[43]

The thoracic outlet syndromes derive from constitutional or acquired morphological alterations; there is also a factor involving traumas or overloads that may trigger the symptoms.

The trigger factors of a TOS are traumas, overload and postural alterations.

There is a constantly increasing amount of evidence showing that traumatic injuries, such as a cervical whiplash, can trigger pathological changes in the muscles of the shoulder girdle that favour the development of a TOS.[8,19,32,88,106-115] The narrowing of the thoracic outlet can be the consequence of the development of muscle changes, such as the scalene, the subclavian and pectoralis minor muscles, as well as the enlargement and fibrosis of the ligamentous and fascial tissues. These changes in the soft tissues, secondary to a trauma, associated with previously asymptomatic anatomical alterations, can trigger a TOS.[6,43,88,116,117] In a review of patients treated with a neurogenic TOS who had a cervical rib or an abnormal first rib, Sanders and Hammond[88] observed that in 80% of the patients, the trigger factor was a trauma.

Work-related activities that involve an overload can trigger the appearance of a TOS, especially in subjects that have structural anomalie.[88,118-123] Sällström and Schmidt[118] observed that the occurrence of the TOS in different work activities that require repeated tasks

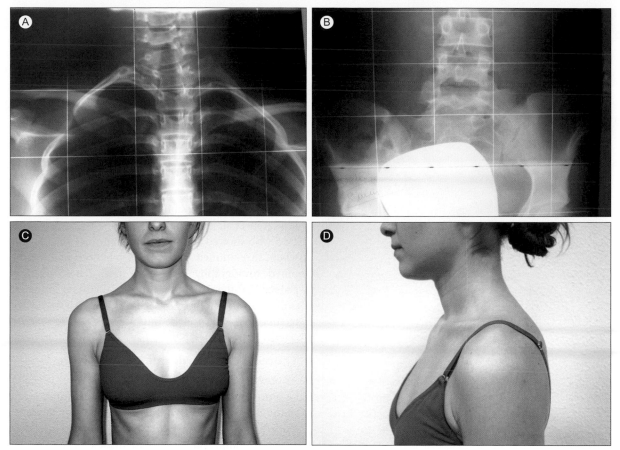

FIGURE 3-12 ■ The association between a cervical rib and lumbosacral transitional anomalies is frequent. In the radiographs an assimilation is seen on the right side between the first and seconds ribs, which articulates with C7 (A). The same subject presents a hemisacralization of L5 (B). In the frontal and profile picture (C) the prominence of the first right rib can be appreciated (D).

involving arm use is very high, amounting to 18% of all injuries. The majority of patients were women who performed repetitive tasks and whose symptoms became evident after a few years. It is therefore recommended to suspect a TOS in young women who have jobs that require continuous upper limb movement and who report a progressive weakening of the hands.[121]

The TOS can also be seen in athletes, especially in sports that require repetitive movements of arm abduction, such as swimming.[1,27,124–130] Furthermore, it has also been found in musicians, presumably due to the positions they adopt.[131]

The development of a TOS is linked to postural aspects that involve a modification of the alignment of the shoulder girdle and the cervical spine, especially with positions that allow for the shortening and loss of the extensibility in the cervicoscapular muscles. These shortened muscles tend to compress the neurovascular structures in the thoracic outlet with minimal stretching. An example of this are subjects with a head in a forward position and shoulders in protraction. These subjects tend to shorten the scalene muscles and the pectoralis minor. Women with TOS seem to have a characteristic typology with a long neck and sloping shoulders.[8,23,25,29,54,132,133] Demondion et al.[49] have also

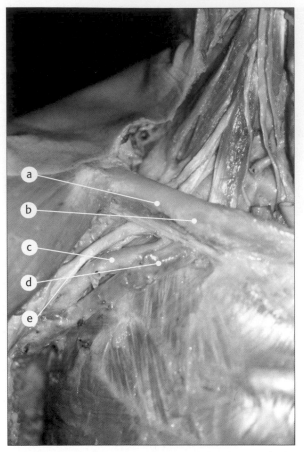

FIGURE 3-13 ■ Costoclavicular space. Clavicle (a) and subclavian muscle (b) and their close relationships with the subclavian artery (c), the subclavian vein (d) and the brachial plexus (e).

observed a higher degree of obliquity of the first rib in women compared to men. This could explain the higher occurrence in women. The rate of occurrence is also higher in overweight females,[23] as well as in those with excessively large breasts.[25,31,39,134] In males, the TOS is usually seen in muscular subjects, whose cervicothoracic muscles, mainly the scalene muscles, are hypertrophic.[29,54,132]

A possible cause of TOS is an alteration in the way the shoulder girdle hangs or how stable it is as a result of an injury of the accessory spinal nerve or the long thoracic nerve. The paresis or paralysis of the serratus anterior or the trapezius and the sternocleidomastoid can trigger neurovascular compression in the thoracic outlet[135] (Fig. 3-15).

Thoracic outlet syndrome and articular dysfunction

In the physiopathology of a TOS, the cervical spine and the shoulder girdle are involved as a functional unit. The TOS not only occurs as a consequence of an anatomical anomaly but also, in most cases, results from an alteration of the function of the articular and muscular structures related to the neurovascular structures.[136,137] Joint dysfunctions can contribute to the appearance of a TOS. The reduction of the normal mobility of the joints of the shoulder girdle or the cervical spine can reduce the space of the thoracic outlet, or limit the possibility of its decompression.[138–140] Lindgren et al.[137] presented the case of a female with TOS who showed an upper subluxation of the first rib when three-dimensional reconstruction with computed tomography (CT) was used. These authors proved that the patient's symptoms could be solved by improving the mobility of the first rib with a stretching technique for the scalene muscles.

Thoracic outlet syndrome and posture

As previously described, a trigger factor for a TOS can be a postural imbalance. The postural attitudes, such as the upper crossed syndrome described by Janda,[141] help the muscles adapt to a rest position while they are shortening. The shortened muscles decrease the length of the sarcomeres and increase the number of the parallel sarcomeres. This morphological change in the muscles increases the stress over the neurovascular structures that are linked to them. In 1994, Mackinnon and Novak[142] developed an integrated hypothesis of the physiopathology of the multiple diffuse disorders of the upper limb, including the TOS. This hypothesis suggests that repetitive movements and alterations in the statics of the head, cervical spine and the upper limb determine two main consequences: nerve compression and muscular imbalance. The deficient statics and the repetitive muscles lead to three effects: (1) they directly increase in the pressure over the nerve where they are more prone to entrapment, and increase the tension they support by creating a chronic compression situation; (2) certain postures keep the muscles in an abnormal shortened position that modifies their length so that when they cross the neurovascular structure, they compress it as they are

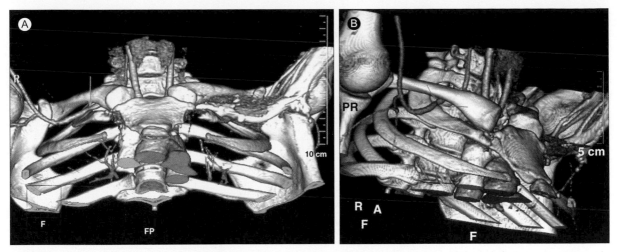

FIGURE 3-14 ■ (A, B) In these three-dimensional reproductions of CTs, the compression of the subclavian artery is seen in the costoclavicular space. *(Courtesy of Mayoral.)*

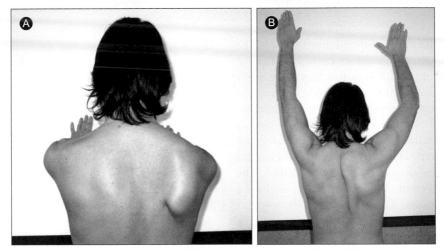

FIGURE 3-15 ■ The injury of the long thoracic nerve and the resulting paresis of the serratus anterior muscle can trigger a neurovascular compression in the thoracic outlet. (A) The descent and flapping of the scapula is seen. (B) The limitation of the active abduction of the upper limb is shown.

stretched; and (3) the situation of shortening of these muscles induces the lengthening of other muscles, thus causing muscular imbalance. The muscular imbalance favours the forward position of the head and the thoracic kyphosis. This leads to an abnormal pattern of scapular movement with weakness of the middle and lower trapezius and the serratus anterior. The weakness of these muscles leads to the excessive demand of others, such as the upper trapezius and the levator scapulae. A repetitive activity in subjects with

an abnormal postural pattern leads to a progression of the nerve compression and the cycle of muscular imbalance–neural compression becomes chronic (Fig. 3-16).

Thoracic outlet syndrome and alteration of the motor control of the shoulder girdle

One of the paradigms that can help to explain the development of a TOS, and that constitutes a development of the previously explained postural imbalance

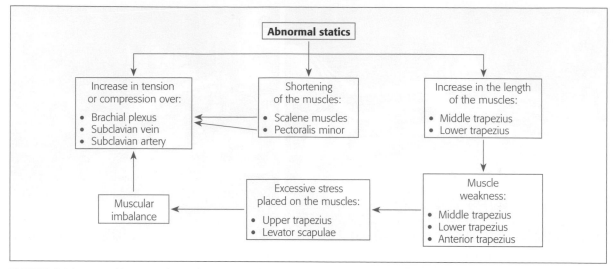

FIGURE 3-16 ■ Mackinnon and Novak's integrated hypothesis suggest that the alterations in the statics of the cervical spine and the upper limb can favour a thoracic outlet syndrome. *(Adapted from Mackinnon and Novak.[142])*

concepts, is the alteration of the motor control of the shoulder girdle. Dynamic stability control is essential in order for the upper limbs to function correctly.[143] The scapula should be directed properly, placing the glenoid in the adequate position for each shoulder movement, and it should simultaneously become a stable base that enables the movements of the upper limb. An insufficient scapular stability alters the correct functioning of the shoulder girdle and leads to the appearance of different clinical symptoms, such as a subacromial syndrome. This alteration of the scapular control can be the most important trigger factor in the development of a TOS.

The main important scapular muscles used for stabilization are the trapezius and the serratus anterior. The upper and lower trapezius and the serratus anterior work together, creating a superior rotation of the scapula associated with the elevation of the distal end of the clavicle.

The muscles primarily involved in the movement of the scapula are the levator scapulae, the major and minor rhomboid muscles, the pectoralis minor and the latissimus dorsi.

The levator scapulae lifts the scapula, brings it closer and rotates it in the inferior direction. The pectoralis minor pulls the coracoid process in an anterior direction, causing a protraction and lower rotation of

the scapula. The latissimus dorsi, especially if it is hyperactive, can excessively abduct the scapula during the elevation of the upper limb.

There are suspicions of changes to neuromuscular control when an abnormal rest position of the scapula is observed and is shown by rising and lowering movements from the upper limb.

Thoracic outlet syndrome and double entrapment

One of the hypotheses that best explains the physiopathology of the TOS, as well as its confusing clinical manifestations, is the *double crush syndrome* or the *two-level compression hypothesis* devised by Upton and McComas[144] in 1973. This hypothesis argues that the existence of a neural compression situation at the proximal level, as it occurs with the TOS, increases the vulnerability of the distal portions of the nerve, making it more susceptible to compression. Although the magnitude of the compression is not significant, the accumulative effect of minor compressions, at different levels, along the same nerve, leads to pathological changes in neural tissue and the subsequent appearance of symptoms (Fig. 3-17). In their review, the authors observed the high occurrence of carpal and ulnar tunnel syndromes in subjects with radicular compression. They suggested that

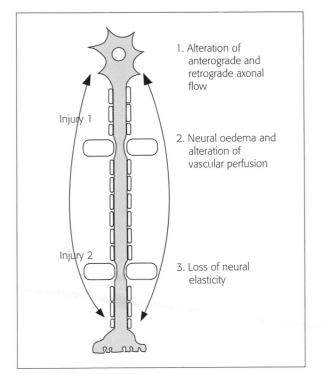

1. Alteration of anterograde and retrograde axonal flow

Injury 1

2. Neural oedema and alteration of vascular perfusion

Injury 2

3. Loss of neural elasticity

FIGURE 3-17 ■ The hypothesis of the double entrapment or two-level compression affirms that the existence of a neural compression situation at the proximal level (Injury 1) and increases the vulnerability of the distal portions of the nerve (Injury 2) by different mechanisms: alteration of the anterograde and retrograde axonal flow (1), oedema and alteration of neural blood perfusion (2), loss of nerve elasticity (fibrosis and adherence in Injury 1 increase the stretching of the injury 2) (3).

the alteration of the axoplasmic flow, responsible for maintaining the nutrition and functionality of the nerve cells, was a mechanism involved in this susceptibility of the neural tissue. Lundborg[145] described the double inverse crushing, in which a compression in a distal point can alter the retrograde axoplasmic transport, favouring the neural compression in the more proximal areas. Subsequently, the possibility of a multiple crush was described by Mackinnon and Dellon.[146] As indicated by Sunderland,[147] Mackinnon,[148,149] Dellon and Mackinnon[150] and Butler,[151] once an injury or irritation occurs in a point of the neural tissue in the upper limb, there is a very high probability that neuropathies will develop in other multiple locations.[152]

■ One of the phenomena that can explain the physiopathology of the TOS is the double crush syndrome or two-level compression.

■ Neural compression that occurs at the proximal level, as in the TOS, increases the vulnerability of the distal portions of the nerve, making it more susceptible to compression.

This relationship between the TOS and the double crushing is supported by several studies in which a compression of the carpal tunnel or ulnar neuropathy is observed simultaneously with TOS.[13,46,87,146,153–158] The overlapping of the symptoms deriving from different entities, such as the TOS, cervical radiculopathy or neuropathies due to distal compression, is one of the common causes of diagnostic errors.[156] In these cases of double or multiple crush, it is crucial to identify and treat the structure responsible for the higher degree of compression, considering also that a treatment of the other areas involved in the double crush can contribute to the improvement of the patient.

However, the development of the double crush hypothesis was undoubtedly linked to an insufficient interpretation of referred and neuropathic pain. Surely, for many patients diagnosed with double crush syndrome, the symptoms away from the source were not linked with a second area of compression, but with the referred pain itself.

SYMPTOMS OF THE THORACIC OUTLET SYNDROME

The clinical manifestations of the TOS depend on the affected neurovascular structures.[39,41,159] The TOS is usually divided into two clinical patterns: neurogenic and vascular. This division is useful when deciding upon a treatment method; however, the close proximity between these different structures often leads to a link being made between nerve compression and vascular compression symptoms, although to a different degree of extension and severity (59).

The clinical spectrum is extremely wide and can go from a serious compression, with vascular and/or nerve permanent injury, to intermittent symptoms related to certain postures or activities without any organ damage.[160]

Most TOS cases are neurogenic: this category amounts to between 70% and 95% of all cases.[2,24,49,100,161–163] The vascular TOS, with objective findings of subclavian artery or vein compression, makes up between 5% and 30% of all patients.[41,164]

In the vascular TOS, an affected vein is more common than the artery.[24,27,161,163–165] The vascular TOS can occur more frequently in its bilateral form than the truly neurogenic TOS.[101,154,166,167]

Neurogenic syndrome

The neurogenic syndrome is divided into two categories: the truly neurogenic TOS and the presumably neurogenic or non-specific TOS.

Roos[6] classifies the TOS according to the level of compression of the brachial plexus and makes three categories: superior, if it affects the portion of the plexus that depends on the C5, C6 and C7 roots; inferior, if it affects the roots that depend on C8 and T1; and combined, when it affects all of them.[168]

The classic and most common frequent form of the neurogenic syndrome is the inferior type, and it manifests itself with symptoms of the C8–T1 root. The most common symptoms are paraesthesiae in the upper limb, which are noticed on the ulnar side of the forearm and the two ulnar fingers.[1,8,41] In a superior TOS, the pain and the paraesthesiae are referred to the shoulder, arm and the area metamerically corresponding to the median nerve. The symptoms are also referred to the cervical spine and the head.[1,2,169,170]

Paraesthesiae appear frequently at night in relation to changes in the position of the shoulder girdle, although they can be triggered by daily activities. Pain is usually dull and intermittent, and it is aggravated by certain postures, such as lying down at night, or by activities that increase the compression of the brachial plexus.

The effect on motor ability in the lower TOS is manifested as a progressive weakness and atrophy of the muscles innervated by the lower trunk of the brachial plexus. Atrophy is more serious in the muscles of the thenar eminence that depend on the median nerve than in the intrinsic muscles that depend on the ulnar nerve. This is because the fibres that come from the T1 roots, which contain the motor fibres of the median nerve, usually suffer higher compression than the roots of C8, which contain the fibres of the ulnar nerve.[1,2,10,41,152,171,172] This amyotrophy characteristic of

the thenar, hypothenar and interosseous muscles, associated frequently to a hyperaesthesia in the distribution of the medial cutaneous nerve of the forearm, is also known as *Gilliatt–Sumner hand*.[86,173]

The sensitive deficit is manifested in the ulnar portion of the hand and forearm.[8,10] As a result of the uncommon nature of the truly neurogenic TOS, these symptoms tend to be interpreted as being caused by a cervical radiculopathy or a ulnar neuropathy at the level of the elbow or the wrist.

The presumably neurogenic or non-specific TOS is the most common type.[8–11,30–33,36,42,168,174–176] In these cases, the patient refers the complaints characteristic of the neurogenic TOS, such as pain and paraesthesiae, and it is not possible to confirm that the plexus has been affected[177] with objective tests such as electrophysiological studies. This is the most controversial form of the TOS, and some authors even question its existence.[10] Therefore, the diagnosis of this form of TOS is based exclusively on the patient's subjective symptoms.[11]

The TOS is seen more frequently on the dominant side, and in approximately 70% of cases it coincides with the right arm.[46]

Other common symptoms are the intolerance to cold and thoracic pain. If this thoracic pain appears on the left side it can be interpreted as having cardiac origin, and many of these patients often avail of urgent care facilities.[38,178–180]

The symptoms are usually aggravated during the day with activities that imply an elevation of the limb, when driving a vehicle or carrying heavy objects with the arms.[172]

The compression of the sympathetic fibres of the brachial plexus can lead to vasomotor changes in the upper limb and Raynaud's phenomenon.[4,38] The sympathetic compromise can manifest itself in trophic disorders, such as the thinning of the skin and hand oedema. Furthermore, in some subjects, the cardiac sympathetic nerve can also be affected, and it can be manifested as a tachycardia.[181,182] This phenomenon could be explained by the compression of the stellate ganglion. This structure is located on the lateral edge of the longissimus cervicis, between the base of the transverse process of C7 and the first rib, and in front of this process, the prevertebral fascia is located. The stellate ganglion or its postganglionic fibres can be compressed by a cervical rib, although the most common causes are the fibrous bands that expand from the transverse process of C7 and the first rib.[182] Tachycardia can be triggered with Roos' test.[182]

Venous syndrome

The venous syndrome is much more common than the arterial syndrome, and it is estimated to be present in 1.5–10% of all patients with TOS.[27,183] The causes of venous compression are primarily the subclavian muscle and the costoclavicular ligament. To a lesser extent, the presence of supernumerary muscles, such as the subclavius posticus, are also responsible.[59,183,184] The most typical symptoms are oedema in the upper limb, cyanosis, collateral circulation, superficial venous dilatation and heavy sensation.[35,183,185,186] Among all these symptoms, the earliest and most common is the oedema in the upper limb, which is aggravated by activity.[59,186]

There are two possible ways in which the venous syndrome can manifest itself[187]: acute deep vein thrombosis of the subclavian vein that is linked to mechanical stress and, more often, intermittent chronic venous obstruction.

The acute thrombosis of the subclavian vein may appear after the upper limb is subjected to intense activity. It is known as effort thrombosis or Paget–von Schroetter syndrome.[188,189] It typically affects young males that perform intense activities with the arms.[10,27,35,122,125,127,130,183,190–196]

Arterial syndrome

The arterial syndrome is less frequent than all the other types of TOS, and it does not even amount to 5% of all cases.[165] Arterial complications are usually associated with a cervical rib or a rudimentary first rib. According to Durham et al.,[197] of the patients with arterial symptoms, 56–67% of the cases involve a cervical rib. However, in 12% of cases, it can occur without any type of bone anomaly.[165] Another frequent cause is the compression of the subclavian artery caused by the hypertrophic scalenus anterior or fibrous bands associated with it.[33]

The physiopathological mechanisms begin with the compression of the subclavian artery, which leads to stenosis, poststenotic dilatation, formation of an aneurysm, thrombosis and embolism.[10,129,158,198,199] According to Reid et al.,[44] more than 64% of patients with arterial TOS have an aneurysm or poststenotic

dilatation of the subclavian artery. The ischaemic symptoms of the arteries of the fingers and the palmar arch can go from a Raynaud's phenomenon to an extremely serious ischaemia, which can lead to necrosis of the hand.[8] Depending on the severity of the condition, some authors differentiate between a major and a minor TOS.[171]

The symptoms deriving from an arterial insufficiency are weakness, which can lead to an intermittent claudication of the upper limb, coldness and ischaemic pain.[100] The examination can show differences in the temperature of the limb in relation to the contralateral limb, as well as in the pulse.

The arterial compromise can occur in two different groups of subjects: young adults, who often present anatomical anomalies such as a cervical rib; and patients of over 40 years of age, who suffer from degenerative arterial changes, possibly as a result of the turbulent flow caused by the extrinsic compression.[27]

DIAGNOSIS

The diagnosis of a TOS is complex, and consists primarily of a clinical diagnosis, based on a detailed medical history and a complete physical examination.[5,8,13,25,120,172,200–203]

The diagnosis of a neurogenic TOS is relatively easy when the subject has a predominant sensitive alteration in the ulnar distribution of the hand and forearm, which is aggravated with activity, and linked to the weakness and atrophy of the intrinsic muscles of the hand; a cervical rib can be seen in radiographs and can be confirmed by neurophysiological studies.[204] However, most of the patients with a supposed neurogenic TOS do not show such a clear clinical setting. The presence of an acute amyotrophy of the hand can only be seen in patients with a history of long development, who have an anomaly of the bones or soft parts. Although different complementary tests can, in some cases, be of great help, in most patients these tests usually produce negative or unclear results.

- ▪ The diagnosis of the TOS is primarily clinical, since complementary tests tend to produce negative or unclear results with the majority of patients.
- ▪ The diagnosis requires a detailed history and a complete physical examination.

The first diagnostic problem is the fact that the clinical presentation of the TOS is very similar to other pathologies; for example, cervical radiculopathy; different peripheral nerve entrapment syndromes, such as carpal tunnel and the ulnar neuropathy; the subacromial syndrome; and the pattern of referred pain of certain axial muscles and the upper limb.[7,205] It is therefore important to perform a detailed medical history, which should include history of traumas, the duration and the gravity of the symptoms.[8,98] Because different entities can simulate the clinical presentation of the TOS, the diagnosis is often made by a process of exclusion.[10,160]

Some entities with which it is also necessary to use the differential diagnosis are Raynaud's syndrome, multiple sclerosis,[8,27] and tumours.[206–209] In subjects over the age of 50 years old with a history of smoking, it is imperative to rule out the presence of Pancoast's tumour.[210–213]

Physical examination

The cervical spine and the shoulder girdle should be examined to rule out an articular pathology, together with the muscles that can be related to the TOS. When a neurogenic TOS is suspected, a neurological examination of the upper limb is required to differentiate a TOS from any other peripheral nerve compression. A TOS should be suspected when the most significant aspect of the clinical presentation is pain, the neurological symptoms correspond mainly to the C8–T1 levels and they worsen when the arm is raised.[48] Furthermore, the presence of vascular signs should be observed: changes in the temperature of the upper limb, hand oedema, changes in the pigmentation of the hand, venous dilation, differences in the pulse of the two upper extremities, etc.

A TOS should be suspected when the most significant aspect of the clinical presentation is pain, the neurological symptoms correspond mainly to the C8–T1 levels and they worsen when raising the arm.

Provocation tests

Regarding the provocation manoeuvres, it is important to highlight that none of them provide a diagnosis themselves, as false positives are frequent. In order to

consider that a test is positive, it is not sufficient to detect abolition of the pulse in the wrist during the elevation of the arm or the descent of the shoulder. However, the symptoms of the patient should also be reproduced and the clinical picture should be compatible with a TOS.[8,51,160,214] It has been demonstrated with photoplethysmography that in 60% of normal subjects an arterial occlusion is detected during the provocation manoeuvres, such as Adson's, the costoclavicular or hyperabduction manoeuvres.[215] Therefore, given the frequency of false positives, these tests have a limited diagnostic value.[200]

No provocation test is a diagnosis on itself due to the frequent false negatives.

Adson's manoeuvre. Adson's manoeuvre is used to detect a stenosis in the interscalene space, during the simultaneous contraction and stretching of the scalene muscles. For this purpose, the radial pulse is taken while the patient, keeping the cervical spine in a contralateral side-bending position and ipsilateral rotation, takes a deep breath; the test is positive when there is a clear diminution of the radial pulse and/or it reproduces the patient's symptoms. The ipsilateral rotation displaces the anterior scalene in the posterior direction. This moves the anterior edge of the interscalene space closer to the neurovascular bundle. The interscalene space can also be reduced by taking the scalenus posterior forwards, placing the cervical spine in contralateral rotation (Fig. 3-18). It is very common to have a positive test in subjects with no pathology of the thoracic outlet.[51] This test, as well as Wright's test (hyperabduction manoeuvre), should last between 1 and 2 minutes.

Test for the costoclavicular space. In order to evaluate this outlet, the shoulder girdle is pushed downwards and backwards, which reduces the space between the clavicle and the first rib, while the subclavian artery and vein and the brachial plexus are compressed (Fig. 3-19). The test is considered positive when the radial pulse is obliterated and the symptoms are triggered, during or immediately after the compression.[94] A similar manoeuvre is Halsted's, in which the patient is asked to adopt a similar position, with the arms pushed back and down, while the radial pulse is palpated.

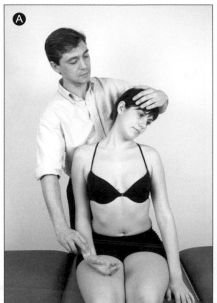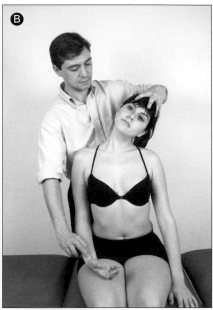

FIGURE 3-18 ■ ■ Adson's manoeuvre with contralateral (A) and ipsilateral (B) rotation.

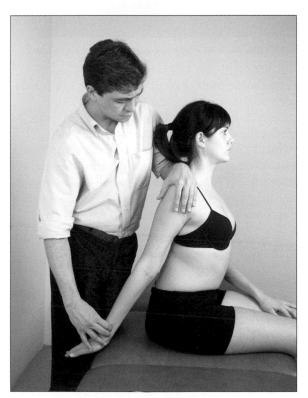

FIGURE 3-19 ■ Costoclavicular space test.

Eden's manoeuvre. Eden's manoeuvre is also similar; it involves palpating the radial pulse during the compression of the clavicle in the inferior and posterior direction (Fig. 3-20).

Wright's hyperabduction manoeuvre. This test involves the passive and progressive elevation of the upper limb in the maximum horizontal abduction. By directing the shoulder girdle in the posterior direction, this causes the pectoralis minor to tense up and induces leaning of the neurovascular structures below the coracoid process.[61] The manoeuvre is positive when an abolition of the radial pulse is detected and the patient's symptoms are provoked (Fig. 3-21).

Pectoralis minor compression test. Another manoeuvre for this space is the direct compression of the pectoralis minor, just below the coracoid, for a few minutes, as well as its rapid release (Fig. 3-22). The test is considered positive when a response in the form of a 'flood of paraesthesiae' appears.

Ross' test. This test is performed by asking the patient to open and close the hand for 3 minutes, keeping the

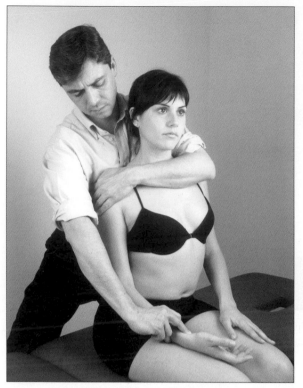

FIGURE 3-20 ■ Eden's manoeuvre.

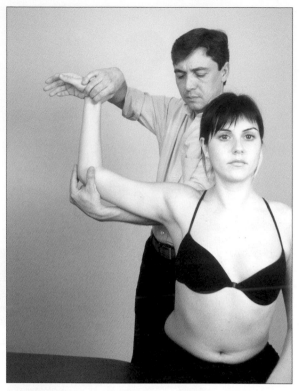

FIGURE 3-21 ■ Wright's hyperabduction manoeuvre.

arms at an angle of 90° of abduction, external rotation and maximum horizontal abduction[6,51] (Fig. 3-23). In order to sensitize the test, the therapist can add caudal and posterior compression to the clavicle (Fig. 3-24). This test affects the interscalene triangle, the costoclavicular and the retropectoral space. The test is positive when the patient is unable to perform the test for that time and the symptoms get aggravated. Although, according to Roos,[6,50,51] this test is highly reliable, since it is never positive in entities with a similar presentation, such as a discogenic or spondylotic cervical radiculopathy, different authors question its sensitivity and specificity.[216] According to Leffert,[8] Roos' test should be considered positive when the limping and cramping symptoms of the forearm muscles appear within 30 seconds.

Palpation of the supraclavicular fossa and Tinel's sign. The sensitivity of the supraclavicular fossa to palpation should be explored, as well as Tinel's sign.[50,157,163] Often it is possible to reproduce the

paraesthesiae of the patient with four or five percussions on the supraclavicular fossa (Fig. 3-25).

Several studies have been performed in order to analyse the clinical value of the provocation tests.[215–220] Whereas some authors value greatly Roos' and Tinel's tests,[15,50] others consider them to have little use in clinical practice.[200] Although, as we have discussed, specificity of provocation tests is low, it increases when associated with several provocation tests.[215,217]

> In general, provocation tests for TOS have an acceptable sensitivity level, but a low specificity.
>
> The specificity improves when several provocation tests are linked.

Gillard et al.[160] have conducted a specific study in order to understand the sensitivity and specificity of these provocation tests. They analysed five manoeuvres: Adson's, hyperabduction with abolition of the pulse, hyperabduction with reproduction of the symptoms, Wright's test with reproduction of the symptoms, and Roos' and Tinel's tests. In general, all these

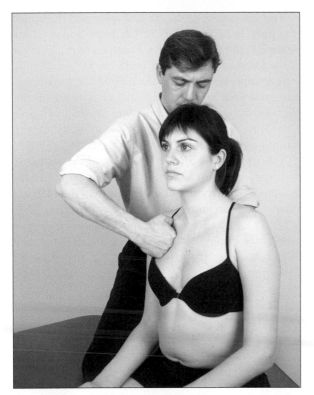

FIGURE 3-22 ■ Compression test of the pectoralis minor.

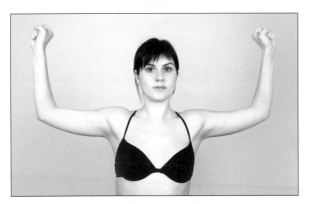

FIGURE 3-23 ■ Roos' test.

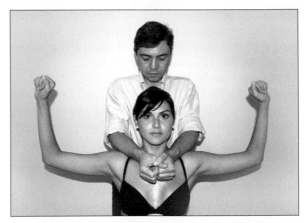

FIGURE 3-24 ■ Roos' test plus clavicular compression.

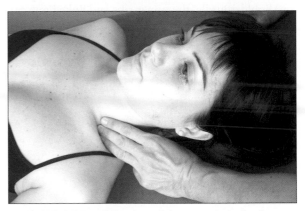

FIGURE 3-25 ■ Palpation of the supraclavicular fossa.

70%; Roos' test, 84%), but a very low specificity. The manoeuvres that have a higher positive predictive value are Adson's test (85%) and hyperabduction with abolition of the pulse (92%). When these five tests are positive, the sensitivity and specificity is 84%.

Neurodynamic tests

Neurodynamic tests evaluate the mechanosensitivity of the neural tissues, making it easy to identify when a response is abnormal. These tests have clinically demonstrated their reliability.[221–228] Recently, Shack-lock[229] has demonstrated with ecographic studies the significant movement of the brachial plexus in the thoracic outlet, chiefly with cervical side-bending and the upper limb neurodynamic test 1 (ULNT1), and how this mobility can be limited by a depression of the scapula or an elevation of the first rib. The

manoeuvres have an acceptable sensitivity (72%), but their specificity is low (53%). Tinel's test has a low sensitivity (46%) and an equally low specificity (56%). Adson's test has a better sensitivity (79%) and specificity (76%). Roos' and Wright's tests have a very high sensitivity (Wright's test with reproduction of symptoms, 90%; Wright's test with abolition of the pulse,

cranial-caudal displacement of the plexus during breathing movements has also been shown, as well as how a pronounced propping of the plexus occurs against the first rib when breathing in.

The most useful tests in the diagnosis of the TOS are the ULNT1 (Fig. 3-26), the ULNT1a and the ULNT3 (Fig. 3-27), because the lower portion of the plexus is affected more frequently. During the neurodynamic test, the radial pulse can be palpated to see if it is cancelled out.

Assessment of the mechanical interphase

The assessment of the mechanical interphase in the TOS involves the examination of the mobility and the posture of the cervical and cervicothoracic spine, the shoulder girdle, the upper ribs and linked muscular structures.

The assessment of the cervical spine and the upper ribs have been explained in Chapters 8 and 12 of Volume 1, and therefore a few examples of exploration of the joints of the shoulder girdle are shown.

It is important to assess the mobility of the sternoclavicular joint and the possibility of opening up the costoclavicular space: examples are shown in Figures 3-28–3-30. Some examples of the mobility of the acromioclavicular joint are shown in the Figure 3-31.

The mobility of the first rib should be evaluated with the respiratory mobility test and with passive manoeuvres, analysing the movement in the inferior, anteroposterior and posteroanterior direction (Fig. 3-32). These manoeuvres are aimed at detecting hypomobility or hypermobility in the costal joints that may be involved in the development of the patient's symptoms.

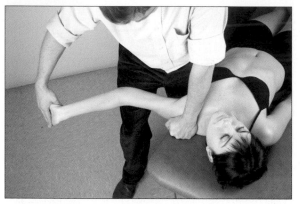

FIGURE 3-26 ■ Upper limb neurodynamic test 1 (ULNT1).

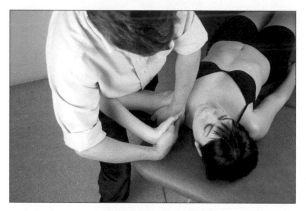

FIGURE 3-27 ■ ULNT3.

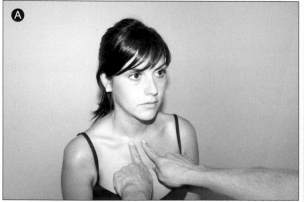

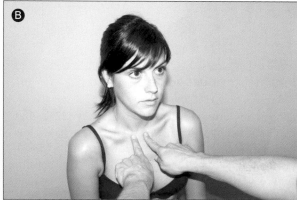

FIGURE 3-28 ■ Assessment of the active mobility of the sternoclavicular joint in horizontal abduction (A) and adduction (B).

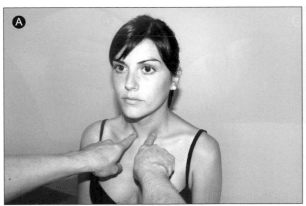
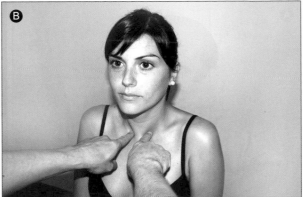

FIGURE 3-29 ■ Assessment of the active mobility in elevation (A) and descent (B) of the sternoclavicular joint.

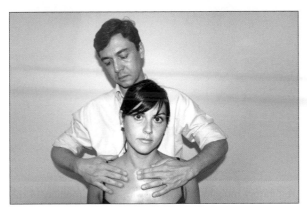

FIGURE 3-30 ■ Assessment of the ability of distraction of the sternoclavicular joint.

Assessment of the motor control of the shoulder girdle. In addition to performing a complete postural assessment,[230] it is crucial to evaluate the motor control of the cervical spine and the shoulder girdle. The evaluation tests of the motor control of the cervical spine are explained in Chapters 5 and 6 of volume 1.

The evaluation of an alteration of the motor control is performed starting with the scapular resting position, and with the movements of elevation and lowering of the upper limb.

Although there is a wide individual variability, the ideal resting position of the scapula is the following. It should be attached to the thorax, 7.6 cm from the middle line and with an anterior rotation of approximately 30° in relation to the coronal plane. The upper

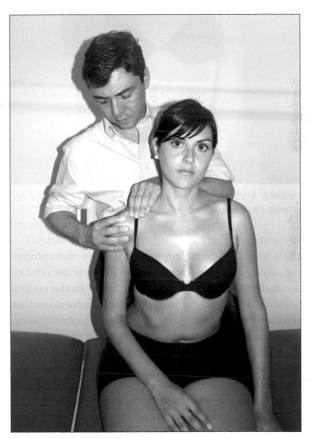

FIGURE 3-31 ■ Assessment of the anteroposterior mobility of the acromioclavicular joint.

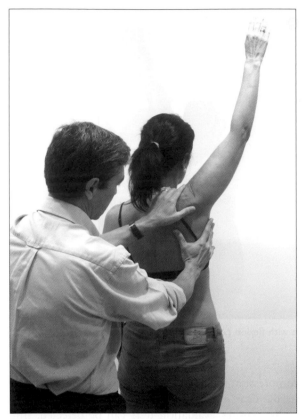

FIGURE 3-34 ■ The patient is asked to perform an arm abduction and a record is made of the moment when the symptoms begin to appear or the abduction level at which the Wright test is positive. The therapist places his left hand along the superior border of the scapula, while placing the thumb of his right hand along the medial border of the scapula near its inferior third. The patient is again asked to elevate the arm, adding a small component of scapular upward rotation. This correction is maintained for 60 seconds. A positive response is a significant improvement in symptoms.

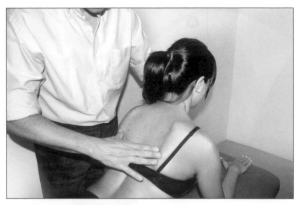

FIGURE 3-35 ■ Assessment of the serratus anterior in the sphinx position.

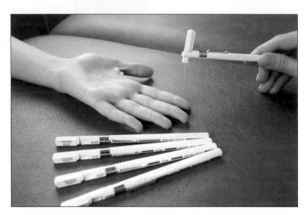

FIGURE 3-36 ■ Semmes–Weinstein monofilaments.

Complementary tests

Imaging tests

Conventional radiographs of the cervical spine are more interesting in the diagnosis of the TOS, providing that the first rib and the clavicle can be seen properly. In order to rule out a Pancoast tumour, it is sometimes advisably recommended to have a screening of the thorax that clearly displays the apex of the lungs. To obtain precise images of the anatomy of the bones, the preferred technique is a CT.[236,237]

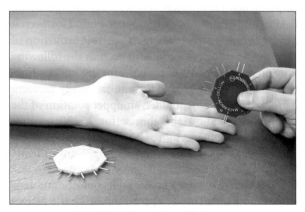

FIGURE 3-37 ■ Disk-Criminator.

Different complementary tests can be used to diagnose the vascular TOS. Doppler ultrasound allows for the detection of haemodynamic alterations in the subclavian artery and vein.[48,160,238] Plethysmography can be used to evaluate venous TOS, as it offers high sensitivity and specificity[239] and has the advantages of being non-invasive, inexpensive and allowing obstruction to be quantified.[164]

Magnetic resonance imaging (MRI) can be used to evaluate the anatomy and pathology of the brachial plexus, and the presence of tumours or other expansive injuries can be ruled out, as well as to detect a neurovascular compression.[49,240–242] During the exploration with MRI, provocation manoeuvres can be performed in order to observe changes and modifications in the vascular circulation.

Using MRI, angiography and venography enable us to carry out a relatively quick evaluation of the vascular structures, both in the neutral position and in abduction, within a single examination.[199,243,244]

Electrophysiological studies

The use of electrophysiological studies for diagnosis varies, depending on the type of TOS and the duration and severity of the symptoms.[5,13,36,38,97,174,175,245–255] Since the entrapment is intermittent and it affects a segment of the neural tissue that is extremely short, the electrophysiological studies are frequently normal. Another factor that contributes to the high proportion of normal findings is the fact that the access to the area of the thoracic outlet is complex. Therefore, the sensitivity of these tests in the diagnosis of the TOS is low and they only serve to confirm the clinical diagnosis.[6,11,48,97,175,177,252,256]

CONSERVATIVE TREATMENT

Conservative treatment is the preferred treatment method for most patients for whom physiotherapy plays an essential role.[2,8,26,38,131,137,163,205,257–275] A conservative treatment performed early can prevent the need of surgery.[265,276,277] According to Roos,[6] only 10% of patients with acute symptoms require surgical decompression. Although in some cases conservative treatment may not lead to a complete cure, it can significantly improve the symptoms and has far less risks than surgical treatment.[30,262,276,278,279]

The surgical treatment is recommended in cases of significant vascular compromise that have oedema or signs of ischaemia, progressive neurological deterioration and refractory pain as a result of the conservative treatment.[1,27,257,280]

Indications that surgical treatment is the preferred treatment:

- Important vascular compromise, with oedema or signs of ischaemia.
- Progressive neurological deterioration.
- Pain resistant to the conservative treatment.

The conservative treatment is intended to increase the functional space of the thoracic outlet and to decrease the compression of the neurovascular structures and its possible adherence to the surrounding tissues. To enlarge the spaces that are crossed by the neurovascular structures, it is imperative to normalize the articular relationships between the neck and the upper limb, as well as to increase the extensibility of the muscles related to the TOS.[131] This treatment of the mechanical interphase should be accompanied by the mobilization of the neurovascular tissues and, in this regard, neural gliding techniques are crucial.[149,152,281–284]

The treatment should be specifically targeted at the anatomical or functional defect responsible for this compromise situation: therefore, there is no single protocol to handle these patients on its own, trusting that the problem will solve itself.[8]

The treatment can be outlined in three stages. In the first stage, the goal is to control and reduce the symptoms; in the second stage, the tissues responsible for the compression are normalized and complete mobility of the neural tissues is obtained; and in the third stage, the aim is postural re-education and the training in work-related and daily activities.[27,257,285]

Stages of the conservative treatment:

1. Control and reduction of symptoms.
2. Normalization of the tissues responsible for the compression, and obtaining complete tissue mobility.
3. Postural re-education and training in work-related and daily activities.

In the first stage, and especially if the condition is irritable, the patient is taught those positions that allow for the maximum opening of the mechanical interphase and minimum strain of the brachial plexus. The cervical flexion associated with an elevation and protraction of the shoulder girdle increases the distance between the clavicle and the first rib and eliminates the tension on the brachial plexus. The patient should avoid activities that trigger the symptoms, especially repetitive activities that reduce the space available in the thoracic outlet, such as carrying heavy objects or activity that involves lifting the upper limbs.

In this distension position, deep but unforced breathing exercises have an interesting effect. By decreasing the activity of the scalene muscles and causing the first rib to lower, they prevent the neurovascular bundle from bending over the rib (Fig. 3-38). Patients can perform these exercises by resting their flexed elbows on pillows in order to make the costoclavicular clamp open up.

In the second stage, the intensity of the articular normalization manoeuvres is increased, and oscillatory or high-velocity manoeuvres can be used to lower the first rib. In this stage, neural gliding exercises can be used without leading to a worsening of symptoms. It can be interesting to stretch the scalene and pectoralis minor muscles, due to their relationship with the neurovascular bundle of the upper limb, once the irritability of the symptoms has been reduced.

The third stage is targeted at helping the patients return to their daily and work activities. At this this stage, postural re-education exercises become increasingly important.

Articular treatment

The cervical spine and the shoulder girdle form a functional unit. The treatment should be aimed at all the articular elements of this unit that may be potentially involved in a TOS,[34] with the purpose of normalizing the articular relationships of the cervical region and the shoulder girdle. In the first stage of the treatment, the mobilizations are performed in a gentle and progressive manner, to avoid aggravating the patient's symptoms.

It is possible to use manoeuvres that are directed at the bone structures that comprise the thoracic outlet, such as the scapula, the clavicle or the first rib. The aim of the techniques is to obtain complete articular mobility of the different bone elements involved in the TOS, in order to achieve an effective opening of the spaces of the thoracic outlet, while simultaneously acting on the muscles and soft tissues that link them together.

To improve the opening of spaces where neurovascular structures are compromised in the TOS, it is possible to mobilize sternoclavicular and acromioclavicular joints as well as use movements aimed at mobilizing the clavicle and the costoclavicular and retropectoral spaces (Figs 3-39–3-49).

The shoulder girdle can be mobilized globally in order to obtain the relaxation of the soft tissues and the muscles of the shoulder girdle. The scapula can be mobilized in different directions: in abduction and

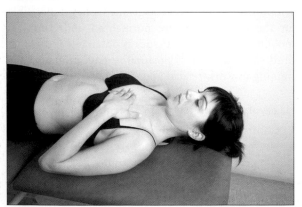

FIGURE 3-38 ■ Deep breathing exercises.

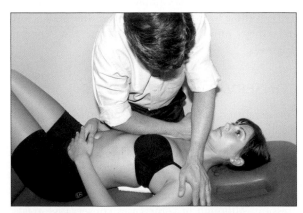

FIGURE 3-39 ■ Sternoclavicular joint distraction manoeuvre. The therapist holds the patient's shoulder and, pushing rhythmically in the lateral and posterior direction, causes a distraction of the sternoclavicular joint.

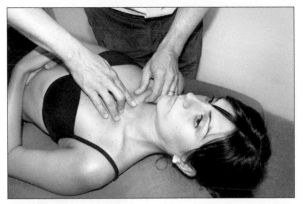

FIGURE 3-40 ■ Craniocaudal mobilization of the sternoclavicular joint. The therapist holds the proximal end of the clavicle and applies a craniocervical rhythmic mobilization, monitoring the movement of the joint with the fingers of the other hand.

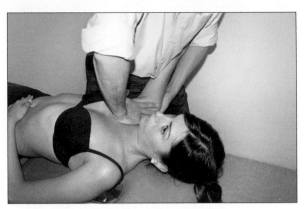

FIGURE 3-42 ■ Mobilization in circumduction of the shoulder girdle, applying rhythmic mobilizations on the costoclavicular space.

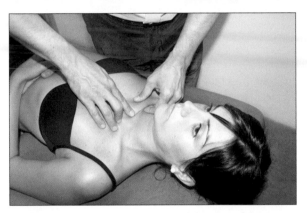

FIGURE 3-41 ■ Anteroposterior mobilization of the sternoclavicular joint. The therapist applies an anteroposterior rhythmic mobilization on the proximal end of the clavicle, while monitoring the movement with the fingers of the other hand.

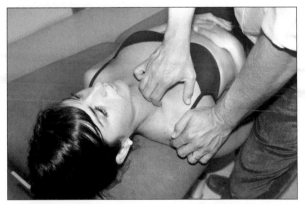

FIGURE 3-43 ■ Anterior mobilization of the clavicle. The therapist keeps the patient's shoulder in the lateral and posterior direction with the external hand, in order to open the sternoclavicular joint, while, with the fingers of the other hand, performs an anterior pull over the proximal end of the clavicle.

horizontal abduction, upper on lower rotation and circumduction (Fig. 3-50).

Costal mobilization techniques

Both the mobilization techniques of the costal rack and those focused directly on the first rib can aid in the treatment of the TOS, since they act on the interphases that are related to the neural structures involved.

Superior costal pumping manoeuvre

The patient is in the supine position, with the therapist by the head of the table facing the patient's feet. With the aid of the external arm, the therapist holds, with the hand on the shoulder, the patient's upper limb. With the inner hand, the therapist applies a rhythmic thrust over the upper costal rack. The upper costal pumping manoeuvres produce an interesting mechanical effect on the costoclavicular and retropectoral space (Fig. 3-51).

First rib techniques

Oscillatory techniques can be applied in the inferior, anteroposterior and posteroanterior directions in order to lower the first rib (Fig. 3-52). Lindgren

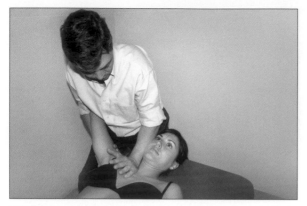

FIGURE 3-44 ■ Traction on the scapular girdle with rhythmical pressure on the costoclavicular clavicle.

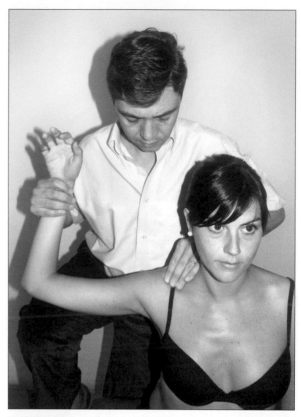

FIGURE 3-45 ■ Outward shoulder movements in order to mobilize the costoclavicular and retropectoral spaces.

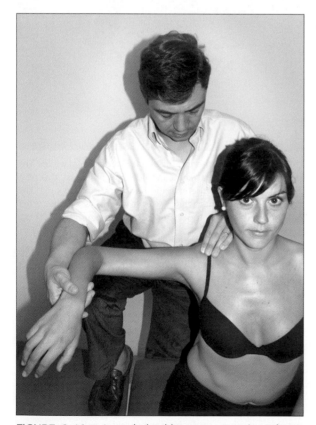

FIGURE 3-46 ■ Inward shoulder movements in order to mobilize the costoclavicular and retropectoral spaces.

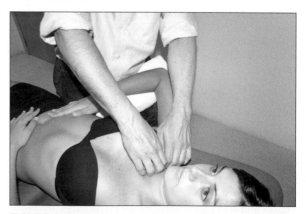

FIGURE 3-47 ■ Opening manoeuvre of the costoclavicular clamp. The therapist holds the patient's clavicle with both hands, applying a rhythmic movement in the anterior and caudal direction, in order to obtain the opening of the costoclavicular clamp.

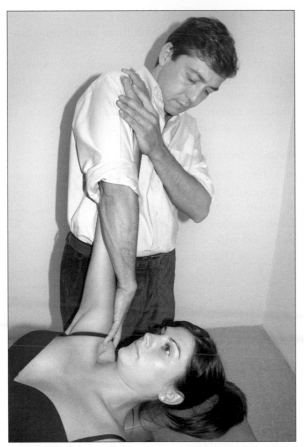

FIGURE 3-48 ■ Rhythmic traction of the arm. The therapist embraces the patient's upper limb, making wide contact with the shoulder and, with the other hand, pulls the patient's arm in a rhythmic manner from different angles.

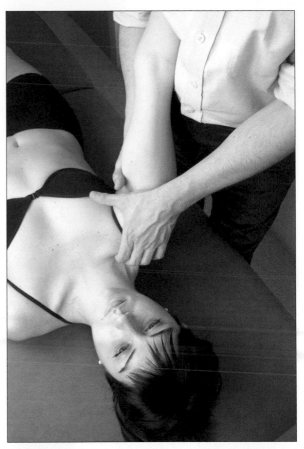

FIGURE 3-49 ■ Opening of the costoclavicular clamp and circumduction of the shoulder girdle. The therapist holds the patient's shoulder and, with the fingers of the other hand, holds the clavicle with a hook grip. This manoeuvre involves a rhythmic circular motion of the patient's upper limb associated with an anterior traction of the clavicle

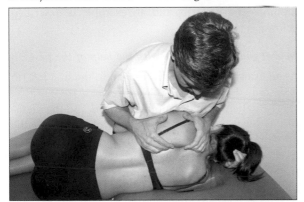

FIGURE 3-50 ■ Mobilization of the scapulothoracic joint. The scapula can be mobilized in different directions: in the superior, inferior, in abduction and horizontal abduction, superior and inferior rotation and circumduction.

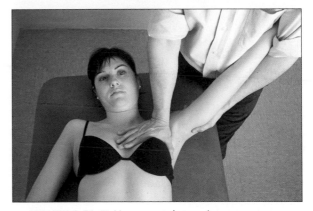

FIGURE 3-51 ■ Upper costal pumping manoeuvres.

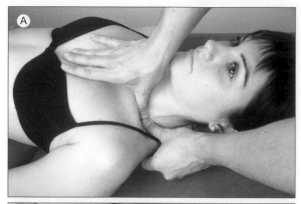

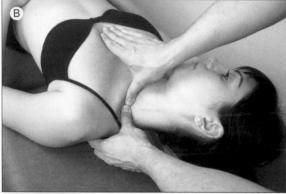

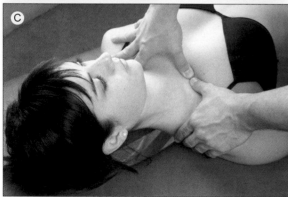

FIGURE 3-52 ■ (A–C) Oscillatory manoeuvres for the descent of the first rib.

et al.[138-140,286,287] have published several works that link the TOS and the stiffness of the first rib. The treatment involved restoring the normal mobility of the first rib through contraction–relaxation isometric techniques. In order to lower the first rib, and if the patient's clinical condition allows for it, manipulative techniques

can be used (Fig. 3-53). It is very important not to irritate the neural tissues with these neural mobilization and manipulation techniques.

Furthermore, to improve the costal mobility, it is important to act on the joints that link the ribs to the thoracic spine, using both general and thoracic flexibilization manoeuvres, and oscillatory techniques, as well as manipulative techniques.

Muscular treatment

In order to free up the interscalene space, techniques are targeted at improving the extensibility of the group of scalene muscles by stretching the anterior and middle scalenus[288] (Fig. 3-54). This stretching can be associated with a position of neural tension of the upper limb (Fig. 3-55). Furthermore, the stretching of the scalene muscles can return mobility to the first rib.[288] The muscular treatment of the retropectoral space is intended to stretch the pectoralis minor muscle (Fig. 3-56).

Neurodynamic treatment

The neurodynamic techniques that may be useful in a TOS are similar to those used in the treatment of a cervical radiculopathy and are not described in this chapter (see Chapters 1 and 2 of this volume). The purpose of these techniques is to restore the mobility of the neural tissues, acting on the mechanisms of intrinsic vascularization and axonal transport and reducing neural mechanosensitivity. Neurodynamic techniques can be associated with manoeuvres that mobilize the first rib, and an example is described below.

Neural gliding manoeuvre with the help of the first rib

As an example, a technique applied to the first left rib is described.

The patient is in the supine position, and the therapist is by the head of the table while touching the upper portion of the first rib with both thumbs, at the level of the supraclavicular space (Fig. 3-57). Keeping the patient's head in slight contralateral inclination, the therapist applies a downward force with the thumbs over the first rib. The patient is asked to flex the right elbow as the first rib lowers. The patient is then asked to perform an extension of the elbow when the therapist releases the pressure over the first rib. In

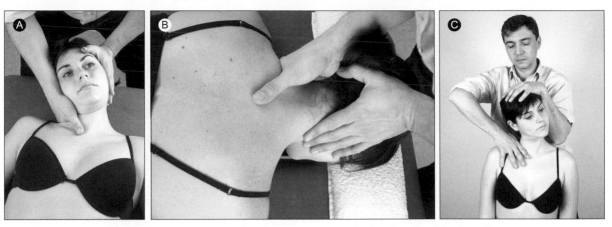

FIGURE 3-53 ■ (A–C) High-velocity manoeuvres for the descent of the first rib.

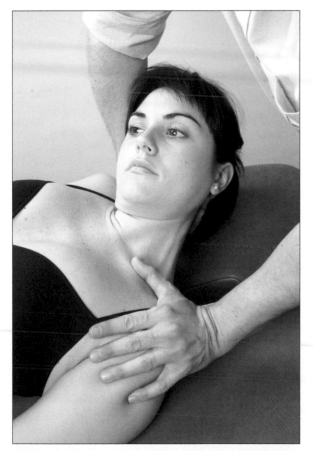

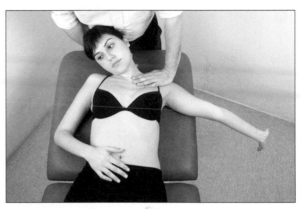

FIGURE 3-55 ■ Stretching of the scalene muscles associated with a neural tension position.

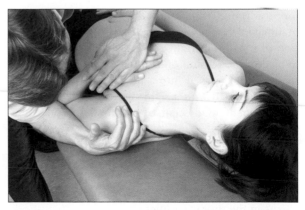

FIGURE 3-54 ■ Stretching of the scalene muscles. Using the contraction–relaxation technique, the therapist stabilizes the shoulder girdle with one hand and takes the cervical spine to a lateral inclination progressively.

FIGURE 3-56 ■ Stretching of the pectoralis minor. Stabilizing the scapula while the patient exhales, the therapist induces a descent of the upper ribs.

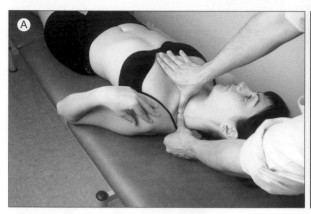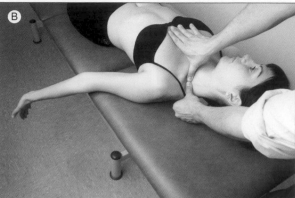

FIGURE 3-57 ■ Neural gliding manoeuvre with descent of the first rib. During the descent phase of the first rib, the patient flexes the elbow (A) and, when the therapist releases the pressure over the first rib, the patient extends the elbow (B).

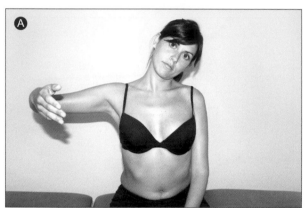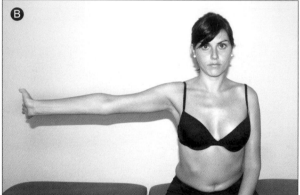

FIGURE 3-58 ■ Stretching exercise for the scalene muscles and neural mobilization. Self-stretching of the scalene muscles associated with an elbow flexion (A) and neural tensioner starting with an extension of the elbow and the wrist with the cervical spine in the neutral position (B).

more advanced phases of the treatment, the same manoeuvre can be performed starting from the position of maximum right cervical inclination, in order to place more tension on the neural tissues. This technique can be turned into a neural tension technique when combined with a right cervical inclination with a component of descent of the first rib and elbow extension.

Finally, the therapist can apply exercises that exert a certain degree of tension over the neural tissue. A treatment that is intended to release the possible areas of neural entrapment can decrease the tension of the plexus in the thoracic outlet.

It is important for the patient to perform exercises several times a day in order to mobilize the interphase and the neural tissue several times a day. Some of the exercises described in Chapter 1 can be used. Some examples are explained in Figures 3-58–3-61.

Re-education of the motor control of the shoulder girdle

Re-education of the control of the neutral scapular position

The patient can be trained to place the scapula in its optimal neutral position and to maintain this position actively and consciously, with a low-intensity contraction for 10–15 seconds, and with no substitutions.[143]

Mottram[143] recommends that when performing the right scapular movement, the patient should place a

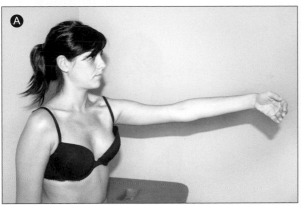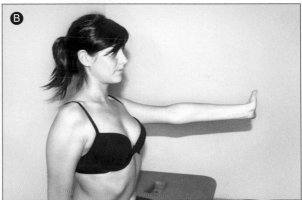

FIGURE 3-59 ■ Horizontal opening exercise of the costoclavicular clamp and neural mobilization. The patient performs a protraction of the shoulder, which causes the opening of the costoclavicular clamp, and flexes the wrist simultaneously (A). During the movement of the return of the shoulder to its neutral position, the patient extends the wrist (B).

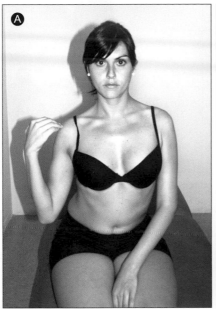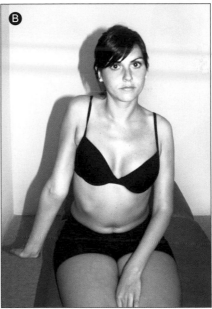

FIGURE 3-60 ■ Vertical opening exercise of the costoclavicular clamp and neural mobilization. The patient performs an elevation of the shoulder girdle, associated with an extension of the elbow and the wrist (B). During the return movement, simultaneously with the descent of the scapular girdle, the patient flexes the elbow and the wrist (A).

finger (index or middle) of the contralateral hand on the coracoid process, with the hand following the orientation of the pectoralis minor. Starting from this position, the patient should attempt to move the coracoid away from the finger (Fig. 3-62).

If the patient is unable to perform this exercise with the arm resting along the body, she can unload the upper limb by supporting it on a table with a 60–70° shoulder abduction, maintaining the scapula in a 30° horizontal abduction. In this position, it is usually easier for the patient to obtain an adequate neutral position of the scapula. After obtaining the neutral position, the patient should raise the elbow 1 cm from the table, controlling the scapular position. The

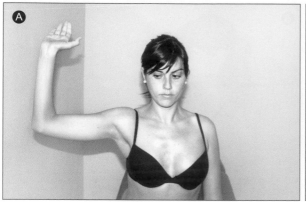
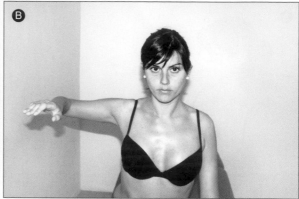

FIGURE 3-61 ■ (A, B) Stretching exercise for the pectoralis minor and neural mobilization.

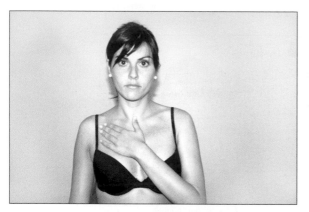

FIGURE 3-62 ■ Re-training of the control of the neutral scapular position.

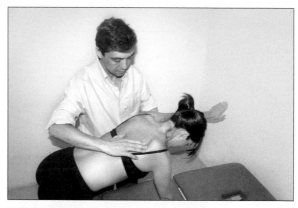

FIGURE 3-63 ■ Recruitment exercise of the serratus anterior in a closed kinetic chain.

difficulty of the exercise can be increased by reducing the shoulder abduction and performing low-amplitude abduction–adduction movements.

Once the patient is able to maintain an ideal scapular position, a higher degree of difficulty can be added by requiring a 90° glenohumeral flexion or a 60° abduction, while maintaining the scapular neutral position. The control of the scapular position should be maintained during both the concentric contraction phase, and the eccentric phase of return to the starting position.

Exercise of recruitment for the serratus anterior in the closed kinetic chain

The same test described to evaluate the serratus anterior in the sphinx or kneeling on four points can be used as an exercise. The progression of this exercise would involve an adequate scapular neutral position, while the patient is in four-point kneeling, supported only by an arm (Fig. 3-63).

Some recruitment exercises for the serratus anterior can be performed using loads while in the supine position or while unloading the body weight on an arm in different degrees of elevation and moving the subject gradually further away from the wall (Fig. 3-64).

Exercise to control the shoulder girdle while sitting down

The patient is sitting down on a stool facing a table. The arms are in 90° of abduction and 30° of horizontal abduction. With both hands holding the edge of the table, the patient places the scapula in a slight upper

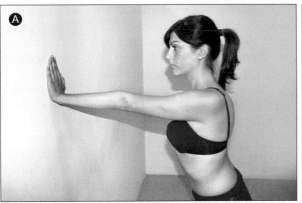 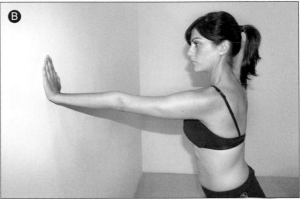

FIGURE 3-64 ■ (A, B) Recruitment exercise of the serratus anterior.

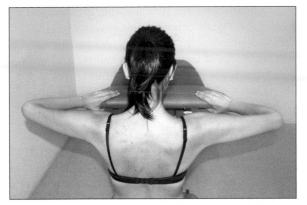 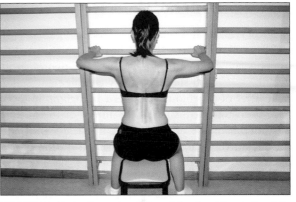

FIGURE 3-65 ■ Control exercise of the shoulder girdle while sitting down.

FIGURE 3-66 ■ Control exercise of the shoulder girdle while sitting down with a load.

rotation, and keeps it attached to the thorax, while performing rhythmic stabilizations of low intensity in abduction–adduction–horizontal adduction and flexion–extension (Fig. 3-65).

Exercise of control of the shoulder girdle while sitting down with loads

The starting position is identical to the previous exercise, but in this case the patient holds a set of wall bars with both hands. Once the position of the scapula has been controlled correctly, the patient moves 1 cm from the chair (Fig. 3-66). The hands can be placed at different heights to improve the scapular control in the different degrees of elevation of the upper limb.

Protraction exercise for the shoulder girdle while lying down

The patient is in the supine position, keeping a correct alignment of the head and the entire spine. Then, the patient lowers the upper ribs while breathing out and, with the arms in a position of shoulder, elbow and wrist flexion, performs a protraction of both shoulders (Fig. 3-67). This exercise causes the costoclavicular clamp to open and increases the mobility of the neurovascular tissues. The exercise can be also performed while sitting down. The training of the motor control of the shoulder girdle requires an adequate re-training of the alignment of the entire spine.

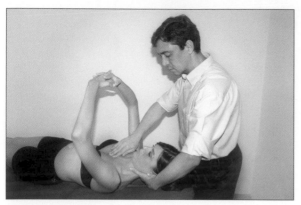

FIGURE 3-67 ■ Protraction exercise of the shoulder girdle in the supine position.

SURGICAL TREATMENT

Surgical treatment should be only used on patients for whom conservative treatment has been unsuccessful, or who show a significant vascular or neurological deficit.[8,10,39,88] TOS surgery is very complex and has a high level of morbidity. Different iatrogenic injuries have been reported, such as the injury of the plexus, the phrenic nerve and the long thoracic nerve, the subclavian vein and artery and the perforation of the pleura.[27,289–294] Therefore, it is necessary to have experts in peripheral nerve surgery and, in some cases, experts in vascular and thoracic surgery.[26,39,88,295] There is a high level of surgical failure: 28% of first surgery interventions are unsuccessful.[88]

Vascular TOS requires a decompressive surgical treatment, usually involving the resection of the first rib or of a cervical rib, associated with a medical treatment with anticoagulants and fibrinolytics and, in some cases, vascular surgery is necessary.[38,90,100,129,164,183,186,194,296–299] This surgery is recommended when the alteration of the bone or of the soft parts cause a deformity in the subclavian vessels, even when the patient is asymptomatic. Surgery is urgent in cases of ischaemia, and should be performed early when there is *a risk* of ischaemia.

With truly neurogenic TOS, involving the typical Gilliatt–Sumner hand, surgery is clearly recommendable, although the chances of complete recovery are limited.[86–204] The surgical treatment is also recommended to reduce the painful symptoms.[204]

Three types of approaches are used: transaxillary,[8,59,87,162,163,290,300–304] anterior[8,195,301,305–309] and posterior.[41] At present, the most commonly used techniques are the resection of the first rib with a transaxillary approach and anterior scalenotomy.[8,38,100,310]

Patients that have undergone this decompressive surgery have a 60–90% chance of improvement in the initial symptoms, depending on the severity and evolution of the clinical *profile*, with a variable chance of returning to their previous activity.[46,82,303,311] The recurrence of TOS after surgery is due to the formation of scar tissue and the adherence of the neurovascular tissues to the surrounding tissues. Consequently, it is essential to begin physical therapy within 24 hours.[2,52,312] The gradual mobilization techniques of the shoulder girdle and the cervical spine, as well as the mobilization techniques for the neural tissue, are necessary to achieve these goals. It is advisable to continue with the gliding exercises of the brachial plexus and the subclavian vessels for at least 6 months, and preferably for a year.[52] Often, the subject can return to normal activities within a period of 8–10 weeks.[27]

CONCLUSION

The TOS is currently one of the most controversial clinical e. Although some authors consider that TOS is diagnosed too often, others consider it to be an insufficiently diagnosed pathology.

TOS is one of the more difficult neurovascular compressive conditions to handle, because of its diagnostic complexity. The clinical manifestations can be very diverse and, therefore, there is no single clinical condition that is easy to identify. In the development of a TOS, congenital anatomical anomalies of the bone structures or soft tissues of these anatomical narrowing spaces are often involved, although not always. TOS is a dynamic entity, in such a way that the alteration of the static and dynamic balance of the shoulder girdle and the cervical and thoracic spine are frequently involved in its establishment. The diagnosis of a TOS is primarily clinical, since complementary tests in most patients usually produce negative or unclear results. With the majority of patients, it is preferable to use conservative treatments, and the aim is to increase the functional space of the thoracic outlet and to decrease the compression of the neurovascular structures and their possible adherence to the surrounding tissues. The surgical treatment should be reserved for patients who have not had any success with conservative treatment, or who may present a significant vascular or neurological deficit and untreatable pain. As in other painful conditions that tend to acquire a chronic character, the psychosocial aspects play a role both in the pathogenesis and the prognosis. It is therefore necessary in some cases to adopt a multidimensional approach with these patients.[313]

REFERENCES

1. Nichols AW. The thoracic outlet syndrome in athletes. J Am Board Fam Pract 1996;9(5):346–55.
2. Athanassiadi K, Kalavrouziotis G, Karydakis K, et al. Treatment of thoracic outlet syndrome: long-term results. World J Surg 2001;25(5):553–7.
3. Atasoy E. History of thoracic outlet syndrome. Hand Clin 2004;20(1):15–16, v.
4. Atasoy E. Thoracic outlet compression syndrome. Orthop Clin North Am 1996;27(2):265–303.
5. Novak CB, Mackinnon SE. Thoracic outlet syndrome. Orthop Clin North Am 1996;27(4):747–62.
6. Roos DB. Thoracic outlet syndrome is underdiagnosed. Muscle Nerve 1999;22(1):126–9, discussion 137–8.
7. Oates SD, Daley RA. Thoracic outlet syndrome. Hand Clin 1996;12(4):705–18.
8. Leffert R. The conundrum of thoracic outlet surgery. Tech Should Elb Surg 2002;3(4):262–70.
9. Naidu S, Kothari M. Thoracic outlet syndrome: does fiction outweigh facts? Curr Opin Orthop 2003;14:209–14.
10. Huang JH, Zager EL. Thoracic outlet syndrome. Neurosurgery 2004;55(4):897–902, discussion 902–3.
11. Wilbourn AJ. Thoracic outlet syndrome is overdiagnosed. Muscle Nerve 1999;22(1):130–6, discussion 136–7.
12. Cherington M, Happer I, Machanic B, et al. Surgery for thoracic outlet syndrome may be hazardous to your health. Muscle Nerve 1986;9(7):632–4.
13. Novak CB, Mackinnon SE, Patterson GA. Evaluation of patients with thoracic outlet syndrome. J Hand Surg Am 1993;18(2):292–9.
14. Hendler NH, Kozikowski JG. Overlooked physical diagnoses in chronic pain patients involved in litigation. Psychosomatics 1993;34(6):494–501.
15. Roos DB. Historical perspectives and anatomic considerations. Thoracic outlet syndrome. Semin Thorac Cardiovasc Surg 1996;8(2):183–9.
16. Parziale JR, Akelman E, Weiss AP, et al. Thoracic outlet syndrome. Am J Orthop 2000;29(5):353–60.
17. Edwards DP, Mulkern E, Raja AN, et al. Trans-axillary first rib excision for thoracic outlet syndrome. J R Coll Surg Edinb 1999;44(6):362–5.
18. Shukla PC, Carlton FB Jr. Diagnosis of thoracic outlet syndrome in the emergency department. South Med J 1996;89(2):212–17.
19. Schenardi C. Whiplash injury. TOS and double crush syndrome. Forensic medical aspects. Acta Neurochir Suppl 2005;92:25–7.
20. Birch R, Bonney G, Parry CW. Surgical disorders of the peripheral nerves. London: Churchill Livingstone; 1998.
21. Wilbourn AJ. Thoracic outlet syndromes: a plea for conservatism. Neurosurg Clin N Am 1991;2(1):235–45.
22. Yanaka K, Asakawa H, Matsumaru Y, et al. Diagnosis of vascular compression at the thoracic outlet using magnetic resonance angiography. Eur Neurol 2004;51(2):122–3.
23. Clarys JP, Barbaix E, Van Rompaey H, et al. The muscular arch of the axilla revisited: its possible role in the thoracic outlet and shoulder instability syndromes. Man Ther 1996;1(3):133–9.
24. Whitenack S, Hunter J, Jaeger S, et al. Thoracic outlet syndrome: a brachial plexopathy. In: Hunter J, Mackin E, Callahan A, editors. Rehabilitation of the hand: surgery and therapy. St Louis: Mosby; 1995. p. 857–84.
25. Leffert RD. Thoracic outlet syndromes. Hand Clin 1992;8(2):285–97.
26. Mackinnon SE, Patterson GA, Novak CB. Thoracic outlet syndrome: a current overview. Semin Thorac Cardiovasc Surg 1996;8(2):176–82.
27. Anthony M. Thoracic outlet syndrome. In: Clark G, editor. Hand rehabilitation. A practical guide. 2nd ed. New York: Churchill Livingstone; 1997. p. 195–212.
28. Lord JW Jr. Critical reappraisal of diagnostic and therapeutic modalities for thoracic outlet syndromes. Surg Gynecol Obstet 1989;168(4):337–40.
29. Swift TR, Nichols FT. The droopy shoulder syndrome. Neurology 1984;34(2):212–15.
30. Wilbourn AJ. The thoracic outlet syndrome is overdiagnosed. Arch Neurol 1990;47(3):328–30.
31. Le Forestier N, Moulonguet A, Maisonobe T, et al. True neurogenic thoracic outlet syndrome: electrophysiological diagnosis in six cases. Muscle Nerve 1998;21(9):1129–34.
32. Kai Y, Oyama M, Kurose S, et al. Neurogenic thoracic outlet syndrome in whiplash injury. J Spinal Disord 2001;14(6):487–93.
33. Konuskan B, Bozkurt MC, Tagil SM, et al. Cadaveric observation of an aberrant left subclavian artery: a possible cause of thoracic outlet syndrome. Clin Anat 2005;18(3):215–16.
34. Becker F. Thoracic outlet syndrome. Rev Med Suisse 2005;1(4):306, 308–11.
35. Green RM. Vascular manifestations of the thoracic outlet syndrome. Semin Vasc Surg 1998;11(2):67–76.
36. Felice KJ, Butler KB, Druckemiller WH. Cervical root stimulation in a case of classic neurogenic thoracic outlet syndrome. Muscle Nerve 1999;22(9):1287–92.
37. Redenbach DM, Nelems B. A comparative study of structures comprising the thoracic outlet in 250 human cadavers and 72 surgical cases of thoracic outlet syndrome. Eur J Cardiothorac Surg 1998;13(4):353–60.

38. Urschel HC Jr, Razzuk MA. Neurovascular compression in the thoracic outlet: changing management over 50 years. Ann Surg 1998;228(4):609–17.

39. Leffert RD. Thoracic outlet syndrome. J Am Acad Orthop Surg 1994;2(6):317–25.

40. Le Forestier N, Mouton P, Maisonobe T, et al. True neurological thoracic outlet syndrome. Rev Neurol (Paris) 2000;156(1): 34–40.

41. Urschel HC, Patel A. Thoracic outlet syndromes. Curr Treat Options Cardiovasc Med 2003;5(2):163–8.

42. Naidu S, Khotari M. Thoracic outlet syndrome: does fiction outweigh facts? Curr Opin Orthop 2003;14:209–14.

43. Makhoul RG, Machleder HI. Developmental anomalies at the thoracic outlet: an analysis of 200 consecutive cases. J Vasc Surg 1992;16(4):534–42, discussion 542–5.

44. Reid JR, Morrison SC, DiFiore JW. Thoracic outlet syndrome with subclavian aneurysm in a very young child: the complementary value of MRA and 3D-CT in diagnosis. Pediatr Radiol 2002;32(1):22–4.

45. Yang J, Letts M. Thoracic outlet syndrome in children. J Pediatr Orthop 1996;16(4):514–17.

46. Nannapaneni R, Marks SM. Neurogenic thoracic outlet syndrome. Br J Neurosurg 2003;17(2):144–8.

47. Sällström J, Thulesius O. Non-invasive investigation of vascular compression in patients with thoracic outlet syndrome. Clin Physiol 1982;2(2):117–25.

48. Cooke RA. Thoracic outlet syndrome – aspects of diagnosis in the differential diagnosis of hand-arm vibration syndrome. Occup Med (Lond) 2003;53(5):331–6.

49. Demondion X, Bacqueville E, Paul C, et al. Thoracic outlet: assessment with MR imaging in asymptomatic and symptomatic populations. Radiology 2003;227(2):461–8.

50. Roos DB. Congenital anomalies associated with thoracic outlet syndrome. Anatomy, symptoms, diagnosis, and treatment. Am J Surg 1976;132(6):771–8.

51. Roos DB. Pathophysiology of congenital anomalies in thoracic outlet syndrome. Acta Chir Belg 1980;79(5):353–61.

52. Atasoy E. Thoracic outlet syndrome: anatomy. Hand Clin 2004;20(1):7–14, v.

53. Collins JD, Disher AC, Miller TQ. The anatomy of the brachial plexus as displayed by magnetic resonance imaging: technique and application. J Natl Med Assoc 1995;87(7):489–98.

54. Pang D, Wessel HB. Thoracic outlet syndrome. Neurosurgery 1988;22(1 Pt 1):105–21.

55. Lusskin R, Weiss CA, Winer J. The role of the subclavius muscle in the subclavian vein syndrome (costoclavicular syndrome) following fracture of the clavicle. A case report with a review of the pathophysiology of the costoclavicular space. Clin Orthop Relat Res 1967;54:75–83.

56. Hama H, Matsusue Y, Ito H, et al. Thoracic outlet syndrome associated with an anomalous coracoclavicular joint. A case report. J Bone Joint Surg Am 1993;75(9):1368–9.

57. Molina JE. Need for emergency treatment in subclavian vein effort thrombosis. J Am Coll Surg 1995;181(5):414–20.

58. Hasan SS, Romeo AA. Thoracic outlet syndrome secondary to an anomalous subclavius muscle. Orthopedics 2001;24(8): 793–4.

59. Sanders RJ, Hammond SL. Subclavian vein obstruction without thrombosis. J Vasc Surg 2005;41(2):285–90.

60. Wayman J, Miller S, Shanahan D. Anatomical variation of the insertion of scalenus anterior in adult human subjects: implications for clinical practice. J Anat 1993;183(Pt 1): 165–7.

61. Wright I. The neurovascular syndrome produced by hyperabduction of the arm. Am Heart J 1945;29:1–19.

62. Miguel M, Llusa M, Ortiz JC, et al. The axillopectoral muscle (of Langer): report of three cases. Surg Radiol Anat 2001;23(5):341–3.

63. Yuksel M, Yuksel E, Surucu S. An axillary arch. Clin Anat 1996;9(4):252–4.

64. Vischi S, Roesel R, Capriata G, et al. The axillo-pectoral muscle and Karl Langer: an anatomical variation and a rather unknown great anatomist. Minerva Chir 2003;58(6):833–7.

65. Suzuma T, Sakurai T, Yoshimura G, et al. Magnetic resonance axillography for preoperative diagnosis of the axillopectoral muscle (Langer's axillary arch): a case report. Breast Cancer 2003;10(3):281–3.

66. Daniels IR, della Rovere GQ. The axillary arch of Langer – the most common muscular variation in the axilla. Breast Cancer Res Treat 2000;59(1):77–80.

67. Turgut HB, Peker T, Gulekon N, et al. Axillopectoral muscle (Langer's muscle). Clin Anat 2005;18(3):220–3.

68. Bergman RA. Doubled pectoralis quartus, axillary arch, chondroepitrochlearis, and the twist of the tendon of pectoralis major. Anat Anz 1991;173(1):23–6.

69. Ucerler H, Ikiz ZA, Pinan Y. Clinical importance of the muscular arch of the axilla (axillopectoral muscle, Langer's axillary arch). Acta Chir Belg 2005;105(3):326–8.

70. Keshtgar MR, Saunders C, Ell PJ, et al. Langer's axillary arch in association with sentinel lymph node. Breast 1999;8(3): 152–3.

71. Bonastre V, Rodriguez-Niedenfuhr M, Choi D, et al. Coexistence of a pectoralis quartus muscle and an unusual axillary arch: case report and review. Clin Anat 2002;15(5): 366–70.

72. Babu ED, Khashaba A. Axillary arch and its implications in axillary dissection – review. Int J Clin Pract 2000;54(8): 524–5.

73. Petrasek AJ, Semple JL, McCready DR. The surgical and oncologic significance of the axillary arch during axillary lymphadenectomy. Can J Surg 1997;40(1):44–7.

74. Dharap A. An unusually medial axillary arch muscle. J Anat 1994;184(Pt 3):639–41.

75. Serpell JW, Baum M. Significance of 'Langer's axillary arch' in axillary dissection. Aust N Z J Surg 1991;61(4):310–12.

76. Brantigan CO, Roos DB. Etiology of neurogenic thoracic outlet syndrome. Hand Clin 2004;20(1):17–22.

77. Naffziger H, Grant W. Neuritis of the brachial plexus mechanical in origin. The escalenus syndrome. Surg Gynecol Obstet 1938;67:722–30.

78. Ochsner A, Gage M, DeBakey M. Scalenus anticus (Naffziger) syndrome. Am J Surg 1935;28:669–95.

79. Keller T. Howard Christian Naffziger: the surgeon and his syndrome. Am Surg 1998;64(4):376–7.

80. Thomas GI, Jones TW, Stavney LS, et al. The middle scalene muscle and its contribution to the thoracic outlet syndrome. Am J Surg 1983;145(5):589–92.

81. Sanders RJ, Jackson CG, Banchero N, et al. Scalene muscle abnormalities in traumatic thoracic outlet syndrome. Am J Surg 1990;159(2):231–6.

82. Sanders RJ. Results of the surgical treatment for thoracic outlet syndrome. Semin Thorac Cardiovasc Surg 1996;8(2):221–8.

83. Machleder HI, Moll F, Verity MA. The anterior scalene muscle in thoracic outlet compression syndrome. Histochemical and morphometric studies. Arch Surg 1986;121(10):1141–4.

84. Juvonen T, Satta J, Laitala P, et al. Anomalies at the thoracic outlet are frequent in the general population. Am J Surg 1995;170(1):33–7.

85. Leffert R. Thoracic outlet syndrome. In: Gelberman R, editor. Operative nerve repair and reconstruction. Philadelphia: Lippincott; 1991. p. 1177–95.

86. Tender GC, Thomas AJ, Thomas N, et al. Gilliatt-Sumner hand revisited: a 25-year experience. Neurosurgery 2004;55(4):883–90, discussion 890.

87. Wood VE, Twito R, Verska JM. Thoracic outlet syndrome. The results of first rib resection in 100 patients. Orthop Clin North Am 1988;19(1):131–46.

88. Sanders RJ, Hammond SL. Management of cervical ribs and anomalous first ribs causing neurogenic thoracic outlet syndrome. J Vasc Surg 2002;36(1):51–6.

89. Roos DB. The place for scalenectomy and first-rib resection in thoracic outlet syndrome. Surgery 1982;92(6):1077–85.

90. Whitenack S, Hunter J, Jaeger S, et al. Thoracic outlet syndrome: a brachial plexopathy. In: Hunter J, Mackin E, Callahan A, editors. Rehabilitation of the hand: surgery and therapy. Philadelphia: Mosby; 1995. p. 857–84.

91. Gruber W. Ueber die Halsrippen des Menschen mit vergleichend-anatomischen Remerkungen. Mem Acad Imper Sci St Petersburg 1869;7 Ser:No 2.

92. Sargent P. Lesions of the brachial plexus associated with rudimentary ribs. Brain 1921;44:95–124.

93. Erken E, Ozer HT, Gulek B, et al. The association between cervical rib and sacralization. Spine 2002;27(15):1659–64.

94. Falconer M, Weddell G. Costo-clavicular compression of the subclavian artery and vein. Relation to scalenus syndrome. Lancet 1943;ii:539–43.

95. Forcada P, Rodríguez-Niedenführ M, Llusá M, et al. Subclavius posticus muscle: supernumerary muscle as a potencial cause for thoracic outlet syndrome. Clin Anat 2001;14:55–7.

96. Akita K, Tsuboi Y, Sakamoto H, et al. A case of muscle subclavius posticus with special reference to its innervation. Surg Radiol Anat 1996;18(4):335–7.

97. Gillard J. Diagnosing thoracic outlet syndrome: contribution of provocative test, ultrasonography, electrophysiology, and helical computed tomography in 48 patients. Joint Bone Spine 2001;68:416–24.

98. Chen DJ, Chuang DC, Wei FC. Unusual thoracic outlet syndrome secondary to fractured clavicle. J Trauma 2002;52(2):393–8, discussion 398–9.

99. Hill JM, McGuire MH, Crosby LA. Closed treatment of displaced middle-third fractures of the clavicle gives poor results. J Bone Joint Surg Br 1997;79(4):537–9.

100. Davidovic LB, Kostic DM, Jakovljevic NS, et al. Vascular thoracic outlet syndrome. World J Surg 2003;27(5):545–50.

101. Hughes AW, Sherlock DA. Bilateral thoracic outlet syndrome following non-union of clavicles, associated with radio-osteodystrophy. Injury 1988;19(1):40–1.

102. Kitsis CK, Marino AJ, Krikler SJ, et al. Late complications following clavicular fractures and their operative management. Injury 2003;34(1):69–74.

103. Subramonia S, Holdsworth D. Neurogenic thoracic outlet syndrome secondary to non-union os unrecognised first rib fracture. EJVES 2004;7:40–2.

104. Merida-Velasco JR, Rodriguez Vazquez JF, Merida Velasco JA, et al. Axillary arch: potential cause of neurovascular compression syndrome. Clin Anat 2003;16(6):514–19.

105. Sachatello CR. The axillopectoral muscle (Langer's axillary arch): a cause of axillary vein obstruction. Surgery 1977;81(5):610–12.

106. Capistrant TD. Thoracic outlet syndrome in cervical strain injury. Minn Med 1986;69(1):13–17.

107. Ellison DW, Wood VE. Trauma-related thoracic outlet syndrome. J Hand Surg [Br] 1994;19(4):424–6.

108. Magnusson T. Extracervical symptoms after whiplash trauma. Cephalalgia 1994;14(3):223–7, discussion 181–2.

109. Mailis A, Papagapiou M, Vanderlinden RG, et al. Thoracic outlet syndrome after motor vehicle accidents in a Canadian pain clinic population. Clin J Pain 1995;11(4):316–24.

110. Casbas L, Chauffour X, Cau J, et al. Post-traumatic thoracic outlet syndromes. Ann Vasc Surg 2005;19(1):25–8.

111. Mulder DS, Greenwood FA, Brooks CE. Posttraumatic thoracic outlet syndrome. J Trauma 1973;13(8):706–15.

112. Evans RW. Some observations on whiplash injuries. Neurol Clin 1992;10(4):975–97.

113. Ferrari R, Bohr T, Wilbourn AJ. Thoracic outlet syndrome (TOS) is one of the traumatic complications of whiplash injury. J Spinal Disord Tech 2002;15(4):334–5.

114. Kai Y, Oyama M, Kurose S, et al. Neurogenic thoracic outlet syndrome in whiplash injury [see comment]. J Spinal Disord 2001;14(6):487–93.

115. Alexandre A, Coro L, Azuelos A, et al. Thoracic outlet syndrome due to hyperextension-hyperflexion cervical injury. Acta Neurochir Suppl 2005;92:21–4.

116. Carty NJ, Carpenter R, Webster JH. Continuing experience with transaxillary excision of the first rib for thoracic outlet syndrome. Br J Surg 1992;79(8):761–2.

117. Hempel GK, Rusher AH Jr, Wheeler CG, et al. Supraclavicular resection of the first rib for thoracic outlet syndrome. Am J Surg 1981;141(2):213–15.

118. Sällström J, Schmidt H. Cervicobrachial disorders in certain occupations, with special reference to compression in the thoracic outlet. Am J Ind Med 1984;6(1):45–52.

119. Sheon RP. Repetitive strain injury. 2. Diagnostic and treatment tips on six common problems. The Goff Group. Postgrad Med 1997;102(4):72–8, 81, 85 passim.

120. Sheth RN, Belzberg AJ. Diagnosis and treatment of thoracic outlet syndrome. Neurosurg Clin N Am 2001;12(2):295–309.

121. Tilki HE, Stalberg E, Incesu L, et al. Bilateral neurogenic thoracic outlet syndrome. Muscle Nerve 2004;29(1):147–50.

122. Fiorentini C, Mattioli S, Graziosi F, et al. Occupational relevance of subclavian vein thrombosis in association with thoracic outlet syndrome. Scand J Work Environ Health 2005;31(2):160–3.

123. Pratikto TH, Zwetschke V, Goyen M, et al. Recurrent exercise induced subclavian vein thrombosis in a conductor. Vasa 2002;31(3):209–11.

124. Strukel RJ, Garrick JG. Thoracic outlet compression in athletes a report of four cases. Am J Sports Med 1978;6(2):35–9.

125. Esposito MD, Arrington JA, Blackshear MN, et al. Thoracic outlet syndrome in a throwing athlete diagnosed with MRI and MRA. J Magn Reson Imaging 1997;7(3):598–9.

126. Feugier P, Aleksic I, Salari R, et al. Long-term results of venous revascularization for Paget-Schroetter syndrome in athletes. Ann Vasc Surg 2001;15(2):212–18.

127. Koffler KM, Kelly JD 4th. Neurovascular trauma in athletes. Orthop Clin North Am 2002;33(3):523–34, vi.

128. Richardson AB. Thoracic outlet syndrome in aquatic athletes. Clin Sports Med 1999;18(2):361–78.

129. Casey RG, Richards S, O'Donohoe M. Exercise induced critical ischaemia of the upper limb secondary to a cervical rib. Br J Sports Med 2003;37(5):455–6.

130. Chaudhry MA, Hajarnavis J. Paget-von Schrötter syndrome: primary subclavian-axillary vein thrombosis in sport activities. Clin J Sport Med 2003;13(4):269–71.

131. Lederman RJ. Neuromuscular and musculoskeletal problems in instrumental musicians. Muscle Nerve 2003;27(5):549–61.

132. Clein LJ. The droopy shoulder syndrome. Can Med Assoc J 1976;114(4):343–4.

133. Leffert RD. Thoracic outlet syndrome and the shoulder. Clin Sports Med 1983;2(2):439–52.

134. Kaye BL. Neurologic changes with excessively large breasts. South Med J 1972;65(2):177–80.

135. Al-Shekhlee A, Katirji B. Spinal accessory neuropathy, droopy shoulder, and thoracic outlet syndrome. Muscle Nerve 2003;28(3):383–5.

136. Lindgren KA. TOS (thoracic outlet syndrome) – a functional disease? Duodecim 1994;110(12):1131–9.

137. Lindgren KA, Manninen H, Rytkonen H. Thoracic outlet syndrome – a functional disturbance of the thoracic upper aperture? Muscle Nerve 1995;18(5):526–30.

138. Lindgren KA. Thoracic outlet syndrome with special reference to the first rib. Ann Chir Gynaecol 1993;82(4):218–30.

139. Lindgren KA. Reasons for failures in the surgical treatment of thoracic outlet syndrome. Muscle Nerve 1995;18(12):1484–6.

140. Lindgren KA, Leino E. Subluxation of the first rib: a possible thoracic outlet syndrome mechanism. Arch Phys Med Rehabil 1988;69(9):692–5.

141. Janda V. Muscle strength in relation to muscle length, pain and muscle imbalance. In: Harms-Ringdahl K, editor. Muscle strength. Edinburgh: Churchill Livingstone; 1993. p. 83–91.

142. Mackinnon SE, Novak CB. Clinical commentary: pathogenesis of cumulative trauma disorder. J Hand Surg Am 1994;19(5):873–83.

143. Mottram SL. Dynamic stability of the scapula. Man Ther 1997;2(3):123–31.

144. Upton AR, McComas AJ. The double crush in nerve entrapment syndromes. Lancet 1973;2(7825):359–62.

145. Lundborg G. Nerve injury and repair. New York: Churchill Livingstone; 1988.

146. Mackinnon SE, Dellon AL. Surgery of the peripheral nerve. New York: Thieme; 1988.

147. Sunderland S. Nerve and nerve injuries. New York: Churchill Livingstone; 1978.

148. Mackinnon SE. Double and multiple 'crush' syndromes. Double and multiple entrapment neuropathies. Hand Clin 1992;8(2):369–90.

149. Mackinnon SE. Pathophysiology of nerve compression. Hand Clin 2002;18(2):231–41.

150. Dellon AL, Mackinnon SE. Chronic nerve compression model for the double crush hypothesis. Ann Plast Surg 1991;26(3):259–64.

151. Butler D. Mobilisation of the nervous system. New York: Churchill Livingstone; 1991.

152. Mackinnon SE, Novak CB. Thoracic outlet syndrome. Curr Probl Surg 2002;39(11):1070–145.

153. Lord JW Jr, Rosati LM. Thoracic-outlet syndromes. Clin Symp 1971;23(2):1–32.

154. Putters JL, Kaulesar Sukul DM, Johannes EJ. Bilateral thoracic outlet syndrome with bilateral radial tunnel syndrome: a double-crush phenomenon. Case report. Arch Orthop Trauma Surg 1992;111(4):242–3.

155. Narakas AO. The role of thoracic outlet syndrome in the double crush syndrome. Ann Chir Main Memb Super 1990;9(5):331–40.

156. Wood VE, Biondi J. Double-crush nerve compression in thoracic-outlet syndrome. J Bone Joint Surg Am 1990;72(1):85–7.

157. Sucher BM. Palpatory diagnosis and manipulative management of carpal tunnel syndrome: Part 2. 'Double crush' and thoracic outlet syndrome. J Am Osteopath Assoc 1995;95(8):471–9.

158. Abe M, Ichinohe K, Nishida J. Diagnosis, treatment, and complications of thoracic outlet syndrome. J Orthop Sci 1999;4(1):66–9.

159. Blanchard B, Blanchard G, Forcier P, et al. The thoracic outlet: true syndromes, disputed syndrome (TOS, thoracic outlet syndrome). Current status 1991. Rev Med Suisse Romande 1992;112(3):253–66.

160. Gillard J, Perez-Cousin M, Hachulla E, et al. Diagnosing thoracic outlet syndrome: contribution of provocative tests, ultrasonography, electrophysiology, and helical computed tomography in 48 patients. Joint Bone Spine 2001;68(5):416–24.

161. Aburahma AF, White JF 3rd. Thoracic outlet syndrome with arm ischemia as a complication of cervical rib. W V Med J 1995;91(3):92–4.

162. Roos DB. Transaxillary approach for first rib resection to relieve thoracic outlet syndrome. Ann Surg 1966;163(3):354–8.
163. Jamieson WG, Chinnick B. Thoracic outlet syndrome: fact or fancy? A review of 409 consecutive patients who underwent operation. Can J Surg 1996;39(4):321–6.
164. Coletta JM, Murray JD, Reeves TR, et al. Vascular thoracic outlet syndrome: successful outcomes with multimodal therapy. Cardiovasc Surg 2001;9(1):11–15.
165. Sanders RJ, Haug C. Review of arterial thoracic outlet syndrome with a report of five new instances. Surg Gynecol Obstet 1991;173(5):415–25.
166. Basile C, Giordano R, Montanaro A, et al. Bilateral venous thoracic outlet syndrome in a haemodialysis patient with long-standing body building activities. Nephrol Dial Transplant 2001;16(3):639–40.
167. Thomas de Montpreville V, Dulmet E, Ponlot R, et al. Giant bilateral fibrous dysplasia of first ribs: compression of mediastinum and thoracic outlet. Eur Respir J 1995;8(6):1028–9.
168. Wilbourn AJ. 10 most commonly asked questions about thoracic outlet syndrome. Neurologist 2001;7(5):309–12.
169. Raskin NH, Howard MW, Ehrenfeld WK. Headache as the leading symptom of the thoracic outlet syndrome. Headache 1985;25(4):208–10.
170. Matsuyama T, Okuchi K, Goda K. Upper plexus thoracic outlet syndrome – case report. Neurol Med Chir (Tokyo) 2002;42(5):237–41.
171. Brower R. Differential diagnosis of cervical radiculopathy and myelopathy. In: Clark C, editor. The cervical spine. Philadelphia: Lippincott Williams & Wilkins; 2005. p. 995–1008.
172. Mackinnon SE, Novak CB. Evaluation of the patient with thoracic outlet syndrome. Semin Thorac Cardiovasc Surg 1996;8(2):190–200.
173. Gilliatt RW, Le Quesne PM, Logue V, et al. Wasting of the hand associated with a cervical rib or band. J Neurol Neurosurg Psychiatry 1970;33(5):615–24.
174. Cakmur R, Idiman F, Akalin E, et al. Dermatomal and mixed nerve somatosensory evoked potentials in the diagnosis of neurogenic thoracic outlet syndrome. Electroencephalogr Clin Neurophysiol 1998;108(5):423–34.
175. Kothari MJ, Macintosh K, Heistand M, et al. Medial antebrachial cutaneous sensory studies in the evaluation of neurogenic thoracic outlet syndrome. Muscle Nerve 1998;21(5):647–9.
176. Sobey AV, Grewal RP, Hutchison KJ, et al. Investigation of non-specific neurogenic thoracic outlet syndrome. J Cardiovasc Surg (Torino) 1993;34(4):343–5.
177. Komanetsky RM, Novak CB, Mackinnon SE, et al. Somatosensory evoked potentials fail to diagnose thoracic outlet syndrome. J Hand Surg Am 1996;21(4):662–6.
178. Urschel HC Jr, Razzuk MA, Hyland JW, et al. Thoracic outlet syndrome masquerading as coronary artery disease (pseudoangina). Ann Thorac Surg 1973;16(3):239–48.
179. Campbell PT, Simel DL. Left arm pain isn't always angina. N C Med J 1988;49(11):564–7.
180. Yoshikawa H, Ueno Y, Nakamura N, et al. Hands up for angina. Lancet 1998;352(9129):702.
181. Gockel M, Lindholm H, Vastamaki M, et al. Cardiovascular functional disorder and distress among patients with thoracic outlet syndrome. J Hand Surg [Br] 1995;20(1):29–33.
182. Kaymak B. A novel finding in thoracic outlet syndrome: tachycardia. Joint Bone Spine 2004;71:430–2.
183. Sanders RJ, Haug C. Subclavian vein obstruction and thoracic outlet syndrome: a review of etiology and management. Ann Vasc Surg 1990;4(4):397–410.
184. Akita K, Ibukuro K, Yamaguchi K, et al. The subclavius posticus muscle: a factor in arterial, venous or brachial plexus compression? Surg Radiol Anat 2000;22(2):111–15.
185. Heis HA, Bani-Hani KE. Effort thrombosis of the subclavian-axillary vein. Saudi Med J 2002;23(10):1199–202.
186. Sanders RJ, Hammond SL. Venous thoracic outlet syndrome. Hand Clin 2004;20(1):113–18, viii.
187. Parry E, Eastcott H. Cervical rib and thoracic outlet syndrome. In: Eastcott H, editor. Arterial surgery. Edinburgh: Churchill Livingstone; 1992. p. 333–53.
188. Paget J. Practice among the out-patients of St Bartholomew's Hospital: III, on some affections on voluntary muscles. Med Times Gazette 1858;16:260–1.
189. Schröetter LV. Erkrankungen der Gafabe. In: Nothnagel H, editor. Specielle Pathologie und Therapie, XV, II, Theil II. Halfe: Erkrankungen der Venen. Vienna: Holder; 1899. p. 533–5.
190. Judy KL, Heymann RL. Vascular complications of thoracic outlet syndrome. Am J Surg 1972;123(5):521–31.
191. Shuttleworth RD, van der Merwe DM, Mitchell WL. Subclavian vein stenosis and axillary vein 'effort thrombosis'. Age and the first rib bypass collateral, thrombolytic therapy and first rib resection. S Afr Med J 1987;71(9):564–6.
192. Fantini GA. Reserving supraclavicular first rib resection for vascular complications of thoracic outlet syndrome. Am J Surg 1996;172(2):200–4.
193. Hood DB, Kuehne J, Yellin AE, et al. Vascular complications of thoracic outlet syndrome. Am Surg 1997;63(10):913–17.
194. Azakie A, McElhinney DB, Thompson RW, et al. Surgical management of subclavian-vein effort thrombosis as a result of thoracic outlet compression. J Vasc Surg 1998;28(5):777–86.
195. Maxey TS, Reece TB, Ellman PI, et al. Safety and efficacy of the supraclavicular approach to thoracic outlet decompression. Ann Thorac Surg 2003;76(2):396–9, discussion 399–400.
196. Urschel HC Jr, Patel AN. Paget-Schroetter syndrome therapy: failure of intravenous stents. Ann Thorac Surg 2003;75(6):1693–6, discussion 1696.
197. Durham JR, Yao JS, Pearce WH, et al. Arterial injuries in the thoracic outlet syndrome. J Vasc Surg 1995;21(1):57–69, discussion 70.
198. Maisonneuve H, Planchon B, de Faucal P, et al. Vascular manifestation of thoracic outlet syndrome. Prospective study of 104 patients. J Mal Vasc 1991;16(3):220–5.
199. Hagspiel KD, Spinosa DJ, Angle JF, et al. Diagnosis of vascular compression at the thoracic outlet using gadolinium-enhanced high-resolution ultrafast MR angiography in abduction and adduction. Cardiovasc Intervent Radiol 2000;23(2):152–4.

200. Warrens AN, Heaton JM. Thoracic outlet compression syndrome: the lack of reliability of its clinical assessment. Ann R Coll Surg Engl 1987;69(5):203–4.

201. Kelly TR. Thoracic outlet syndrome: current concepts of treatment. Ann Surg 1979;190(5):657–62.

202. Jamieson WG, Merskey H. Representation of the thoracic outlet syndrome as a problem in chronic pain and psychiatric management. Pain 1985;22(2):195–200.

203. Brantigan CO, Roos DB. Diagnosing thoracic outlet syndrome. Hand Clin 2004;20(1):27–36.

204. Donaghy M, Matkovic Z, Morris P. Surgery for suspected neurogenic thoracic outlet syndromes: a follow up study. J Neurol Neurosurg Psychiatry 1999;67(5):602–6.

205. Lindgren KA. Conservative treatment of thoracic outlet syndrome: a 2-year follow-up. Arch Phys Med Rehabil 1997;78(4):373–8.

206. Chon S, Lee C, Oh Y. Calcifying fibrous pseudotumor causing thoracic outlet syndrome. Eur J Cardiothorac Surg 2005;27: 353–5.

207. Sergeant G, Gheysens O, Seynaeve P, et al. Neurovascular compression by a subpectoral lipoma. A case report of a rare cause of thoracic outlet syndrome. Acta Chir Belg 2003;103(5): 528–31.

208. Nakazawa H, Terada S, Nozaki M, et al. Unusual case of thoracic outlet syndrome caused by a neurilemmoma in the pectoralis minor space. Acta Orthop Belg 2005;71(3):357–60.

209. Melliere D, Ben Yahia NE, Etienne G, et al. Thoracic outlet syndrome caused by tumor of the first rib. J Vasc Surg 1991;14(2):235–40.

210. Jones DR, Detterbeck FC. Pancoast tumors of the lung. Curr Opin Pulm Med 1998;4(4):191–7.

211. Villas C, Collia A, Aquerreta JD, et al. Cervicobrachialgia and Pancoast tumor: value of standard anteroposterior cervical radiographs in early diagnosis. Orthopedics 2004;27(10):1092–5.

212. Pitz CC, de la Riviere AB, van Swieten HA, et al. Surgical treatment of Pancoast tumours. Eur J Cardiothorac Surg 2004;26(1):202–8.

213. Kichari JR, Hussain SM, Den Hollander JC, et al. MR imaging of the brachial plexus: current imaging sequences, normal findings, and findings in a spectrum of focal lesions with MR-pathologic correlation. Curr Probl Diagn Radiol 2003;32(2):88–101.

214. Rayan GM. Thoracic outlet syndrome. J Shoulder Elbow Surg 1998;7(4):440–51.

215. Gergoudis R, Barnes RW. Thoracic outlet arterial compression: prevalence in normal persons. Angiology 1980;31(8):538–41.

216. Rayan GM, Jensen C. Thoracic outlet syndrome: provocative examination maneuvers in a typical population. J Shoulder Elbow Surg 1995;4(2):113–17.

217. Plewa MC, Delinger M. The false-positive rate of thoracic outlet syndrome shoulder maneuvers in healthy subjects. Acad Emerg Med 1998;5(4):337–42.

218. Roos DB. Thoracic outlet syndromes: update 1987. Am J Surg 1987;154(6):568–73.

219. Barsotti J, Chiaroni DP, Chiaroni P. Thoracic outlet syndrome. Diagnosis by Roos' test. Presse Med 1984;13(21):1335.

220. Vin F, Koskas F, Levy D, et al. Thoracic outlet syndrome. Value of non-invasive arterial studies. Presse Med 1986;15(34): 1709–11.

221. Selvaratnam PJ, Matyas TA, Glasgow EF. Noninvasive discrimination of brachial plexus involvement in upper limb pain. Spine 1994;19(1):26–33.

222. Coppieters M, Stappaerts K, Janssens K, et al. Reliability of detecting 'onset of pain' and 'submaximal pain' during neural provocation testing of the upper quadrant. Physiother Res Int 2002;7(3):146–56.

223. Kleinrensink GJ, Stoeckart R, Mulder PG, et al. Upper limb tension tests as tools in the diagnosis of nerve and plexus lesions. Anatomical and biomechanical aspects. Clin Biomech (Bristol, Avon) 2000;15(1):9–14.

224. Quintner JL. A study of upper limb pain and paraesthesiae following neck injury in motor vehicle accidents: assessment of the brachial plexus tension test of Elvey. Br J Rheumatol 1989;28(6):528–33.

225. Shacklock MO. Positive upper limb tension test in a case of surgically proven neuropathy: analysis and validity. Man Ther 1996;1(3):154–61.

226. Wainner RS, Fritz JM, Irrgang JJ, et al. Reliability and diagnostic accuracy of the clinical examination and patient self-report measures for cervical radiculopathy. Spine 2003;28(1):52–62.

227. Coppieters MW, Stappaerts KH, Wouters LL, et al. Aberrant protective force generation during neural provocation testing and the effect of treatment in patients with neurogenic cervicobrachial pain. J Manipulative Physiol Ther 2003;26(2): 99–106.

228. Coppieters MW, Kurz K, Mortensen TE, et al. The impact of neurodynamic testing on the perception of experimentally induced muscle pain. Man Ther 2005;10(1):52–60.

229. Shacklock M. Clinical neurodynamics. Philadelphia: Elsevier Butterworth Heinemann; 2005.

230. Sucher BM, Heath DM. Thoracic outlet syndrome – a myofascial variant: Part 3. Structural and postural considerations. J Am Osteopath Assoc 1993;93(3):334, 340–5.

231. Sobush DC, Simoneau GG, Dietz KE, et al. The Lennie Test for measuring scapular position in healthy young adult females: a reliability and validity study. J Orthop Sports Phys Ther 1996;23(1):39–50.

232. Sahrmann S. Diagnóstico y tratameinto de las alteraciones del movimiento. Badalona: Paidotribo; 2006.

233. Kibler WB. The role of the scapula in athletic shoulder function. Am J Sports Med 1998;26(2):325–37.

234. Kibler WB, McMullen J. Scapular dyskinesis and its relation to shoulder pain. J Am Acad Orthop Surg 2003;11(2):142–51.

235. Watson LA, Pizzari T, Balster S. Thoracic outlet syndrome part 1: clinical manifestations, differentiation and treatment pathways. Man Ther 2009;14(6):586–95.

236. Matsumura JS, Rilling WS, Pearce WH, et al. Helical computed tomography of the normal thoracic outlet. J Vasc Surg 1997;26(5):776–83.

237. Remy-Jardin M, Doyen J, Remy J, et al. Functional anatomy of the thoracic outlet: evaluation with spiral CT. Radiology 1997;205(3):843–51.

238. Wadhwani R, Chaubal N, Sukthankar R, et al. Color Doppler and duplex sonography in 5 patients with thoracic outlet syndrome. J Ultrasound Med 2001;20(7):795–801.

239. Gardner GP, Cordts PR, Gillespie DL, et al. Can air plethysmography accurately identify upper extremity deep venous thrombosis? J Vasc Surg 1993;18(5):808–13.

240. van Es HW. MRI of the brachial plexus. Eur Radiol 2001;11(2):325–36.

241. Smedby O, Rostad H, Klaastad O, et al. Functional imaging of the thoracic outlet syndrome in an open MR scanner. Eur Radiol 2000;10(4):597–600.

242. Demondion X, Boutry N, Drizenko A, et al. Thoracic outlet: anatomic correlation with MR imaging. AJR Am J Roentgenol 2000;175(2):417–22.

243. Charon JP, Milne W, Sheppard DG, et al. Evaluation of MR angiographic technique in the assessment of thoracic outlet syndrome. Clin Radiol 2004;59(7):588–95.

244. Pedrosa I, Aschkenasi C, Hamdan A, et al. Effort-induced thrombosis: diagnosis with three-dimensional MR venography. Emerg Radiol 2002;9(6):326–8.

245. Urschel HC Jr, Razzuk MA, Wood RE, et al. Objective diagnosis (ulnar nerve conduction velocity) and current therapy of the thoracic outlet syndrome. Ann Thorac Surg 1971;12(6):608–20.

246. Yiannikas C, Walsh JC. Somatosensory evoked responses in the diagnosis of thoracic outlet syndrome. J Neurol Neurosurg Psychiatry 1983;46(3):234–40.

247. Wilbourn AJ, Lederman RJ. Evidence for conduction delay in thoracic-outlet syndrome is challenged. N Engl J Med 1984;310(16):1052–3.

248. Veilleux M, Stevens JC, Campbell JK. Somatosensory evoked potentials: lack of value for diagnosis of thoracic outlet syndrome. Muscle Nerve 1988;11(6):571–5.

249. Baran E. Somatosensory evoked potentials: utility is assessing brachial plexopathies and thoracic outlet syndrome. In: Hunter J, Mackin E, Callahan A, editors. Rehabilitation of the hand: Surgery and therapy. 4th ed. St Louis: Mosby; 1995. p. 843–55.

250. Urschel JD, Hameed SM, Grewal RP. Neurogenic thoracic outlet syndromes. Postgrad Med J 1994;70(829):785–9.

251. Hurtevent JF. Neurophysiological explorations of thoracic outlet syndrome. Rev Med Interne 1999;20(Suppl. 5):494S–6S.

252. Passero S, Paradiso C, Giannini F, et al. Diagnosis of thoracic outlet syndrome. Relative value of electrophysiological studies. Acta Neurol Scand 1994;90(3):179–85.

253. Cuevas-Trisan RL, Cruz-Jimenez M. Provocative F waves may help in the diagnosis of thoracic outlet syndrome: a report of three cases. Am J Phys Med Rehabil 2003;82(9):712–15.

254. Seror P. Medial antebrachial cutaneous nerve conduction study, a new tool to demonstrate mild lower brachial plexus lesions. A report of 16 cases. Clin Neurophysiol 2004;115(10):2316–22.

255. Haghighi SS, Baradarian S, Bagheri R. Sensory and motor evoked potentials findings in patients with thoracic outlet syndrome. Electromyogr Clin Neurophysiol 2005;45(3):149–54.

256. Rousseff R, Tzvetanov P, Valkov I. Utility (or futility?) of electrodiagnosis in thoracic outlet syndrome. Electromyogr Clin Neurophysiol 2005;45(3):131–3.

257. Walsh MT. Therapist management of thoracic outlet syndrome. J Hand Ther 1994;7(2):131–44.

258. Novak CB. Conservative management of thoracic outlet syndrome. Semin Thorac Cardiovasc Surg 1996;8(2):201–7.

259. Molina JE. Combined posterior and transaxillary approach for neurogenic thoracic outlet syndrome. J Am Coll Surg 1998;187(1):39–45.

260. Sellke FW, Kelly TR. Thoracic outlet syndrome. Am J Surg 1988;156(1):54–7.

261. Fernandez E, Pallini R, Marchese E, et al. Neurosurgery of the peripheral nervous system: entrapment syndromes of the brachial plexus. Surg Neurol 2000;53(1):82–5.

262. Novak CB, Collins ED, Mackinnon SE. Outcome following conservative management of thoracic outlet syndrome. J Hand Surg Am 1995;20(4):542–8.

263. Dobrusin R. An osteopathic approach to conservative management of thoracic outlet syndromes. J Am Osteopath Assoc 1989;89(8):1046–50, 1053–7.

264. Huffman JD. Electrodiagnostic techniques for and conservative treatment of thoracic outlet syndrome. Clin Orthop Relat Res 1986;207:21–3.

265. Lindgren KA. TOS (thoracic outlet syndrome) – a challenge to conservative treatment. Nord Med 1997;112(8):283–7.

266. Köknel Talu G. Thoracic outlet syndrome. Agri 2005;17(2):5–9.

267. Coccia MR, Satiani B. Thoracic outlet syndrome. Am Fam Physician 1984;29(2):121–6.

268. Daskalakis MK. Thoracic outlet compression syndrome: current concepts and surgical experience. Int Surg 1983;68(4):337–44.

269. Lindgren KA, Oksala I. Long-term outcome of surgery for thoracic outlet syndrome. Am J Surg 1995;169(3):358–60.

270. Crotti FM, Carai A, Carai M, et al. TOS pathophysiology and clinical features. Acta Neurochir Suppl 2005;92:7–12.

271. Crawford FA Jr. Thoracic outlet syndrome. Surg Clin North Am 1980;60(4):947–56.

272. Young HA, Hardy DG. Thoracic outlet syndrome. Br J Hosp Med 1983;29(5):457, 459, 461.

273. Buonocore M, Manstretta C, Mazzucchi G, et al. The clinical evaluation of conservative treatment in patients with the thoracic outlet syndrome. G Ital Med Lav Ergon 1998;20(4):249–54.

274. Beer S, Schlegel C, Hasegawa A. Conservative therapy in thoracic outlet syndrome. Literature review and pathogenetic considerations. Schweiz Med Wochenschr 1997;127(15):617–22.

275. Nathan PA. Outcome following conservative management of thoracic outlet syndrome. J Hand Surg Am 1996;21(3):528–9.

276. Aligne C, Barral X. Rehabilitation of patients with thoracic outlet syndrome. Ann Vasc Surg 1992;6(4):381–9.

277. Pratt NE. Neurovascular entrapment in the regions of the shoulder and posterior triangle of the neck. Phys Ther 1986;66(12):1894–900.

278. Kenny RA, Traynor GB, Withington D, et al. Thoracic outlet syndrome: a useful exercise treatment option. Am J Surg 1993;165(2):282–4.

279. Wehbe MA, Leinberry CF. Current trends in treatment of thoracic outlet syndrome. Hand Clin 2004;20(1):119–21.

280. Narakas A, Bonnard C, Egloff DV. The cervico-thoracic outlet compression syndrome. Analysis of surgical treatment. Ann Chir Main 1986;5(3):195–207.

281. Wehbe MA, Schlegel JM. Nerve gliding exercises for thoracic outlet syndrome. Hand Clin 2004;20(1):51–5, vi.

282. Orset G. Evaluation of the cervicothoracobrachial outlet and results of conservative treatment. Chir Main 2000;19(4):212–17.

283. Totten PA, Hunter JM. Therapeutic techniques to enhance nerve gliding in thoracic outlet syndrome and carpal tunnel syndrome. Hand Clin 1991;7(3):505–20.

284. Crosby CA, Wehbe MA. Conservative treatment for thoracic outlet syndrome. Hand Clin 2004;20(1):43–9, vi.

285. Berthe A. Considerations on rehabilitation of cervicothoracobrachial outlet syndrome. Chir Main 2000;19(4):218–22.

286. Lindgren KA, Leino E, Hakola M, et al. Cervical spine rotation and lateral flexion combined motion in the examination of the thoracic outlet. Arch Phys Med Rehabil 1990;71(5):343–4.

287. Lindgren KA, Leino E, Manninen H. Cervical rotation lateral flexion test in brachialgia. Arch Phys Med Rehabil 1992;73(8):735–7.

288. Lindgren KA, Leino E, Manninen H. Cineradiography of the hypomobile first rib. Arch Phys Med Rehabil 1989;70(5):408–9.

289. Wilbourn AJ. Thoracic outlet syndrome surgery causing severe brachial plexopathy. Muscle Nerve 1988;11(1):66–74.

290. Han S, Yildirim E, Dural K, et al. Transaxillary approach in thoracic outlet syndrome: the importance of resection of the first-rib. Eur J Cardiothorac Surg 2003;24(3):428–33.

291. Sharp WJ, Nowak LR, Zamani T, et al. Long-term follow-up and patient satisfaction after surgery for thoracic outlet syndrome. Ann Vasc Surg 2001;15(1):32–6.

292. Jakubietz MG, Jakubietz RG, Gruenert JG, et al. Bilateral non-traumatic second rib fracture after bilateral first rib resection for TOS. Thorax 2005;60(3):259–60.

293. Leffert RD. Complications of surgery for thoracic outlet syndrome. Hand Clin 2004;20(1):91–8.

294. Pupka A, Rucinski A, Skora J, et al. The treatment of subclavian artery compression with the use of ringed polytetrafluoroethylene vascular prostheses. Polim Med 2004;34(4):53–61.

295. Melliere D, Becquemin JP, Etienne G, et al. Severe injuries resulting from operations for thoracic outlet syndrome: can they be avoided? J Cardiovasc Surg (Torino) 1991;32(5):599–603.

296. Schneider DB, Dimuzio PJ, Martin ND, et al. Combination treatment of venous thoracic outlet syndrome: open surgical decompression and intraoperative angioplasty. J Vasc Surg 2004;40(4):599–603.

297. Machleder HI. Evaluation of a new treatment strategy for Paget-Schroetter syndrome: spontaneous thrombosis of the axillary-subclavian vein. J Vasc Surg 1993;17(2):305–15, discussion 316–17.

298. Schneider DB, Curry TK, Eichler CM, et al. Percutaneous mechanical thrombectomy for the management of venous thoracic outlet syndrome. J Endovasc Ther 2003;10(2):336–40.

299. Angle N, Gelabert HA, Farooq MM, et al. Safety and efficacy of early surgical decompression of the thoracic outlet for Paget-Schroetter syndrome. Ann Vasc Surg 2001;15(1):37–42.

300. Wood VE, Ellison DW. Results of upper plexus thoracic outlet syndrome operation. Ann Thorac Surg 1994;58(2):458–61.

301. Degeorges R, Reynaud C, Becquemin JP. Thoracic outlet syndrome surgery: long-term functional results. Ann Vasc Surg 2004;18(5):558–65.

302. Samarasam I, Sadhu D, Agarwal S, et al. Surgical management of thoracic outlet syndrome: a 10-year experience. ANZ J Surg 2004;74(6):450–4.

303. Yavuzer S, Atinkaya C, Tokat O. Clinical predictors of surgical outcome in patients with thoracic outlet syndrome operated on via transaxillary approach. Eur J Cardiothorac Surg 2004;25(2):173–8.

304. Leffert RD, Perlmutter GS. Thoracic outlet syndrome. Results of 282 transaxillary first rib resections. Clin Orthop 1999;368:66–79.

305. Adson A. Surgical treatment of symptoms produced by cervical ribs and the scalenus anticus muscle. Surg Gynecol Obstet 1947;85:687.

306. Sanders RJ, Pearce WH. The treatment of thoracic outlet syndrome: a comparison of different operations. J Vasc Surg 1989;10(6):626–34.

307. Sanders RJ, Hammond SL. Supraclavicular first rib resection and total scalenectomy: technique and results. Hand Clin 2004;20(1):61–70.

308. Toso C, Robert J, Berney T, et al. Thoracic outlet syndrome: influence of personal history and surgical technique on long-term results. Eur J Cardiothorac Surg 1999;16(1):44–7.

309. Mattson RJ. Surgical approach to anterior scalenectomy. Hand Clin 2004;20(1):57–60.

310. Atasoy E. Recurrent thoracic outlet syndrome. Hand Clin 2004;20(1):99–105.

311. Ambrad-Chalela E, Thomas GI, Johansen KH. Recurrent neurogenic thoracic outlet syndrome. Am J Surg 2004;187(4):505–10.

312. Wishchuk JR, Dougherty CR. Therapy after thoracic outlet release. Hand Clin 2004;20(1):87–90, vii.

313. Snider HC, King GD. Minnesota Multiphasic Personality Inventory as a predictor of operative results in thoracic outlet syndrome. South Med J 1986;79(12):1527–30.

4

CLINICAL APPROACH TO CERVICAL FACET JOINT SYNDROME

RAFAEL TORRES CUECO

Cervical facet syndrome can be defined as the signs and symptoms derived from the pathology or dysfunction of the facet joints. These joints, despite having own innervation and being a potential source of symptoms, have barely been addressed until recently.[1] From a clinical perspective, there has been a growing interest in the study of zygapophyseal joints in recent years because they are the most prevalent source of neck pain and they may be involved in cervical pain following whiplash injuries.[1–13]

Intervertebral disc pathology has captured the interest of clinicians and surgeons, placing the study of the facet joints in the section of degenerative changes of the cervical spine. Often the signs and symptoms of these joints are wrongly attributed to a number of varying entities, using very non-specific terms such as cervical contracture, if a flattening of the lordosis is observed, or cervical spondylosis, in the event degenerative radiological signs.

These diagnoses are quite unspecific and inappropriate. The diagnosis of cervical contracture is often used when tenderness in the cervical musculature is detected, since the role of the facet joints in the generation of pain is dismissed. Cervical spondylosis refers to degenerative changes suffered by the cervical spine. It is diagnostically inaccurate because there is a direct relationship between degenerative changes and cervical pain. Spondylotic changes are observable both in subjects with pain and in completely asymptomatic subjects.[14] In the event that these degenerative changes are responsible for the symptoms, the term 'spondylosis' fails to identify the structures generating such symptoms.

In recent decades considerable progress has been made in understanding the pathology of the facet joints and their role in the development of post-traumatic and chronic patterns of neck pain. Cervical facet syndrome is currently considered as the most common cause of symptoms in the cervical spine.

Cervical facet syndrome is the most common cause of symptoms in the cervical spine. In clinical practice, however, these symptoms are typically attributed to neck contracture, to disc pathology or cervical spondylosis.

Interest was first shown in the pathology of the facet joints in the early 20th century, attempting to establish a cause for back pain and sciatica, and not until recent decades was this syndrome studied in the cervical spine. The first author who suggested that facet joints could be a cause of pain was Goldthwait[15] in 1911. In 1933, Ghormley[16] published an article that would become famous: *Low back pain with special reference to the articular facets*. However, contrary to what the title of the paper gave to understand, it addressed a case of a subject with sciatica due to an arthritic hypertrophy of the posterior joints. Steindler and Luck[17] in 1938 injected local anaesthetic percutaneously into the area of the facets, showing that these joints could be responsible for the low back pain (LBP). Badgley[18] in 1941 and Pedersen et al.[19] in 1956 confirmed the major role of the facet joints in the patterns of LBP and sciatica. In 1956, Lazorthes[20,21] described the articular division of the posterior primary ramus of the spinal nerve, and its close contact with the articular pillars, which, according to this

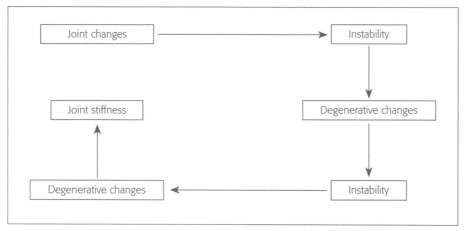

FIGURE 4-13 ■ Evolution of joint changes from a phase of joint instability to stiffness.

develops differently.[83] One of the causes of the asymmetrical degeneration of the facets is the greater traumatic injury or articular stress affecting one of the facet joints. Another cause may be the degenerative loss of morphological symmetry in the intervertebral disc, which, inducing a lateral tilt, causes asymmetrical pressure on the facet joints, which favours earlier degeneration in one of them. This pathophysiological fact explains why unilateral facet syndrome is so common. Mechanically, this asymmetrical degeneration has consequences, because in view of one joint being more unstable than the other, the asymmetric mobility favours the degenerative process (Fig. 4-14).

Facet joints in the cervical spine, because of their relative size with respect to the disc and distinctive orientation nearer to the horizontal plane, are subjected to a considerable load. This pressure per unit of surface area increases significantly when the intervertebral disc begins to show a decrease in height as a result of degenerative changes. The progressive degeneration of the intervertebral disc has a considerable influence on the development of cervical facet syndrome, favouring facet degeneration and hypertrophy and the thickening of the ligamentum flavum, of the pedicles and laminae, in an attempt to absorb increased pressure transmitted by these posterior elements.

The above description shows the existence of different stages in the evolution of facet syndrome. Yong-Hing and Kirkaldy-Willis,[86] in 1983, divided the

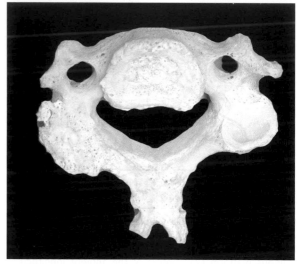

FIGURE 4-14 ■ In this vertebra we note the changes undergone by the subchondral bone and the arthritic hypertrophy of the right facet joint.

evolution of the facet degenerative process into three stages: a first stage or phase of dysfunction; a second stage or phase of instability; and a third stage or phase of stabilization (Box 4.1).

Clinically, in the first temporary dysfunction phase, the patient suffers episodes of neck pain. The instability phase is the result of changes both in the facet joint and in the intervertebral disc. The changes undergone by one joint exacerbate the changes of the other. The degeneration of articular cartilage, and its decreased height, induce laxity in the joint capsule and ligaments, increasing stress on the intervertebral disc. In turn, the changes undergone by the intervertebral disc, such as the decrease of proteoglycans and dehydration of the disc, lead to a decrease in disc height, which in turn leads to an increase in mobility between adjacent vertebrae and increased stress experienced by the facet joints.

The cervical segmental instability can be classified into two types: angular instability and translatory instability.

Previously, angular instability was considered in the event of a sagittal rotation greater than 11° and translatory instability, when this was over 3.5 mm.[87] However, Reitman et al.[88] recently demonstrated that normal cervical mobility is much higher, especially in the mid-cervical region, where sagittal rotation exceeds 15°. Angular instability should only be considered when this movement exceeds 20°. Likewise, previously translatory instability was considered when this movement was over 3.5 mm.[87] However, translation in segments C2–C3, C3–C4 and C5–C6 may be considered normal up to 4.5 mm and in segment C4–C5, up to 5.5 mm.[88]

Cervical segmental instability is classified into two types:

- angular instability, when sagittal rotation is greater than 20°.
- translatory instability, when greater than 4.5 mm.

Segmental instability is observed in the disc with grade 1 and 2 degeneration, while grades 0, 3 and 4 degeneration are less common.[89]

The duration and extent of the period of instability are entirely individualized, with a progressive trend towards the arthritic stabilization of joints. Some patients show a slight joint hypermobility, but never evolve towardS instability, while other patients develop severe instability and degenerative spondylolisthesis.

Instability implies the existence of excess, abnormal or asymmetrical mobility of the vertebral segment. These changes in joint mobility are also characteristic of a situation of joint dysfunction. Therefore, these findings on examination should raise the suspicion that the subject has a facet syndrome and not merely a joint dysfunction.

The last phase of stabilization relates to the reduction of joint mobility, which may lead to a spontaneous arthrodesis. The degenerative evolution in a triarticular complex involves the development of hypertrophic changes that will lead to stabilization. In this phase, the symptoms are generally caused by adjacent segments, which develop compensating hypermobility or is associated with degenerative stenosis of the lateral or central canal (Box 4-2).

CLINICAL PATTERN OF CERVICAL FACET SYNDROME

Degenerative disc disease and facet pathology quite often coexist in the same patient, and it is sometimes difficult to distinguish which structure is responsible for the clinical condition. Bogduk and Aprill[46] established which structure was responsible for the pain in 56 patients who had suffered trauma, noting that in 41% of them, both the facet joints and the discs were symptomatic in the same segment.

Cervical facet syndrome, as in other regions of the spine, can present two clinical patterns described as articular dysfunction and intra-articular dysfunction. Joint dysfunction is the consequence of a functional disorder or post-traumatic degenerative changes, globally affecting the joint elements, while intra-articular dysfunction involves an alteration of the meniscoid tissue interposed between the normal articular surfaces, such as synovial folds or intra-articular, or pathological articular surfaces, such as intra-articular loose bodies. Besides these two clinical patterns, the degenerative pathology of the facet joints can lead to lateral canal stenosis and cervical radiculopathy.[84]

Joint dysfunction

Patients with facet syndrome may refer different symptoms, the most common being cervical pain and stiffness, subjective sensation of cervical unsteadiness, headache and pain referred to the upper thoracic spine and upper arm. These symptoms are non-specific and, alone, do not tell us whether the origin really lies in these joints or in the intervertebral disc, so that without proper examination these two clinical situations cannot be differentiated.

As in other somatic pains, facet pain is typically dull and diffuse, perceived locally, and very often accompanied by referred pain. This diffuse nature is probably due to the dual-type innervation of the cervical facets – namely, segmental and multisegmental innervation[32] – and the very nature of referred pain (see Chapter 5 of Volume 1).

A typical feature of facet pain that helps in the differential diagnosis is its one-sidedness. Just as discogenic pain may be unilateral or bilateral, depending on where the disc tissue injury[90] is located, facet pain is perceived always on one side and is ipsilateral to the affected facet joint.[1,24,25,46,91]

Typically, facet pain during the acute phase is always experienced locally and intensely, whereas during the chronic phase, local pain may be absent and the patient may only experience referred pain in a localized area away from the joint.[92]

Facet pain patterns

Thanks to the work of Bogduk and Marsland,[24] Dwyer et al.,[25] Aprill et al.[26] and Fukui et al.[93] we are able to identify the patterns of referred pain from the facet joints.[94]

The first facet pain maps were described by Dwyer et al.[25] The results of this study were similar to those previously obtained by Bogduk and Marsland[24] in 1988 (Fig. 4-15). Subsequently, Aprill et al.[26] showed how they were clinically useful to predict the location of the symptomatic segment in subjects with facet

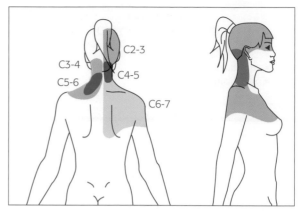

FIGURE 4-15 ■ Patterns of referred facet joint pain described by Bogduk and Marsland. *(Adapted from Bogduk and Marsland.[24])*

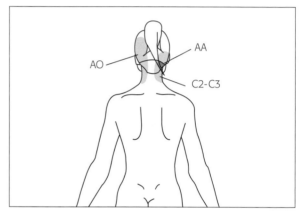

FIGURE 4-16 ■ Referred pain patterns of the atlanto-occipital (AO) and atlantoaxial (AA) joints. *(Adapted from Dreyfuss et al.[96])*

neck pain. These pain patterns were later confirmed by Fukui et al.[93] These authors determined the area of referred pain from the facet joints C0–C1 to C7–T1 in 61 patients with cervicalgia, using the infiltration of a contrast medium, and electrical stimulation of the medial branch of the posterior ramus of the spinal nerve. Subsequently, Fukui et al.[95] studied the pattern of referred pain in the upper thoracic region. The results of this work are also mentioned because the pattern of referred pain in this region overlaps considerably with those of the lower cervical levels. We also include referred pain patterns of atlantoaxial and atlanto-occipital joints described by Dreyfuss et al.[96] (Fig. 4-16). However, it should be noted how often referred pain of facet origin reaches the elbow and even more distally, mainly in the lower segments.

Referred pain patterns are schematically shown below[93] (Fig. 4-17):

- The referred pain pattern of joint C0–C1 and lateral joints C1–C2 are similar to those of the occiput and superior posterolateral cervical region.
- C2–C3 facet joints often refer pain to the frontotemporal region of the same side; however, pain tends to concentrate and be more intense in the occipital region.
- Pain from the C3–C4 facet joints normally concentrates in the posterolateral region of the neck.
- Pain from the C4–C5 facet joints tends to focus and be more intense at the base of the neck.
- Pain from the facet joints C5–C6 concentrates in the supraspinous fossa.
- Pain from the facet joints C6–C7 tends to concentrate in the upper medial border of the scapula.
- Pain from the facet joints C7–T1 tends to focus on the medial border of the scapula.
- The T1–T2 joint may also refer pain to the suprascapular region, the superior angle of the scapula and to the mid-scapular region.
- The T2–T3 joint refers pain exclusively to the mid-scapular region.

These pain patterns correspond to those frequently shown by subjects with persistent neck pain and may be useful to identify symptomatic posterior joints in patients with neck pain.[24]

According to some authors, when interpreting these maps of referred pain, the area to which the pain spreads is not important, yet the point where the patient feels pain more consistently and more intensely. This point where the pain seems to be concentrated is to be compared with maps of pain to identify the cervical segment involved[97] (Fig. 4-18). It is important to note that the maps obtained in the subject after stimulation of the facet joints do not appear to fully correspond to those observed in symptomatic patients. As shown recently by Cooper et al.,[98] the area of patients' referred pain is more variable than in normal subjects.

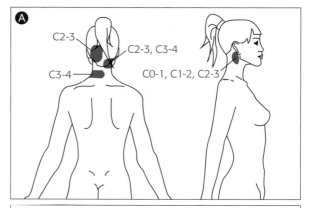

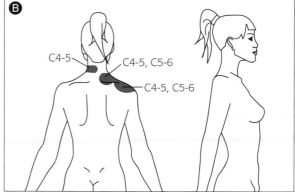

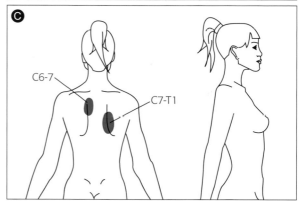

FIGURE 4-17 ■ Patterns of referred facet joint pain described by Fukui et al.[93] Upper and middle cervical spine (A), middle cervical spine (B) and lower cervical spine (C).

Also, as with any map of referred pain, one should be very cautious when determining that the referred pain comes from a specific joint segment. Referred pain is a manifestation of central sensitization and, therefore, depends on the magnitude of neuroplastic changes suffered by a subject.

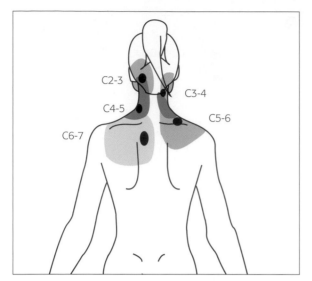

FIGURE 4-18 ■ Patterns of referred facet joint pain and circled areas where pain is felt more consistently and more extensively. *As amended by Bogduk and McGuirk.*[97]

In addition, these pain patterns alone are not able to demonstrate that the source of pain is in the facet joints and are merely a guide which roughly indicates the cervical region where symptoms originate. Recent studies using discography have shown that pain patterns of the cervical intervertebral discs are essentially the same as those of the facet joints of the same segmental level.[90,99–101] Hence, the advantage of the maps of referred pain does not lie in establishing what structure is responsible for referred pain, but only in pointing out the approximate area of the cervical region where it originates.[98,102] Likewise, a patient with chronic pain may present a considerably variable and more widely distributed pattern of referred pain.

Trigger factors

The factors that trigger or aggravate the pain are all those postures and movements involving extension or rotation and side-bending: for example, when the subject performs repetitive movements or sustained positions involving any of these movements. Sustained sitting, as in other dysfunctional or pathological situations, tends to be poorly tolerated. Very often patients have difficulty getting comfortable in bed at night and often 'fight with their pillow'. When this happens, the patient wakes up with a painful stiff neck.

Movements or positions that alleviate symptoms are typically those involving a facet divergence and decreased articular pressure. The subject, if not in an acute and irritable phase at the time, finds relief in movements or positions such as flexion or side-bending to the non-painful side. Some patients adopt the habit of rubbing their neck, which momentarily may produce a sense of relief but can eventually lead to joint hypermobility and joint hypersensitivity. Pain is initially episodic but can develop into persistent pain.

Pain patterns of facet origin vary, such as acute joint dysfunction, intra-articular joint dysfunction, convergence joint dysfunction, divergence joint dysfunction, hyperconvergence joint dysfunction or mixed dysfunction pattern. All these patterns are described in Chapter 6 of Volume 1. Whether joint dysfunction is associated with functional instability or motor control deficits should be further analysed.

Intra-articular dysfunctions

A common clinical situation in the cervical spine is the acute block or wry neck. This situation is often the result of a mechanical malfunction of the posterior joint.[103] This clinical pattern, which can be termed as intra-articular dysfunction, corresponds to a mechanical alteration of the tissue interposed between the articular surfaces, such as meniscoid structures or synovial folds. These structures, despite their small size, have a significant clinical significance in the cervical spine,[104] the mechanical block in this region being more frequent than in the lumbar region. Because of the innervation, they can trigger neck pain patterns.[57,104] It has been shown that cervical facet meniscoids have a nociceptive innervation,[57] which has been previously noted in the lumbar spine,[105–111] and may therefore be involved in cervical pain patterns.[57,104] At present, these structures are believed to be responsible for acute wry neck,[112,113] and they could be involved in joint stiffness.[113]

The clinical manifestation of an intra-articular dysfunction is an acute attack of unilateral cervical pain associated with a sudden restriction of mobility, after a sudden head movement. The individual, following a rapid and uncontrolled movement, perceives a sharp pain localized posterolaterally at the height of a joint pillar, which immediately or after a few hours, causes the blocking of cervical mobility. The patient shows an antalgic attitude in flexion, side-bending and rotation in the opposite direction to the injured side, and a singular pain appears at any attempt to correct this antalgic position.

The explanation proposed for acute cervical block is specifically an entrapment or distortion of the fibroadipose meniscoid. This meniscoid, due to its proportionally large size and to the fact that it projects into the joint, may be pinched or compressed between the joint surfaces. Although according to Grieve[114] this acute block is more frequent in the C2–C3 segment, we believe that it is also common in the middle cervical region, characterized by its considerable mobility in flexion–extension and rotation. Hence, there seems to be a relationship between mobility and acute cervical blocking, which would explain their greater frequency in children and women, probably because of their greater laxity.

Previously, authors like Koss and Wolf,[115] Scher,[116] and Giles[117] proposed that the cause of these sudden blocks was the entrapment or pinching of the meniscus between the two joint surfaces. According to Kos and Wolf,[115] when the meniscus is trapped between the joint surfaces, due to the collagen density at the ends, it can deform the articular cartilage, which prevents it from being released during the physiological movement of the cervical spine. The meniscus also undergoes changes in its structure, so that its end becomes progressively more fibrous, which further hinders its release.

However, authors like Bogduk and Jull[118] consider that this interpretation is mistaken, since this structure is able to withstand compression. They propose that articular facet divergence movements, especially when unilateral, as in coupled bending and ipsilateral rotation movements, result in the meniscus sliding out of the joint. The return movement to neutral should be accompanied by sliding of the meniscus within the joint. Blocking occurs because during this return movement, the meniscus is unable to re-enter the joint, remaining folded between the joint capsule and the margin of the joint (Fig. 4-19). This could trigger the pain by direct compression of the articular meniscus and the increased pressure of the capsule, accompanied by a reflex muscle spasm.[118–120] This explanation is consistent with the fact that blocking does not occur during movements that induce articular divergence, but rather in return movements to the neutral position requiring convergence.

Any movement that quickly causes the gapping and opening of the joint space enables the reinsertion of the meniscus. This action can be effectively achieved with high-speed manipulation. This technique, always observing the analgesic pattern in slight flexion, uses as main parameters contralateral bending and ipsilateral rotation, wherein a thrust in rotation associated with a small translation is recommended, allowing a wide articular gapping that is capable of releasing the menisci, enabling its reinsertion into the joint. This technique is described below. Although there are still not sufficiently precise imaging tests that allow us to visualize the articular meniscus lock, this is an attractive theory because it is consistent with the effectiveness of joint manipulation.[118,120]

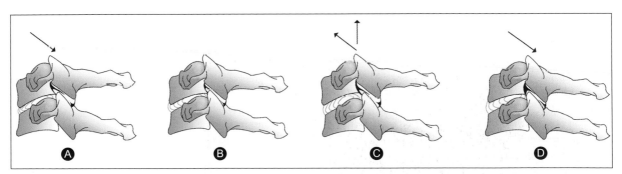

FIGURE 4-19 ■ Acute cervical blocking occurs because during a movement of facet convergence (A) the intra-articular meniscus is unable to re-enter the joint (B), becoming retracted between the joint capsule and the joint margin. A gapping and divergence manipulation (C) is able to release the meniscoid and reinsert it into the joint space (D).

Regarding the role of menisci in cervical stiffness, Mercer[113] suggests that, in addition, they may favour the development of intra-articular adhesions following an injury due to the proliferation of adipose tissue, as in other joints. They could, therefore, be related to cervical rigidity clinically observed, which could cause a hypomobile joint dysfunction.[121] Stiffness may obviously also be the result of a joint haemorrhage due to a dilaceration of the joint capsule or a subchondral fracture.[122]

When a subject frequently suffers from these acute blocks, the existence of a situation of dysfunctional joint hypermobility should be suspected, which must be treated with a muscular stabilization programme.

Differential diagnosis between facet cervical and discogenic

Whenever a patient reports a wry neck, a differential diagnosis must be conducted to distinguish between that resulting from a facet intra-articular dysfunction and that resulting from an acute discogenic syndrome. Distinguishing between facet and discogenic wry neck is critical because treatment differs considerably. For example, manipulation in some cases may be an appropriate treatment for facet pain, while this procedure may aggravate symptoms of discogenic origin.[123] Although the antalgic position is similar in both cases, it is not difficult to differentiate them, as they differ in some aspects (Table 4-2).

The nature of the pain may help in the differential diagnosis. While discogenic pain is typically deep, diffuse and difficult to locate, facet pain is much more localized, and the patient may even point out the responsible joint. In both cases the pain can be intense; however, discogenic pain takes on a different nature – it is accompanied by a feeling of discomfort, being more unpleasant and difficult to bear.

The onset of facet torticollis is directly related to a sudden or quick movements or a posture, while in the case of discogenic wry neck there is not necessarily a prior history of mechanical stress.

Facet symptoms appear immediately, but become worse after a few hours, with postures or movements that irritate the facet-affected joint, while in the case of discogenic pain there is a characteristic latency period between the irritative movement and the onset of pain. For facet torticollis, the severe symptoms begin to subside after approximately 48 hours, although complete remission in some cases may take several weeks. In discogenic torticollis, symptoms worsen progressively, reaching maximum severity after a few days of onset of symptoms.

Facet torticollis typically involves a sharp restriction when the movement exceeds a certain extent, while in the discogenic type, restriction of mobility is the result of a pain-avoidance attitude resulting from the intensity of symptoms and does not always occur in the same joint range amplitude.

TABLE 4-2		
Differentiating facet and discogenic torticollis		
	Facet torticollis	**Discogenic torticollis**
Pain quality	Localized	Deep, diffuse and difficult to locate
Intensity	Variable from mild to severe	Intense, hard to bear, associated with a feeling of discomfort
Settling of pain	Rapid, associated with a movement or posture	Progressive, prior history of mechanical stress not necessary
Onset of pain	Immediate	Latency period
Remission of symptoms	After 48 hours	Sometimes lasting several weeks
Cause of restricted movement	Mechanical	Severity of pain
Location of the joint segment responsible	Simple Response to provocation tests in facet joints	Complex No painful response to palpation or to provocation tests in facet joints
Distribution of symptoms	Unilateral	Unilateral or bilateral and always diffuse

On clinical examination of a facet syndrome, it is not particularly difficult to locate the facet joint responsible, whereas discogenic disorders are typically not painful on palpation or in provocation tests of the posterior joints.

The distribution of symptoms differs in an acute facet syndrome, wherein although referred pain is not uncommon, focal joint pain is more severe. The patient with acute facet pain can often point out the exact joint responsible. Conversely, as discogenic pain is diffuse, the patient tends to point out a large area of the upper trapezius and shoulder region, usually without any cervical pain. While an attempt to correct the analgesic pattern in a subject with facet pain cause the local joint pain to be immediately reproduced, in a subject with discogenic pain, the pain response is often distally referred to the thoracic region.

Facet syndrome and radiculopathy

The facet joints may be responsible for radiculopathy resulting from joint hypertrophy and subsequent stenosis, which has already been discussed in Chapter 1. But this clinical situation may also be due, though less frequently, to the development of a synovial cyst from the joint capsule of the cervical facets.[124,125]

Synovial cysts usually grow gradually, allowing an adaptation of the neural tissue, and only if this is large and grows rapidly will it result in radiculopathy,[124,126,127] and even in cervical myelopathy.[128,129] These synovial cysts can appear in any area of the cervical spine, including the upper portion,[130,131] although they are much more prevalent in the lower portion[125,132–140] and, specifically, in the C7–T1 segment.[125,133,134,139] This is probably due to the mechanical stress suffered by these joints in being located in a transition region between an extremely mobile and a less mobile area. The cause of the formation of synovial cysts is interpreted by some authors as secondary to excessive articular movement,[141] while other authors believe that it is the result of degenerative changes experienced by the joint.[125,135]

Facet syndrome and headache

The pathology or dysfunction of the facet joints can also manifest clinically as a headache (Fig. 4-20). The concept of headache as a result of a disorder of these joints was introduced by Bogduk, Marsland, Dwyer, Bovim, Lord and Barnsley et al.[25,29,142–144] These authors

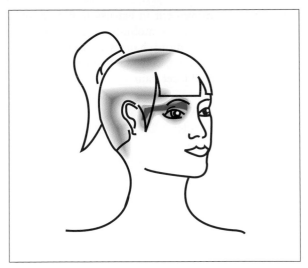

FIGURE 4-20 ■ Headache is a common manifestation of a facet syndrome of the first cervical segments.

demonstrated the remission of chronic headache patterns after the selective blocking of the third cervical nerve. Since then the relationship between headache and facet pathology has been widely studied.[1,28,36,52,142,143,145–155] According to Drottning et al.,[156] 85% of patients with chronic cervicogenic headaches had suffered whiplash. Characteristically, headache appears in the first 3 days after the accident.[1] The facet joint most often responsible for the headache is C2–C3, followed by C3–C4.[25,29,36,52,151,153,157] The relationship between headache and facet joints is discussed in Chapter 7. Importantly, cervicogenic headache corresponds to a referred pain and, as such, it implies the presence of functional neuroplastic changes in the CNS.

PHYSICAL EXAMINATION

Clinical examination of facet syndrome is not particularly difficult. Examination of the regional and segmental mobility, provocation tests and palpation of the articular pillars easily reveals the joint responsible for the clinical pattern.[158]

The following clinical findings, although not diagnostic, are indicative of facet neck pain: locating an articular pillar with maximum sensitivity to pressure; onset of pain with segment provocation tests; decreased range of active movement in extension and/or rotation,; restriction of joint mobility or hypermobility upon manual examination; changes in soft tissues such as increased muscle tone; and pain that corresponds to the areas of referred facet pain.

Facet syndrome clinical findings:

1. Location of articular pillar with maximum sensitivity to pressure.
2. Pain with a segmental provocation test.
3. Reduced active mobility range in extension and/or rotation.
4. Restriction of joint mobility or hypermobility upon manual examination.
5. Changes in soft tissues such as increased muscle tone.
6. Pain corresponding to areas of referred facet pain.

Identifying the facet joint(s) responsible for the patient's symptoms is achieved by assessing active mobility of the cervical spine, assisted active mobility by subregion, the use of combined movements, physiological and accessory passive mobility tests and palpation of the articular pillars. The accumulation of information obtained with each of these tests allows a fairly reliable diagnosis of the facet joint responsible for the symptoms.

The exploration begins with the assessment of the overall active mobility of the cervical spine. Initially, we assessed the movements in all three planes separately, then completing the movement passively to its maximum amplitude. Active mobility usually shows a decrease in extension and rotation movements towards the affected side, which corresponds to a standard compression or closure pattern. However, although this presentation is the most common, facet pain can be expressed with a divergence pattern due to the retraction of the joint capsule following an inflammatory situation, which will determine pain in the opening movements, not being uncommon for the subject to experience discomfort during sustained bending. If the joint has undergone degenerative changes, a mixed dysfunctional pattern can also be observed.

A joint rotation and extension movement to the painful side can be used as a provocation test, finally applying caudal overpressure. This test demonstrates a painful response to facet convergence. To locate the symptomatic joint we induce the mobility of the upper, middle and lower cervical spine separately. Initially, an isolated movement followed by rotation, side-bending and finally extension components jointly. We differentially focus the stress in convergence on the upper, middle and lower cervical spine (Fig. 4-21). This test allows us to focus the exploration on the segments likely to be responsible for the symptoms.

The identification of the facet joint responsible for the symptoms may be more accurate if we put our fingers on the articular pillar which is sensitive to palpation and we focus the extension, side-bending and rotation movements on that specific point. This test, in addition to reproducing the patient's symptoms, attempts to establish the perceived strength in our fingers, especially at the end of the movement and the emergence of muscle responses.

In order to confirm which facet joint is the source of symptoms, the patient can be asked to reproduce the position or movement that aggravates the symptoms. Starting from this position, we add and remove movement components to ultimately detect the joint responsible. For example, if the patient feels pain when extending the cervical spine, in order to establish whether the facet joint responsible is located in the middle or lower cervical spine, these movement can be performed while keeping the middle cervical spine neutral. If the patient still refers symptoms, it is deduced that the facet joint responsible is located in the lower cervical spine.

If the patient reports symptoms in the upper thoracic region during cervical and trunk rotation to the right, trunk rotation can be increased while holding this position, thus increasing symptoms if they originate in this region and decreasing them if coming from the cervical spine. Confirmation is obtained in this position by derotating the thoracic spine, whereby symptoms will decrease if coming from this region or will remain if coming from the cervical spine (Fig. 4-22).

It is interesting to analyse the painful response to *compression* (Fig. 4-23). Compression can be performed at different amplitudes of extension or extension–rotation, which allows us to evaluate the clinical situation and the evolution of facet syndrome, as well as its improvement after treatment.

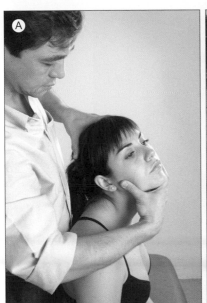
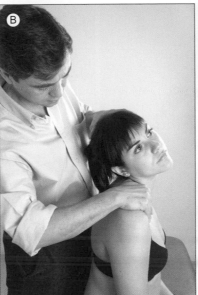
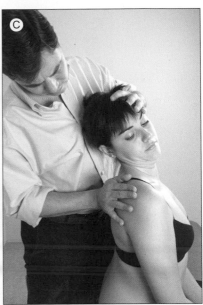

FIGURE 4-21 ■ A provocation test of facet syndrome can be a joint rotation and extension movement towards the painful side, applying an overpressure caudally at the end. Test for upper (A), middle (B) and lower (C) cervical spine.

Manual analysis of segmental mobility plays a key role in the clinical identification of the facet joint responsible for the symptoms. For manual examination it is interesting to use both joint mobility tests and auxiliary mobility tests. This type of exploration is not only important from a diagnostic point of view but also allows us to design the most appropriate type of treatment based on the information obtained.[159]

Passive segmental mobility tests must assess the amount and quality of movement, as well as symptom behaviour throughout the movement. Passive segmental mobility is evaluated in flexion–extension, side-bending and rotation. The test can be performed both in the sitting position (Fig. 4-24) and supine (Fig. 4-25). The aim is to detect if the joint responsible for the symptoms is hypo- or hypermobile. If the joint shows hypermobility, we must establish if this is due to an excessive range of motion or to an increase in the neutral zone. In the case of a hypermobile joint, it is essential to determine whether there is a local or regional hypomobility predisposing or perpetuating such excess mobility. In the event of a hypomobile joint, we must assess the direction(s) of restricted movement.

Equally important as the amount of movement is its quality: the presence of a restriction during movement, rough joint movement, cracking sounds or crepitus, the end feeling of the movement and the appearance of a pain during or at the end of the movement.

There is a significant difference in mobility and facet pain between a case of joint dysfunction and one of intra-articular dysfunction. Diagnosing intra-articular dysfunction is not at all complex. The patient shows a clear antalgic attitude with a pattern of closure, so that any attempt to correct it immediately aggravates symptoms. All movements that produce minimum convergence of the affected joint rapidly reproduce pain. Pain is commonly present throughout the range of motion and not only at end-range. Symptoms severely increase when applying minimal compression between the articular surfaces. Palpation shows an extremely sensitive soft capsular thickening

Accessory mobility tests are a useful tool in the diagnosis of facet syndrome. The relatively superficial location of these joints and the possibility of almost direct palpation means that much information can be obtained in accessory movement tests. These allow us

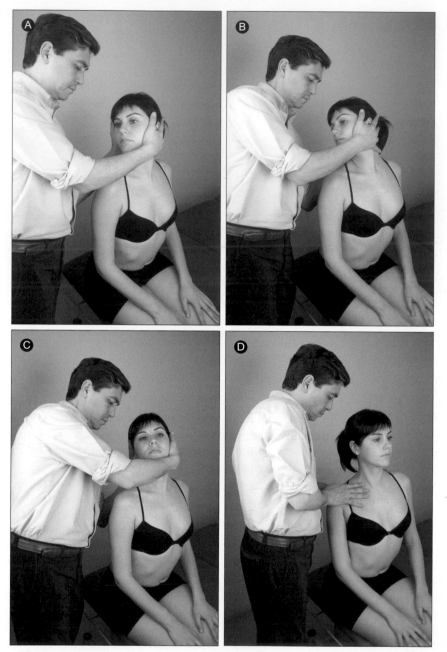

FIGURE 4-22 ■ Distinguishing symptoms between the cervical spine and the upper thoracic spine. Initially, the patient is asked to perform a maximal cervical rotation, no thoracic movement (A), and then is prompted to continue the movement using the thoracic spine (B); thoracic rotation is increased while reducing rotation in the thoracic spine (C) and, finally, the rotation is maintained only in the thoracic spine (D).

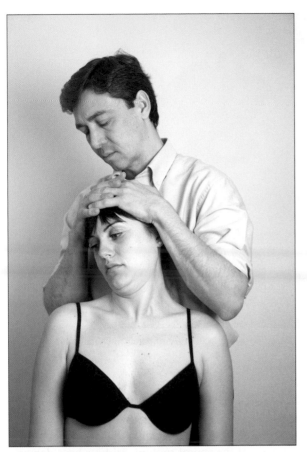

FIGURE 4-23 ■ Compression test. Before applying compression, its effect is focused with a rotation and inclination to the side of the facet joint responsible.

an appreciation of both the amount of movement and various aspects of its quality, such as resistance during the trajectory, quality at end-range, muscle spasm, allowing direct stimulation, and thus ideal for the provocation test. The most useful accessory movement test is the unilateral posteroanterior movement over the facet joint (Fig. 4-26).

The diagnostic criteria for identifying the facet joint responsible for the symptoms are (1) altered amount of perceived movement, either reduced or excessive, (2) abnormal resistance to movement, (3) abnormal quality at the end of the movement and (4) reproduction of pain reported by the patient. The onset of a muscle spasm while performing the tests may confirm that the joint is symptomatic.

Palpation

Palpation of the facet joints gives us two types of information: first, the capsular tissue texture and, secondly, its tenderness to palpation. Palpation of the articular pillars, depending on the stage of evolution, may be from a soft thickening and extremely sensitive in the case of synovitis to a hard and firm consistency in the event of articular hypertrophy (Fig. 4-27). Although the texture and resistance to palpation of tissues can provide some information, a more relevant factor is the infliction of the patient's symptoms. Palpation for tenderness of the articular pillars of the cervical zygapophyseal joints is a reasonably reliable diagnostic tool for cervical facet syndrome.[160]

Reliability of manual scan of the cervical spine

The reliability of various procedures of manual exploration of the cervical spine have been studied, such as global mobility, cervical spine joint play, tenderness over the articular pillars and passive intervertebral movements.[160–168] The range of overall mobility of the cervical spine is more reliable than the range of segmental mobility.[165,169] The only sign with a good interobserver agreement is tenderness over the articular pillars.[160]

Provocation tests are the most reliable, and palpation of changes in the soft tissues are the least reliable. However, the interobserver agreement for the manual exploration test of the cervical spine was considered poor, or at best fair.[167,170] It has also been argued that this method of examination is highly subjective, so it would not accurately detect symptomatic vertebral segments and differentiate them from asymptomatic segments.[171,172] Jull, Bogduk and Marsland[173] in 1988 conducted a study that has been widely discussed and referenced on the accuracy of a manual examination to detect and recognize a symptomatic cervical facet joint dysfunction. This study compared the accuracy of manual examination with the diagnosis obtained by an anaesthetic block. This work showed that this type of exploration is 100% specific and sensitive in diagnosing the source of facet joint pain in the hands of an experienced physiotherapist in spinal manual therapy, and can be as accurate as a diagnostic anaesthetic block.[173] However, some authors stated that the

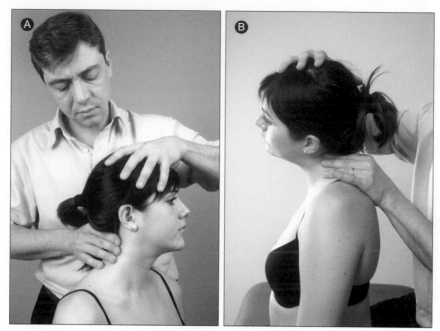

FIGURE 4-24 ■ Assessment of passive segmental mobility in the sitting position: evaluation of rotation (A) and side-bending (B).

results of this study cannot be generalized because it only demonstrated that Gwen Jull was very accurate in diagnosing facet joint pain with manual examination, and furthermore, the diagnostic blocks which at that time were conducted were not controlled diagnostic blocks.[97,167,174]

Recently, however, Schneider et al.[175] have developed a clinical decision guide in the diagnosis of cervical facet joint pain that validates the manual diagnostic procedures in cervical facet pain. In this study, four experienced physiotherapists with 10–25 years of clinical experience assessed 125 subjects prior to the diagnostic blocks. Comparative medial branch controlled blocks were used on two occasions with two different anaesthetics to reduce the high false-positive rate associated with single block procedures. For the identification of patients with pain, manual spinal examination (MSE), palpation for segmental tenderness (PST) and the extension rotation (ER) test were used.

The MSE was performed using unilateral posteroanterior accessory movements over the articular pillars from C2–C3 to C6–C7. Resistance to motion and pain was assessed. The PST of the articular pillars

was performed in the same prone position. For the ER test, the subjects were asked to fully extend their head, followed by rotation to both sides. Patients reported any pain at the end of motion. All tests have demonstrated moderate-to-excellent intrarater and interrater reliability in patients with neck pain referred for diagnostic facet joint blocks.[175]

This study found that when a patient tests positive on the MSE, PST and ER test or a combination of either the MSE/ER test or PST/ER test, the magnitude of the positive likelihood ratio provides the clinician with a small-to-moderate shift in probability that the patient has facet joint-mediated pain. In particular, a positive cluster of the MSE, PST and ER test improves the likelihood of targeting facet joint blocks to the proper candidates. A positive stand-alone finding on any of these three test lacks the diagnostic accuracy to diagnose facet joint-mediated pain. Interestingly, the lowest negative likelihood ratio was associated with the PST test, which means that if a patient tests negative in this test, there is a large and notable shift in probability that the patient does not have facet joint-mediated pain.

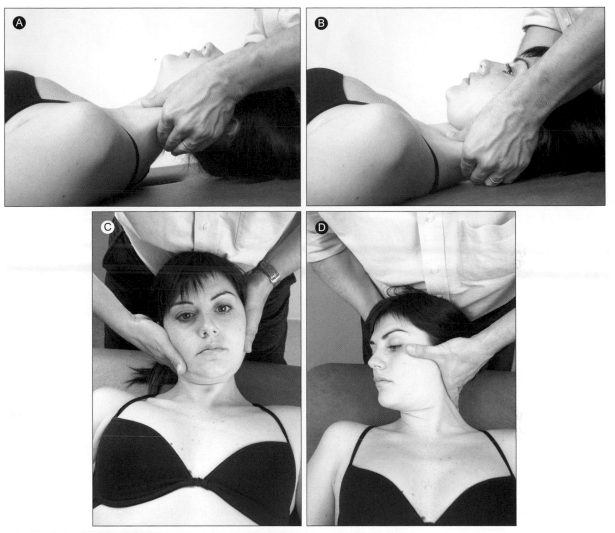

FIGURE 4-25 ■ Assessment of supine passive segmental mobility: evaluation of flexion and extension (A) and (B) side-bending (C) and rotation (D).

Understanding the development of facet syndrome requires an analysis of the possible regional and postural predisposing factors. It is essential to analyse the regional balance of the cervical spine and of the thoracic spine. Knowledge of the characteristic pattern of facet pain and accurate scanning techniques are suitable tools that enable a therapist to perform a reliable diagnosis.

IMAGING TECHNIQUES

Mechanical dysfunctions, as well as traumatic or degenerative diseases of the facet joints, may be a common cause of persistent neck pain in the absence of objective signs shown in an X-ray or through other diagnostic imaging techniques. A number of clinical and experimental studies have shown that, following

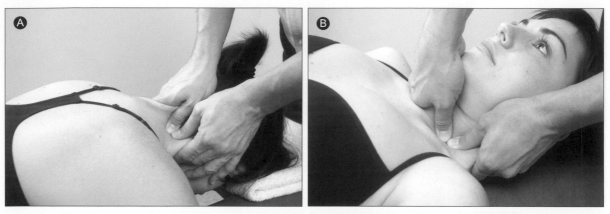

FIGURE 4-26 ■ Accessory movement tests: unilateral pressure posteroanterior (A), and the unilateral pressure anteroposterior on the facet joint (B).

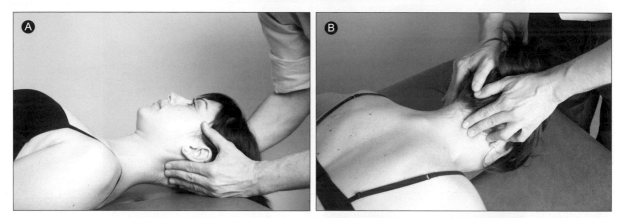

FIGURE 4-27 ■ Palpation of the facet joints supine (A) and prone (B).

traumatic accidents such as whiplash, various injuries of the facet joints occur, such as rupture of the joint capsule, haemarthrosis and fractures of the articular cartilage and subchondral bone, which are not detected by diagnostic imaging methods.[3,5,7,60,176–178]

The information on facet joints obtained from X-ray, CT and MRI is scarce in relation to facet syndrome, except in its last stage, in which degenerative changes of the joint are significant.[27,46,172,178,179] We must insist, however, that there is no correspondence between these degenerative changes and the presence of symptoms.

In radiographic studies, the oblique projection allows us to better visualize the facet joints (Fig. 4-28). The articular changes that can be observed correspond to the evolution of a degenerative process:

pinching of the joint space, subchondral bone sclerosis and joint osteophytes. These changes can also be observed in the lateral projection (Figs 4-29 and 4-30). Signs of joint disease found in the X-ray, CT and MRI are scarcity of the joint line, synovial cysts, yellow ligament hypertrophy, osteophytes, vacuum bubbles and geodes. MRI shows articular hypertrophy, thickening of the joint capsule and ligamentum flavum. We insist that these degenerative changes can occur without the origin of the pain necessarily being in the facet joints.

INVASIVE DIAGNOSTIC TECHNIQUES

The limited diagnostic usefulness of imaging techniques, and distrust of the diagnostic possibilities

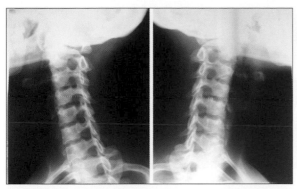

FIGURE 4-28 ■ The oblique projection is useful for observing the articular facets and their possible involvement in a lateral canal stenosis.

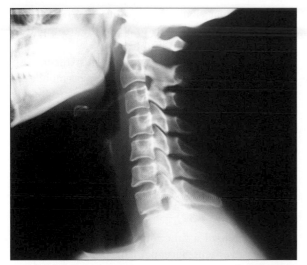

FIGURE 4-29 ■ A lateral radiograph showing the morphology of facet joints.

of methods of manual scan, has led some authors to consider that the only reliable methods in the diagnosis of cervical facet pain are anaesthetic blocks and articular infiltration.[29,46,102,153,179–182] However, these techniques do not have the specificity from a diagnostic point of view and are not usually considered.[183–185]

The diagnosis is made either by infiltrating anaesthetic into the facet joint[157] (Fig. 4-31) or by an anaesthetic block of the medial division of the posterior branch.[29,172,184] Full pain relief implies that its origins lies in the facet joints. However, this procedure, in practice, has some problems, such as false positives and negatives following a technical failure, the placebo component and administration of medication during the technique. For a diagnostic confirmation, controlled comparative diagnostic blocks are required. For this purpose, two blocks are performed randomly, one using a short-duration anaesthetic (2% lidocaine) and another using a long-duration anesthestic (0.5% bupivacaine).[31,36,52,179,180,184] The response is considered positive when full pain relief for at least 2 hours is obtained with lidocaine and for least 3 hours with bupivacaine. When no comparative blocks are used, the percentage of false positives can be quite high. Specifically, the percentage of false-positive diagnosis using a single block can reach 27%.[184] These techniques require certain technical means not always available and trained physicians.

Anaesthetic block is currently preferred to articular infiltration, as it is a simpler procedure than accessing the interior of the joint with a needle, particularly when the joint presents degenerative changes that tighten it.[27,46,172,178]

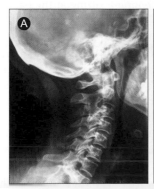

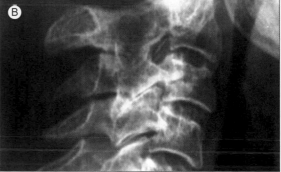

FIGURE 4-30 ■ This lateral radiograph shows degenerative changes in the C3–C4 segment (A). A larger image (B).

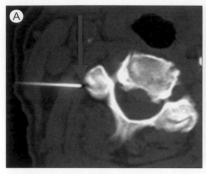 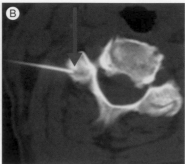 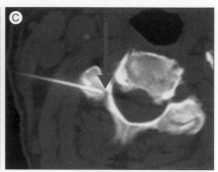

FIGURE 4-31 ■ (A–C) The diagnosis of a cervical facet syndrome can be confirmed with an anaesthetic infiltrated into the facet joint.

CONSERVATIVE TREATMENT

Despite the development of invasive techniques in recent decades, conservative treatment is still the choice for most patients with pain of facet origin. Invasive techniques should be reserved for cases that do not respond to conservative treatment, or to reduce the patient's symptoms and starting treatment promptly. This section addresses some treatment techniques that can be used in cases of non-complex cervical facet pain. The management of patients with symptoms suggestive of facet pain but with a complex clinical pattern or whiplash-associated disorders is discussed in Chapters 9 and 11.

The aim of manual therapy techniques depends on the exploratory findings. First, it is essential to detect the cervical segments responsible for the symptoms. The second aim is to establish if it is a hypomobile or hypermobile dysfunction, and ultimately to determine the specific pattern of joint dysfunction presented by the patient: divergence, convergence, hyperconvergence or combined. Faced with a hypermobile dysfunction, we must establish whether it is secondary or perpetuated by the existence of stiffness in adjacent segments. The management of motor deficits that may be associated with cervical facet pain is discussed in Chapters 5 and 6. Also, somatosensory deficits that may be present in this type of patient are discussed in Chapter 8.

Manual therapy of articular dysfunctions

Facet joint dysfunction treatment must adapt to the chronic, acute or subacute condition. The fact that the articular pillars are accessible to palpation allows us to identify articular changes and joint tenderness. These palpatory findings allow us to adapt the treatment to the patient's clinical condition.

As already discussed above, we must distinguish whether the dysfunction is hypo- or hypermobile. In the case of a hypomobile joint, choice of technique depends on the patient's clinical condition. If the subject has a moderate-to-severe pain and high irritability, physiological movement and accessory movement techniques in moderate amplitude and without pain (grades I and II) are suitable.

Example of articular technique for pain modulation (Fig. 4-32)

As an example of a functional technique that can be used in cases of acute facet pain, the following has been chosen: the patient reported pain in the right facet joint C4–C5 during rotational movements and right side-bending.

Therapist's position: sitting at the patient's head.
Patient's position: supine.
Procedure: the therapist places the ball of the second finger on the right C4–C5 facet joint. With his left hand, with a fronto-temporal grip, he slowly directs the patient's cervical spine to left rotation and bending in a moderate amplitude, trying to focus this movement on the C4–C5 segment. Then, he makes small changes in the position of the head, seeking a decrease in the palpable tension in the right facet joint, optionally adding a slight compression. All these adjustments should entail an improvement in patient symptoms. This position should be maintained for between 1 and

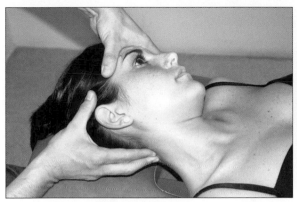

FIGURE 4-32 ■ Articular technique for pain modulation.

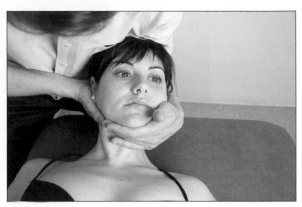

FIGURE 4-34 ■ Technique of physiological motion in rotation for an ipsilateral facet divergence.

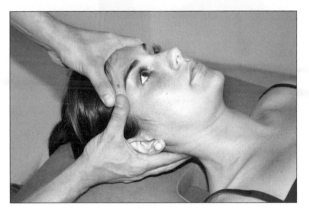

FIGURE 4-33 ■ Articular and compression technique on the articular pillar for pain modulation.

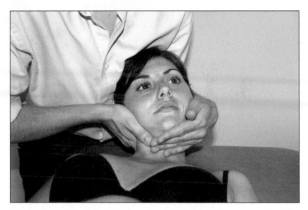

FIGURE 4-35 ■ Technique of physiological motion in side-bending for a contralateral facet divergence.

3 minutes. Finally, while monitoring with the second finger of the right hand and avoiding any symptoms, the therapist slowly and progressively takes the patient's cervical spine to a neutral position.

Subsequently, a technique that can used is to induce a modulation of the facet joint symptoms by performing a low-intensity compression, while gradually and painlessly taking the facet joint towards its motion barrier (Fig. 4-33).

In cases with prevailing stiffness, it is necessary to use techniques aimed at obtaining full and painless mobility. Initially, always start with a physiological and accessory movement applied in the direction of the restriction or motor barrier, adapted to the patient's clinical condition.

Dysfunctional patterns involving a facet joint vary widely: convergence joint dysfunction, divergence joint dysfunction pattern, hyperconvergence joint dysfunction pattern and mixed dysfunction pattern. The manipulative procedures applied to each clinical situation are discussed in Volume 1, Chapter 12, so each of the techniques will not be described in detail here and we merely mention some of the therapeutic possibilities by way of example.

In order to obtain facet divergence, physiological movements can be used in rotation (Fig. 4-34) or contralateral bending (Fig. 4-35), whose amplitude is determined by the patient's clinical condition.

To treat both an excess of lack of articular convergence or divergence, a unilateral facet sliding

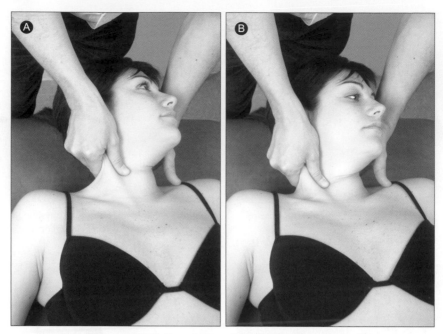

FIGURE 4-36 ■ (A,B) Unilateral facet sliding manoeuvre to treat divergence.

manoeuvre can be used. For divergence, the patient is positioned in contralateral cervical rotation (Fig. 4-36) and, for convergence, in ipsilateral cervical rotation (Fig. 4-37). In both cases, the therapist applies a repetitive sliding movement in the plane of the facet joints: in the first case, in the anterior cranial direction, while in the second, in the posterior caudal direction. This technique usually results in a significant improvement in both range of motion and pain.

In the treatment of painful hyperconvergence dysfunction, mobilization manoeuvres with movement can be used. Taking the example of a painful convergence on the left facet joint of C3–C4, the procedure consists of two parts.

In the first part, the therapist, situated opposite and slightly to the right of the patient, stabilizes with the third finger of his right hand the left articular pillar of C3 and asks the patient to perform between one and three movements of progressive cervical rotation to the right, finally reaching the maximum pain-free range. During this movement, the therapist applies a cranial and anterior pressure, respecting the plane of the joint, over the left pillar of C3, thus accompanying the patient's active rotation.

In the second part, the patient is asked to perform various rotation movements to the left until reaching its maximum amplitude. During these movements, the therapist prevents posterior slippage of the left articular pillar of C3 (Fig. 4-38).

Accessory movement techniques that obtain a direct mobilization of the facet joint are unilateral posteroanterior (Fig. 4-39) and anteroposterior (Fig. 4-40) mobilization. The starting position and the direction of motion can be modified to increase the amplitude of the desired movement and to influence pain.

High-speed manipulation for a divergence dysfunction is the rotation technique that can be performed in the supine position (Fig. 4-41) or in a sitting position (Fig. 4-42).

For a facet convergence, a manipulative technique in laterality can be used following the oblique plane of the zygapophyseal joints, thrusting medially and inferiorly (Fig. 4-43).

In order to obtain facet joint gapping, a laterality-rotation technique can be performed, acting from the side opposite to the dysfunctional facet, both in a sitting position and supine (Fig. 4-44).

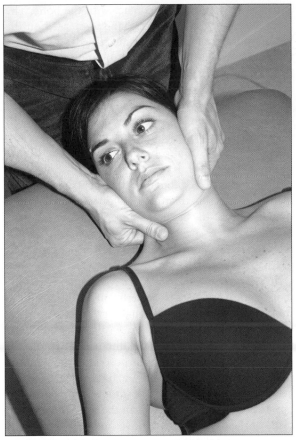

FIGURE 4-37 ■ Unilateral facet sliding manoeuvre to treat convergence.

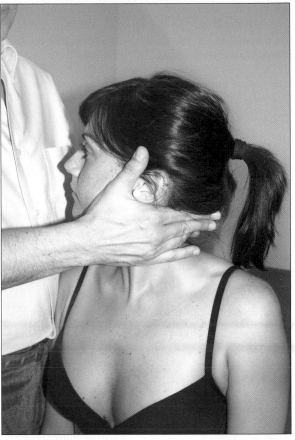

FIGURE 4-38 ■ Manoeuvre in the plane of the facets to treat articular hyperconvergence.

In an acute condition, if a high-speed manipulative technique is applied, it is preferable to initially use a gapping manoeuvre. Frequently, once obtained, the subsequent treatment of convergence or divergence is easier.

Manipulative treatment of intra-articular dysfunction

Note that, except in the case of intra-articular dysfunction, it is advisable to conduct a treatment on the soft tissue before adding manipulative techniques.

This manoeuvre aims to achieve joint gapping by thrusting in laterality and rotation in order to release the intra-articular menisci structures. This technique should be perfectly tolerated by the patient. If the pain

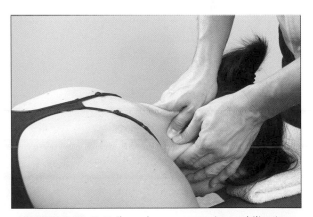

FIGURE 4-39 ■ Unilateral posteroanterior mobilization.

is severe and the necessary parameters for a manipulative technique cannot be achieved, it is preferable to use a low-speed mobilization with movement or physiological motion technique.

Example of manoeuvre to achieve gapping of the left facet joint C4 (Fig. 4-45)

Therapist's position: standing at the patient's left.
Patient's position: sitting position.
Procedure: the therapist places the palmar aspect of the middle or proximal phalanx of the middle finger of the left hand on the anterolateral part of the right facet joint of C4. To improve the contact made by the middle finger and to prevent it from slipping during the manoeuvre, the cervical tissue is folded back

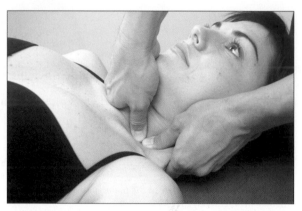

FIGURE 4-40 ■ Unilateral anteroposterior mobilization.

anteriorly before making contact with the bone. The palm and fingers of the right hand are placed on the left temporal region, holding the patient's head. The therapist places a slight lateral translation component from right to left on the right facet of C4 and then applies the left cervical rotation parameter until feeling tension in the facet. A thrust in laterality is applied from the tensioning position, medially and cranially, perpendicular to the plane of the left facet joint of C4. This technique can also be performed in the supine position (Fig. 4-46).

The results of manipulative treatment are often not maintained, if this treatment is not associated with a stabilization of the cervical spine. Since the facet syndrome may be associated with functional instability, it is imperative to work on this aspect, which is discussed in Chapters 5 and 6.

It is advisable also to train the patient in self-mobilization exercises to be performed at home. If the subject reports facet pain during cervical extension, he can be taught a two-step exercise of self-mobilization in divergence. In the first step, the patient places the edge of a towel on the spinous process of the symptomatic vertebra and performs a bending movement, helped with the towel, which she pulls forwards and upwards, attempting to perform the movement in the plane of the facet joints. In the second step, the patient performs several progressive extension movements of a growing amplitude, while stabilizing the dysfunctional segment with the towel (Fig. 4-47).

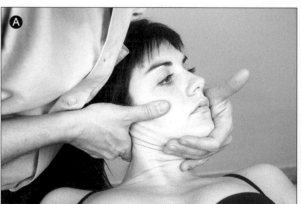
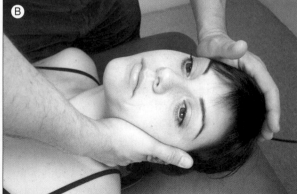

FIGURE 4-41 ■ High-speed manipulative technique in rotation, supine: (A) behind the patient and (B) facing the patient mobilization with movement (MWM).

When the subject reports a painful hyperconvergence, a similar mobilization with movement exercise can be performed. A painful convergence towards the left is chosen as an example. In the first step, the subject places the left edge of the towel over the articular pillar of the vertebra with the painful dysfunction and the right edge is obliquely directed to the next lower segment. The patient performs various rotation movements to the right, finally reaching the maximum painless amplitude, while simultaneously pressing the left edge of the towel forward and upward along the plane of the articular facet. In the second step, while continuing to push in that direction with the towel, the patient performs various movements of rotation to the left trying to achieve the maximum amplitude (Fig. 4-48).

INVASIVE TREATMENT

Facet infiltration and anaesthetic blocking of the medial division of the posterior primary ramus

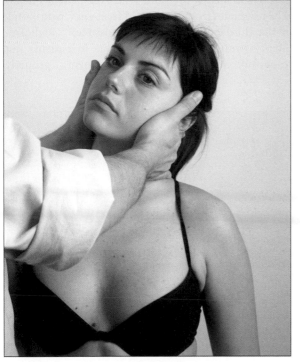

FIGURE 4-42 ■ High-speed manipulative technique in rotation in a sitting position.

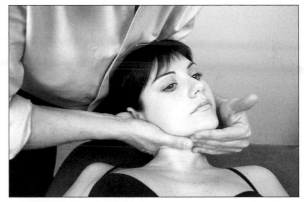

FIGURE 4-43 ■ High-speed manipulative technique in convergence.

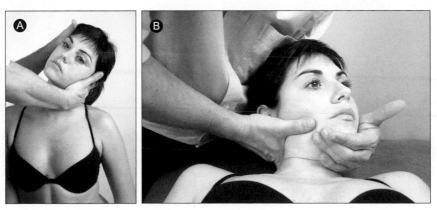

FIGURE 4-44 ■ High-speed manipulative technique in gapping in a sitting position (A) and supine (B).

are procedures that may be especially suitable when symptoms are severe and prevent manual treatment.[29,31,157,186–191]

Recently, radiofrequency neurotomy has become popular for the treatment of facet pain and cervicogenic headache.[91,192–200] This technique consists of a facet joint denervation through the thermocoagulation of the medial division. When the patient's headache originates from the C2–C3 facet joint, neurotomy of the third occipital nerve is possible.[199] Radiofrequency neurotomy may be suitable in patients not responsive to conservative treatment, properly

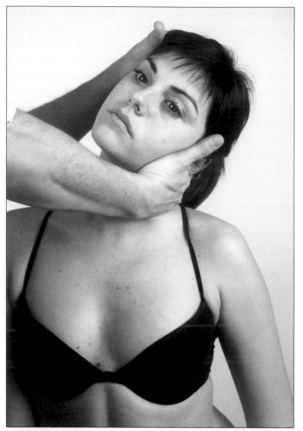

FIGURE 4-45 ■ Manipulative treatment of intra-articular dysfunction in a sitting position.

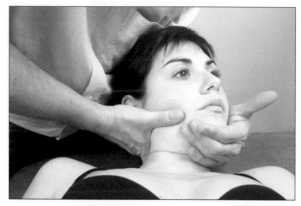

FIGURE 4-46 ■ Manipulative treatment of intra-articular dysfunction in supine.

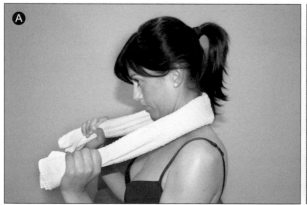
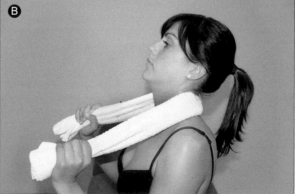

FIGURE 4-47 ■ Self-mobilization in case of facet pain in extension. In the first step, the subject pulls the edge of the towel in the plane of the facet joints while performing flexion (A), and in the second step, she takes the cervical spine to extension, maintaining the towel pressure (B).

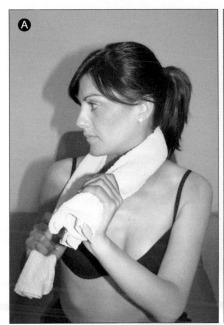
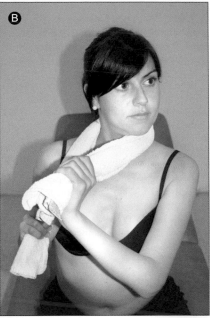

FIGURE 4-48 ■ Self-mobilization in a subject having a painful convergence on the left side. The patient performs various movements of rotation to the right, simultaneously pressing the left edge of the towel in the plane of the facets (A). In the second step, continuing to push in that direction with the towel, the patient performs several movements to the left, trying to achieve the maximum amplitude (B).

designed and provided that complete relief of symptoms has been previously obtained with controlled diagnostic blocks.[200,201]

CONCLUSIONS

Facet syndrome is the most frequent clinical condition in subjects who report neck pain. Facet syndrome is often the result of a traumatic injury such as whiplash, or the result of degenerative joint changes that may affect the intervertebral disc. The facet pathology is the most frequent cause of chronic neck pain and cervico genic headache.

The diagnosis of facet syndrome is not particularly difficult. However, in order to establish that a treatment adapted to the patient is necessary, we must analyse in detail the articular relationships of the affected joint and the mechanical and postural factors that may contribute to the perpetuation of symptoms. Conservative treatment, whenever it suits the patient's clinical situation, renders very good results. Based on this clinical condition, we can use many procedures.

Manual therapy techniques are the treatment of choice. In order to maintain the results, the motor control of the cervical and cervicoscapular muscles needs to be trained, while accounting for the somatosensory deficits, if any.

REFERENCES

1. Lord SM, Barnsley L, Wallis BJ, et al. Chronic cervical zygapophysial joint pain after whiplash. A placebo-controlled prevalence study. Spine 1996;21(15):1737–44, discussion 1744–5.
2. Barnsley L, Lord SM, Wallis BJ, et al. The prevalence of chronic cervical zygapophysial joint pain after whiplash. Spine 1995;20(1):20–5, discussion 26.
3. Jonsson H Jr, Bring G, Rauschning W, et al. Hidden cervical spine injuries in traffic accident victims with skull fractures. J Spinal Disord 1991;4(3):251–63.
4. Taylor JR, Twomey LT. Acute injuries to cervical joints. An autopsy study of neck sprain. Spine 1993;18(9):1115–22.
5. Stabler A, Eck J, Penning R, et al. Cervical spine: postmortem assessment of accident injuries – comparison of radiographic, MR imaging, anatomic, and pathologic findings. Radiology 2001;221(2):340–6.
6. Bogduk N, Yoganandan N. Biomechanics of the cervical spine. Part 3: minor injuries. Clin Biomech (Bristol, Avon) 2001;16(4): 267–75.

7. Taylor J, Taylor M. Cervical spinal injuries: an autopsy study of 109 blunt injuries. J Musculoskel Pain 1996;4(4):61–79.
8. Manchikanti L, Manchikanti KN, Pampati V. The prevalence of facet-joint-related chronic neck pain in postsurgical and nonpostsurgical patients: a comparative evaluation. Pain Pract 2008;8(1):5–10.
9. Falco FJ, Erhart S, Wargo BW, et al. Systematic review of diagnostic utility and therapeutic effectiveness of cervical facet joint interventions. Pain Physician 2009;12(2):323–44.
10. Klessinger S. Radiofrequency neurotomy for the treatment of therapy-resistant neck pain after ventral cervical operations. Pain Med 2010;11(10):1504–10.
11. Chua NH, van Suijlekom HA, Vissers KC, et al. Differences in sensory processing between chronic cervical zygapophysial joint pain patients with and without cervicogenic headache. Cephalalgia 2011;31(8):953–63.
12. Curatolo M, Bogduk N, Ivancic PC, et al. The role of tissue damage in whiplash-associated disorders: discussion paper 1. Spine 2011;36(Suppl. 25):S309–15.
13. Falco FJ, Datta S, Manchikanti L, et al. An updated review of the diagnostic utility of cervical facet joint injections. Pain Physician 2012;15(6):E807–38.
14. Gore DR, Sepic SB, Gardner GM. Roentgenographic findings of the cervical spine in asymptomatic people. Spine 1986;11(6):521–4.
15. Goldthwait J. The lumbosacral articulation: an explanation of many cases of 'lumbago, sciatica y paraplegia'. Boston Med Surg J 1911;164:356–72.
16. Ghormley R. Low back pain with special reference to the articular facets, with presentation of an operative procedure. JAMA 1933;101:1773–7.
17. Steindler A, Luck J. Differential diagnosis of pain in the low back: allocation of the source of pain by procaine hydrochloride method. JAMA 1938;110:106–13.
18. Badgley C. The articular facet in relations to low back pain and sciatic radiation. J Bone Joint Surg 1941;23:481.
19. Pedersen HE, Blunck CF, Gardner E. The anatomy of lumbosacral posterior rami and meningeal branches of spinal nerve (sinu-vertebral nerves); with an experimental study of their functions. J Bone Joint Surg Am 1956;38-A(2):377–91.
20. Lazorthes G. La branche postérieure des nerfs rachidiens. L'innervation des articulations interapophysaires, vertébrales. In: 42nd réunion de l'Association des Anatomistes, 1956; Lisboa.
21. Lazorthes G, Gaubert J. Le syndrome de la branche postérieure des nerfs rachidiens. Presse Médicale 1956;64:2022.
22. Mixter W, Barr J. Rupture of the intervertebral disk with involvement of the spinal canal. N Engl J Med 1934;64:20–2.
23. Mooney V, Robertson J. The facet syndrome. Clin Orthop 1976;115:149–56.
24. Bogduk N, Marsland A. The cervical zygapophysial joints as a source of neck pain. Spine 1988;13(6):610–17.
25. Dwyer A, Aprill C, Bogduk N. Cervical zygapophyseal joint pain patterns. I: A study in normal volunteers. Spine 1990;15(6):453–7.

26. Aprill C, Dwyer A, Bogduk N. Cervical zygapophyseal joint pain patterns. II: A clinical evaluation. Spine 1990;15(6):458–61.
27. Aprill C, Bogduk N. The prevalence of cervical zygapophyseal joint pain. A first approximation. Spine 1992;17(7):744–7.
28. Barnsley L, Lord SM, Wallis BJ, et al. The prevalence of chronic cervical zygapophysial joint pain after whiplash. Spine 1995;20(1):20–5, discussion 26.
29. Bovim G, Berg R, Dale LG. Cervicogenic headache: anesthetic blockades of cervical nerves (C2-C5) and facet joint (C2/C3). Pain 1992;49(3):315–20.
30. Manchikanti L, Boswell MV, Singh V, et al. Prevalence of facet joint pain in chronic spinal pain of cervical, thoracic, and lumbar regions. BMC Musculoskelet Disord 2004;5(1):15.
31. Manchikanti L, Manchikanti KN, Damron K, et al. Effectiveness of cervical medial branch blocks in chronic neck pain: a prospective outcome study. Pain Physician 2004;7:195–201.
32. Ohtori S, Takahashi K, Chiba T, et al. Sensory innervation of the cervical facet joints in rats. Spine 2001;26(2):147–50.
33. Ohtori S, Moriya H, Takahashi K. Calcitonin gene-related peptide immunoreactive sensory DRG neurons innervating the cervical facet joints in rats. J Orthop Sci 2002;7(2):258–61.
34. Ohtori S, Takahashi K, Moriya H. Calcitonin gene-related peptide immunoreactive DRG neurons innervating the cervical facet joints show phenotypic switch in cervical facet injury in rats. Eur Spine J 2003;12(2):211–15.
35. Bogduk N. The clinical anatomy of the cervical dorsal rami. Spine 1982;7(4):319–30.
36. Lord S, Bogduk N. The cervical synovial joints as sources of post-traumatic headaches. J Musculoskel Pain 1996;4:81–94.
37. Kallakuri S, Singh A, Chen C, et al. Demonstration of substance P, calcitonin gene-related peptide, and protein gene product 9.5 containing nerve fibers in human cervical facet joint capsules. Spine 2004;29(11):1182–6.
38. Crosby ND, Gilliland TM, Winkelstein BA. Early afferent activity from the facet joint after painful trauma to its capsule potentiates neuronal excitability and glutamate signaling in the spinal cord. Pain 2014;155(9):1878–87.
39. Hallgren RC, Greenman PE, Rechtien JJ. Atrophy of suboccipital muscles in patients with chronic pain: a pilot study. J Am Osteopath Assoc 1994;94(12):1032–8.
40. McPartland JM, Brodeur RR, Hallgren RC. Chronic neck pain, standing balance, and suboccipital muscle atrophy – a pilot study. J Manipulative Physiol Ther 1997;20(1):24–9.
41. Elliott J, Jull G, Noteboom JT, et al. Fatty infiltration in the cervical extensor muscles in persistent whiplash-associated disorders: a magnetic resonance imaging analysis. Spine 2006;31(22):E847–55.
42. McLain RF. Mechanoreceptor endings in human cervical facet joints. Iowa Orthop J 1993;13:149–54.
43. McLain RF. Mechanoreceptor endings in human cervical facet joints. Spine 1994;19(5):495–501.
44. Holm S, Indahl A, Solomonow M. Sensorimotor control of the spine. J Electromyogr Kinesiol 2002;12(3):219–34.

45. Feng FL, Schofferman J. Chronic neck pain and cervicogenic headaches. Curr Treat Options Neurol 2003;5(6):493–8.

46. Bogduk N, Aprill C. On the nature of neck pain, discography and cervical zygapophysial joint blocks. Pain 1993;54(2):213–17.

47. Bogduk N. The anatomical basis for spinal pain syndromes. J Manipulative Physiol Ther 1995;18(9):603–5.

48. Bogduk N, Lord SM. Cervical spine disorders. Curr Opin Rheumatol 1998;10(2):110–15.

49. Barnsley L, Lord S, Bogduk N. Whiplash injury. Pain 1994;58(3):283–307.

50. Cusick JF, Pintar FA, Yoganandan N. Whiplash syndrome: kinematic factors influencing pain patterns. Spine 2001;26(11):1252–8.

51. Yoganandan N, Cusick JF, Pintar FA, et al. Whiplash injury determination with conventional spine imaging and cryomicrotomy. Spine 2001;26(22):2443–8.

52. Lord SM, Barnsley L, Wallis BJ, et al. Third occipital nerve headache: a prevalence study. J Neurol Neurosurg Psychiatry 1994;57(10):1187–90.

53. Stemper BD, Yoganandan N, Pintar FA. Gender- and region-dependent local facet joint kinematics in rear impact: implications in whiplash injury. Spine 2004;29(16):1764–71.

54. Siegmund GP, Myers BS, Davis MB, et al. Mechanical evidence of cervical facet capsule injury during whiplash: a cadaveric study using combined shear, compression, and extension loading. Spine 2001;26(19):2095–101.

55. Panjabi MM, Cholewicki J, Nibu K, et al. Capsular ligament stretches during in vitro whiplash simulations. J Spinal Disord 1998;11(3):227–32.

56. Winkelstein BA, Nightingale RW, Richardson WJ, et al. The cervical facet capsule and its role in whiplash injury: a biomechanical investigation. Spine 2000;25(10):1238–46.

57. Inami S, Shiga T, Tsujino A, et al. Immunohistochemical demonstration of nerve fibers in the synovial fold of the human cervical facet joint. J Orthop Res 2001;19(4):593–6.

58. Kotani Y, Abumi K, Ito M, et al. Cervical spine injuries associated with lateral mass and facet joint fractures: new classification and surgical treatment with pedicle screw fixation. Eur Spine J 2005;14(1):69–77.

59. Lee KE, Franklin AN, Davis MB, et al. Tensile cervical facet capsule ligament mechanics: failure and subfailure responses in the rat. J Biomech 2006;39(7):1256–64.

60. Uhrenholt L, Grunnet-Nilsson N, Hartvigsen J. Cervical spine lesions after road traffic accidents: a systematic review. Spine 2002;27(17):1934–41, discussion 1940.

61. Bogduk N, Teasell R. Whiplash: the evidence for an organic etiology. Arch Neurol 2000;57(4):590–1.

62. Macnab I. The 'whiplash syndrome'. Orthop Clin North Am 1971;2(2):389–403.

63. Kahane C. An evaluation of head restraints. Federal Motor Vehicle Safety Standard 202. In: NHTSA Report Number DOT HS 806 108. Springfield: National Technical Information Service; 1982.

64. O'Neill B, Haddon W Jr, Kelley AB, et al. Automobile head restraints – frequency of neck injury claims in relation to the presence of head restraints. Am J Public Health 1972;62(3):399–406.

65. Luan F, Yang KH, Deng B, et al. Qualitative analysis of neck kinematics during low-speed rear-end impact. Clin Biomech (Bristol, Avon) 2000;15(9):649–57.

66. Kaneoka K, Ono K, Inami S, et al. Motion analysis of cervical vertebrae during whiplash loading. Spine 1999;24(8):763–9, discussion 770.

67. Bogduk N. Point of view. Spine 2002;27(17):1940–1.

68. Grauer JN, Panjabi MM, Cholewicki J, et al. Whiplash produces an S-shaped curvature of the neck with hyperextension at lower levels. Spine 1997;22(21):2489–94.

69. Yoganandan N, Pintar FA, Klienberger M. Cervical spine vertebral and facet joint kinematics under whiplash. J Biomech Eng 1998;120(2):305–7.

70. Winkelstein BA, McLendon RE, Barbir A, et al. An anatomical investigation of the human cervical facet capsule, quantifying muscle insertion area. J Anat 2001;198(Pt 4):455–61.

71. Yoganandan N, Pintar FA, Cusick JF. Biomechanical analyses of whiplash injuries using an experimental model. Accid Anal Prev 2002;34(5):663–71.

72. Panjabi MM, Pearson AM, Ito S, et al. Cervical spine curvature during simulated whiplash. Clin Biomech (Bristol, Avon) 2004;19(1):1–9.

73. Pearson AM, Ivancic PC, Ito S, et al. Facet joint kinematics and injury mechanisms during simulated whiplash. Spine 2004;29(4):390–7.

74. Ito S, Ivancic PC, Panjabi MM, et al. Soft tissue injury threshold during simulated whiplash: a biomechanical investigation. Spine 2004;29(9):979–87.

75. Muhlbauer M, Eichberger A, Geigl B, et al. Analysis of kinematics and acceleration behaviour of the head and neck in experimental rear-impact collisons. Neuro-Orthopaedics 1999;25:1–17.

76. Ono K, Kanno M. Influences of the physical parameters on the risk to neck injuries in low impact speed rear-end collisions. Accid Anal Prev 1996;28(4):493–9.

77. Yoganandan N, Pintar FA, Sances A, et al. Inertial flexion-extension loading of the human neck. Adv Bioeng 1995;31:45–6.

78. Yoganandan N, Pintar FA. Facet joint local component kinetics in whiplash trauma. ASME Adv Bioeng 1997;36:221–2.

79. Panjabi MM, Cholewicki J, Nibu K, et al. Simulation of whiplash trauma using whole cervical spine specimens. Spine 1998;23(1):17–24.

80. Matsushita T, Sato T, Hirabayashi K, et al. X-ray study of the human neck motion due to head inertia loading. In: 38th Stapp Car Crash Conference 1994; Fort Lauderdale; p. 55-64.

81. Stemper BD, Yoganandan N, Gennarelli TA, et al. Localized cervical facet joint kinematics under physiological and whiplash loading. J Neurosurg Spine 2005;3(6):471–6.

82. Taylor JR, Kakulas BA. Neck injuries. Lancet 1991;338(8778):1343.

83. Fernandez Iruegas J. Lumbociática de origen degenerativo. Su tratamiento actual. Madrid: Jarpyo Editores; 1993.

84. Boyd-Clark LC, Briggs CA, Galea MP. Segmental degeneration in the cervical spine and associated changes in dorsal root ganglia. Clin Anat 2004;17(6):468–77.

85. Kirkaldy-Willis WH, Wedge JH, Yong-Hing K, et al. Pathology and pathogenesis of lumbar spondylosis and stenosis. Spine 1978;3(4):319–28.

86. Yong-Hing K, Kirkaldy-Willis WH. The pathophysiology of degenerative disease of the lumbar spine. Orthop Clin North Am 1983;14(3):491–504.

87. White AA 3rd, Johnson RM, Panjabi MM, et al. Biomechanical analysis of clinical stability in the cervical spine. Clin Orthop 1975;109:85–96.

88. Reitman CA, Mauro KM, Nguyen L, et al. Intervertebral motion between flexion and extension in asymptomatic individuals. Spine 2004;29(24):2832–43.

89. Dai L. Disc degeneration and cervical instability. Correlation of magnetic resonance imaging with radiography. Spine 1998;23(16):1734–8.

90. Schellhas KP, Smith MD, Gundry CR, et al. Cervical discogenic pain. Prospective correlation of magnetic resonance imaging and discography in asymptomatic subjects and pain sufferers. Spine 1996;21(3):300–11, discussion 311-12.

91. Sapir DA, Gorup JM. Radiofrequency medial branch neurotomy in litigant and nonlitigant patients with cervical whiplash: a prospective study. Spine 2001;26(12):E268–73.

92. Maitland G, Hengeveld E, Banks K, et al. Maitland's vertebral manipulation. 6th ed. London: Butterworth-Heinemann; 2001.

93. Fukui S, Ohseto K, Shiotani M, et al. Referred pain distribution of the cervical zygapophyseal joints and cervical dorsal rami. Pain 1996;68(1):79–83.

94. Bogduk N. Cervical zygapophysial joint pain and percutaneous neurotomy. In: Gunzburg R, Szpalski M, editors. Whiplash injuries: current concepts in prevention, diagnosis, and treatment of the cervical whiplash syndrome. Philadelphia: Lippincott-Raven; 1998.

95. Fukui S, Ohseto K, Shiotani M. Patterns of pain induced by distending the thoracic zygapophyseal joints. Reg Anesth 1997;22(4):332–6.

96. Dreyfuss P, Michaelsen M, Fletcher D. Atlanto-occipital and lateral atlanto-axial joint pain patterns. Spine 1994;19(10):1125–31.

97. Bogduk N, McGuirk B. Management of acute and chronic neck pain. An evidence-based approach. Edinburgh: Elsevier; 2006.

98. Cooper G, Bailey B, Bogduk N. Cervical zygapophysial joint pain maps. Pain Med 2007;8(4):344–53.

99. Grubb SA, Kelly CK. Cervical discography: clinical implications from 12 years of experience. Spine 2000;25(11):1382–9.

100. Schellhas KP, Pollei SR. The role of discography in the evaluation of patients with spinal deformity. Orthop Clin North Am 1994;25(2):265–73.

101. Schellhas KP. Diskography. Neuroimaging Clin N Am 2000;10(3):579–96.

102. Bogduk N. The neck. Baillières Clin Rheumatol 1999;13(2):261–85.

103. Maitland GD. Acute locking of the cervical spine. Aust J Physiother 1978;24:103–9.

104. Inami S, Kaneoka K, Hayashi K, et al. Types of synovial fold in the cervical facet joint. J Orthop Sci 2000;5(5):475–80.

105. Giles LG, Taylor JR. Human zygapophyseal joint capsule and synovial fold innervation. Br J Rheumatol 1987;26(2):93–8.

106. Giles LG. Human lumbar zygapophyseal joint inferior recess synovial folds: a light microscope examination. Anat Rec 1988;220(2):117–24.

107. Giles LG, Harvey AR. Immunohistochemical demonstration of nociceptors in the capsule and synovial folds of human zygapophyseal joints. Br J Rheumatol 1987;26(5):362–4.

108. Gronblad M, Korkala O, Konttinen YT, et al. Silver impregnation and immunohistochemical study of nerves in lumbar facet joint plical tissue. Spine 1991;16(1):34–8.

109. Giles LG. Innervation of zygapophyseal joint synovial folds in low-back pain. Lancet 1987;2(8560):692.

110. Giles LG, Taylor JR, Cockson A. Human zygapophyseal joint synovial folds. Acta Anat (Basel) 1986;126(2):110–14.

111. Giles LG, Taylor JR. Innervation of lumbar zygapophyseal joint synovial folds. Acta Orthop Scand 1987;58(1):43–6.

112. Mercer S, Bogduk N. Intra-articular inclusions of the cervical synovial joints. Br J Rheumatol 1993;32(8):705–10.

113. Mercer S. The menisci of the cervical synovial joints. In: Boyling J, Palastanga N, editors. Grieve's modern manual therapy. The vertebral column. 2nd ed. London: Churchill Livingstone; 2000. p. 69–72.

114. Grieve G. Common vertebral joint problems. 2nd ed. Edinburgh: Churchill Livingstone; 1988.

115. Koss J, Wolf J. Les ménisques intervértebraux et leur rôle possible dans les blockages vertébraux. Ann Med Phys 1972;15:2003.

116. Scher AT. Unilateral locked facet in cervical spine injuries. AJR Am J Roentgenol 1977;129(1):45–8.

117. Giles LG. Pressure related changes in human lumbosacral zygapophyseal joint articular cartilage. J Rheumatol 1986;13(6):1093–5.

118. Bogduk N, Jull G. The theoretical pathology of acute locked back: a basis for manipulative therapy. Man Med 1985;1:78–82.

119. Bogduk N, Engel R. The menisci of the lumbar zygapophyseal joints. A review of their anatomy and clinical significance. Spine 1984;9(5):454–60.

120. Bogduk N. Clinical anatomy of the lumbar spine and sacrum. 4 ed. Edinburgh: Elsevier Churchill Livingstone; 2005.

121. Jones TR, James JE, Adams JW, et al. Lumbar zygapophyseal joint meniscoids: evidence of their role in chronic intersegmental hypomobility. J Manipulative Physiol Ther 1989;12(5):374–85.

122. Schonstrom N, Twomey L, Taylor J. The lateral atlanto-axial joints and their synovial folds: an in vitro study of soft tissue injuries and fractures. J Trauma 1993;35(6):886–92.

123. Trott P. Management of selected cervical syndromes. In: Grant R, editor. Physical therapy of the cervical and thoracic spine. 3rd ed. Edinburgh: Churchill Livingstone; 2002. p. 273–94.

124. Miwa M, Doita M, Takayama H, et al. An expanding cervical synovial cyst causing acute cervical radiculopathy. J Spinal Disord Tech 2004;17(4):331–3.

125. Cartwright MJ, Nehls DG, Carrion CA, et al. Synovial cyst of a cervical facet joint: case report. Neurosurgery 1985;16(6): 850–2.

126. Stoodley MA, Jones NR, Scott G. Cervical and thoracic juxta-facet cysts causing neurologic deficits. Spine 2000;25(8): 970–3.

127. Found E, Bewyer D. Cervical synovial cyst: case report. Iowa Orthop J 2011;31:215–18.

128. Kim DS, Yang JS, Cho YJ, et al. Acute myelopathy caused by a cervical synovial cyst. J Korean Neurosurg Soc 2014;56(1): 55–7.

129. Attwell L, Elwell VA, Meir A. Cervical synovial cyst. Br J Neurosurg 2014;28(6):813–14.

130. Aksoy FG, Gomori JM. Symptomatic cervical synovial cyst associated with an os odontoideum diagnosed by magnetic resonance imaging: case report and review of the literature. Spine 2000;25(10):1300–2.

131. Chang H, Park JB, Kim KW. Synovial cyst of the transverse ligament of the atlas in a patient with os odontoideum and atlantoaxial instability. Spine 2000;25(6):741–4.

132. Chaoui FM, Njee-Bugha T, Figarella-Branger D, et al. [Synovial cyst of cervical spine]. Neurochirurgie 2000;46(4):391–4.

133. Cudlip S, Johnston F, Marsh H. Subaxial cervical synovial cyst presenting with myelopathy. Report of three cases. J Neurosurg Spine 1999;90(1):141–4.

134. Epstein NE, Hollingsworth R. Synovial cyst of the cervical spine. J Spinal Disord 1993;6(2):182–5.

135. Jabre A, Shahbabian S, Keller JT. Synovial cyst of the cervical spine. Neurosurgery 1987;20(2):316–18.

136. Kao CC, Winkler SS, Turner JH. Synovial cyst of spinal facet. Case report. J Neurosurg 1974;41(3):372–6.

137. Kayser F, Divano L, Vermer JF. [Ganglion cyst of the cervical spine causing radiculopathy]. J Radiol 1998;79(7):687–9.

138. Patel SC, Sanders WP. Synovial cyst of the cervical spine: case report and review of the literature. AJNR Am J Neuroradiol 1988;9(3):602–3.

139. Shima Y, Rothman SL, Yasura K, et al. Degenerative intraspinal cyst of the cervical spine: case report and literature review. Spine 2002;27(1):E18–22.

140. Takano Y, Homma T, Okumura H, et al. Ganglion cyst occurring in the ligamentum flavum of the cervical spine. A case report. Spine 1992;17(12):1531–3.

141. Holtzman RN, Dubin R, Yang WC, et al. Bilateral symptomatic intraspinal T12-L1 synovial cysts. Surg Neurol 1987;28(3): 225–30.

142. Bogduk N. Headaches and the cervical spine. Cephalalgia 1984;4(1):7–8.

143. Bogduk N, Marsland A. On the concept of third occipital headache. J Neurol Neurosurg Psychiatry 1986;49(7):775–80.

144. Michler RP, Bovim G, Sjaastad O. Disorders in the lower cervical spine. A cause of unilateral headache? A case report. Headache 1991;31(8):550–1.

145. Bogduk N. Neck pain. Aust Fam Physician 1984;13(1):26–30.

146. Bogduk N. Anatomy and physiology of headache. Biomed Pharmacother 1995;49(10):435–45.

147. Bogduk N. Cervical causes of headache and dizziness. In: Boyling J, Palastanga N, editors. Grieve's modern manual therapy. 2nd ed. London: Churchill Livingstone; 2000. p. 317–31.

148. Bogduk N. The neck and headaches. Neurol Clin 2004; 22(1):151–71, vii.

149. Bogduk N, Corrigan B, Kelly P, et al. Cervical headache. Med J Aust 1985;143(5):202, 206-7.

150. Hinderaker J, Lord SM, Barnsley L, et al. Diagnostic value of C2-3 instantaneous axes of rotation in patients with headache of cervical origin. Cephalalgia 1995;15(5):391–5.

151. Bogduk N. Cervicogenic headache: anatomic basis and pathophysiologic mechanisms. Curr Pain Headache Rep 2001;5(4): 382–6.

152. Bogduk N. The anatomical basis for cervicogenic headache. J Manipulative Physiol Ther 1992;15(1):67–70.

153. Bogduk N. Distinguishing primary headache disorders from cervicogenic headache: clinical and therapeutic implications. Headache Currents 2005;2(2):27–36.

154. Bogduk N. Mechanisms and pain patterns of the upper cervical spine. In: Vernon H, editor. The cranio-cervical syndrome. Mechanisms, assessment and treatment. London: Butterworth-Heinemann; 2001. p. 110–16.

155. Uthaikhup S, Sterling M, Jull G. Cervical musculoskeletal impairment is common in elders with headache. Man Ther 2009;14(6):636–41.

156. Drottning M, Staff PH, Sjaastad O. Cervicogenic headache (CEH) after whiplash injury. Cephalalgia 2002;22(3): 165–71.

157. Slipman CW, Lipetz JS, Plastaras CT, et al. Therapeutic zygapophyseal joint injections for headaches emanating from the C2-3 joint. Am J Phys Med Rehabil 2001;80(3):182–8.

158. Cole A, Dreyer S, Dreyfuss P, et al. Zygapophyseal (facet) joint pain: a functional approach. In: Windsor R, Lox D, editors. Soft tissue injuries: diagnosis and treatment. Philadelphia: Hanley & Belfus; 1998. p. 47–64.

159. Grimshaw DN. Cervicogenic headache: manual and manipulative therapies. Curr Pain Headache Rep 2001;5(4):369–75.

160. Hubka MJ, Phelan SP. Interexaminer reliability of palpation for cervical spine tenderness. J Manipulative Physiol Ther 1994;17(9):591–5.

161. Deboer KF, Harmon R Jr, Tuttle CD, et al. Reliability study of detection of somatic dysfunctions in the cervical spine. J Manipulative Physiol Ther 1985;8(1):9–16.

162. Mior S, King R, McGregor M, et al. Intra and interexaminer reliability of motion palpation in the cervical spine. J Can Chiro Assoc 1985;29:195–8.

163. Nansel DD, Peneff AL, Jansen RD, et al. Interexaminer concordance in detecting joint-play asymmetries in the cervical spines of otherwise asymptomatic subjects. J Manipulative Physiol Ther 1989;12(6):428–33.

164. Youdas JW, Carey JR, Garrett TR. Reliability of measurements of cervical spine range of motion – comparison of three methods. Phys Ther 1991;71(2):98–104, discussion 105-6.

165. Fjellner A, Bexander C, Faleij R, et al. Interexaminer reliability in physical examination of the cervical spine. J Manipulative Physiol Ther 1999;22(8):511–16.
166. Smedmark V, Wallin M, Arvidsson I. Inter-examiner reliability in assessing passive intervertebral motion of the cervical spine. Man Ther 2000;5(2):97–101.
167. King W, Lau P, Lees R, et al. The validity of manual examination in assessing patients with neck pain. Spine J 2007;7(1):22–6.
168. Siegenthaler A, Eichenberger U, Schmidlin K, et al. What does local tenderness say about the origin of pain? An investigation of cervical zygapophysial joint pain. Anesth Analg 2010;110(3):923–7.
169. Seffinger MA, Najm WI, Mishra SI, et al. Reliability of spinal palpation for diagnosis of back and neck pain: a systematic review of the literature. Spine 2004;29(19):E413–25.
170. Gross AR, Aker PD, Quartly C. Manual therapy in the treatment of neck pain. Rheum Dis Clin North Am 1996;22(3):579–98.
171. Edmeads J. The cervical spine and headache. Neurology 1988;38(12):1874–8.
172. Speldewinde GC, Bashford GM, Davidson IR. Diagnostic cervical zygapophyseal joint blocks for chronic cervical pain. Med J Aust 2001;174(4):174–6.
173. Jull G, Bogduk N, Marsland A. The accuracy of manual diagnosis for cervical zygapophysial joint pain syndromes. Med J Aust 1988;148(5):233–6.
174. Bogduk N, Govind J. Cervicogenic headache: an assessment of the evidence on clinical diagnosis, invasive tests, and treatment. Lancet Neurol 2009;8(10):959–68.
175. Schneider GM, Jull G, Thomas K, et al. Derivation of a clinical decision guide in the diagnosis of cervical facet joint pain. Arch Phys Med Rehabil 2014;95(9):1695–701.
176. Smith GR, Beckly DE, Abel MS. Articular mass fracture: a neglected cause of post-traumatic neck pain? Clin Radiol 1976;27(3):335–40.
177. Woodring JH, Goldstein SJ. Fractures of the articular processes of the cervical spine. AJR Am J Roentgenol 1982;139(2):341–4.
178. Barnsley L, Bogduk N. Medial branch blocks are specific for the diagnosis of cervical zygapophyseal joint pain. Reg Anesth 1993;18(6):343–50.
179. Barnsley L, Lord S, Bogduk N. Comparative local anaesthetic blocks in the diagnosis of cervical zygapophysial joint pain. Pain 1993;55(1):99–106.
180. Lord SM, Barnsley L, Bogduk N. The utility of comparative local anesthetic blocks versus placebo-controlled blocks for the diagnosis of cervical zygapophysial joint pain. Clin J Pain 1995;11(3):208–13.
181. Martelletti P, van Suijlekom H. Cervicogenic headache: practical approaches to therapy. CNS Drugs 2004;18(12):793–805.
182. Bogduk N. Diagnostic nerve blocks in chronic pain. Best Pract Res Clin Anaesthesiol 2002;16(4):565–78.
183. Schwarzer AC, April CN, Derby R, et al. The false-positive rate of uncontrolled diagnostic blocks of the lumbar zygapophysial joints. Pain 1994;58(2):195–200.
184. Barnsley L, Lord S, Wallis B, et al. False-positive rates of cervical zygapophysial joint blocks. Clin J Pain 1993;9(2):124–30.
185. Solomon S. Chronic post-traumatic neck and head pain. Headache 2005;45(1):53–67.
186. Dussault RG, Nicolet VM. Cervical facet joint arthrography. J Can Assoc Radiol 1985;36(1):79–80.
187. Dory MA. Arthrography of the cervical facet joints. Radiology 1983;148(2):379–82.
188. Roy DF, Fleury J, Fontaine SB, et al. Clinical evaluation of cervical facet joint infiltration. Can Assoc Radiol J 1988;39(2):118–20.
189. Hove B, Gyldensted C. Cervical analgesic facet joint arthrography. Neuroradiology 1990;32(6):456–9.
190. Barnsley L, Lord SM, Wallis BJ, et al. Lack of effect of intraarticular corticosteroids for chronic pain in the cervical zygapophyseal joints. N Engl J Med 1994;330(15):1047–50.
191. Kwan O, Fiel J. Critical appraisal of facet joints injections for chronic whiplash. Med Sci Monit 2002;8(8):RA191–5.
192. Lord SM, Barnsley L, Bogduk N. Percutaneous radio-frequency neurotomy in the treatment of cervical zygapophysial joint pain: a caution. Neurosurgery 1995;36(4):732–9.
193. Lord SM, Barnsley L, Wallis BJ, et al. Percutaneous radio-frequency neurotomy for chronic cervical zygapophyseal-joint pain. N Engl J Med 1996;335(23):1721–6.
194. Wallis BJ, Lord SM, Bogduk N. Resolution of psychological distress of whiplash patients following treatment by radiofrequency neurotomy: a randomised, double-blind, placebo-controlled trial. Pain 1997;73(1):15–22.
195. van Suijlekom HA, van Kleef M, Barendse GA, et al. Radiofrequency cervical zygapophyseal joint neurotomy for cervicogenic headache: a prospective study of 15 patients. Funct Neurol 1998;13(4):297–303.
196. McDonald GJ, Lord SM, Bogduk N. Long-term follow-up of patients treated with cervical radiofrequency neurotomy for chronic neck pain. Neurosurgery 1999;45(1):61–7, discussion 67-8.
197. van Suijlekom HA, Weber WE, van Kleef M, et al. Radiofrequency cervical zygapophyseal joint neurotomy for cervicogenic headache: a short term follow-up study. Funct Neurol 1998;13(1):82–3.
198. van Suijlekom JA, Weber WE, van Kleef M. Cervicogenic headache: techniques of diagnostic nerve blocks. Clin Exp Rheumatol 2000;18(2 Suppl. 19):S39–44.
199. Govind J, King W, Bailey B, et al. Radiofrequency neurotomy for the treatment of third occipital headache. J Neurol Neurosurg Psychiatry 2003;74(1):88–93.
200. Bogduk N. Cervicogenic headache. Cephalalgia 2004;24(10):819–20.
201. Smith AD, Jull G, Schneider G, et al. Cervical radiofrequency neurotomy reduces central hyperexcitability and improves neck movement in individuals with chronic whiplash. Pain Med 2014;15(1):128–41.

5

CLINICAL APPROACH TO CRANIOVERTEBRAL INSTABILITY

RAFAEL TORRES CUECO

Cervical instability is among the causes of neck pain and can be related to different clinical conditions, such as the cervical zygapophyseal joint syndrome, articular degenerative disease, cervicogenic headache,[1,2] whiplash-associated disorders[3] and discogenic syndrome.[4] Instability can be of congenital, inflammatory, traumatic and degenerative origin, and it can occur in different degrees. Therefore, from a conceptual point of view, it is possible to talk about a major or minor instability. Major instability is one of the situations that contraindicate the use of manual therapy techniques and other conservative therapeutic procedures.

The aetiology of instability can be congenital, inflammatory, traumatic and degenerative.

Major instability often involves the disruption of the craniocervical ligaments. It is usually detected radiographically and can cause a compression of the neural and vascular structures. It is imperative to be able to identify this type of instability, especially for those that work with the manual therapy of the cervical spine, not just due to its increasing prevalence, which is in part due to car accidents, but also because an incorrect diagnosis can result in the onset or aggravation of a neurological deficit and even have fatal consequences.

Minor instability involves an altered dynamic control of the cervical spine, causing pain and dysfunction, without leading to significant disruption of the ligaments or a neurovascular compromise. This second category of instability is not associated with the

risks of major instability; however, it does appear to be a significant factor that may contribute to chronic neck pain chronicity[5] and is usually overlooked in the diagnosis. Consequently, the evaluation of motor control, and treatment aimed at improving it, forms an integral part of diagnosis and management of musculoskeletal disorders affecting the cervical spine.[6]

Major instability:

- Frequent disruption of the craniocervical ligaments.
- It is usually detected radiographically.
- It can cause a compression of the neural and vascular structures.
- Its diagnosis is crucial, given the serious consequences of the application of a manipulative treatment

---

DEFINITION OF INSTABILITY

Before describing the pathogeny of craniovertebral instability, the term 'instability' requires some definition as it can be interpreted in different ways. It is also necessary to differentiate between instability and hypermobility, since the concept of instability implies a pathological situation, while this is not the case in hypermobility. However, this difference does not seem to be clear in literature and both terms have been used interchangeably.[7]

From a mechanical point of view, instability can be defined as an abnormal response to the forces that are applied to the spine, resulting in an increase of segmental mobility beyond the physiological limits. Yet,

169

in clinical practice, this definition is insufficient, since many subjects with an articular mobility beyond the normal limits are completely asymptomatic.

For this reason, attempts have been made to create different definitions of clinical instability. Frymoyer[8] defines it as the 'loss of spinal motion segment stiffness, in such a way that force application to that motion segment produces greater displacement(s) than would be seen in a normal structure, resulting in a painful condition, possible progressive deformity that endanger neurological structures'.

White et al.[9] define clinical stability as the loss of the ability of the spine to maintain its pattern of displacement under physiological loads. Consequently, there is incapacity and/or pain due to the resulting structural changes.

Kirkaldy-Willis and Farfan[10] developed a definition of instability that is not linked to the biomechanical behaviour of the joint, but which is solely linked to the patient's symptoms. According to these authors, segmental instability occurs in patients with low back problems whose clinical status is unstable and who have symptoms fluctuating between mild and severe, even in response to minor provocations. This definition provides the concept of unstable balance. The patient is able to maintain a functional situation, but has a precarious clinical condition so that a minimal mechanical perturbation can trigger a significant incapacity. It is evident that this definition does not necessarily relate to a biomechanical instability. However, from a practical point of view, instability defined as a precarious functional situation is one of the usual characteristics of patients with symptomatic mechanical instability.

Panjabi made an important advance to the concept of instability by pointing out that articular instability is more attributable to changes in the range of the neutral zone than it is to an excessive range of mobility. This division in the range is based on the biomechanical behaviour of the articular system determined by its passive and active elements. The neutral zone is the initial portion of segmental range of motion during which spinal motion is produced against minimal internal resistance. The elastic portion of range of motion is the portion nearer to the end-range of movement that is produced against substantial internal resistance (Fig. 5-1). Panjabi defines clinical instability as a significant decrease in the capacity of the stabilizing system of the spine to maintain spinal neutral zones within physiological limits so there is no neurological deficit, no major deformity and no incapacitating pain. This hypothesis posits that a

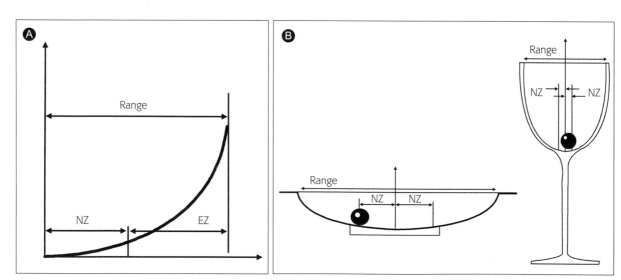

FIGURE 5-1 ■ The neutral zone (NZ) is the part of the range of movement of a joint, near its rest position, in which the joint expresses its maximum capacity of movement with minimum internal resistance. The elastic zone (EZ) is the range of intervertebral mobility from the end of the neutral area to the end of the physiological movement (A). In the analogy between a ball and its container, the cup would represent an intervertebral segment with a reduced neutral zone and, therefore, it is very stable (B); the wide plate would represent an intervertebral segment with a very wide neutral zone and, therefore, it is relatively unstable.

significant increase in the neutral zone can indicate a clinical instability, and it goes against the classical hypothesis that defines instability as an increase in the range of movement.[11] Panjabi[12,13] suggests that an increase in the size of the neutral zone may be a better indicator of segmental instability than an increase in total range of motion. This definition emphasizes the quality of motion more so than the quantity of motion. Moreover, patients who are suspected of suffering from instability of the cervical spine frequently complain of pain within the mid-ranges of spinal motion than at the end-ranges.[14] In fact, in a spine with degenerative changes, there can be an increase in the neutral zone without an increase in the total range of motion. The deep stabilizing muscles play a crucial role in controlling the neutral zone.

This definition emphasizes the quality as opposed to the quantity of motion and appears to fit the clinical observation that many patients with suspected segmental instability have greater movement difficulties.

Instability and neutral zone:

- The neutral zone is the initial portion of segmental range of motion during which spinal motion is produced against minimal internal resistance.
- Joint instability is more attributable to changes in the range of the neutral zone than it is to an excessive range of mobility.
- Clinical instability involves a significant decrease in the capacity of the spine to maintain the neutral intervertebral zone within the physiological limits

It has also been proposed that instability may be linked to the quality or pattern of movement.[15] Thus, the instability would be the consequence of a loss of proportion between the components of rotation and translation of a vertebra. A segment would express, for instance, a disproportional sagittal translation in relation to the component of sagittal rotation.

When treating instability, the elements responsible for the decrease in stiffness, the increase of the neutral zone or the onset of a pattern of abnormal segmental mobility should be known.[15]

A complete definition of instability should also refer to an alteration of the articular mechanics. The different definitions that include the mechanical aspect involve the existence of excessive mobility, an increase

in the neutral zone, or an alteration of the pattern of movement.

In order to understand the concept of clinical instability, Panjabi[13] pointed out that vertebral instability depends on three interactive subsystems: passive, active and control. The passive subsystem is made up of the morphology of the articular surfaces and the capsuloligamentous system; the active subsystem is composed of the intrinsic stabilizing muscles; and the control subsystem is composed of the articular proprioception and the central mechanisms of control joint movement.

The vertebral stability depends on three interactive subsystems:

- Passive subsystem: articular morphology and capsuloligamentous system.
- Active subsystem: local and global stabilizing muscles.
- Control subsystem: articular proprioception and central mechanisms of control of the position and articular movement.

These three subsystems work together in order to provide dynamic stability to the vertebral segment during the application of external forces. Instability can appear, not only when the passive subsystem is insufficient but also when the active and control subsystems are unable to maintain control of the neutral zone.

CHARACTERISTICS OF INSTABILITY

The three defining characteristics of instability are:

1. Instability results in a clinical situation.
2. The patient has a precarious balance: relatively lower mechanical stress results in a significant disability.
3. There is abnormal mobility in response to physiological forces due to the excess of the range of movement or the increase of the neutral zone, or the alteration of the pattern of movement.

Minor cervical instability

The concept of minor cervical instability involves the presence of a cervical instability associated with pain and dysfunction due to an altered cervical neuromuscular control. It can determine the loss of control of the neutral zone.[16] It can also be classified as cervical movement control dysfunction and can be defined as the presence of aberrant or uncontrolled movements of the cervical spine which are observed during prescribed active movements of the neck and/or upper limb.[17]

This clinical situation can manifest itself with very subtle signs and symptoms, which makes the diagnosis more difficult. The clinical symptoms that can be associated with minor cervical instability are cervical pain, a catching/locking sensation, weakness, muscular control deficit, altered range of mobility and history of greater trauma or repetitive microtrauma. This condition can be associated with a series of signs and symptoms, with the exception of a severe disabling pain, cord compression symptoms of and disruption of the vertebral artery.[16]

MINOR instability:

- Loss of control of the neutral articular zone, without disruption of the ligaments or neurovascular compromise.
- It is manifested with very subtle signs and symptoms, such as cervical pain, catching/locking sensation, weakness, deficit of muscular control or altered range of mobility.
- It is a common cause of persistent cervical pain and is often overlooked in the diagnosis.

ELEMENTS RESPONSIBLE FOR CRANIOVERTEBRAL INSTABILITY

The craniovertebral spine is responsible for directing head movement in all directions. The extraordinary mobility of this joint complex, and the necessity to maintain its stability, mean that the bone, ligament and articular structures are subject to important functional demands.[7] Due to the *lack of* bone stability, especially in the C1–C2 segment, the ligaments of this region, especially the transverse ligament, the alar ligaments and the tectorial membrane, play a crucial biomechanical role.[18]

Atlanto-occipital joint (C0–C1)

The stability of the atlanto-occipital joint is based on the pronounced concave configuration of the upper joints of the atlas, which enable the adaptation of the occipital condyles (Fig. 5-2). The lateral walls of the

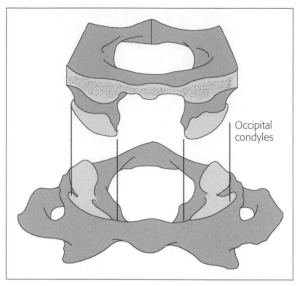

FIGURE 5-2 ■ The instability of C0–C1 depends in part on the bone configuration of the joint that helps the occipital condyles to be deeply introduced into the lateral masses of the atlas.

articular facets of the atlas prevent the lateral gliding of the occipital, and its anterior and posterior walls prevent the anteroposterior movement. This joint is more unstable in the sagittal plane than in the coronal plane.

The stability of the region also depends on the ligamentous connections between the occipital and the axis, thanks to the tectorial membrane and the alar ligaments. The articular capsules and the anterior and posterior atlanto-occipital membranes offer additional stabilization, although it is of less importance.

During childhood, the stability of this joint is precarious,[19] and it increases as adulthood approaches, thanks to the decrease in the elasticity of the ligaments. The dislocation of this joint usually has fatal consequences.

In order to objectivize the sagittal instability of the occipital in a lateral radiograph, the distance between the anterior edge of the foramen magnum (basion) and the vertex of the odontoid process can be measured. When this distance is greater than 4 or 5 mm, we must suspect the presence of instability (Fig. 5-3).

Another way to show atlanto-occipital instability in a lateral radiography is using Powers index[20,21] (Fig. 5-4).

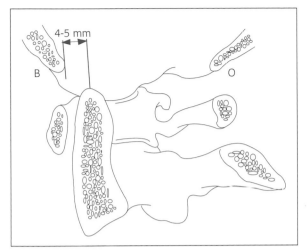

FIGURE 5-3 ■ The sagittal instability of the occipital can be objectivize by measuring the edge of the foramen magnum (basion) (B) and the vertex of the odontoid process (O). When this distance is greater than 4 or 5 mm, it is possible to suspect instability.

The axial rotation of the occipital usually does not tend to exceed 4°, and is limited by the alar ligaments. The rotatory instability of the occipital is confirmed when, in a CT performed in rotation, this movement is greater 8°.[22]

Atlantoaxial joint

The lateral atlantoaxial joints, due to their biconvex configuration and the significant *laxity* of their articular capsule necessary to allow for wide mobility, barely contribute to the stability of this segment. The stability of this joint comes primarily from the ligaments that are related to the odontoid, such as the transverse ligament and the alar ligaments. Injury to any of these elements can result in serious neurological problems.

The instability in C1–C2 is much more common than in C0–C1, and can appear as a consequence of a trauma, a rheumatoid arthrosis or a tumour.

The transverse ligament is the main stabilizing element of the medial atlantoaxial joint. The attenuation or rupture of this ligament enables the atlas to be displaced forward in relation to the odontoid, especially during cervical flexion[23] (Fig. 5-5). Therefore, often, the problem is not objectivized in a lateral radiography in the neutral position. The studies of Fielding[24] show that, when the transverse ligament is

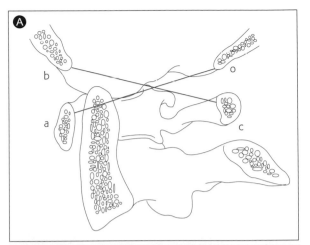

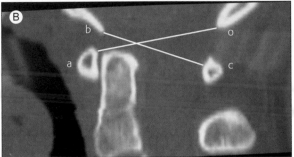

FIGURE 5-4 ■ Powers index: graphic (A) and CT (B). (a) Anterior arch of the atlas, (b) basion, (c) posterior arch of the atlas and (o) opisthion. The bc/oa index usually equals 1. A larger index indicates the sagittal instability of the occipital.

intact, the anterior displacement of C1 in relation to the odontoid is less than 3 mm. The tectorial membrane reinforces the stabilizing action of the transverse ligament. The anterior displacement of the atlas can significantly reduce the anteroposterior diameter of the central canal. The two ligaments that emerge from the transverse ligament, the transverso-occipital and transversoaxial ligaments do not seems to have much significance in the control of the craniocervical stability.

The relationship between the odontoid process, the atlas and the central canal follows Steel's rule of thirds.[25] The odontoid process occupies one-third, the spinal cord another third, and the last third is occupied by the safety area, located in front of and behind the spinal cord (Fig. 5-6).

In order to radiologically evaluate the competence of the transverse ligament, the anterior

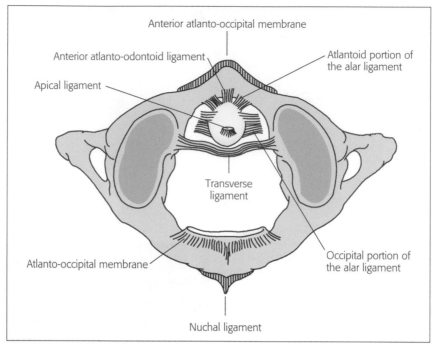

FIGURE 5-5 ■ The transverse ligament is the main stabilizing element of the medial atlantoaxial joint. Its reduction of rupture displaces the atlas forward in relation to the odontoid.

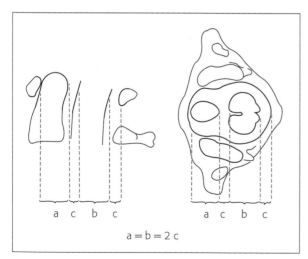

FIGURE 5-6 ■ Steel's rule of thirds: (a) odontoid process, (b) spinal cord and (c) safety zone: a = b = 2c. The odontoid process occupies a third, the cord another third, and the last third is the free safety zone, in front of and behind the cord.

atlanto-odontoid interval is measured, which corresponds to the distance between the posterior margin of the anterior arch of the atlas and the anterior face of the odontoid. A distance greater than 3 mm indicates the attenuation of the transverse ligament and, when the translation is greater than 5 mm, implies a rupture[26,27] (Fig. 5-7). The measurement if this interval does not have high reliability.[28]

The alar ligaments play a crucial role in the craniovertebral stability. These ligaments limit the flexion and the side-bending and are responsible mainly for the control of the craniocervical rotation. The flexion is limited by the tension of both ligaments; the side-bending is limited by the tension of the ipsilateral atlantoid portion and the contralateral occipital portion; the rotation, by the tension of both ligaments, although more intensely by the contralateral ligament.[23,29–33] (Fig. 5-8). The alar ligaments are therefore fundamental for controlling the rotation of the atlas[22,23,30] and their traumatic rupture determines the rotatory subluxation of the atlas (Fig. 5-9).

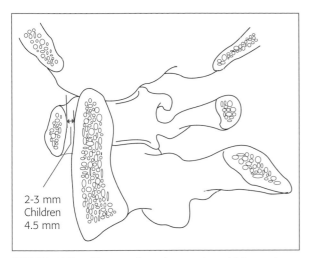

FIGURE 5-7 ■ The anterior atlanto-odontoid interval corresponds to the distance between the posterior margin of the anterior arch of the atlas and the anterior face of the odontoid. This interval should not be higher than 3 mm in adults or 4 mm in children. A distance higher than 3 mm indicates a reduction of the transverse ligament and when the translation is higher than 5 mm, it indicates its rupture.

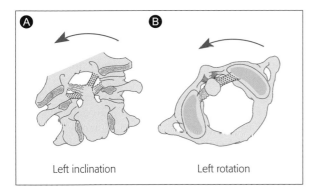

FIGURE 5-8 ■ The alar ligaments limit flexion and lateral inclination, and they are chiefly responsible for the control of the craniocervical rotation. (A) The lateral inclination is limited by the tension of the homolateral atlantoid portion and the contralateral occipital portion. (B) The rotation is limited by the tension of both ligaments, although more intensely by the contralateral ligament.

The confirmation of the rupture of the alar ligament can only be achieved with a CT in the neutral position and rotation. In normal subjects, the rotation of the atlas does not exceed 43° (standard deviation 5.5°). An axial rotation toward one side that is greater

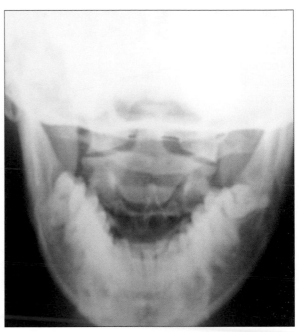

FIGURE 5-9 ■ In this subject, with this transoral projection, a rotatory subluxation of the atlas can be suspected. However, the confirmation can only be performed with a CT scan in rotation. The images of a CT of the same patient correspond to Figure 5-35.

than 56° indicates a pathological hypermobility due to the rupture of the contralateral alar ligament.[22]

Krakenes et al.[34] have shown that lesions of the alar ligament can be detected with high-resolution proton-weighted magnetic resonance imaging (MRI).

The injury of the alar ligament can manifest itself through an increase in the neutral zone in rotation. The alar ligaments can be injured during a trauma, such as a cervical whiplash, a mechanism of rotation or contralateral side-bending that may or may or may not be linked to flexion. Alar ligament injuries are suspected when the subject suffers a lateral impact of the head against the vehicle in car accidents.

The articular capsules have a role to play in atlantoaxial stability, although not to the same extent as the transverse and alar ligaments. They limit the rotation and the lateral flexion.[23,35] The disruption of an articular capsule causes an increase in the contralateral rotation, while the lateral flexion only increases if both capsules are divided.[35] The capsular ligaments suffer

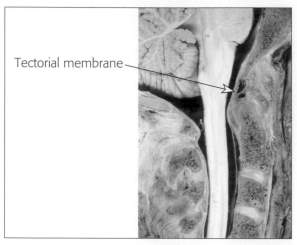

Tectorial membrane

FIGURE 5-10 ■ The tectorial membrane limits flexion of the head and is an important vertical stabilizer of the head, limiting its cranial translation in relation to C1 and C2.

significant stress during the mobility of that segment, and are often injured.

The tectorial membrane limits the flexion of the head and plays an important vertical stabilization role for it, limiting cranial translation in relation to C1 and C2[18,19,36] (Fig. 5-10).

The posterior atlanto-occipital and atlantoaxial membranes, which connect the posterior arch of the occipital with the posterior arch of C1 and C2, do not provide stability to the craniocervical spine. The lesions of the tectorial membrane and of the posterior atlanto-occipital membranes can be identified MRI.[34]

The nuchal ligament or dorsal raphe, although it can restrict the cervical flexion in some patients, does not participate in the stability of the cervical spine.

AETIOLOGY OF THE INSTABILITY

The causes of craniovertebral instability can be divided into congenital, inflammatory, traumatic and degenerative. In this chapter, only the first three causes are explained, since the last one has already been discussed in Chapter 2.

Congenital instability

Congenital malformations of the base of the skull, the atlas and the odontoid process are very diverse and can be manifested clinically in many ways. While some of them can cause an acute or progressive neurological deterioration, others remain completely asymptomatic.[37] In most cases, a direct relationship cannot be established between a particular malformation and specific signs and symptoms.

Basilar impression

The basilar impression is the most common cervico-occipital malformation and it involves the hypoplasia of the occipital, with the shortening of the clivus, associated with an invagination of the bone contour of the foramen magnum towards the inner part of the posterior cranial fossa. The foramen magnum is reduced in size as it is displaced upward inside the cranial cavity. The odontoid process tends to protrude inside the foramen magnum, which in turn leads to a greater narrowing of the foramen magnum and a decrease of the volume of the posterior fossa. Frequently, the basilar impression is accompanied by other anomalies, such as the assimilation of the atlas, the occipital vertebra, the anterior and posterior spina bifida of the atlas, the posterior translation of the odontoid, Klippel-Feil syndrome, malformation of Arnold–Chiari malformation and syringomyelia.[38,39]

The basilar impression can also be secondary to bone diseases, such as Paget's disease, imperfect osteogenesis, achondroplasia or rheumatoid arthritis.

The importance of this anomaly is linked to its compressive effects on the nervous system. The usual signs and symptoms associated with this deformity are muscular weakness, spasticity, alteration of gait, cervical pain and alteration of vesical or intestinal function. Some of the patients show signs suggesting the presence of this anomaly, such as a low hair line, short neck or stiff neck or restricted cervical mobility.[39]

The basilar impression can be defined radiologically by the quantity of protrusion of the vertex of the odontoid in the foramen magnum. In order to objectivize it, different lines can be drawn in a lateral projection of the cervical spine with conventional radiology, computed tomography (CT) or MRI, such as McRae's line (Fig. 5-11), Chamberlain's line (Fig. 5-12) or McGregor's line (Fig. 5-13); all of these link the distance of the odontoid with the base of the skull (Figs 5-14 and 5-15).

In order to detect this malformation, the bidigastric line (Fig. 5-16) and the basilar line of Wackenheim

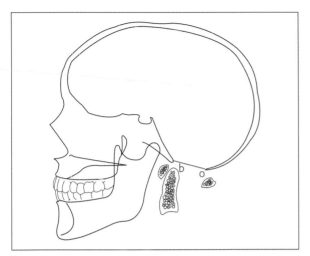

FIGURE 5-11 ■ McRae's line. It is drawn from the anterior edge of the foramen magnum (basion) (b) to its posterior edge (opisthion) (o). The odontoid should be located below this line. If this is not the case, it is a basilar impression.

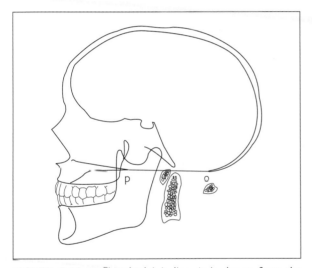

FIGURE 5-12 ■ Chamberlain's line. It is drawn from the posterior edge of the hard palate (p) to the opisthion (o). The vertex of the odontoid should not be projected more than 2.5 mm above this line.

(Fig. 5-17) can be drawn in an anteroposterior projection.

Anomalies in the upper cervical segmentation

There are various possible anomalies in the segmentation of the craniocervical spine and they include the

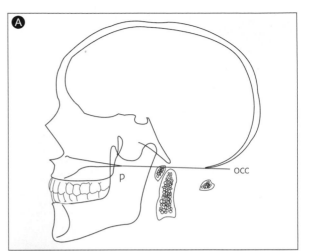

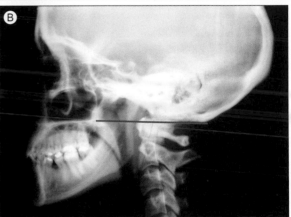

FIGURE 5-13 ■ McGregor's line. This is the easiest method used to measure the relationship between the odontoid and the base of the skull in a conventional radiograph. It touches the posterior edge of the hard palate (p) with the most caudal portion of the occipital (occ). The vertex of the odontoid should not extend more than 4.5 mm above this line. Graphic (A) and radiographic projection (B).

occipitalization of the atlas, the vertebralization of the occipital and the Klippel–Feil syndrome. The most common anomaly is the occipitalization of the atlas, either totally or partially. The anomalies in the bone configuration are accompanied by morphological anomalies in the ligaments responsible for the possible craniocervical instability.

Assimilation of the atlas. The assimilation or occipitalization of the atlas is one of the most common

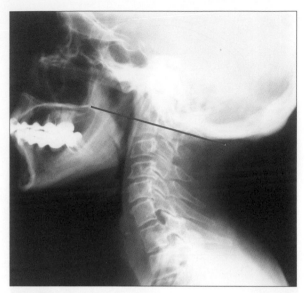

FIGURE 5-14 ■ Basilar impression secondary to an assimilation of the atlas.

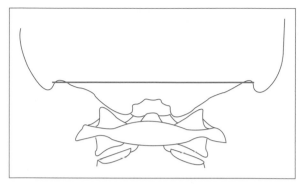

FIGURE 5-16 ■ Bidigastric line (Metzger and Fischgold). This line joins the two openings where the digastric muscle is inserted in the internal face of the base of the mastoid. This line crosses above the vertex of the odontoid. Due to the difficulty, in many cases, of the visualization of the digastric openings, another way to detect a basilar impression in an anteroposterior projection is to draw Wackenheim's line.

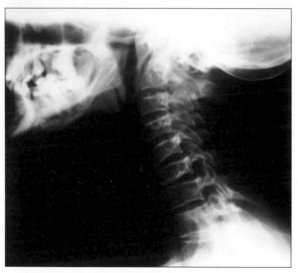

FIGURE   5-15 ■ Basilar   impression   secondary   to hyperparathyroidism,

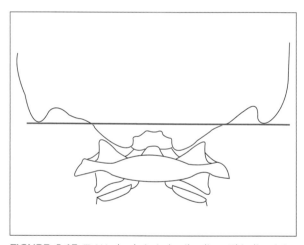

FIGURE 5-17 ■ Wackenheim's basilar line. This line joins the inferior edge of both mastoid processes. It is usually located 1 cm below the bidigastric line.

congenital anomalies of the craniovertebral spine[40] and is the result of a segmentation error between the last occipital and the first cervical sclerotoma, partially or completely. In most cases, it occurs between the anterior part of the arch of the atlas and the anterior edge of the foramen magnum and it can be associated with other malformations[41,42] (Fig. 5-18).

The assimilation of the occipital, as with other defects of the segmentation of the spine, causes greater stress in the adjacent segments.[43] Furthermore, if this anatomical anomaly is accompanied by a congenital block of the second and third cervical vertebrae, the result is atlantoaxial instability. The instability can lead to the proliferation of granulation tissue, which in turn aggravates the stenosis of the central canal.

Some subjects with assimilation of the atlas have clinical signs similar to the Klippel–Feil syndrome,

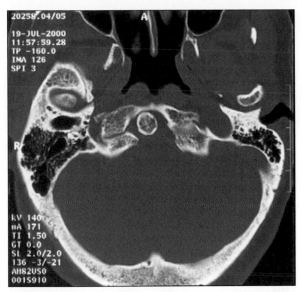

FIGURE 5-18 ■ CT showing assimilation of the atlas. The anterior arch of the atlas can be seen; the posterior arch is assimilated in the occipital.

such as a low hair line, short neck, restricted cervical mobility and occasional stiffness of the neck.

This anomaly can sometimes be identified using lateral radiography of the cervical spine and the possible instability of C1–C2, with dynamic projections. CT makes it possible to visualize the bone deformity and possible atlantoaxial instability, while MRI helps evaluate the formation of the granulation tissue and the degree of involvement of the neuroaxis.

In conclusion, the assimilation of the atlas is not usually symptomatic, but associated malformations can be symptomatic, such as the instability of C1–C2, the basilar invagination, the formation of granulation tissue or the fusion of C2–C3.

Klippel–feil syndrome. The most serious segmentation defect of the cervical spine is the Klippel–Feil syndrome. It is characterized by a congenital fusion of two or more cervical vertebrae, which can lead to increased instability between the mobile segments and those that are fused. It occurs as a consequence of an alteration in the embryonic development between 3 and 8 weeks of pregnancy. Klippel and Feil described a characteristic triad of the syndrome: short neck, low implantation of hair on the back of the neck and neck stiffness; this triad of signs and symptoms are present in only half of the cases.[44]

The fusion between C2 and C3 is the most common in the Klippel–Feil syndrome, and is not frequent in the C1–C2 and C0–C2 segments.[42,45,46]

The anomalies that are most often associated with the Klippel–Feil syndrome are the skeletal alterations (basilar invagination, skull asymmetry, scoliosis, etc.), deterioration of hearing, congenital heart conditions, eye malformations, facial asymmetry, cleft palate,[47,48] genitourinary malformations[49] and mirror movements.[44,50,51] Subjects with this syndrome can develop a spinal compression condition due to instability and anatomical alterations suffered by the central canal.[52]

Anterior and posterior spina bifida of the atlas. The dehiscence of the atlas can appear both in the anterior and posterior arch, and is more common in the posterior arch.[37] The defects of the posterior arch can be expressed in the form of complete aplasia, hemiaplasia or, more frequently, nonunion.[37,53] The congenital hyploplasia of the posterior arch can be associated with segmentation defects of the cervical spine[54] and, occasionally, this anomaly can be detected with a transoral projection, although the preferred diagnosis method is a CT scan with bone window.

The anomalies in the fusion of the atlas, anterior and posterior, are not manifested clinically, unless they are linked to other malformations or an atlantoaxial subluxation. Therefore, they do not usually require surgical stabilization, except for when they are accompanied by other anomalies, such as the Klippel–Feil syndrome, the basilar impression, the atlantoaxoid subluxation or the assimilation of the atlas. However, the presence of this type of anomalies contraindicates manual therapy treatment.

Os odontoideum. Os odontoideum can be defined as a separation of the odontoid process of the body of the axis. Patients with this anomaly can be asymptomatic or have a local mechanical irritation (neck pain and neck stiffness), a progressive myelopathy or transitory symptoms secondary to the compression of the vertebral artery.

Its pathogenesis is controversial. While some authors argue that, at least in some cases, its origin is congenital,[55,56] by observing a certain familial trend,[57,58] the majority consider that it is the consequence of a fracture of the synchondrosis of the odontoid caused in the intrauterine phase or before its closure, at the age of 5 or 6.[59-61] In this case, the tension exerted by the alar ligaments on the fragment of the odontoid causes the loss of its vascular irrigation and the subsequent bone reabsorption, leaving the characteristic round ossicle (Fig. 5-19). Regardless of its origin, this anomaly is of clinical importance, given that a mobile or insufficient odontoid causes incompetence of the transverse ligament of the atlas, and can lead to a compression of the cervical cord.

It was previously believed that the os odontoideum was the consequence of a failure in the fusion of the secondary ossification centre of the odontoid. This secondary ossification centre is merged with the odontoid during adolescence[62] and when this lack of ossification occurs, the anomaly is known as persistent ossiculum terminale, and has no relationship with the os odontoideum. This ossiculum terminale is different to than the os odontoideum, in the sense that it is smaller, and is located at the level of the ring of the atlas, above the transverse ligament and, unlike the os odontoideum, it does not cause atlantoaxial instability.

The os odontoideum is also different from a fracture of the odontoid process. In the first case, a round, conical or oval ossicle appears, with a smooth and uniform cortical, separated from the base of the axis by a wide space.[63] It can be associated with a hypoplasia of the posterior arch of the atlas and a hypertrophy of the anterior arch, which appears secondary due to a bone reaction to the atlantoaxial instability.[64-66] On the contrary, the characteristic image of an odontoid fracture associates irregular lower edges without being delimited by a cortical.

The prevalence of the os odontoideum is unknown, although it is not very common. Patients with this anomaly can be asymptomatic, and can detect its presence accidentally, or can have acute or progressive symptoms after a trauma. The more common symptoms are cervicalgia or neck stiffness, but in some cases this entity can be manifested as a compressive myelopathy or neurovascular symptoms due to the compression of the vertebral artery.[67-70]

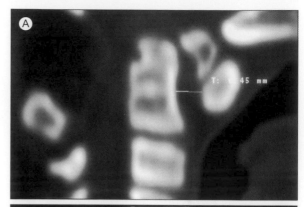

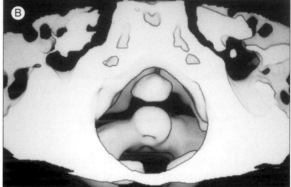

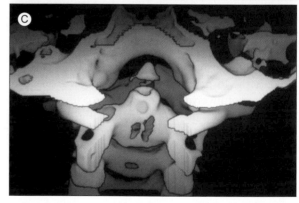

FIGURE 5-19 ■ Os odontoideum that has been displaced in the anterior direction in a CT scan (A) and its three-dimensional reconstruction (B and C).

The os odontoideum can be in a normal position in relation to the odontoid process (orthotopic), cranially displaced (dystopic) or fused with the clivus.[40]

It can be diagnosed in a lateral or transoral projection or by using a CT scan with bone window and three-dimensional reconstruction. The MRI helps to

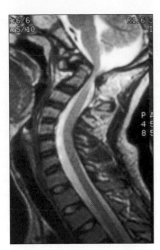

FIGURE 5-20 ■ In this MRI, a significant stenosis of the central canal can be seen as a consequence of an odontoid bone.

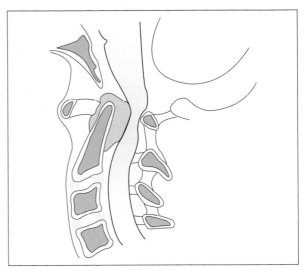

FIGURE 5-21 ■ In this diagram, an anterior subluxation of C2, it is possible to see the formation of the synovial pannus around the odontoid process and erosion of this process. The subluxation and growth of the synovial pannus determines the compression of the cervical spinal cord against the posterior arch of C1.

visualize the cervical cord and the possible myelomalacia secondary to atlantoaxial instability (Fig. 5-20). The majority of symptomatic patients show instability in dynamic radiographies, with an average displacement of 1 cm, generally in the anteroposterior direction, although it can be multidirectional.[68]

When the displacement of the os odontoideum leads to a reduction in the central canal (≤13 mm) and the patient has a clinical history of myelopathy or progressive neurological changes, surgical stabilization is recommended.[71] The management of this type of patient is similar to that of rheumatic patients with a subluxation of C1–C2.

Down syndrome. Atlantoaxial instability has a high occurrence in patients with Down syndrome, since this is the most frequent cause of congenital instability. There is an incidence rate of between 20% and 40% in subjects with this syndrome.[72–76] This instability is due to the ligament laxity that is characteristic of Down syndrome and to the higher prevalence of congenital defects, such as the hypoplasia of the odontoid and the os odontoideum.[76,77] In most cases, this instability is asymptomatic[76] and, although the neurological risk diminishes with age, it can ultimately result in myelopathy in adults.[78]

In 1–2% of subjects with Down syndrome, instability leads to spinal compression by the posterior displacement of the odontoid.[79] The joint mobilization techniques are therefore not recommended for these patients.

Inflammatory instability

Inflammatory conditions, specifically, rheumatoid arthritis, can be responsible for a serious instability of the craniocervical spine.

The clinical manifestations of rheumatoid arthritis are the result of an autoimmune process that affects the synovial joint. The release of cytokines stimulates an inflammatory reaction, with the development of a synovial pannus that results in joints being destroyed and the erosion of the bone structures.[80–82]

The craniocervical spine is very often affected by its high mobility and the several synovial structures. The subluxation of the craniocervical segments and the direct compression of the synovial pannus and the fibrous tissue that is formed in response to hypermobility can finally cause the compression of the spinal cord or the brainstem[82,83] (Fig. 5-21). The involvement of these joints increases mortality due to rheumatoid arthritis.[84]

In 43–86% of patients with rheumatoid arthritis, it is possible to radiologically observe cervical instability[85,86] and the atlantoaxial joint is the most commonly affected in 50–70% of all subluxations of the cervical spine.[86–90] This instability is very often caused by involvement of the synovial bursa, located between the posterior wall of the odontoid process and the transverse ligament of the atlas.[91] The progression of the atlantoaxial subluxation is also related to other factors, such as the involvement of multiple peripheral joints, the prolonged used of corticosteroids or the early onset of the disorder.[87,92,93]

The majority of subluxations are caused by an anterior displacement of the atlas, although they can also be due to lateral, posterior and rotatory subluxations[86,94–96] (Fig. 5-22). Approximately, 20% of rheumatoid subluxations are linked to a basilar invagination, due to the progressive destruction of the atlantoaxial and atlanto-occipital joints, and the lateral masses of the atlas. The basilar invagination is the most serious of all subluxations.[88,97,98] However, different studies have shown that, although patients with rheumatoid arthritis tend to suffer a radiological progression of their disorder in the cervical spine, the majority of them do not develop neurological deficits.[85,89,97,98]

Changes that emerge alongside rheumatoid arthritis in the cervical spine can be very subtle. Typically, patients report pain, especially in the upper cervical region, accompanied by a suboccipital headache. There may also be facial pain due to the compression of the trigeminal nerve. The neurological symptoms are multiples, and they range from hand paraesthesias to Lhermitte's sign. In some cases, basilar invagination can lead to a vertebrobasilar insufficiency.

The palpation of the craniocervical spine enables the detection of crepitation and, on occasion, a dull noise may indicate the presence of atlantoaxial instability. It is difficult to interpret the physical examination as slight neurological changes can be masked and be mistaken for other musculoskeletal manifestations of the disease. In these patients, it is important not to provoke either a cervical flexion or a retraction of the head, since they aggravate the anterior subluxation of the atlas.[99]

Radiographic examination

A simple radiograph facilitates the first evaluation of the articular disorder and the instability in a rheumatoid arthritis.

The anterior atlantoaxial subluxation can be objectified with the measurement of the anterior atlanto-odontoid interval. When this interval is greater than 3 mm in adults or 4 mm in children, it can be at risk[100] (Fig. 5-23). The interval increases with flexion, so that in a dynamic projection, it is possible to see if there is

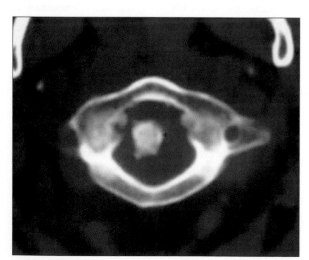

FIGURE 5-22 ■ Atlanto-occipital instability due to rheumatoid arthritis.

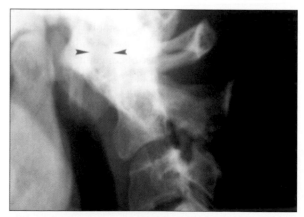

FIGURE 5-23 ■ Increase in the anterior atlanto-odontoid interval.

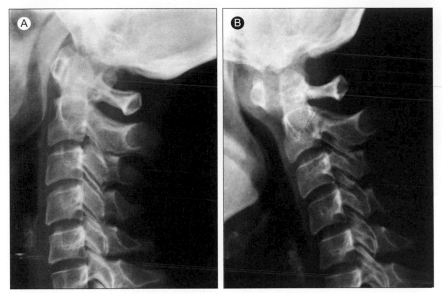

FIGURE 5-24 ■ Lateral radiographs of a patient with rheumatoid arthritis (A) in which an increase in the anterior atlanto-odontoid interval cannot be seen. However, a projection in flexion shows atlanto-odontoid instability (B).

excessive mobility (Fig. 5-24). The measurement of the difference of the atlanto-odontoid interval between the positions of flexion and extension is more clinically relevant than the measurement of the maximum flexion interval.

The method that seems to have higher specificity and sensitivity in the evaluation of the atlantoaxial subluxation is the measurement of the posterior atlanto-odontoid interval. This interval is defined as the distance that separates the posterior wall of the odontoid from the anterior margin of the lamina of C1. Its value should not be lower than 13 mm (Figs 5-25 and 5-26). This space, although it corresponds to the diameter of the canal, in patients with rheumatoid arthritis, does not represent the available space for the spinal cord, since the retro-odontoid synovial pannus can occupy between 1 and 3 mm.[88,97,101]

The vertical migration of the odontoid can be evaluated radiographically in different ways. It is possible to measure the position of the vertex of the odontoid in relation to the McRae, Chamberlain or McGregor lines. Since the vertex of the odontoid can be difficult to identify, due to the osteopenia and bone destruction associated with rheumatoid arthritis, other methods

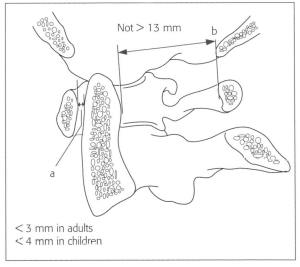

FIGURE 5-25 ■ Anterior and posterior atlanto-odontoid interval. The anterior atlanto-odontoid interval should not be higher than 3 mm in adults or 4 mm in children (a). The posterior atlanto-odontoid interval should not be lower than 13 mm (b).

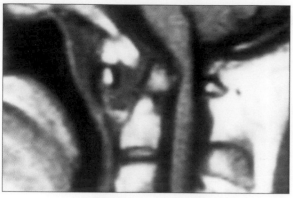

FIGURE 5-26 ■ In this MRI, a significant decrease in the space between the posterior wall of the odontoid and the posterior arch of the atlas in a subject with rheumatoid arthritis can be seen.

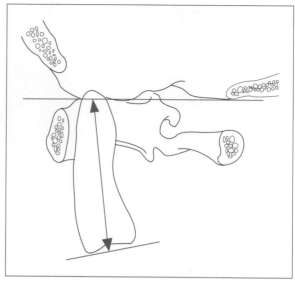

FIGURE 5-28 ■ Redlund-Johnell and Pettersson method. In a lateral radiography the distance between the McGregor line and the lower platform of the body of C2 is measured. The normal values are ≥34 mm in males and ≥ 29 mm in females. This method is useful when the visualization of the odontoid process is poor.

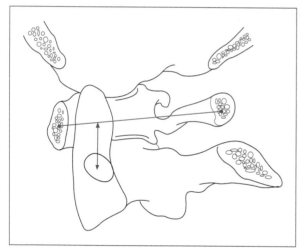

FIGURE 5-27 ■ Ranawat's method. A lateral radiograph measures the distance from the centre of the pedicles of C2 and a line drawn between the centre of the anterior and posterior arches of C1. The normal values should be ≥15 mm in males and ≥13 mm in females.

BOX 5-1

RISK FACTORS IN SPINAL COMPRESSION

- ADI > 9 mm
- PADI < 14 mm
- Basilar invagination, especially if combined with atlantoaxial subluxation
- Diameter of the central canal in the subaxial cervical spine < 14 mm

---

ADI, anterior atlanto-odontoid interval; PADI, posterior atlantoodontoid interval.

---

have been developed in order to quantify the intrusion of the odontoid in the foramen magnum.[102] These include the Ranawat method (Fig. 5-27), the Redlund-Johnell and Pettersson method[103] (Fig. 5-28) or the Kauppi method.[104]

The Redlund-Johnell and Pettersson method is highly reliable.[95,102] However, MRI is the preferred technique to show a possible spinal compression, as it makes it possible to directly observe the hypertrophy of the soft tissues, the secondary stenosis of the central canal and the changes in intensity of the spinal signal, secondary to compression.[105] At present, some authors are showing interest in using dynamic MRI to diagnose this pathology.[106,107]

The risk factors of the spinal compression are shown in Box 5-1.

Grisel syndrome

The Grisel syndrome is an uncommon condition that primarily affects the paediatric population, with 70%

of cases seen in children younger than 12 years old.[108] It is defined as a rotatory luxation of the atlas in relation to C2, maintaining normal anatomical relationships between the occipital and C2. Its origin is not usually traumatic, and it is seen after an infection of the upper respiratory tract.[11,109–113] The pharynx has lymphatic connections with the atlantoaxial region, so that a tooth, nasal, tonsil or middle ear infection can be drained into the craniocervical region. The secondary inflammation or hyperaemia can lead to an attenuation of the transverse ligament and the articular capsules, facilitating the luxation of the atlas.[109,114]

The characteristic presentation of the Grisel syndrome is a child with neck stiffness and painful limitation to movement, which appears spontaneously after an infection or a surgery of the upper respiratory tract.[111,115,116] The infection may have been overlooked, or perhaps the parents did not see the connection between it and the clinical condition. Therefore, the existence of a previous respiratory infection is a crucial aspect of the diagnosis.[109]

The confirmation of this injury is obtained with a CT or MRI[117,118] and early diagnosis is important to avoid the irreducibility of the luxation[119,120] (Fig. 5-29)

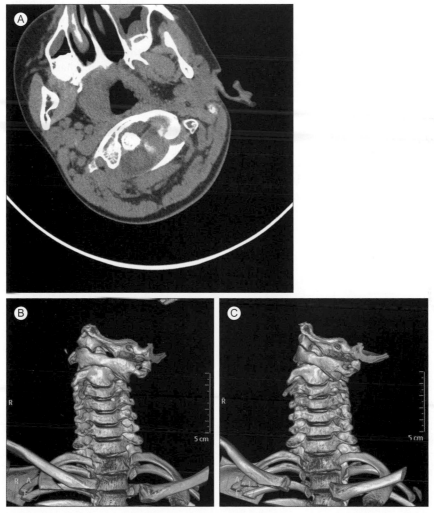

FIGURE 5-29 ■ Rotational subluxation of the atlas secondary to Grisel syndrome in a girl of 12 years old. Axial CT (A), CT 3D in left (B) and right rotation (C).

The initial treatment can involve an immobilization for 1 or 2 weeks and the use of anti-inflammatory medication or muscle relaxants. If the symptoms do not improve, a soft cervical traction and physical therapy should be applied.[109,121] If there is no improvement to symptoms or if new neurological symptoms appear, then it is necessary to have surgical reduction and stabilization.[122]

It is important to take this condition into account, since if the instability is acute, the neurological risk is high and if no spontaneous reduction occurs, it becomes more complicated to manage.

Traumatic instability

Craniocervical instability resulting from trauma, such as fractures and ligament ruptures, is often associated with high-energy mechanism, such as car accidents.[123–125] Injuries caused by high-velocity traumas can be bone injuries, such as the fracture of the occipital condyles and of the lateral masses of the atlas, the odontoid and the posterior arch of the axis. Many of the fractures of the craniocervical spine are accompanied by an injury of the ligaments. It is important to point out that a significant proportion of subjects with cervical fractures do not receive a correct diagnosis. In fact, up to 23% of patients are affected by delays diagnosing these fractures.[21] The problem is that these patients can request manual treatment for symptoms such as cervical pain and headaches.

Craniocervical spine fractures

The fractures of the occipital condyles are caused by direct impacts to the skull. The severity of the impact can lead to a loss of consciousness, in such a way that the fracture is not identified in some cases. Often, the only symptoms that the patient reports are suboccipital pain and headaches.[126] There have been some reports of subjects with chronic suboccipital pain having a non-diagnosed fracture of the occipital condyle.[127] The fractures of the occipital condyles can cause, due to their proximity, the rupture of the alar ligaments.

The fracture of the atlas is caused primarily by an axial compression mechanism or by hyperextension[128] (Fig. 5-30). It can be an isolated fracture of the anterior or posterior arch, or it can also affect both arches, in which case it is known as Jefferson's fracture (Fig. 5-31). In this fracture there is a lateral sliding of the fragments of the atlas. It can be seen in a transoral projection, since the margins of the lateral masses of the atlas exceed those of the lateral masses of the axis.

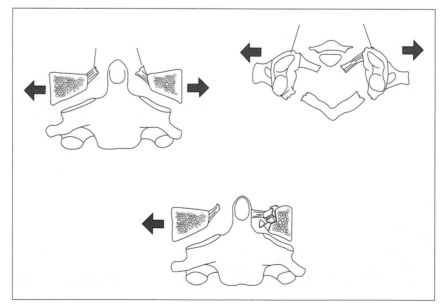

FIGURE 5-30 ■ In this fracture of the atlas, a lateral gliding of the fragments has occurred.

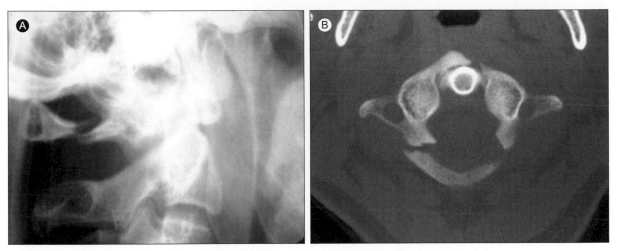

FIGURE 5-31 ■ Jefferson's fracture. Lateral radiograph (A) and CT scan (B).

The fracture of the odontoid process is quite common, occurring in more than 20% of the acute fractures of the cervical spine,[129–131] and 90–95% of the fractures of the odontoid are caused by a serious trauma, mainly due to traffic accidents.[132] Some of the fractures of the odontoid cause high atlantoaxial instability and constitute a significant risk of serious spinal injury.[133]

The fractures of the odontoid process are classified into three types[134] (Fig. 5-32):

- Type I: fracture of the apical portion of the odontoid. These fractures are very rare, and normally they are considered stable, although in some cases they are accompanied by the avulsion of the alar ligament and, therefore, of craniocervical instability.[131]
- Type II: fracture of the neck of the odontoid. This fracture is the most common type and it leads to atlantoaxial instability.
- Type III: fracture of the odontoid that extends to the body of C2 (Fig. 5-33).

Traumatic spondylolisthesis of the axis

Aside from fracturing of the odontoid, this is the most frequent traumatic injury of the axis.[131,135] In a traumatic spondylolisthesis, the fracture occurs in the articular isthmus of C2 (Fig. 5-34). This injury, classically known as hangman's fracture, usually occurs in car accidents, and it is rarely linked to a neurological deficit.[131]

Ligament injuries

Ligament injuries, such as the rupture or attenuation of the alar ligaments, the transverse ligament or the tectorial membrane, can appear by themselves, without having an associated fracture. This means that they are sometimes not detected by conventional radiographic examinations.

They are serious injuries that can go unnoticed, as the symptoms reported by the patients, such as headaches or pain in the suboccipital region, are common to other minor injuries.[126,127] Therefore, any patient with an injury caused by a high-energy mechanism should be considered to have a high risk of craniocervical injury, and a complete neurological evaluation should be carried out.[136]

> Any patient with a medical record listing an injury caused by a high-energy mechanism should be considered to have a high risk of craniocervical injury, and a complete neurological evaluation should be carried out.

Injuries of the alar ligaments.

The alar ligaments are the most important elements in the control of rotation. In fact, an axial rotation of C1 towards one side higher than 56° is indicative of pathological hypermobility caused by the rupture of the contralateral alar ligament.[22]

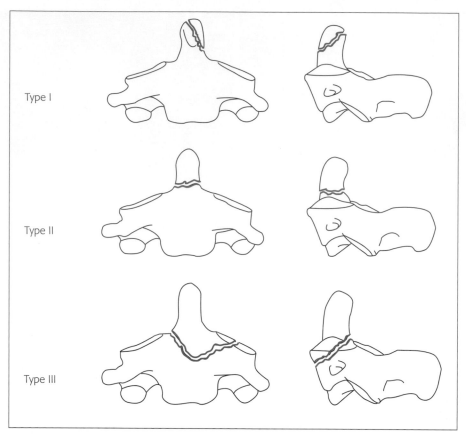

FIGURE 5-32 ■ The fractures of the odontoid process are classified into three types: type I, fracture of the apical portion of the odontoid; type II, fracture of the neck of the odontoid; and type III, fracture of the odontoid that extends to the body of C2.

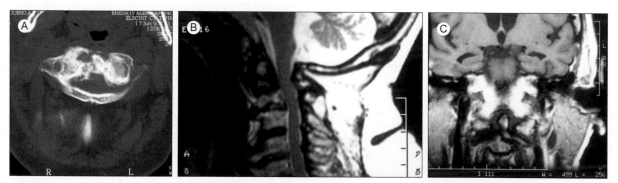

FIGURE 5-33 ■ Type III odontoid fracture. A reduction of the anteroposterior diameter of the central canal can be seen. CT (A), sagittal MRI (B) and coronal MRI (C).

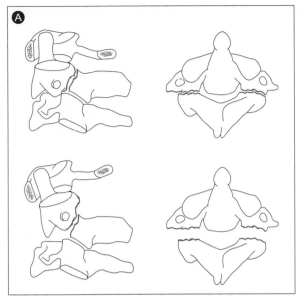

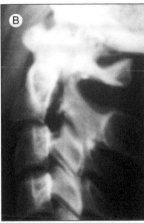

FIGURE 5-34 ■ Fracture of the posterior arch of C2. Diagram (A) and radiographic image (B).

An isolated injury of the alar ligament can occur after a forced lateral flexion or rotation.[30] The trauma should be high energy, and it is more likely to occur, for example, when the subject hits his head against the vehicle in a car accident.

Rupturing of the alar ligaments is confirmed with a functional CT in left and right rotation, in which an abnormal displacement of the atlas is shown (Fig. 5-35). The injuries of the alar ligament can be identified with high-resolution proton density-weighted MRI.[137] The injuries of these ligaments can go unnoticed, since often patients have a minimal symptomatology, leading to chronic pain by instability.

Injuries of the transverse ligament. The injury of the transverse ligament is caused by an anterior translation or rotation mechanism.[24,138] The most frequent injury involves an impact on the posterior part of the head, which usually leads to a forced flexion. The acute traumatic rupture of the transverse ligament can be associated with a shatter fracture of C1 (Jefferson's fracture).[129,139,140]

This serious injury is usually accompanied by brain trauma, but the neurological signs and symptoms vary from a normal function to a temporary tetraparesis (Fig. 5-36).[141] The spasm of the muscles of the neck causes a limitation of the cervical mobility, and if there is an associated injury of the vertebral artery, it is possible to observe symptoms of vertebrobasilar insufficiency.

The rupture of the transverse ligament of the atlas can be diagnosed by measuring the anterior atlanto-odontoid interval in a lateral radiography, which should not be greater than 3 mm in adults, or 4 mm in children.[88,100,141]

In the same way, a posterior atlanto-odontoid interval lower than 17 mm indicates atlantoaxial instability, and if it is lower than 14 mm, it points to possible spinal compression.

In order to detect an atlantoaxial instability, the Thiebaut–Vrousos–Wackenheim line can be drawn (Fig. 5-37), or a measurement can be made of the vertex–clivus distance of the odontoid (Fig. 5-38). Krakenes et al.[142] have shown that the injuries of the transverse ligament can be identified with high-resolution proton-weighted MR sequences.

DIAGNOSIS OF CRANIOVERTEBRAL INSTABILITY

Subjective examination

Major instability

The subjective examination can indicate that there is instability, and the review of a traumatic history, as well as the behaviour of the symptoms, can lead us to suspect its presence.

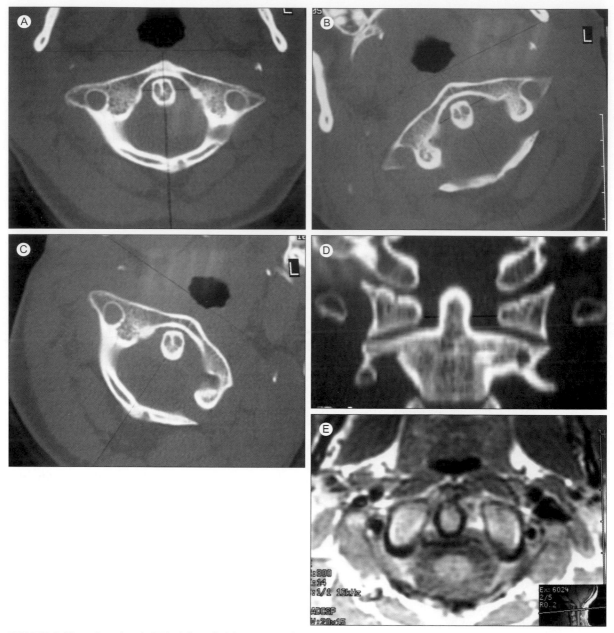

FIGURE 5-35 ■ Functional CT in left and right rotation for a rupture of the alar ligaments. In this patient, a left rotatory subluxation of the atlas can be seen. CT in neutral rotation (A), right rotation (B) and left rotation (C) in which the displacement of the odontoid can be seen. The coronal CT (D) and the MRI (E) show an increase in the distance of the odontoid in relation to the left lateral mass of the atlas.

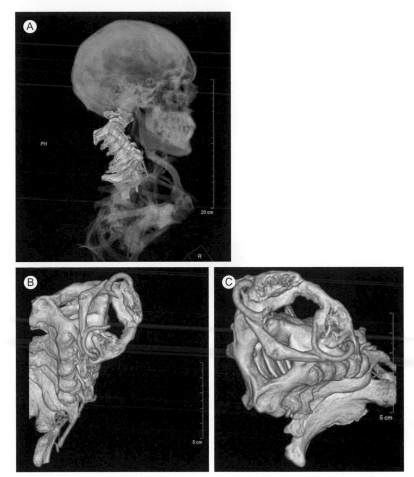

FIGURE 5-36 ■ (A–C) Complete rupture of the basioccipital ligamentary complex. A 34-year-old male came to a hospital 3 months following a traffic accident. He stated that he has had difficulty looking at the computer screen over the last month. The only symptom that the patient reported was a slight sporadic tingling pain in his right hand. In the 3D reconstruction with a CT scan, it was possible to observe complete anterior movement of C1 onto C2. This happened in such a way that the posterior arc of C1 was supported on the odontoides.

The first measure that should be adopted with patients that have suffered a cervical trauma is to rule out the existence of ligament fractures or injuries. The diagnosis of cervical whiplash often conceals serious ligament fractures or injuries.

There is some information obtained from the subjective examination that can make us suspect a fracture or a serious injury. In an injury caused by a cervical whiplash, the symptoms do not usually appear immediately, but after a few hours. Therefore, when the patient reports severe pain immediately after the accident, there could be a serious trauma. Serious injury is also suspected if the subject has suffered loss of consciousness.

In a cervical whiplash, the injuries are potentially more serious when the subject suffers a head impact on the dashboard or the car window.

During the patient's examination, a serious injury can be suspected when the patient has a significant limitation of the mobility in all directions. A patient with serious instability, especially after a fracture, usually holds his head to avoid any movement.

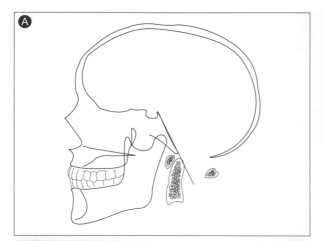

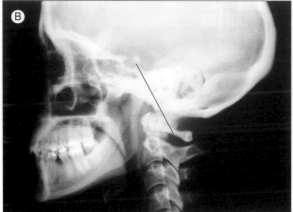

FIGURE 5-37 ■ Thiebaut–Vrousos–Wackenheim's line. This line is directed towards the prolongation of the clivus and should cross in the posterior direction of the odontoid. When this line cuts through the odontoid, there is a displacement of the odontoid, secondary to atlantoaxial instability. Diagram (A) and radiographic projection (B).

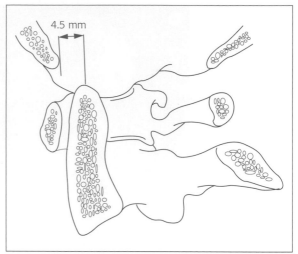

FIGURE 5-38 ■ Clivus–vertex distance of the odontoid. This distance in normal adults should not be higher than 4.5 mm. A higher distance can indicate atlanto-odontoid instability due to an injury of the transverse ligament.

When there is any indication of instability, it is necessary to request adequate diagnostic imaging tests. It should be remembered that dynamic projections should never be requested without a prior static projection. Some serious injuries, seen in a conventional radiography, contraindicate the use of dynamic projections. It is worth noting that, in some cases, muscular spasms can conceal instability in a dynamic radiography.

Indications to suspect serious traumatic instability:

- Intense traumatic accident.
- Direct head impact against the dashboard or car window.
- Severe pain that appears immediately.
- Loss of consciousness.
- Haematomas on the face, neck and behind the mastoid process.
- Significant limitation of mobility in all directions.
- Muscle weakness in all directions.
- Dysphagia in the days following the accident.

Minor instability

The diagnosis of major cervical instability is performed by considering the history and clinical presentation of the patient and, generally, it can be confirmed

Another sign that may lead to suspicions is the presence of haematomas on the face or neck, and on occasions the fractures of the bones of the base of the skull lead to a haematoma behind the mastoid process (Battle's sign).

When there is a fracture, the patient normally shows an inhibition of muscular contraction, with a pronounced weakness in all directions.[143] In these cases, patients are often unable to raise their head from the pillow without using their hands to help them.

A serious injury of the bones or soft tissues can lead to a retropharyngeal haematoma, which manifests itself as a dysphagia in the days following the accident.

with the aid of imaging techniques. However, when diagnosing minor instability, it is necessary to take a series of signs and symptoms into consideration and some of these are very subjective.

The first thing to find out is whether the patient's medical record contains any previous trauma or activity that can place a repeated overload on an articular segment.

On occasion, the patient reports a history of frequent wry neck or neck stiffness or a catching/locking sensation that occurs when performing rapid or large movements of the cervical spine. The same patients tend to limit the mobility of the head in order to avoid pain, and they often report a subjective sensation of weakness and a lack of control over the cervical spine. Holding positions that require cervical stabilization are done with difficulty, and the smallest amount of mechanical stress causes the appearance of serious symptoms that take several days to disappear.

Niere and Torney[16] have conducted a study with the aim of recognizing the signs of minor instability in the cervical spine by consulting with physiotherapists who are experts at managing the pathology of the cervical spine. The clinical findings that more than 50% of the consulted physical therapists considered suggestive of minor instability were the following: history of serious trauma or repeated microtrauma, sensation of catching/locking/giving way, poor muscular control, radiographic signs of hypermobility, excessively free end-feel with palpation and unpredictable symptoms.

In this study, the different findings possibly related to instability were grouped into four factors: passive dysfunction, active dysfunction, pattern of involvement of the craniovertebral spine and alteration of the mobility. Table 5-1 displays these four factors.

The authors recommend that therapists who treat patients with cervical pathology should consider the possible presence of a minor instability in the cervical spine when one of the six findings described or one of the group factors identified by the analysis of the factors are present.[16]

Cook et al.[144] conducted a Delphi study with the purpose of obtaining identifiers that suggest cervical instability, which included both symptoms suggestive of instability and findings in the physical examination. The symptoms suggestive of instability were classified into five conceptual areas: movements, descriptive components, postures, neurological phenomena and headaches.

Regarding the movements, it was found:

- Sharp pain, possibly with sudden movements.
- Neck gets stuck, or locks, with movement.
- Minor movements provoke symptoms.
- Unwillingness, apprehension, or fear of making movements.

As descriptive components, the following are described:

- Past history of neck dysfunction or trauma.
- Improvement with an external support, such as the hands or collar.
- Frequent need for self-manipulation.

TABLE 5-1
Signs of minor instability in the cervical spine

Factor 1	Factor 2	Factor 3	Factor 4
Passive dysfunction	Active dysfunction	Pattern of involvement of the craniocervical spine	Alteration of mobility
Traction spurs	Insufficient muscle control	Headache	Excessively free end-feel with palpation
Signs of hypermobility on X-ray	Subjective sensation of neck weakness	Neck pain	Altered range of motion
Spondylolisthesis	Unpredictable symptoms	Muscle spasm	History of major trauma
History of repeated microtrauma	Catching/locking/giving way	Muscle atrophy	
History of major trauma	Muscular atrophy		

- Feeling of instability, shaking, or loss of control.
- Frequent episodes of acute attacks.
- Head feels heavy.
- Catching, clicking, clunking and popping sensation.
- Muscles feel tight or stiff.
- Temporary improvement with manipulation.
- The symptoms worsen as the day progresses.

Related to posture:

- Intolerance to prolonged static postures.
- Improvement in unloaded position such as lying down.

Among the findings of the physical examination, the most frequent were:

- Poor coordination/neuromuscular control (poor recruitment and dissociation of cervical segments with movement).
- Abnormal joint play.
- Motion that is not smooth throughout the range of movement.
- Aberrant movement.
- Catching, clicking, clunking and popping sensation heard during movement assessment.
- Apprehension and fear or decreased willingness to move during examination.
- Disparity between amplitude active range of motion and passive range of motion.
- Decreased active range of motion in weight bearing.

No consensus was obtained with regard to the articular integrity tests.

Instability tests

Before a cervical manual therapy intervention, it is recommended to screen patients for upper cervical instability to minimize the risk of complications.[145–147] Clinical craniocervical instability tests are advised when the subjective examination indicates that there may be a prior history of trauma, or when the symptoms of the patients point to an instability. Some of the instability tests described are the Sharp–Purser test,[148–152] the clunking test,[151] the palate sign,[151] the sagittal stress test of the atlanto-occipital joint and atlantoaxial joint,[36] the lateral stress for the atlanto-axial joint,[36] the alar ligament test,[153] the transverse ligament test,[153] the tectorial membrane test[36,153] and the posterior atlanto-occipital membrane test.[153]

The majority of the instability tests involve performing a translatory movement of a joint in order to notice any abnormal movement or reproduce the symptoms in a controlled manner.[154] The reliability of these tests has been questioned recently.[155,156] Moreover, all manual instability tests require very skilled assessment, and have not been corroborated by simultaneous diagnostic measurement.[144]

At the moment there are few studies that have assessed the diagnostic accuracy of upper cervical instability screening tests.[148,150–153]

In a recent systematic review, Hutting et al.[157] analysed the diagnostic accuracy of some upper cervical spine instability tests: the clunking test, the palate sign, the transverse ligament test, the tectorial membrane test, the alar ligament test, the atlanto-occipital membrane test and the Sharp–Purser test. The specificity of almost all the tests was sufficient, so they can be used to rule in patients with upper cervical spine instability, but confidence intervals of the likelihood ratios were very wide, indicating precision. The sensitivity for most tests was insufficient when it came to detecting upper cervical spine instability. They concluded that screening for upper cervical instability using instability tests cannot be carried out accurately at the moment. However, the atlanto-axial membrane test and the tectorial membrane test have shown good diagnostic accuracy in patients with whiplash-associated disorders (WAD). In conclusion, the role of these tests in diagnosing upper cervical spine instability as screening tools has yet to be confirmed. However, when the subjective examination suggests a prior trauma history and/or the symptoms of cervical instability, the clinician should carry out these tests carefully and interpret the results with caution. As always, the patient's clinical profile should have a greater bearing on the clinical examination.

The tests described in this section are considered positive when an abnormal movement is perceived and/or the patient experiences one or more of the following symptoms[36]:

1. Loss of balance in relation to head movements, history of drop attacks.

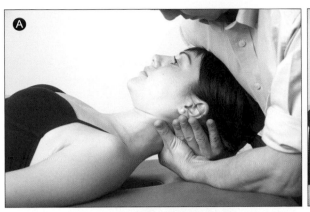
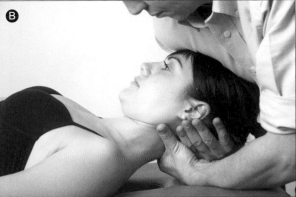

FIGURE 5-39 ▪ Distraction test (A) and distraction test in flexion (B).

2. Facial and lip paraesthesia, reproduced by active or passive movements.
3. Bilateral or quadrilateral limb paraesthesia, either constant or reproduced/aggravated by movements of the head or neck.
4. Nystagmus caused by active or passive movement of the head or neck.

Before performing any integrity test of the craniocervical ligaments it is imperative for the patient to perform all the physiological movements. If a significant antalgic patter is seen, these tests are contraindicated. Also, if a clunking noise is felt during active movements, then these tests should not be carried out.

Distraction test

This test evaluates the integrity of the ligaments that are orientated longitudinally. Research conducted on specimens by Pettman[36] shows how, due to their posterior orientation, the ligaments that resist distraction also resist the flexion of the spine. An example of this is the tectorial membrane, which has been shown to be the structure that most limits the distraction of the head in relation to C1 and C2, and is tensed significantly with atlantoaxial flexion.

The test is performed in the following way: with the patient's head and neck in the neutral position, the therapist stabilizes the posterior arch of C2 with the thumb and the index finger, and with the other hand on the occipital, applies progressive traction. The reproduction of symptoms suggests ligament instabil-

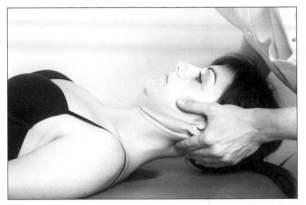

FIGURE 5-40 ▪ Test for the posterior stability of the atlanto-occipital joint.

ity, with particular involvement of the tectorial membrane (Fig. 5-39).

Sagittal stress tests

Test for the posterior stability of the atlanto-occipital joint. The therapist, using the palms of both hands, applies a slight compression to stabilize the skull. Then, anterior force is applied on the posterior arch of C2 with the index fingers, with the purpose of causing an anterior translation of C1 and C2 in relation to the occipital (Fig. 5-40).

Test for the anterior stability of the atlanto-occipital joint. The therapist stabilizes the patient's skull with both hands and, with the aid of both thumbs, pushes

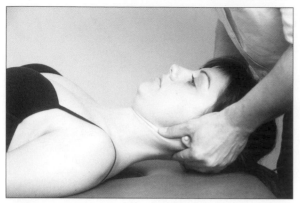

FIGURE 5-41 ■ Test for the anterior stability of the atlanto-occipital joint.

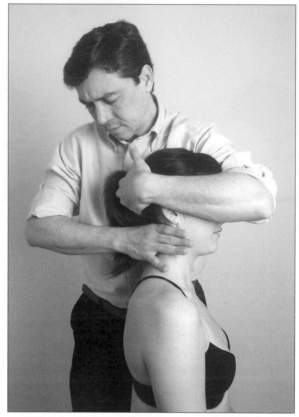

FIGURE 5-42 ■ Test for the anterior stability of the atlanto-axial joint.

the transverse processes of C1 and C2 in the posterior direction and with fingers 2 to 5 in an anterior direction, with the purpose of identifying anterior atlanto-occipital instability (Fig. 5-41).

Test for the anterior stability of the atlantoaxial joint. This test has the purpose of identifying anterior atlantoaxial instability. With the patient sitting down, the therapist fixes the posterior arch of C2 with the thumb and index finger. With the other arm, the therapist holds the patient's head and applies a progressive translatory force in the posterior direction (Fig. 5-42). Under normal conditions, no movement should be noticed. If there is atlantoaxial instability, a movement is noticed, sometimes accompanied by a noise caused by the impact of the anterior arch of C1 with the odontoid process. This test does not attempt to reproduce the patient's symptoms.

Sharp–purser test[149]. This test also has the aim of identifying atlantoaxial instability. Therefore, it analyses the appearance of signs and symptoms with the flexion of the cervical spine and their disappearance when a posterior translation of the occipital and the atlas is applied.

With the subject sitting down, the head and the neck are flexed gently and checks are made to see if the patient refers symptoms. If any symptoms appear, the spinous process of C2 is stabilized with the index and the thumb of one hand, and with the other hand the patient's forehead is pushed in the posterior

direction. The test is positive when the symptoms appear with the flexion of the head and neck, and when they disappear with the posterior translation of the head (Fig. 5-43).

Uitvlugt and Indenbaum[148] showed the clinical validity of this test in the diagnosis of atlantoaxial instability. According to these authors, its sensitivity is 88% when the subluxation is larger than 4 mm. The predictive value is 85% and the specificity level is 95%.

Coronal stress tests

Test of lateral stress for the atlantoaxial joint. This test attempts to objectivize the instability of the atlas in the coronal plane, displacing it from one side to the other. With the patient in the supine position, the therapist holds the occipital with one hand and places the index finger on the lateral face of the posterior arch

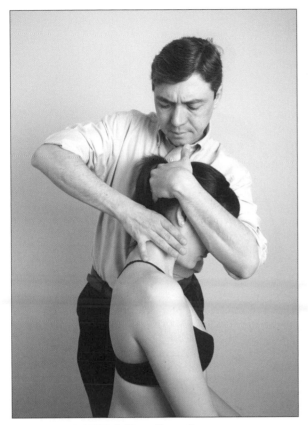

FIGURE 5-43 ■ Sharp–Purser test.

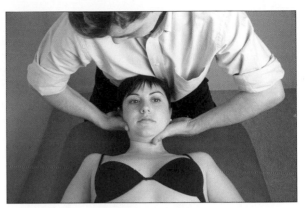

FIGURE 5-44 ■ Lateral stress test for the atlantoaxial joint.

of C1. The index of the other hand is placed on the lateral face of the posterior arch of C2. Then, the test is performed by applying a movement of lateral translation of the atlas, first towards one side and then towards the other (Fig. 5-44). Excessive movement or the reproduction of the patient's symptoms suggests the lateral instability of the joint.

Stress test of the alar ligaments

Tests of the alar ligaments in lateral flexion. This test is based on the coupling pattern of C2 during the lateral flexion of the head in which a rotation of C2 occurs towards the same side of the side-bending necessarily.[158]

With the patient sitting down, the therapist stabilizes the posterior arch of C2 with the thumb and index fingers of one hand and, with the other hand, applies a lateral inclination to the head. If the thumb

and index fingers prevent the rotation of C2, the lateral flexion of the head is not possible, and if this movement occurs, it is possible to suspect a rupture of the contralateral alar ligament (Fig. 5-45).

Tests of the alar ligaments in rotation. This test analyses the resistance offered by the alar ligaments to the rotation movement. With the patient sitting down, the therapist stabilizes, with the thumb and index fingers of one hand, the posterior arch of C2, and with the other hand causes a rotation of the head. Under normal circumstances, it is not possible to have more than 20–30° of rotation. If the mobility exceeds this range, it is necessary to suspect a rupture of the alar ligament of the opposite side of the rotation (Fig. 5-46).

Despite the fact that, as some studies have shown,[156] these tests have a low level of reliability, they are currently the only clinical tools that help detect possible craniocervical instability.

Motor control tests

The description of the motor control tests is shown with a sequence that is considered to be the most comfortable for the patient. Many of the tests described below correspond to active movements that are part of the basic active examination of the spinal column. They are included in this chapter in order to highlight aspects that may indicate poor motor control of the neck when carrying out tests. The evaluation of movement control disorders and its direct treatment is

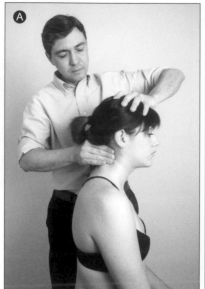
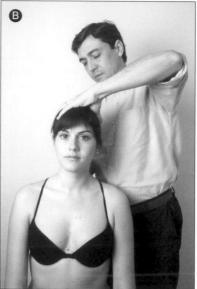

FIGURE 5-45 ■ Test of the alar ligaments in lateral flexion. The therapist stabilizes the posterior arch of C2 with the index finger and the thumb of one hand (A), and with the other hand applies a lateral inclination to the head (B).

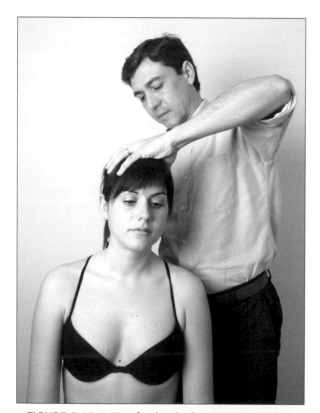

FIGURE 5-46 ■ Test for the alar ligaments in rotation.

considered to be an integral part of diagnosis and management of cervical musculoskeletal disorders.[6,159,160] The validity[161,162] and reliability[163,164] of the craniocervical flexion test and the deep neck flexor endurance test have been demonstrated. Recently, the inter- and intra-tester reliability of a battery of cervical movement control dysfunction tests has been analysed and are described in this section comparing expert and novice examiners with subjects that have chronic neck pain (15 subjects) and a control group (17 subjects).[165] Specifically, the tests looked at active bilateral arm flexion in standing,[17] active unilateral arm flexion in standing,[166] active cervical extension in sitting,[6] active return to neutral from cervical extension in sitting,[6] active cervical rotation in sitting,[166] active cervical flexion in 4 point kneeling,[166] active cervical extension in 4 point kneeling,[6] rocking backwards in 4 point kneeling[166] and active upper cervical rotation in 4 point kneeling.[6]

Intra- and inter-tester reliability for the complete battery of these tests was shown to be substantial to excellent. Intra-rater reliability values for the expert and novice were overall comparable. This suggests that novices can achieve good accuracy with the battery of tests, if trained.

Frequency of impaired performances for the complete battery of tests and for most tests individually was comparable between groups (neck pain and healthy). A greater number of impaired ratings was only identified in the neck pain group for two individual cervical movement control dysfunction tests (i.e. active cervical extension in 4-point kneeling and active cervical rotation in sitting). This suggests that cervical movement control dysfunction tests, although reliable, when used in isolation may not be helpful for distinguishing between the neck and non-neck pain groups.

When carrying out motor control tests, it is important to note that a positive test does not necessarily mean that there is a lack of motor control. Many subjects can carry out functional movements in different ways, which can involve different learned movement strategies. Furthermore, a positive motor control test does not dictate a mean of treatment; in many cases, these alterations to voluntary movement are adaptive strategies that the subject has developed in response to acute pain. Therefore, first of all we have to determine if the alteration to motor control has any relevance to the patient's clinical condition. Secondly, it is essential to consider if the alteration to motor control is adaptive or not, as if it is adaptive, then treatment is not initially recommended.

Active bilateral arm flexion in standing. This test, described by Comerford and Mottram,[17] assesses the flexor activation and extensor muscle co-contraction. The clinician asks the patient to elevate both arms at the same time. The cervical spine should remain still during 180° of bilateral arm flexion. The test is positive if the patient shows a compensatory/excessive forward head movement or extension of the cervical spine during bilateral arm flexion (Fig. 5-47).[17]

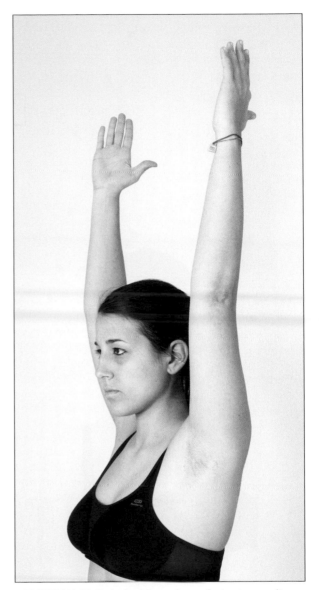

FIGURE 5-47 ■ Active bilateral arm flexion in standing.

Active unilateral arm flexion in standing. This test, described by Sahrmann,[166] assesses the flexor activation and extensor muscle co-contraction. The clinician asks the patient to elevate one arm. The cervical spine should remain still during single-arm 180° flexion. The test is positive if the patient shows a compensatory motion of cervical rotation/side-bending during arm flexion (Fig. 5-48).

Active cervical extension in sitting. This test, described by Jull et al.,[6] assesses the eccentric control of flexor muscles. The clinician asks the patient to do a neck extension movement. Ideally, the head moves backwards in extension behind the frontal plane of the shoulders to within 15–20° from horizontal. A pattern of smooth and even neck extension should be observed. There should be concurrent upper and lower cervical

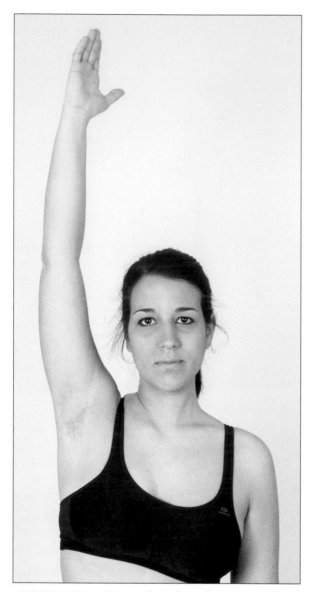

FIGURE 5-48 ■ Active unilateral arm flexion in standing.

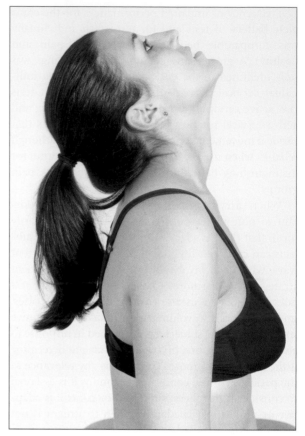

FIGURE 5-49 ■ Active cervical extension in sitting.

movement. The test is positive if the clinician observes one or two possible dysfunctional movements. In one of them, the patient shows a dominant upper cervical spine extension with minimal, if any, posterior head movement. In the other, the patient's head moves backward but then reaches a point of extension where it appears to drop or tilt backwards. This is often quite uncomfortable for the patient who wants to return

immediately to the upright position, occasionally by using their hands. Patients may describe pain or feeling of loss of control of their head at this point (Fig. 5-49).

Assisted cervical extension in sitting. We also do an assisted test when the patient shows a dominant upper cervical spine extension with minimal or no lower cervical spine extension (Fig. 5-50). This test can help to know if the lack of lower neck extension is due to a joint stiffness or to a lack of eccentric control of the cervical spine flexors. It also helps us to identify an apprehension or fear-avoidance behaviour to this movement.

Active return to neutral from cervical extension in sitting. The clinician asks the patient to return to neutral position, starting with craniocervical flexion

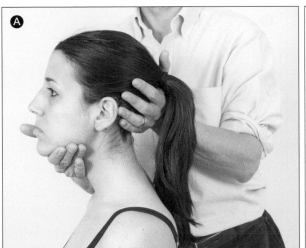 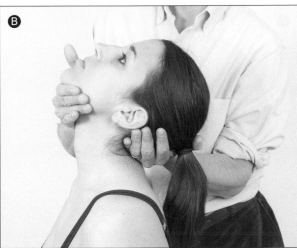

FIGURE 5-50 ■ (A, B) Assisted cervical extension in sitting.

followed by lower cervical flexion. This test, described by Jull et al.,[6] assesses the concentric control of the flexor muscles. The test is positive if the patient initiates the return to neutral position with lower cervical flexion but not upper craniocervical flexion. Craniocervical flexion is the last component of the pattern of movement and not the first as it should be. This normally occurs because of an excessive activation of the sternocleidomastoid and anterior scalene muscles (Fig. 5-51).

Active cervical rotation when sitting. The clinician asks the patient to perform a right and then left rotation. This test, described by Sahrmann,[166] evaluates the rotation movement control. A pattern of smooth and even head rotation around a vertical axis of movement should be observed to each side (70–80° rotation to each side). The plane of the face should stay vertical, with the eyes horizontal and with concurrent upper and lower cervical movement. No other components of motion, such as side-bending, extension or flexion, should be observed (Fig. 5-52).

Craniocervical flexion test. This is a specific test, developed by Jull et al.,[6,167] that evaluates the role of the deep cervical flexor muscles longus colli, longus capitis, rectus capitis anterior using a Chattanooga Stabilizer Pressure Biofeedback (Chattanooga Group, NJ, USA). There is a large amount of evidence showing the validity[161,162] and reliability[163,164] of this test. The patient is in the supine crook lying position and the cervical spine in the neutral position, keeping the forehead and the chin in the horizontal plane. Towels can be placed under the occipital in order to keep the cervical spine correctly aligned. In subjects with thoracic kyphosis, some of the layers of the towel are extended on the space between the posterior part of the neck and the surface where the test is performed in order to prevent the Biofeedback device from overinflating. Subjects who rectify the lordosis in this position should be trained to adopt a neutral cervical position.

■ The pressure Biofeedback device is located in the suboccipital region and the system is inflated with an initial base pressure of 20 mmHg.
■ The patient should perform a craniocervical flexion, as if nodding. The activation of the deep cervical flexor muscles is associated with a slight straightening of the cervical lordosis, translated into an increase of the pressure recorded by the Biofeedback device (Fig. 5-53).
■ In the craniocervical flexion test, the pressure should initially increase only 2 mmHg. When the patient is able to perform the test avoiding the replacement of the superficial muscles or with any other motor strategy, the pressure is increased another 2 mmHg. As such, five levels

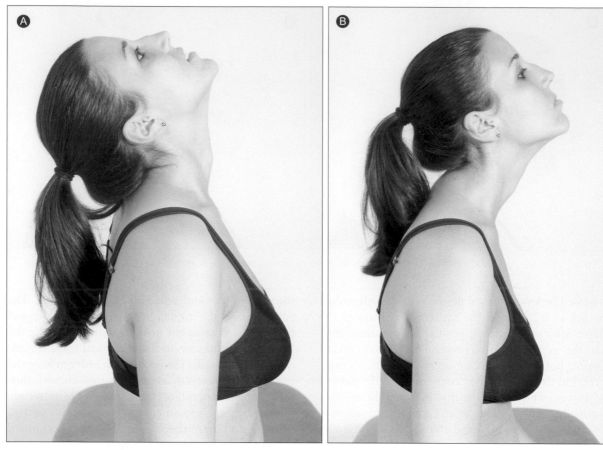

FIGURE 5-51 ■ Active return to neutral from extension in sitting. (A) Correct performance. (B) The patient initiates the return to neutral position with lower cervical flexion but not upper craniocervical flexion.

of progression are taken into consideration (22, 24, 26, 28 and 30 mmHg).

- Normally, the goal is to achieve a pressure increase of at least 26 mmHg, maintaining it for 10 seconds and performing 10 repetitions. The ideal carrying out of the test should achieve and maintain between 28 and 30 mmHg, without a dominant activity of the superficial cervical muscles.

- Therefore, the pressure increases progressively in intervals of 2 mmHg, until the patient is able to maintain a pressure of 28/30 mmHg 10 times for 10 seconds, without a dominant activity of the superficial muscles.

- First, the test attempts to evaluate patients' capacity to activate their deep cervical flexor muscle and, secondly, the capacity to maintain the contraction in time.

- During the test, clinical analysis is carried out on the pattern of mobility of the patient in order to detect the appearance of compensation strategies.

- When the patient can correctly perform the craniocervical flexion, the amount of time when the patient can maintain the contraction of the deep cervical flexors should be evaluated.

- The objective of the test is to check the level of pressure that the patient can reach with a correct craniocervical flexion pattern, while maintaining it for 10 seconds.

The compensation strategies that are seen when the patient is unable to activate adequately the deep cervical flexor muscles are retraction of the head and hyperactivity of the superficial flexors and the suprahyoid and infrahyoid muscles.

A common compensation when the patient is unable to activate the deep cervical flexor muscles correctly is a cervical retraction muscle. The craniocervical flexion is an anterior rotation movement of the skull, which should not involve an increase of the pressure of the head against the table. This pattern of compensation can be detected by placing a hand below the occipital, and in order to avoid it, the patient should be trained to carry out the movement with the eyes. The patient should look at his feet and accompany this eye movement with a slow movement of the head, as if nodding.

The hyperactivity of the superficial flexors manifests itself through dominant activity of the sternocleidomastoid and scalene muscles, which can be detected with an electromyographic biofeedback device. The patient should be taught how to palpate the deep cervical flexor muscles in order to detect this abnormal activity during the exercise.

In order to avoid the hyperactivity of the suprahyoid and infrahyoid muscles, the patient can be asked to touch the tip of the tongue with the palate, while the lips are touching and the teeth are in disocclusion. This strategy prevents the compensation of the platysma and the suprahyoid and infrahyoid muscles.

Active cervical flexion in 4 point kneeling. The patient is asked to perform a cervical full flexion in 4 point kneeling. This test, described by Sahrmann,[166] evaluates the neck extensor muscles. The movement

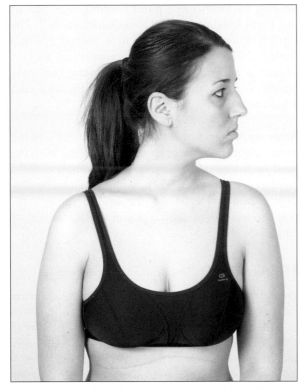

FIGURE 5-52 ■ Active cervical rotation in sitting.

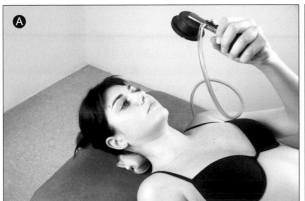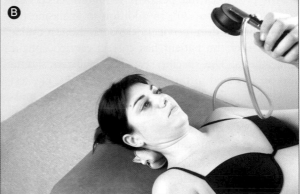

FIGURE 5-53 ■ Craniocervical flexion test with Stabilizer. Starting position (A), and activation of the deep cervical flexors (B).

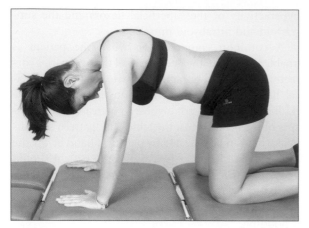

FIGURE 5-54 ■ Active cervical flexion in 4 point kneeling.

should be a predominant anterior sagittal plane rotation of the head and cervical spine during the flexion movement. The most common substitution is an anterior translation movement of the head and the cervical spine, with diminished anterior sagittal plane rotation during the flexion movement (Fig. 5-54).

Active cervical extension in 4 point kneeling. This test, described by Jull et al.,[6] can be performed with the patient in 4 point kneeling or in the sphinx position. Initially, the patient can be asked to maintain the cervical spine in the neutral position for 10 seconds. The patient is asked to move from full neck flexion to an active extension about 20°. The patient should be able to dissociate mid-lower from upper cervical extension. The head should remain in a neutral position while performing mid-lower cervical extension of about 20°. In addition to analysing the activity of the deep cervical extensors, the test evaluates whether the patient has correct cervicocephalic kinaesthesia. The specific scapular stabilizers should also be activated in this position (Fig. 5-55). The test is positive if the patient is unable to dissociate mid-lower from upper cervical extension. Different impairments can be observed. One impairment is when the patient cannot reach 20° of mid-lower extension while keeping the craniocervical region in neutral. Another impairment is when the patient adopts a poor coordination strategy to perform the test and uses superficial cervical muscles in the phase

of the return to the extension position. There is an excessive use of superficial muscles and it can be noted as a poked chin movement and also as an increase in recruitment or hypertonicity of semispinalis capitis muscles, so it can be seen as longitudinal ridges on the back of the neck.

Rocking backwards in 4 point kneeling. The patient in 4 point kneeling is asked to rock backwards.[166] The cervical spine should remain in a neutral position during the movement. The compensatory motion usually is an excessive cervical extension, but some patients compensate with different substitutions such a head retraction (Fig. 5-56).

Active upper cervical rotation[6]. The patient is in the prone sphinx position or in 4 point kneeling. With the head in the neutral position, he introduces a slight craniocervical flexion. Then, while maintaining this slight craniocervical flexion, she slowly performs rotation movements to the right and the left of 40° of amplitude (Fig. 5-57).

TREATMENT

Treatment for major instability. In cases involving major instability, the most important step is to detect it. A correct subjective examination and the use of adequate imaging diagnostic techniques in most cases show major instability. There is no therapeutic protocol applicable to structural anomalies responsible for major instability, and many of them require surgical stabilization. The main objective of this section is to alert the clinician that sometimes, the symptoms of the patient can be linked to a potentially serious instability that contraindicates any form of manual therapy treatment. Those major instabilities that may not be high risk and, therefore, are subject to conservative treatments can benefit from some of the therapeutic proposals described for minor instability.

Treatment for minor instability. The treatment for minor instability seeks to stimulate the neuromuscular control subsystem and increases the strength and resistance of the stabilizer muscles. The treatment should be adapted to the severity and type of instability, since there is no single protocol.

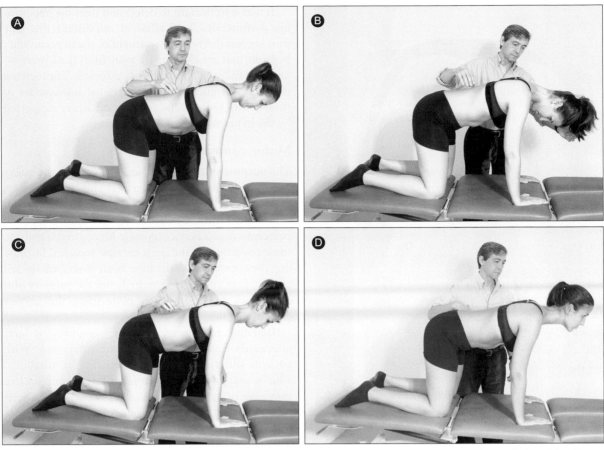

FIGURE 5-55 ■ Active cervical extension in 4 point kneeling. (A) Maintaining the cervical spine in the neutral position for 10 seconds. (B) Controlled flexion of the cervical spine. (C) Return to the neutral position. (D) Excessive activation of the superficial extensor muscles.

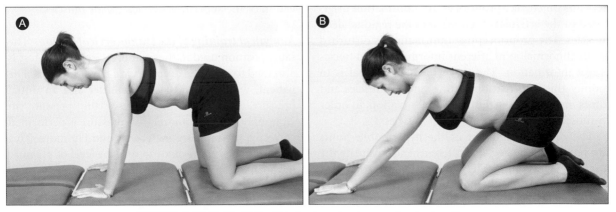

FIGURE 5-56 ■ (A, B) Rocking backwards when on 4 point kneeling.

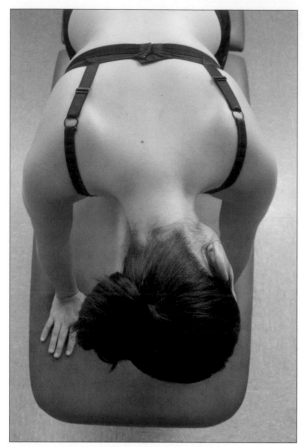

FIGURE 5-57 ■ Active upper cervical rotation in 4 point kneeling (deep suboccipital bias).

The active stability of the craniocervical spine depends on correct proprioceptive information originated in the articular system and in the regional deep muscles. The proprioceptive information is disturbed by an abnormal joint afferent information and nociceptive information. The main therapeutic goal is to modify this information, acting on the muscles and joints involved in the dysfunctional situation, in order to subsequently activate the deep muscles.

The manual treatment of the hypermobile joints can reduce the nociceptive afferents and stimulate the joint proprioception. There are different procedures that are able reduce the nociceptive stimulation, such as the oscillatory mobilization within the joint neutral zone and the physiological and accessory techniques.

It is also important to detect and treat the hypomobile dysfunctions, both adjacent and distant, that may prolong instability. The treatment of the hypomobility in joints that are close or far away from the hypermobile joint follows the availability principle. The increase in the involvement of the functional movements of these joints reduces the mechanical stress supported by the hypermobile or unstable joints.

Motor control exercises

The purpose of these exercises is to activate the stabilizer muscles of the craniocervical and cervical spine, in particular the deep cervical flexor and extensor and suboccipital muscles, which help to improve the proprioception and cervicocephalic kinaesthesia, and the tonic resistance of the deep cervical muscles. In these exercises, most of which have been described by Jull et al.,[167] low intensities are used, and the primary aim is to have precision when performing the correct pattern or movement.

Initially, retraining is done analytically, and afterwards functional activities are integrated. With patients suffering from significant clinical instability, who have significant pain or fear of performing active movements during the first days of treatment, it is possible to perform eye movement exercises in order to stimulate the contraction of the deep stabilizing muscles.

Deep cervical flexors

The functional instability of the cervical spine is characterized by a decrease in the activity and resistance of the deep cervical flexor muscles, with an excessive activation of the superficial cervical flexor muscles.

Analytical training of the craniocervical flexion. The same position used in the craniocervical flexion test is also used to train the deep cervical flexor muscles. The patient, with the aid of the Stabilizer and an initial pressure of 20 mmHg, increases the pressure to 22 mmHg. If the craniocervical pressure is performed correctly, the pressure increases 2 mmHg more. This is how an attempt is made to find the level of pressure in which the patient uses the superficial muscles or any other compensatory strategy for the performance of the craniocervical flexion (e.g. retraction of the head). The level of pressure in the beginning of the training is immediately lower than the level that appeared in the compensation. Then, at this level of pressure, the patient is asked to perform a craniocervical flexion again and to maintain it for 10 seconds. The goal is to perform 10 repetitions each lasting 10 seconds, using a correct pattern of movement. Only when the patient achieves this goal, will the treatment then advance towards a higher level of compression. Pressure is increased in increments of 2 mmHg at a time, and there are five levels of progression (22, 24, 26, 28 and 30 mmHg). The ultimate goal of the training of the deep cervical muscles is to make the patient be able to maintain a pressure of 28/30 mmHg, 10 times for 10 seconds, without a dominant activity of the superficial muscles.

Training of the craniocervical flexion in functional positions. When the patient is able to perform a correct pattern of craniocervical flexion in the supine position, he is asked to perform it sitting down and standing, during daily activities. In order to perform the exercise correctly, it is necessary to train the patient to maintain good postural alignment.

As the patient acquires a correct activation pattern, the craniocervical flexion is added progressively, first in an isometric manner and, then, in an isotonic way (Fig. 5-58).

Holding the chin with one hand, the patient performs a craniocervical flexion against the resistance, while, with the other hand, she palpates the superficial sternocleidomastoid and scalene muscles. It may be of interest to show the patient how to mobilize the hyoid muscle in order to check that the suprahyoid and infrahyoid muscles are not activated. Accordingly, the patient should perform low-intensity contractions of the deep flexor muscles with a minimum activation of the superficial flexors.

Progression can be made with eccentric and concentric control exercises of the craniocervical flexion, in different degrees of cervical extension.

NEUTRAL POSITION TO EXTENSION EXERCISE. The patient should perform, from the neutral position, a harmonic extension of the cervical spine, avoiding an isolated extension pattern of the craniocervical spine. This exercise requires an adequate eccentric control of the movement by the deep craniocervical flexors (Fig. 5-59).

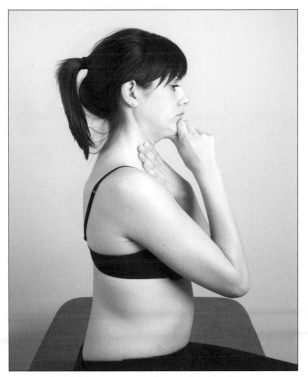

FIGURE 5-58 ■ Training of the deep cervical flexors while sitting down against slight resistance.

EXTENSION TO NEUTRAL POSITION EXERCISE. The patient, starting from an extension position, should reach the neutral position, avoiding an excessive activation of the superficial cervical flexors.

Deep cervical extensors

Training of the craniocervical extension on 4 point kneeling. This exercise involves the same test described for the evaluation of the craniocervical extensors. The patient is asked to maintain the cervical spine in the neutral position for 10 seconds, thus activating the specific scapular stabilizers. Then, the patient should slowly flex the cervical spine and return to the neutral position.

Training of the craniocervical extension in functional positions. When the patient can perform a correct craniocervical extension pattern, she should practice it sitting down and standing up during daily activities. In order to do this, it is imperative to maintain good postural alignment.

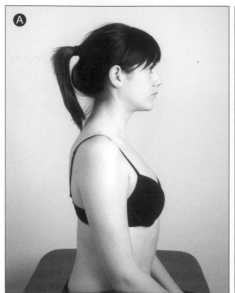
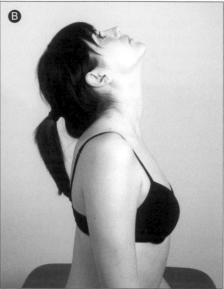

FIGURE 5-59 ■ Exercise from the neutral position (A) to extension (B).

Holding the chin with one hand, the patient performs a craniocervical extension against the resistance, while, with the other hand, she palpates the posterior cervical muscles in order to check that there is no excessive contraction of the superficial extensors (Fig. 5-60).

RHYTHMIC STABILIZATIONS IN FLEXION–EXTENSION. With the head in the neutral position and the cervical spine aligned, the patient holds the chin with one hand and performs low-intensity static contractions of the craniocervical flexors and extensors. With the other hand, she palpates the superficial flexor muscles in order to check that they are not activated during the contraction. The recruitment of the deep muscles can be facilitated with eye movements.

Suboccipital rotator muscles

The patient is in the prone sphinx position. With the head in the neutral position, she introduces a slight craniocervical flexion. Then, while maintaining this slight craniocervical flexion, she slowly performs rotation movements to the right and the left of 40° of amplitude (Fig. 5-61).

The same exercise can be performed while sitting down. The patient should maintain correct postural alignment at all times. First, a slight craniocervical

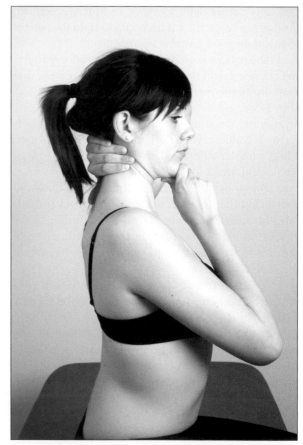

FIGURE 5-60 ■ Training of the craniocervical extension against slight resistance applied to the chin.

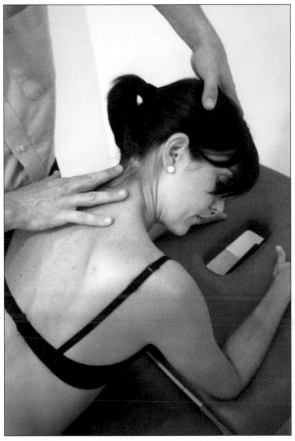

FIGURE 5-61 ■ Training of suboccipital rotator muscles.

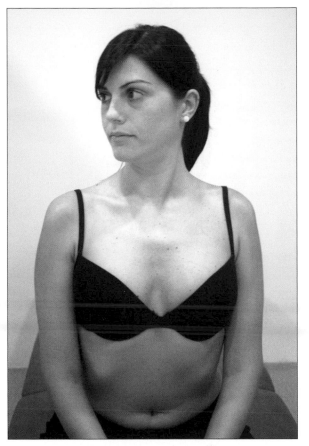

FIGURE 5-62 ■ 'No' exercise.

flexion is introduced, and then a cervical rotation from one side to the other, without exceeding 40° of amplitude (Fig. 5-62). In more advanced phases of the treatment, the same exercise can be performed at a higher speed.

Subsequently, the patient can perform this exercise with different degrees of craniocervical extension and flexion.

In order to use the suboccipital rotators against the resistance, the patient can resist the cervical rotation with one hand, while, with the other hand, she palpates the contralateral sternocleidomastoid to check if it is contracted. The contraction of the suboccipital rotators can be facilitated with directed eye movements. In this way, rhythmic stabilization movements

can be performed in rotation from the neutral position (Fig. 5-63) or in different degrees of rotation, without exceeding 40° of articular amplitude (Fig. 5-64).

Retraining the patterns of craniocervical mobility. Initially, these three exercises are performed in a limited amplitude of movement, and are then gradually increased.

CRANIOCERVICAL PROTRACTION–RETRACTION/ FLEXION–EXTENSION (Fig. 5-65). The purpose of the exercise is to teach the patient to perform specific craniocervical flexion–extension movements and how to differentiate them from the movements of protraction and retraction. Accordingly, the craniocervical

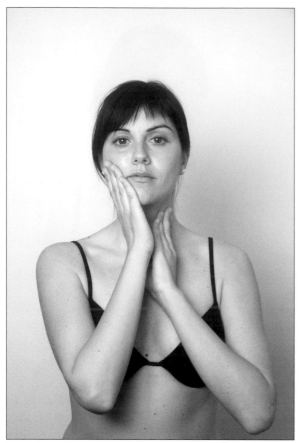

FIGURE 5-63 ■ Exercise against resistance of the suboccipital rotators.

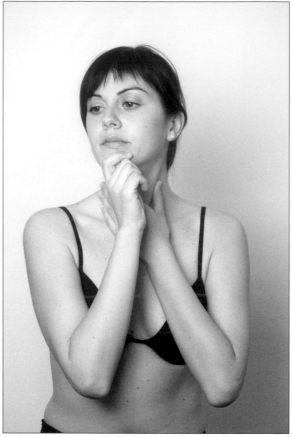

FIGURE 5-64 ■ Rhythmic stabilizations in different rotation degrees.

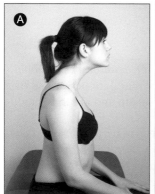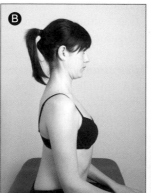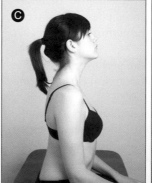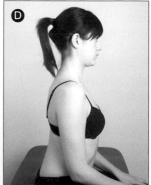

FIGURE 5-65 ■ Protraction (A), retraction (B), extension (C) and craniocervical flexion (D).

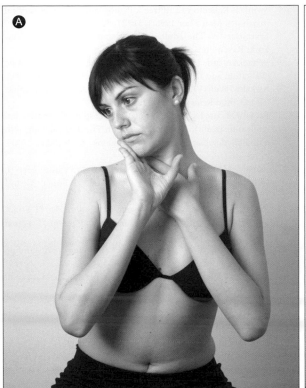
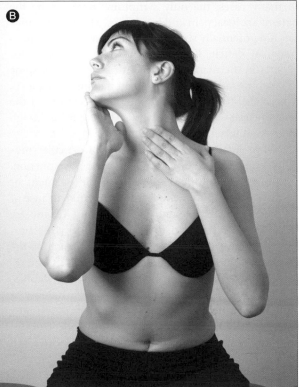

FIGURE 5-66 ■ Ipsilateral pattern of C2 (A) and contralateral pattern (B).

proprioception is improved in the sagittal plane of movement.

IPSILATERAL PATTERN OF C2 (Fig. 5-66A). The patient performs an ipsilateral movement of inclination–rotation, by placing the fingers of the same hand of the inclination–rotation on the lateral face of the mandible, while, with the other hand, she palpates the homolateral superficial muscles. By directing the eyes in the lateral and inferior directions, the patient performs the inclination–rotation, progressively increasing the movement resistance level.

CONTRALATERAL PATTERN (Fig. 5-66B). The patient performs a contralateral movement of inclination–rotation by placing the hand of the same side of the rotation on the lateral face of the mandible, while, with the other hand, she palpates the sternocleidomastoid on the other side. In order to perform the contralateral inclination–rotation movement, the patient directs the eyes upwards and outwards.

Postural re-education exercises. All of these exercises can be performed by adopting different postural re-education positions.

The stabilization exercises can be combined as well with the cervicocephalic kinaesthesia exercises described in Chapter 8.

CONCLUSION

Craniocervical instability is a clinical problem that is often inadequately diagnosed. Its aetiology can be congenital, inflammatory, degenerative and traumatic, and each one of these pathologies causes different modifications to the anatomical elements of the craniocervical spine. Clinically speaking, it is possible to establish a difference between major and minor instability. Major instability involves the disruption of the articular elements and/or craniocervical ligament elements, has a highly variable clinical presentation, and in many cases, the only symptoms reported by the patient are local pain and headaches. Many of the injuries are potentially serious and can cause a severe neurological deficit. Consequently, it is important for experts in the manual treatment of the cervical spine to be able to identify them. When making a diagnosis, it is crucial to have an adequate interpretation of the imaging tests Clinical tests can also be helpful, although their reliability has not been proven.

Minor instability involves a loss of articular mobility control, leading to pain and dysfunction, without a significant disruption of the ligament or neurovascular compromise. It is frequently a cause of chronic cervical pain and is usually not diagnosed, since the diagnosis is usually established by the subjective examination. Some clinical tests, such as the craniocervical flexion test, have been shown to be reliable in determining the activity of the deep stabilizing muscles. The treatment of minor instability is aimed at stimulating the subsystem of neuromuscular control and increasing the strength and resistance of the stabilizing muscles. The proposed techniques are aimed at improving proprioception, decreasing articular and muscular nociceptive afferents and encouraging the activity of the deep stabilizing muscles. The therapeutic possibilities of the instability are described in greater detail in the next chapter.

REFERENCES

1. Jull G, Trott P, Potter H, et al. A randomized controlled trial of exercise and manipulative therapy for cervicogenic headache. Spine 2002;27(17):1835–43, discussion 1843.
2. Petersen SM. Articular and muscular impairments in cervicogenic headache: a case report. J Orthop Sports Phys Ther 2003;33(1):21–30, discussion 30-2.
3. Kristjansson E, Leivseth G, Brinckmann P, et al. Increased sagittal plane segmental motion in the lower cervical spine in women with chronic whiplash-associated disorders, grades I-II: a case-control study using a new measurement protocol. Spine 2003;28(19):2215–21.
4. Dai L. Disc degeneration and cervical instability. Correlation of magnetic resonance imaging with radiography. Spine 1998;23(16):1734–8.
5. O'Leary S, Falla D, Elliott JM, et al. Muscle dysfunction in cervical spine pain: implications for assessment and management. J Orthop Sports Phys Ther 2009;39(5):324–33.
6. Jull G, Sterling M, Falla D, et al. Whiplash, headache, and neck pain: research-based directions for physical therapies. Edinburgh: Churchill Livingstone Elsevier; 2008.
7. Swinkels R, Beeton K, Alltree J. Pathogenesis of upper cervical instability. Man Ther 1996;1(3):127–32.
8. Frymoyer JW. The adult spine, principles and practice. New York: Raven Press; 1991.
9. White AA 3rd, Panjabi MM, Posner I, et al. Spinal stability: evaluation and treatment. Instr Course Lect 1981;30:457–83.
10. Kirkaldy-Willis WH, Farfan HF. Instability of the lumbar spine. Clin Orthop Relat Res 1982;165:110–23.
11. Panjabi M, Yue J, Dvorák J, et al. Cervical spine kinematics and clinical instability. In: Clark C, editor. The cervical spine. 4th ed. Philadelphia: Lippincott Williams & Wilkins; 2005. p. 55–78.
12. Panjabi MM. The stabilizing system of the spine. Part II. Neutral zone and instability hypothesis. J Spinal Disord 1992;5(4):390–6, discussion 397.
13. Panjabi MM. The stabilizing system of the spine. Part I. Function, dysfunction, adaptation, and enhancement. J Spinal Disord 1992;5(4):383–9, discussion 397.
14. Panjabi MM, Lydon C, Vasavada A, et al. On the understanding of clinical instability. Spine 1994;19(23):2642–50.
15. Bogduk N. Clinical anatomy of the lumbar spine and sacrum. 4th ed. Edinburgh: Elsevier Churchill Livinstone; 2005.
16. Niere KR, Torney SK. Clinicians' perceptions of minor cervical instability. Man Ther 2004;9(3):144–50.
17. Comerford M, Mottram S. The management of uncontrolled movement. Australia: Churchill Livingstone; 2012.
18. Harris MB, Duval MJ, Davis JA Jr, et al. Anatomical and roentgenographic features of atlantooccipital instability. J Spinal Disord 1993;6(1):5–10.
19. White AA, Panjabi MM. Clinical biomechanics of the spine. 2nd ed. Philadelphia: Lippincott Williams & Wilkins; 1990.
20. Powers B, Miller MD, Kramer RS, et al. Traumatic anterior atlanto-occipital dislocation. Neurosurgery 1979;4(1):12–17.
21. Richards PJ. Cervical spine clearance: a review. Injury 2005;36(2):248–69, discussion 270.
22. Dvorak J, Hayek J, Zehnder R. CT-functional diagnostics of the rotatory instability of the upper cervical spine. Part 2. An evaluation on healthy adults and patients with suspected instability. Spine 1987;12(8):726–31.
23. Dvorak J, Schneider E, Saldinger P, et al. Biomechanics of the craniocervical region: the alar and transverse ligaments. J Orthop Res 1988;6(3):452–61.
24. Fielding J. Tears of the transverse ligament of the atlas: a clinical and biomechanical study. J Bone Joint Surg 1974;56A: 1683–91.
25. Steel H. Anatomical and mechanical considerations of the atlanto-axial articulation. J Bone Joint Surg 1968;50(A):1481.
26. Fielding JW, Cochran GB, Lawsing JF 3rd, et al. Tears of the transverse ligament of the atlas. A clinical and biomechanical study. J Bone Joint Surg Am 1974;56(8):1683–91.
27. Dvorak J, Panjabi MM, Grob D, et al. Clinical validation of functional flexion/extension radiographs of the cervical spine. Spine 1993;18(1):120–7.
28. Westaway MD, Hu WY, Stratford PW, et al. Intra- and interrater reliability of the anterior atlantodental interval

measurement from conventional lateral view flexion/extension radiographs. Man Ther 2005;10(3):219–23.

29. Panjabi M, Dvorak J, Crisco JJ 3rd, et al. Effects of alar ligament transection on upper cervical spine rotation. J Orthop Res 1991;9(4):584–93.

30. Dvorak J, Panjabi MM. Functional anatomy of the alar ligaments. Spine 1987;12(2):183–9.

31. Dvorak J, Panjabi M, Gerber M, et al. CT-functional diagnostics of the rotatory instability of upper cervical spine. 1. An experimental study on cadavers. Spine 1987;12(3):197–205.

32. Panjabi M, Dvorak J, Crisco J 3rd, et al. Flexion, extension, and lateral bending of the upper cervical spine in response to alar ligament transections. J Spinal Disord 1991;4(2):157–67.

33. Crisco JJ 3rd, Panjabi MM, Dvorak J. A model of the alar ligaments of the upper cervical spine in axial rotation. J Biomech 1991;24(7):607–14.

34. Krakenes J, Kaale BR, Moen G, et al. MRI of the tectorial and posterior atlanto-occipital membranes in the late stage of whiplash injury. Neuroradiology 2003;45(9):585–91.

35. Crisco JJ 3rd, Oda T, Panjabi MM, et al. Transections of the C1-C2 joint capsular ligaments in the cadaveric spine. Spine 1991;16(Suppl. 10):S474–9.

36. Pettman E. Stress tests of the craniovertebral joints. In: Boyling J, Palastanga N, editors. Grieve's modern manual therapy. The vertebral column. 2nd ed. Edinburgh: Churchill Livingstone; 1994. p. 529–37.

37. Dávid K, Crockard A. Congenital malformations of the base of the skull, atlas and dens. In: Clark C, editor. The cervical spine. 4th ed. Philadelphia: Lippincott Williams & Wilkins; 2005. p. 415–26.

38. Royo-Salvador MB. [Platybasia, basilar groove, odontoid process and kinking of the brainstem: a common etiology with idiopathic syringomyelia, scoliosis and Chiari malformations]. Rev Neurol 1996;24(134):1241–50.

39. Goel A, Bhatjiwale M, Desai K. Basilar invagination: a study based on 190 surgically treated patients. J Neurosurg 1998;88(6):962–8.

40. Hensinger RN. Osseous anomalies of the craniovertebral junction. Spine 1986;11(4):323–33.

41. McRae DL, Barnum AS. Occipitalization of the atlas. Am J Roentgenol Radium Ther Nucl Med 1953;70(1):23–46.

42. David DJ, Edwards RM. Klippel-Feil syndrome. Anaesth Intensive Care 1995;23(6):752.

43. Wiesel SW, Rothman RH. Occipitoatlantal hypermobility. Spine 1979;4(3):187–91.

44. Hensinger RN, Lang JE, MacEwen GD. Klippel-Feil syndrome; a constellation of associated anomalies. J Bone Joint Surg Am 1974;56(6):1246–53.

45. David KM, Copp AJ, Stevens JM, et al. Split cervical spinal cord with Klippel-Feil syndrome: seven cases. Brain 1996;119(Pt 6):1859–72.

46. Jeanneret B, Magerl F. Congenital fusion C0-C2 associated with spondylolysis of C2. J Spinal Disord 1990;3(4):413–17.

47. Gunderson CH, Solitare GB. Mirror movements in patients with the Klippel-Feil syndrome. Neuropathologic observations. Arch Neurol 1968;18(6):675–9.

48. Nagib MG, Maxwell RE, Chou SN. Identification and management of high-risk patients with Klippel-Feil syndrome. J Neurosurg 1984;61(3):523–30.

49. Ramsey J, Bliznak J. Klippel-Feil syndrome with renal agenesis and other anomalies. Am J Roentgenol Radium Ther Nucl Med 1971;113(3):460–3.

50. Schott GD, Wyke MA. Congenital mirror movements. J Neurol Neurosurg Psychiatry 1981;44(7):586–99.

51. Whittle IR, Besser M. Congenital neural abnormalities presenting with mirror movements in a patient with Klippel-Feil syndrome. Case report. J Neurosurg 1983;59(5):891–4.

52. Vaidyanathan S, Hughes PL, Soni BM, et al. Klippel-Feil syndrome – the risk of cervical spinal cord injury: a case report. BMC Fam Pract 2002;3:6.

53. Westermeyer RR. Odontoid hypoplasia presenting as torticollis: a discussion of its significance. J Emerg Med 2003;24(1):15–18.

54. Chigira M, Kaneko K, Mashio K, et al. Congenital hypoplasia of the arch of the atlas with abnormal segmentation of the cervical spine. Arch Orthop Trauma Surg 1994;113(2):110–12.

55. Hensinger RN, Fielding JW, Hawkins RJ. Congenital anomalies of the odontoid process. Orthop Clin North Am 1978;9(4):901–12.

56. Truex RC Jr, Johnson CH. Congenital anomalies of the upper cervical spine. Orthop Clin North Am 1978;9(4):891–900.

57. Morgan MK, Onofrio BM, Bender CE. Familial os odontoideum. Case report. J Neurosurg 1989;70(4):636–9.

58. Kirlew KA, Hathout GM, Reiter SD, et al. Os odontoideum in identical twins: perspectives on etiology. Skeletal Radiol 1993;22(7):525–7.

59. Ricciardi JE, Kaufer H, Louis DS. Acquired os odontoideum following acute ligament injury. Report of a case. J Bone Joint Surg Am 1976;58(3):410–12.

60. Fielding JW, Hensinger RN, Hawkins RJ. Os odontoideum. J Bone Joint Surg Am 1980;62(3):376–83.

61. Hawkins RJ, Fielding JW, Thompson WJ. Os odontoideum: congenital or acquired. A case report. J Bone Joint Surg Am 1976;58(3):413–14.

62. Ogden JA, Murphy MJ, Southwick WO, et al. Radiology of postnatal skeletal development. XIII. C1-C2 interrelationships. Skeletal Radiol 1986;15(6):433–8.

63. Matsui H, Imada K, Tsuji H. Radiographic classification of os odontoideum and its clinical significance. Spine 1997;22(15):1706–9.

64. Aksoy FG, Gomori JM. Symptomatic cervical synovial cyst associated with an os odontoideum diagnosed by magnetic resonance imaging: case report and review of the literature. Spine 2000;25(10):1300–2.

65. Holt RG, Helms CA, Munk PL, et al. Hypertrophy of C-1 anterior arch: useful sign to distinguish os odontoideum from acute dens fracture. Radiology 1989;173(1):207–9.

66. Vargas TM, Rybicki FJ, Ledbetter SM, et al. Atlantoaxial instability associated with an orthotopic os odontoideum: a multimodality imaging assessment. Emerg Radiol 2005;11(4):223–5.

67. Sasaki H, Itoh T, Takei H, et al. Os odontoideum with cerebellar infarction: a case report. Spine 2000;25(9):1178–81.

68. Watanabe M, Toyama Y, Fujimura Y. Atlantoaxial instability in os odontoideum with myelopathy. Spine 1996;21(12):1435–9.

69. Choit RL, Jamieson DH, Reilly CW. Os odontoideum: a significant radiographic finding. Pediatr Radiol 2005;35(8):803–7.

70. Fukuda M, Aiba T, Akiyama K, et al. Cerebellar infarction secondary to os odontoideum. J Clin Neurosci 2003;10(5):625–6.

71. Dai L, Yuan W, Ni B, et al. Os odontoideum: etiology, diagnosis, and management. Surg Neurol 2000;53(2):106–8, discussion 108-9.

72. Tredwell SJ, Newman DE, Lockitch G. Instability of the upper cervical spine in Down syndrome. J Pediatr Orthop 1990;10(5):602–6.

73. Cremers MJ, Ramos L, Bol E, et al. Radiological assessment of the atlantoaxial distance in Down's syndrome. Arch Dis Child 1993;69(3):347–50.

74. Murphy J, Hoey HM, Philip M, et al. Guidelines for the medical management of Irish children and adolescents with Down syndrome. Ir Med J 2005;98(2):48–52.

75. Winell J, Burke SW. Sports participation of children with Down syndrome. Orthop Clin North Am 2003;34(3):439–43.

76. Ali FE, Al-Bustan MA, Al-Busairi WA, et al. Cervical spine abnormalities associated with Down syndrome. Int Orthop 2006;30(4):284–9.

77. Menezes AH, Ryken TC. Craniovertebral abnormalities in Down's syndrome. Pediatr Neurosurg 1992;18(1):24–33.

78. Masuda K, Iwasaki M, Seichi A, et al. Cervical myelopathy in an adult due to atlantoaxial subluxation associated with Down syndrome: a case study. J Orthop Sci 2003;8(2):227–31.

79. Pueschel SM, Herndon JH, Gelch MM, et al. Symptomatic atlantoaxial subluxation in persons with Down syndrome. J Pediatr Orthop 1984;4(6):682–8.

80. Goldring SR. Pathogenesis of bone erosions in rheumatoid arthritis. Curr Opin Rheumatol 2002;14(4):406–10.

81. Haugeberg G, Orstavik RE, Kvien TK. Effects of rheumatoid arthritis on bone. Curr Opin Rheumatol 2003;15(4):469–75.

82. O'Brien MF, Casey AT, Crockard A, et al. Histology of the craniocervical junction in chronic rheumatoid arthritis: a clinicopathologic analysis of 33 operative cases. Spine 2002;27(20):2245–54.

83. Shirado O, Azuma H, Takeda N, et al. Quadriparesis complicating atlantoaxial subluxation and ossification of the posterior longitudinal ligament in a patient with rheumatoid arthritis. A case report. J Bone Joint Surg Am 2005;87(6):1354–7.

84. Riise T, Jacobsen BK, Gran JT. High mortality in patients with rheumatoid arthritis and atlantoaxial subluxation. J Rheumatol 2001;28(11):2425–9.

85. Pellicci PM, Ranawat CS, Tsairis P, et al. A prospective study of the progression of rheumatoid arthritis of the cervical spine. J Bone Joint Surg Am 1981;63(3):342–50.

86. Kauppi M, Hakala M. Prevalence of cervical spine subluxations and dislocations in a community-based rheumatoid arthritis population. Scand J Rheumatol 1994;23(3):133–6.

87. Weissman BN, Aliabadi P, Weinfeld MS, et al. Prognostic features of atlantoaxial subluxation in rheumatoid arthritis patients. Radiology 1982;144(4):745–51.

88. Roche CJ, Eyes BE, Whitehouse GH. The rheumatoid cervical spine: signs of instability on plain cervical radiographs. Clin Radiol 2002;57(4):241–9.

89. Bouchaud-Chabot A, Liote F. Cervical spine involvement in rheumatoid arthritis. A review. Joint Bone Spine 2002;69(2):141–54.

90. Tanaka N, Sakahashi H, Hirose K, et al. Results after 24 years of prophylactic surgery for rheumatoid atlantoaxial subluxation. J Bone Joint Surg Br 2005;87(7):955–8.

91. Shen FH, Samartzis D, Jenis LG, et al. Rheumatoid arthritis: evaluation and surgical management of the cervical spine. Spine J 2004;4(6):689–700.

92. Lipson SJ. Rheumatoid arthritis in the cervical spine. Clin Orthop Relat Res 1989;239:121–7.

93. Rasker JJ, Cosh JA. Radiological study of cervical spine and hand in patients with rheumatoid arthritis of 15 years' duration: an assessment of the effects of corticosteroid treatment. Ann Rheum Dis 1978;37(6):529–35.

94. Halla JT, Hardin JG, Vitek J, et al. Involvement of the cervical spine in rheumatoid arthritis. Arthritis Rheum 1989;32(5):652–9.

95. Crockard A, Grob D. Rheumatoid arthritis. Upper cervical involvement. In: Clark C, editor. The cervical spine. 4th ed. Philadelphia: Lippincott Williams & Wilkins; 2005. p. 914–22.

96. Kauppi MJ, Barcelos A, da Silva JA. Cervical complications of rheumatoid arthritis. Ann Rheum Dis 2005;64(3):355–8.

97. Boden SD, Dodge LD, Bohlman HH, et al. Rheumatoid arthritis of the cervical spine. A long-term analysis with predictors of paralysis and recovery. J Bone Joint Surg Am 1993;75(9):1282–97.

98. Cha C, Boden S, Clark C. Rheumatoid arthritis in the cervical spine. In: Clark C, editor. The cervical spine. 4th ed. Philadelphia: Lippincott Williams & Wilkins; 2005. p. 901–13.

99. Maeda T, Saito T, Harimaya K, et al. Atlantoaxial instability in neck retraction and protrusion positions in patients with rheumatoid arthritis. Spine 2004;29(7):757–62.

100. Dickman CA, Mamourian A, Sonntag VK, et al. Magnetic resonance imaging of the transverse atlantal ligament for the evaluation of atlantoaxial instability. J Neurosurg 1991;75(2):221–7.

101. Dvorak J, Grob D, Baumgartner H, et al. Functional evaluation of the spinal cord by magnetic resonance imaging in patients with rheumatoid arthritis and instability of upper cervical spine. Spine 1989;14(10):1057–64.

102. Riew KD, Hilibrand AS, Palumbo MA, et al. Diagnosing basilar invagination in the rheumatoid patient. The reliability of radiographic criteria. J Bone Joint Surg Am 2001;83-A(2):194–200.

103. Redlund-Johnell I, Pettersson H. Radiographic measurements of the cranio-vertebral region. Designed for evaluation of abnormalities in rheumatoid arthritis. Acta Radiol Diagn (Stockh) 1984;25(1):23–8.

104. Kauppi M, Sakaguchi M, Konttinen YT, et al. A new method of screening for vertical atlantoaxial dislocation. J Rheumatol 1990;17(2):167–72.

105. Einig M, Higer HP, Meairs S, et al. Magnetic resonance imaging of the craniocervical junction in rheumatoid arthritis: value, limitations, indications. Skeletal Radiol 1990;19(5):341–6.

106. Karhu JO, Parkkola RK, Koskinen SK. Evaluation of flexion/extension of the upper cervical spine in patients with rheumatoid arthritis: an MRI study with a dedicated positioning device compared to conventional radiographs. Acta Radiol 2005;46(1):55–66.

107. Laiho K, Soini I, Kautiainen H, et al. Can we rely on magnetic resonance imaging when evaluating unstable atlantoaxial subluxation? Ann Rheum Dis 2003;62(3):254–6.

108. Herzka A, Sponseller PD, Pyeritz RE. Atlantoaxial rotatory subluxation in patients with Marfan syndrome. A report of three cases. Spine 2000;25(4):524–6.

109. Fernandez Cornejo VJ, Martinez-Lage JF, et al. Inflammatory atlanto-axial subluxation (Grisel's syndrome) in children: clinical diagnosis and management. Childs Nerv Syst 2003; 19(5–6):342–7.

110. Villas C, Arriagada C, Zubieta JL. Preliminary CT study of C1-C2 rotational mobility in normal subjects. Eur Spine J 1999;8(3):223–8.

111. Meek MF, Hermens RA, Robinson PH. La maladie de Grisel: spontaneous atlantoaxial subluxation. Cleft Palate Craniofac J 2001;38(3):268–70.

112. Gourin CG, Kaper B, Abdu WA, et al. Nontraumatic atlantoaxial subluxation after retropharyngeal cellulitis: Grisel's syndrome. Am J Otolaryngol 2002;23(1):60–5.

113. Ugur HC, Caglar S, Unlu A, et al. Infection-related atlantoaxial subluxation in two adults: Grisel syndrome or not? Acta Neurochir (Wien) 2003;145(1):69–72.

114. Boole JR, Ramsey M, Petermann G, et al. Radiology quiz case. Grisel syndrome with vertebral osteomyelitis and spinal epidural abscess. Arch Otolaryngol Head Neck Surg 2003; 129(11):1247.

115. Tschopp K. Monopolar electrocautery in adenoidectomy as a possible risk factor for Grisel's syndrome. Laryngoscope 2002;112(8 Pt 1):1445–9.

116. Isern AE, Ohlin A, Stromblad LG, et al. Grisel syndrome after velopharyngoplasty. Scand J Plast Reconstr Surg Hand Surg 2004;38(1):53–7.

117. Ono K, Yonenobu K, Fuji T, et al. Atlantoaxial rotatory fixation. Radiographic study of its mechanism. Spine 1985;10(7):602–8.

118. Harth M, Mayer M, Marzi I, et al. Lateral torticollis on plain radiographs and MRI: Grisel syndrome. Eur Radiol 2004;14(9):1713–15.

119. Martinez-Lage JF, Martinez Perez M, Fernandez Cornejo V, et al. Atlanto-axial rotatory subluxation in children: early management. Acta Neurochir (Wien) 2001;143(12):1223–8.

120. Yu KK, White DR, Weissler MC, et al. Nontraumatic atlantoaxial subluxation (Grisel syndrome): a rare complication of otolaryngological procedures. Laryngoscope 2003;113(6):1047–9.

121. Subach BR, McLaughlin MR, Albright AL, et al. Current management of pediatric atlantoaxial rotatory subluxation. Spine 1998;23(20):2174–9.

122. Domínguez-Carrillo L, Trujillo-Dervín M, Segovia A. Síndrome de Grisel, luxación rotatoria atlanto-axoidea. Acta Médica Grupo Ángeles 2005;3(2).

123. Bucholz RW, Burkhead WZ. The pathological anatomy of fatal atlanto-occipital dislocations. J Bone Joint Surg Am 1979;61(2): 248–50.

124. Alker GJ, Oh YS, Leslie EV, et al. Postmortem radiology of head neck injuries in fatal traffic accidents. Radiology 1975;114(3): 611–17.

125. James R, Nasmyth-Jones R. The occurrence of cervical fractures in victims of judicial hanging. Forensic Sci Int 1992;54(1):81–91.

126. Clayman DA, Sykes CH, Vines FS. Occipital condyle fractures: clinical presentation and radiologic detection. AJNR Am J Neuroradiol 1994;15(7):1309–15.

127. Stroobants J, Fidlers L, Storms JL, et al. High cervical pain and impairment of skull mobility as the only symptoms of an occipital condyle fracture. Case report. J Neurosurg 1994;81(1): 137–8.

128. Bernhardt M, Wong W, Panjabi M, et al. Mechanisms of injury in the cervical spine: basic concepts, biomechanical evidence and clinical experience. In: Clark C, editor. The cervical spine. 4th ed. Philadelphia: Lippincott Williams & Wilkins; 2005.

129. Greene KA, Dickman CA, Marciano FF, et al. Acute axis fractures. Analysis of management and outcome in 340 consecutive cases. Spine 1997;22(16):1843–52.

130. Ochoa G. Surgical management of odontoid fractures. Injury 2005;36(Suppl. 2):B54–64.

131. Cusick JF, Yoganandan N. Biomechanics of the cervical spine 4: major injuries. Clin Biomech (Bristol, Avon) 2002;17(1): 1–20.

132. Apfelbaum RI, Lonser RR, Veres R, et al. Direct anterior screw fixation for recent and remote odontoid fractures. J Neurosurg 2000;93(Suppl. 2):227–36.

133. Crockard HA, Heilman AE, Stevens JM. Progressive myelopathy secondary to odontoid fractures: clinical, radiological, and surgical features. J Neurosurg 1993;78(4):579–86.

134. Anderson LD, D'Alonzo RT. Fractures of the odontoid process of the axis. J Bone Joint Surg Am 1974;56(8):1663–74.

135. Arand M, Neller S, Kinzl L, et al. The traumatic spondylolisthesis of the axis. A biomechanical in vitro evaluation of an instability model and clinical relevant constructs for stabilization. Clin Biomech (Bristol, Avon) 2002;17(6):432–8.

136. Dickman CA, Papadopoulos SM, Sonntag VK, et al. Traumatic occipitoatlantal dislocations. J Spinal Disord 1993;6(4): 300–13.

137. Krakenes J, Kaale BR, Moen G, et al. MRI assessment of the alar ligaments in the late stage of whiplash injury – a study of structural abnormalities and observer agreement. Neuroradiology 2002;44(7):617–24.

138. Levine AM, Edwards CC. Traumatic lesions of the occipitoatlantoaxial complex. Clin Orthop Relat Res 1989;(239): 53–68.

139. Lipson SJ. Fractures of the atlas associated with fractures of the odontoid process and transverse ligament ruptures. J Bone Joint Surg Am 1977;59(7):940–3.

140. Spence KF Jr, Decker S, Sell KW. Bursting atlantal fracture associated with rupture of the transverse ligament. J Bone Joint Surg Am 1970;52(3):543–9.

141. Hasharoni A, Errico T. Transverse ligament injury. In: Clark C, editor. The cervical spine. 4th ed. Philadelphia: Lippincott Williams & Wilkins; 2005.

142. Krakenes J, Kaale BR, Nordli H, et al. MR analysis of the transverse ligament in the late stage of whiplash injury. Acta Radiol 2003;44(6):637–44.

143. Meadows J. Diagnóstico diferencial en fisioterapia. Madrid: McGraw-Hill Interamericana; 2000.

144. Cook C, Brismee JM, Fleming R, et al. Identifiers suggestive of clinical cervical spine instability: a Delphi study of physical therapists. Phys Ther 2005;85(9):895–906.

145. Refshauge KM, Parry S, Shirley D, et al. Professional responsibility in relation to cervical spine manipulation. Aust J Physiother 2002;48(3):171–9, discussion 180-5.

146. Hing WA, Reid DA, Monaghan M. Manipulation of the cervical spine. Man Ther 2003;8(1):2–9.

147. Mintken PE, Metrick L, Flynn TW. Upper cervical ligament testing in a patient with os odontoideum presenting with headaches. J Orthop Sports Phys Ther 2008;38(8):465–75.

148. Uitvlugt G, Indenbaum S. Clinical assessment of atlantoaxial instability using the Sharp-Purser test. Arthritis Rheum 1988;31(7):918–22.

149. Sharp J, Purser D. Spontaneous atlanto-axial dislocation in ankylosing spondylitis and rheumatoid arthritis. Ann Rheum Dis 1961;20:47–74.

150. Forrester G, Barlas P. Reliability and validity of the Sharp-Purser test in the assessment of atlato-axial instability in patients with rheumatoid arthritis. Physiotherapy 1999;85:376.

151. Mathews JA. Atlanto-axial subluxation in rheumatoid arthritis. Ann Rheum Dis 1969;28(3):260–6.

152. Stevens JC, Cartlidge NE, Saunders M, et al. Atlanto-axial subluxation and cervical myelopathy in rheumatoid arthritis. Q J Med 1971;40(159):391–408.

153. Kaale BR, Krakenes J, Albrektsen G, et al. Clinical assessment techniques for detecting ligament and membrane injuries in the upper cervical spine region – a comparison with MRI results. Man Ther 2008;13(5):397–403.

154. Aspinall W. Clinical testing for the craniovertebral hypermobility syndrome. J Orthop Sports Phys Ther 1990;12(2):47–54.

155. Swinkels RA, Oostendorp RA. Upper cervical instability: fact or fiction? J Manipulative Physiol Ther 1996;19(3):185–94.

156. Cattrysse E, Swinkels RA, Oostendorp RA, et al. Upper cervical instability: are clinical tests reliable? Man Ther 1997;2(2):91–7.

157. Hutting N, Scholten-Peeters GG, Vijverman V, et al. Diagnostic accuracy of upper cervical spine instability tests: a systematic review. Phys Ther 2013;93(12):1686–95.

158. Derrick L, Chesworth B. Post-motor vehicle accident alar ligament laxity. J Orthop Sports Phys Ther 1992;16(1):6–11.

159. McDonnell MK, Sahrmann SA, Van Dillen L. A specific exercise program and modification of postural alignment for treatment of cervicogenic headache: a case report. J Orthop Sports Phys Ther 2005;35(1):3–15.

160. Childs JD, Cleland JA, Elliott JM, et al. Neck pain: Clinical practice guidelines linked to the International Classification of Functioning, Disability, and Health from the Orthopedic Section of the American Physical Therapy Association. J Orthop Sports Phys Ther 2008;38(9):A1–34.

161. Falla D, Jull G, Dall'Alba P, et al. An electromyographic analysis of the deep cervical flexor muscles in performance of craniocervical flexion. Phys Ther 2003;83(10):899–906.

162. Falla DL, Jull GA, Hodges PW. Patients with neck pain demonstrate reduced electromyographic activity of the deep cervical flexor muscles during performance of the craniocervical flexion test. Spine 2004;29(19):2108–14.

163. James G, Doe T. The craniocervical flexion test: intra-tester reliability in asymptomatic subjects. Physiother Res Int 2010;15(3):144–9.

164. Arumugam A, Mani R, Raja K. Interrater reliability of the craniocervical flexion test in asymptomatic individuals – a cross-sectional study. J Manipulative Physiol Ther 2011;34(4):247–53.

165. Segarra V, Duenas L, Torres R, et al. Inter-and intra-tester reliability of a battery of cervical movement control dysfunction tests. Man Ther 2015;20(4):570–9.

166. Sahrmann S. Movement System Impairment Syndromes of the Extremities, Cervical and Thoracic Spines. St.Louis: Elsevier; 2011.

167. Jull G, Falla D, Treleaven J, et al. A therapeutic exercise approach for cervical disorders. In: Boyling J, Jull G, editors. Grieve's Modern Manual Therapy: The Vertebral Column. 3rd ed. Edinburgh: Elsevier Churchill Livingstone; 2004.

6

SPECIFIC ASSESSMENT AND MANAGEMENT OF PATIENTS WITH LOW CERVICAL INSTABILITY

PIETER WESTERHUIS

INTRODUCTION AND DEFINITIONS

One problem with the concept of instability is that different authors use different definitions.[1,2] Depending on the individual focus, researchers have defined instability in various ways.[3]

Panjabi[4] divides the spinal stabilizing system into three subsystems (Fig. 6-1):

1. The passive subsystem (e.g. form closure of the joints, capsule, ligaments, etc.).
2. The active subsystem (e.g. muscles, strength, endurance).
3. The regulating/controlling subsystem (e.g. proprioception, coordination).

The passive subsystem

The stability of the passive subsystem is influenced by several factors, including form closure of the joints (compare for instance the biconvexity of C1–C2 with the concave–convexity of Occ.–C1), the integrity of the joint capsule and ligaments and the integrity of the discs. Damage to these structures can lead to so-called structural instability.[5–8] In structural instability the emphasis is upon biomechanical aspects. An example would be the performing of an anterior drawer test on a knee with an anterior cruciate ligament insufficiency.

The examiner assesses the following aspects:

1. The available range of motion before first resistance is encountered (= neutral zone = NZ).[4]

2. The behaviour of resistance once the movement is continued into resistance. The so-called 'stiffness' within the elastic zone is evaluated.[9]
3. The overall range of motion (= ROM).
4. Perceived pain and other symptoms.
5. Protective muscle spasm.

Maitland has described so called 'movement diagrams' with which the examiner can depict graphically his findings with passive motion testing.

This movement diagram in Figure 6-2A shows a normal cervical rotation to the right. The A–B line is the normal average ROM, which would be approximately 80°. The examiner feels first onset of resistance at approximately 30°. Initially, the resistance increases only slightly, while at approximately 60° there is an exponential increase of resistance. The patient feels no symptoms and there is no protective muscle spasm.

This movement diagram in Figure 6-2B depicts a hypermobile cervical right rotation. The cervical spine can be rotated beyond B (which is defined as the normal average ROM) to approximately 100°. The first resistance only begins at approximately 50°, which means the neutral zone is enlarged. However, the exponential increase of resistance is normal.

This movement diagram in Figure 6-2C depicts an unstable joint. Normally the A–B line should be approximately 10 mm and the first resistance should begin after 2 or 3 mm. In this case, however, the first resistance begins too late (after approximately 6 mm). Therefore, the neutral zone is enlarged. The total ROM is excessive (approximately 12 mm = beyond B).

217

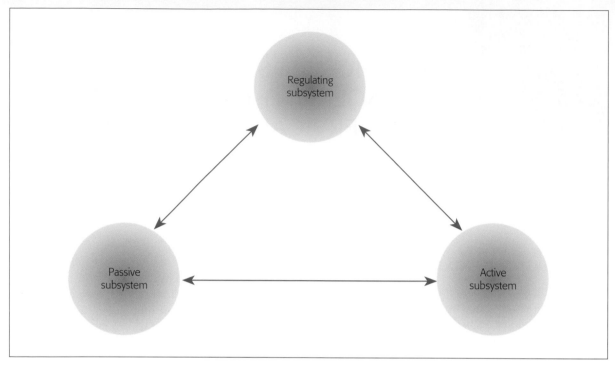

FIGURE 6-1 ■ Stabilizing system of the spine.[4]

Moreover, the exponential increase of resistance is lacking (= loss of 'stiffness'). Typically, in this movement diagram there is also protective muscle spasm (= S) and symptoms (in this case pain = P)

From a biomechanical perspective the following definition can be made:

> *A structural instability is an excessive range of motion in an accessory movement direction, with an abnormal behaviour of resistance through range (loss of stiffness) and an increased neutral zone.*
> **Adapted from Panjabi et al.[10] and Maitland et al.[11]**

According to Panjabi,[12] changes of the neutral zone are more significantly associated with the occurrence of an instability than changes in the ROM. This was confirmed by more recent studies by, for example, Lee et al.,[13] Zhu et al.[5] and Kettler et al.[14] Moreover, in the clinical examination, the evaluation of the total ROM is sometimes difficult due to symptoms and/or muscle spasm. Therefore it is essential to assess the moment of first onset of resistance when structural instability tests are performed.

The most commonly used instability tests primarily evaluate structural rather than functional instability.[15,16]

According to Sanchez Martin,[17] the most common causes of structural instability are:

1. Trauma e.g.
   – massive trauma, like whiplash-associated disorder (= WAD)
   – repetitive microtrauma.
2. Congenital, e.g. Down syndrome.
3. Metastasis.
4. Disease like
   – Ehlers–Danlos syndrome
   – rheumatoid arthritis.

One of the greatest difficulties, however, is that there is no direct correlation between the amount of structural instability and the patient's symptoms.[1,18,19] This is explained by Panjabi[4] by the hypothesis that

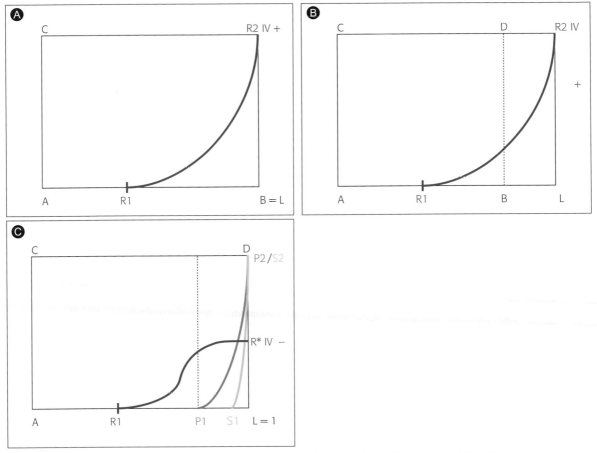

FIGURE 6-2 ■ Movement diagrams. (A) Normal right cervical rotation. (B) Hypermobile right cervical rotation. (C) Instability. A–B line represents the range of movement. B = average normal range of movement. L indicates the individual motion limit. In a normal movement diagram L should equal B. The A–C line shows the intensity of various factors. R stands for resistance (R1 = first resistance, R2 = resistance at the end of the movement, R* = no resistance felt), P for pain (P1 = first pain, P2 = pain at the end of the movement) and S for protective muscular spasm (S1 = first muscular spasm, S2 = muscular spasm at the end of the movement).

insufficiencies in one subsystem may be compensated by the other subsystems.

The active and regulating subsystem

The stability of the active subsystem is dependent upon the capacity of the muscles to generate adequate amounts of force and to be able to maintain it over a prolonged period of time: therefore, adequate strength and endurance play a certain role. It is, however, the regulating subsystem that coordinates the timing and the intensity of the individual muscle contractions.

The afferent input from the other subsystems like the joints,[20] discs[21] and muscles[22] play an important role. The regulating subsystem processes all input to coordinate an adequate muscular reaction.

Dysfunctions of the regulating subsystem can either be caused by dysfunctions within the input system[23] or by dysfunctions within the output system.

According to Panjabi, minor dysfunctions in one of the three subsystems may be compensated by the other subsystems. Therefore, the examiner should assess both the structural instability and the functional instability.

Functional/clinical instability

The clinical instability of the spine has been defined as the loss of ability of the spine under physiological loads to maintain its pattern of displacement so there is no initial or additional neurological deficit, no major deformity and no incapacitating pain.[24]

The emphasis of this definition is upon the ability of the spine to maintain the correct orientation of the vertebrae in relationship with each other under physiological loads. This means that a certain joint may be structurally unstable, but as long as the other subsystems can maintain optimal joint orientation, it is not necessarily functionally unstable. However, a joint may be structurally stable, but if the segment buckles under normal loads, it is functionally unstable.

The examiner may observe functional stability by, for instance, observing control over the cervical spine position when the patient has to lift the arms towards the ceiling or when the patient has to lift a weight. More formal assessment of the active subsystem is with the graded craniocervical flexion test (CCFT).

CLINICAL PRESENTATION OF LOW CERVICAL INSTABILITY

Body chart

During the subjective examination, the location and type of symptoms are recorded on a body chart. Pettman[15] emphasized the importance of so-called 'cardinal symptoms'. These are symptoms indicating serious pathology like spinal cord signs and/or vertebrobasilar insufficiency, which might be caused by marked structural instability. If the patient shows cardinal symptoms, special care should be taken during the physical examination and vigorous testing is contraindicated.

Spinal cord signs

Marked structural instability may compromise the integrity of the spinal cord. This may present with the following symptoms[25,26]:

- insecurity/stumbling with walking
- ataxia
- extrasegmental sensory disturbances in lower and upper extremity
- disturbance of bowel and or bladder function
- muscle spasms.

Normally, therapists working in private practice will rarely come across patients with these symptoms, because they are usually referred for surgery. However, some patients may only show subtle spinal cord signs.

Vertebrobasilar insufficiency

Abnormal translation in the midcervical segments and/or excessive rotation in the upper cervical spine may cause impaired blood flow in the vertebrobasilar system.[27] One of the main symptoms is dizziness. Coman,[28] however, states that dizziness may be caused by many different factors. If the dizziness is caused by impaired blood flow in the vertebrobasilar system, then other parts of the brainstem should also have impaired blood flow. This may be presented as dysphagia, diplopia, dizziness, dysarthria and drop attacks (= a sudden loss of muscle tone without losing consciousness which leads to falling down).

According to Coman,[28] these so-called 5 D's are pathognomonic for vertebrobasilar insufficiency.[29]

Pain

Instability causes abnormal segmental movement patterns, leading to abnormal biomechanical stresses. This may lead to overload of different structures, causing symptoms.[30] Therefore, the patient may, for instance, present with pain due to zygapophyseal joints or intervertebral discs. Additionally, however, nerves may also react to abnormal stretching and/or compression, leading to neural irritation. The patient may also present with a radicular distribution of symptoms.

Insufficient muscular control

Patients may complain: 'The head is too heavy for my neck', 'I cannot control my head', 'I have to hold my neck', 'My neck might break apart any minute' or 'My neck feels so tired'.

Further symptoms

- Movement restrictions.
- Acute cervical locking, which might be due to entrapment of intra-articular meniscoid structures.
- Clicking and/or cracking sounds with movements of the neck.
- Dysphagia /'It feels like there is a lump in my throat'.

■ Associated symptoms like nausea /vomiting, tinnitus or nystagmus /diploplia.

Behaviour of symptoms

The most dominant aspect within the behaviour of the symptoms is its inconsistency. The patients may be able to perform activities that put a lot of stress on the cervical spine without any discomfort, while other activities, which seem to be less stressful, produce symptoms. The patient may, for instance, be able to play tennis without any problems, but a small sudden movement during daily life activities like reversing a car may cause severe symptoms. One of the explanations for this discrepancy is that as long as the muscles are prepared and have appropriate muscle tone adequate stability is supplied.

Usually the patients feel worse as the day continues, because the muscles fatigue.

Another feature is that the patients do not like sustained end-of-range positions. Muscle fatigue in sustained positions, combined with ligamentous creep, may lead to abnormal symptoms. Also, it is quite common for these patients to complain of 'catches of pain' with sudden uncontrolled movements.

History

Again, a dominant feature may be the inconsistency. Quite commonly, the patients have had their symptoms for a long period with recurring episodes. Severe episodes may be triggered by seemingly trivial incidents. Episodes may vary enormously without clear pattern. 'Good' days and 'bad' days may come and go without apparent cause.

It is important to ask for a previous history of trauma. Studies have shown that whiplash injuries may, for instance, cause instabilities.[6,31,32] Normal X-ray reports do not rule out instabilities, as there are often 'false-negative' findings'.[33,34] Furthermore, authors like Foreman and Croft[35] and Delfini et al.[26] have described the so-called 'delayed instability', which only becomes apparent after a certain period of time. Delayed instabilities are defined as patients who do not show any instability on initial X-rays, but who become symptomatic 20 days or more after trauma (see also Ref 36). One explanation for this could be the so-called 'rim lesion'. These have been described by Taylor and Twomey,[34] and are fine tears that run horizontal at the anterior side of the disc, which is being torn off from

its deck plate. Rim lesions cannot be detected on normal X-rays, but may cause degeneration of the disc. The disc loses height and, hence, causes ligamentous laxity.[37]

Instability may also be caused by minor trauma. Especially in patients who are generalized hypermobile, relatively minor trauma, like for instance the placing of a crown for the teeth at the dentist, can precipitate a severe episode.

Sometimes patients describe a trauma that happened many years ago and only caused a short period of discomfort. Now 15 years later, however, without any clear cause there is a recurrence of symptoms. With these patients, one explanation could be that the original trauma triggered a slow degeneration of the movement segment and now this degeneration has progressed from its 'dysfunction phase' into its 'instability phase'.[38,39] An alternative explanation could be that although the segment might have been slightly structurally unstable due to the original trauma, it was still functionally stable. As the patient has grown older, however, adjacent segments have slowly started to stiffen up and that is the reason why the unstable segment has become symptomatic

Finally, the clinician should ask for throat infections just before the onset of the neck symptoms to rule out a Grisel syndrome. Grisel has described how bacteria might use the lymphatic system to reach the C1–C2 segment and destroy the ligamentous stability, causing instability.

PHYSICAL EXAMINATION

Introduction

This part of the chapter will not describe the whole assessment procedure of the cervical spine, but will limit itself to those aspects which are particularly relevant in relationship with instability problems. Also it must be emphasized that one test/observation in isolation cannot prove or disprove the existence of an instability. It is essential that a number of tests/observations confirm each other in relationship with the primary hypothesis from the subjective examination. The clinical pattern evolves throughout the physical examination. To confirm or refute the existence of a cervical instability, the following aspects of the physical examination are particular relevant:

- Inspection.
- Active movements.
- Passive physiological intervertebral movements.
- Linear movements.
- Passive accessory intervertebral movements.
- Muscular control.

The final 'clinical proof', that instability of the cervical spine played a major role in the dysfunction is, if, after appropriate treatment of the instability, the subsequent reassessment shows an improvement of the symptoms.

If the clinician has generated the hypothesis that there might be an instability involved in the generation of the symptoms, this has the following consequences for the physical examination:

- Even if the active movements do not provoke symptoms, one should refrain from performing overpressure, as the unstable segment might inadvertently be pushed beyond normal physiological limits.
- Unstable segments often respond negatively when they are moved too often to their end of range and, therefore, the clinician should limit the amount of test movements to the minimal.
- If the joint has been passively moved to the normal average range of motion and the clinician has felt there is a large increased neutral zone and the normal feeling of resistance end of range is absent (= loss of stiffness) then it may be inadvisable to continue the passive motion in order to assess the total available range of motion.

Inspection

The observation/inspection already begins during the subjective examination. How is the willingness of the patient to move the neck while describing his symptoms? Some patients seem to be moving the neck constantly during the interview ('the patient talks with his neck'). Another contributing factor is those (especially female) patients who have a very long and slender neck ('swan-like'). Conversely, there are those patients who seem to have an accentuated (hypomobile?) cervicot-

horacic kyphosis. This is usually accompanied by a secondary lordotic bend at the C5–C6 region, which may be indicated by a deep skin crease. These patients often have excessive motion in extension in this region.

Active movements

A thorough analysis of the quantity and quality of the active movements is one of the mainstays of the physical examination.

Quantity of motion

For scientific purposes one would need to measure the range of motion with, for instance, a CROM device. In daily practice, however, this would be too time consuming and therefore not practical. As a rough guideline, the clinician can use the frontal plane of the face. In normal sitting, this should be vertical. With the active movements, the clinician can estimate the amount of motion roughly in degrees (Fig. 6-3). Normal values are:

- extension 80° ± 10°
- flexion 80° ± 10°

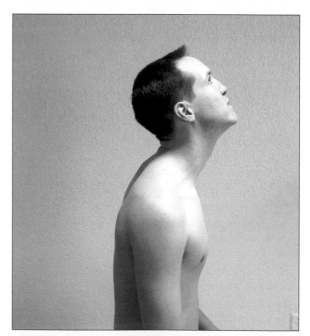

FIGURE 6-3 ■ Active movement extension. This patient shows approximately 40° of cervical extension. There is little movement in the cervicothoracic region and there appears to be slight 'hinging' in the mid-cervical spine.

- rotation 80° ± 10°
- side-flexion 35° ± 10°.

If there are abnormalities in the ROM, it is essential to evaluate the pattern within these 6 movement directions. If a patient only has 40° of extension and the reason for this is a stiff segment, then there usually is an equivalent movement (in this case 50%) restriction in rotation and side-flexion. If, however, an unstable segment is the reason for the restriction in extension, then there usually is only minimal restriction in rotation and side-flexion. A possible explanation for this phenomenon could be that as the head moves into extension, the centre of gravity moves far behind the axis of rotation, leading to a large torque. Therefore the muscles must work much harder with movements in the sagittal plane. As there is 4 to 6 times less muscle mass anterior than posterior, this can especially be seen with extension.

Another typical feature of instability is that although the patient may be very limited in his daily life because of cervical dysfunctions, there is relatively little movement restrictions during the physical examination. This seeming discrepancy can be explained by the fact that during the examination the movements are prepared and not the sudden/uncontrolled movements used in daily life.

Quality of motion

Another important aspect is to assess the quality of motion:

- Are there regions which show too much movement and others which show too little?
- Does the spine show a smooth equal curve, or does it appear to 'hinge' in a particular region?
- Sometimes it appears as if there is excessive translation in a particular segment.
- There may be a painful arc. This could be caused by a discrepancy between the amount of translation and the amount of rotation.
- There may be excessive muscular activity like muscle spasm or a 'shaking' quality of movement.
- Sometimes the patient describes apprehension with certain movements and is unwilling to move beyond a particular point, as he fears he cannot control the head anymore.

It is also important to assess these aspects during return from end-of-range positions. As the head returns from extension, normally there should be a cranial-to-caudal initiation of the movement. This is dependent upon correct activation of the deep cervical flexors. With cervical pathology there may be an inhibition of the deep stabilizing muscles (for a review see Falla[40]). This may lead to an imbalance, with overactivity in the more superficial muscles like for instance the sternocleidomastoid muscle.[41,42] The patient will now initiate the return from extension with a protruding motion of the chin, which leads to excessive mid-cervical shear. A similar abnormal movement pattern may be seen on return from flexion when the patient initiates with an upper cervical extension (which is indicative for loss of control of upper cervical flexion) and then a subsequent pulling back of the head in space.

A final indicator for instability is that when the patient activates his muscles around the neck, there is a marked improvement of the symptoms and/or ROM. In order to achieve this, the patient is asked to press with little force the tip of his tongue against the base of his two upper frontal teeth. This will activate the hyoid muscles, which (although not being the correct stabilizing muscles for the neck) will add to stability of the neck. If the reason for the symptoms is a facet joint that cannot glide sufficiently or an intervertebral foramen that cannot close sufficiently or a spinal nerve that is being compressed, there should be no improvement with this manoeuvre.

Passive physiological intervertebral movements

The passive physiological intervertebral movements (PPIVMs) assess the quantity and the quality of the intersegmental ROM in a physiological movement direction. The following parameters should be evaluated (see also Fig. 6-2C):

- neutral zone (A – R1)
- stiffness (the behaviour of R throughout the range)
- total range of motion (A – L = ROM)
- symptoms like pain, paraesthesia, discomfort, dizziness, etc.
- protective muscular spasm (S).

For a detailed description of the PPIVMs, please refer to Maitland et al.[43]

Linear movements and specific tests for ligamentous integrity

The linear movements, or linear stress tests, are movements whereby one vertebra is fixed and the other is moved. This movement is pure translational, without any concurrent physiological movement. Normally there should be almost no movement possible and the end-feel is hard-elastic. The clinician should also assess symptoms.

Pettman[15] hypothesizes that linear movements cause translational stress on the vertebral artery and/or nervous system in patients with cervical instability, whereas with PPIVMs the stress to these structures is due to excessive length changes. The linear stress tests are comparable with the drawer tests for the knee and the shoulder and are specific tests for structural integrity. A positive result implies a possible segmental instability, but does not point towards any specific structural deficit. The tests have been described by Pettman[15] in detail but, unfortunately, up to date there has been no scientific research done into the reliability and validity of these tests in the mid-cervical spine in patients with symptoms after trauma.

The most important linear stress tests for the mid/low cervical region are:

- Cranial vertebra versus caudal vertebra towards anterior.
- Caudal vertebra versus cranial vertebra towards anterior.
- Transverse stress.

The following section describes these tests for the C2–C3 segment.

Linear stress test C2 on C3 towards anterior (Fig. 6-4)

Starting position: supine, head on the bench.
Position of the therapist: standing or sitting behind the patient.
Fixation: both thumbs carefully fixate the C3 transverse processes from ventral.
Method: with both middle fingers against the laminae, C2 is moved ventrally.
Interpretation: normally, there should be no movement. The same principles apply for instability testing of C3–C7.

Linear stress test C3 on C2 towards anterior (Fig. 6-5)

Starting position: supine, head on the bench.
Position of the examiner: standing or sitting behind the patient.
Fixation: both thumbs carefully hold the C2 transverse processes from ventral.
Method: with the middle fingers against the C3 laminae C3 is moved ventrally.
Interpretation: normally, there should be no movement. Clinically one will frequently reproduce

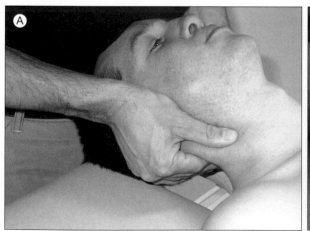
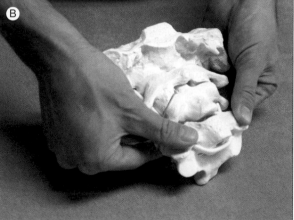

FIGURE 6-4 ■ (A, B) Linear stress test C2 on C3 towards anterior.

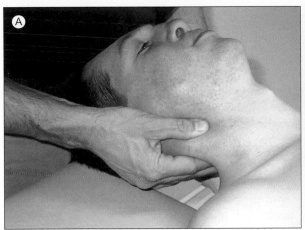
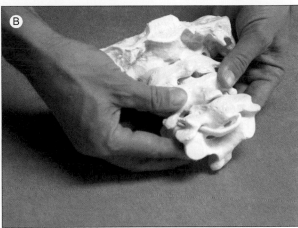

FIGURE 6-5 ■ (A, B) Linear stress test C3 on C2 towards anterior.

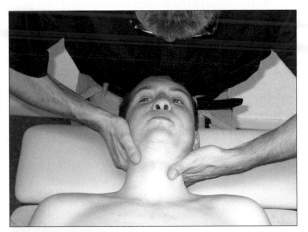

FIGURE 6-6 ■ Transverse stress to the left for C2 on C3.

symptoms with this test in patients with a dorsal extension instability.

Transverse stress test to the left for C2 on C3 (Fig. 6-6)

Starting position: the patient is lying supine.

Position of the examiner: the therapist is sitting or standing behind the patient. The head of the patient is positioned in the right hand and against the stomach of the therapist. The radial side of the metacarpophalangeal joint of the therapist's right index finger is positioned laterally against the C2 transverse process.

Fixation: the radial side of the metacarpophalangeal joint of the therapist's left index finger is positioned laterally against C3 transverse process.

Method: the therapist attempts with his right hand to shift occiput and C2 to the left relative to C3. It is important to take up the soft tissue slack first to avoid false-positive results.

Interpretation: normally, no movement should be possible.

Passive accessory intervertebral movements

Passive accessory intervertebral movements (PAIVMs) examine intersegmental mobility during accessory movements. For a detailed description, please refer to Maitland et al.[43]

A number of studies have confirmed the validity of manual assessment of intersegmental mobility. PPIVM and PAIVM techniques have been compared with discography, facet joint injection and ultrasound.[44–49] However, since most of these studies investigated validity of manual testing on hypomobile joints, one may not assume that the same applies for the examination of hypermobile/unstable joints.

Muscle control

In order to assess muscle control in the cervical spine, one can either perform the craniocervical flexion test or one may examine control over the position of the cervical spine under functional loads.

Graded craniocervical flexion test (Fig. 6-7)

The CCFT is a specific test to evaluate the function of the deep cervical flexors that has been developed by Jull et al.[50] In an impressive series of studies, they have been able to show that the result of this test reflects the ability of the subject to selectively activate the deep cervical neck flexors (for a review see Fallah[40]) Furthermore, they have been able to show that patients after whiplash, with chronic cervical symptoms and those with cervicogenic headache, show poorer results with this test and compensate with overactivity in other muscles like the sternocleidomastoid muscle.

This test is performed using a pressure biofeedback and is described in Chapter 5.

A pressure biofeedback unit (PBU) is placed under the cervical lordosis. The PBU is adjusted to 20 mm Hg. The patient is instructed to perform an upper cervical flexion, a movement similar to the nodding of the head when saying 'yes' (tucking motion).

For the graded craniocervical flexor test, the pressure should first increase by only 2 mmHg to 22 mmHg. If the patient is able to perform this without superficial muscle substitution, an additional 2 mmHg is attempted. The pressure is gradually increased until the patient is able to hold 30 mmHg without substitution 10 times for 10 seconds.

Variation: instead of a PBU, the examiner may place his hand under the patient's head. The examiner's right hand is placed underneath the occiput, the fingers of his left hand supporting the cervical lordosis. His left thumb palpates for SCM activity (Fig. 6-8).

If the patient performs the task correctly, the pressure on the left hand will increase while the pressure on the right hand does not change.

Functional stability test

These tests have originally been described by Sahrmann.[42] The goal of these tests is to evaluate the capacity of the patient to be able to control the position of the cervical spine under functional loads. The following dysfunctions may be seen:

- opening of the jaw leads to an extension movement in the cervical spine
- elevation of the arms is accompanied by a protruding of the head (Fig. 6-9)
- bending forward while standing produces a hinging into extension of the lower cervical spine.

Conclusion

As mentioned before, one test in isolation does not prove the hypothesis of instability. It is essential that a pattern appears whereby the initial hypothesis of the subjective examination is confirmed or disproven by

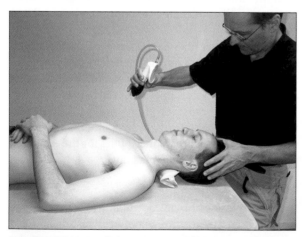

FIGURE 6-7 ■ Graded craniocervical flexion test with a pressure biofeedback unit (PBU).

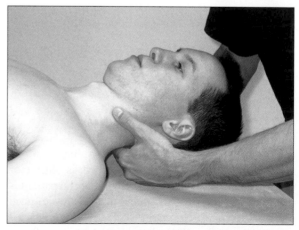

FIGURE 6-8 ■ Variation of the craniocervical flexion test (CCFT).

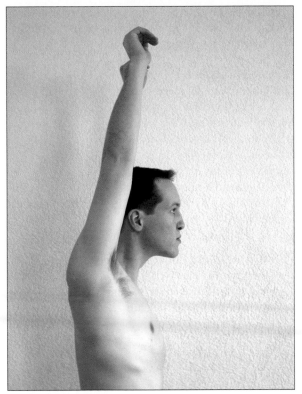

FIGURE 6-9 ■ Elevation of the arms leads to a marked protruding of the head.

subsequent test findings. The features of the different tests have to fit into a clinical pattern. The final clinical proof is if the condition of the dysfunction improves after appropriate treatment.

TREATMENT

When planning treatment, the therapist will need to analyse individual findings and prioritize them. During this process the therapist will need to consider particular hypotheses categories.[51,52]

This section will focus mainly on peripheral nociceptive pain mechanisms. Peripheral nociceptive symptoms are consistently dependent on activities, positions and loading.[52] The primary sources of the symptoms are found in the cervical region and healing has reached the stage of consolidation and reorganiza-

tion (from day 21).[53] The treatment examples will focus on the level of body function and structure of the neck.

For further information on aspects of treatment of patients with predominantly central pain mechanisms or with problems predominantly at the level of participation, refer to Gifford.[54,55]

Treating neuromusculoskeletal dysfunctions

Dysfunctions of the neuromusculoskeletal system cause abnormal movements and may lead to symptoms. Symptoms may again cause abnormal muscle activity.[56] Svensson and Graven-Nielsen[57] described the following musculoskeletal pains in their literature review:

- Increased activity of superficial muscles, e.g. sternocleidomastoid.
- Decreased activity of the deep stabilizing muscles, e.g. longus colli.
- Changes of the neural control of muscles.
- Proprioceptive deficits.

These changes may persist, even after the acute symptoms have subsided.[58] This may be a contributing factor for the persistence of symptoms or for relapses.[59] The result is a *vicious circle*: dysfunction – symptoms – abnormal muscle activity – dysfunction.

The treatment will therefore need to address the various neuromusculoskeletal aspects of the syndrome. Since pain of the motor segments inhibits physiological muscle function, the joints should be approached before muscular control exercises are attempted.[60]

Sterling et al.[61] demonstrated how mobilization of the lower cervical spine in patients with unilateral cervical pain decreases sternocleidomastoid activity in the graded craniocervical flexor test. The management of an instability problem will therefore need to include the following components:

a. Treatment of the joints.
b. Treatment of the muscles.
c. Treatment of neurodynamics.
d. Contributing factors.

Treating joint dysfunctions

For a detailed description of joint mobilization techniques, please refer to Maitland et al.[11] Functional cervical instabilities are commonly found in combination with these joint dysfunctions:

- hypomobile painful joints
- hypomobile adjacent joints
- unstable painful joints.

Hypomobile painful joints. Figure 6-10 shows a movement diagram of side-flexion of the mid-cervical spine towards the right.

Applicable treatment techniques are grade IV mobilizations, being a small-amplitude oscillation at the limit of range of movement. As the intensity of the pain at the limit is quite high, the initial techniques should not provoke any symptoms. If the reassessment does not show any improvement, mobilization can be progressed until some discomfort is produced. It is important that the pain comes and goes in the rhythm with the oscillation and that its intensity does not increase. One possible technique is PAIVM. For example, left unilateral posteroanterior mobilization of the appropriate mid-cervical segment. Sterling et al.[61] demonstrated that unilateral posteroanterior mobilization of the lower cervical segments decreased local pain perception and also decreased symptoms on end-of-range rotation. If local hypersensitivity does not allow for direct techniques, one might prefer indirect techniques like right side-flexion to avoid manual contact with the painful segments.

If the patient has been assessed for contraindications, manipulations like transverse thrust to the left might also be appropriate.

Hypomobile adjacent joints. Hypomobility of adjacent joints causes an increased load and hypermobility of the neighbouring segments. To reduce the load, hypomobility should be treated by manual therapy. One needs to be careful not to accidentally load the adjacent hypermobile joints.

Example: patient A has hypomobility of the cervicothoracic junction on extension and rotation to the right and instability/hypermobility in the mid-cervical segments.

The following techniques might be beneficial:

- Anteroposterior mobilization through the sternum (Fig. 6-11).
- Localized rotation to the right. The right hand holds the seventh cervical segment and is primarily responsible for the rotation/mobilization.

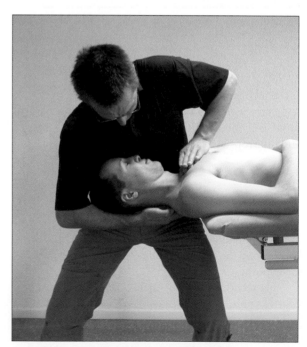

FIGURE 6-11 ■ Upper thoracic anteroposterior mobilization through the sternum.

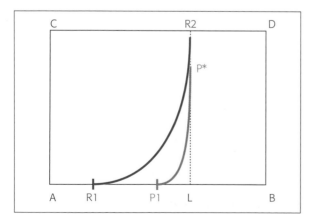

FIGURE 6-10 ■ Movement diagram of side-flexion to the right.

■ Automobilization of the craniothoracic junction:

The patient is sitting on a chair with his fourth–sixth thoracic segments against the backrest of the chair. He folds his hands behind his neck and the craniocervical area. He then draws in his tummy to avoid compensatory movements of the lumbar spine and mobilizes his upper thoracic spine into extension.

Another example: patient B has hypomobility of the upper two cervical segments on rotation to the left. He also shows compensatory hypermobility of the lower cervical segments on extension and rotation to the left. Since rotation to the left is coupled with lateroflexion to the right, the therapist may decide to mobilize the upper segments by lateroflexion to the right. This would lead to an increase in upper cervical rotation to the left without overstressing the lower segments.

For the automobilization technique, the patient will need a big towel. The patient is sitting on a chair with the towel behind his back. His hands are crossed in such a manner that the right hand holds the left end of the towel and is positioned underneath the left hand, which holds the right end of the towel. The edge of the towel is placed on the left side of the dorsal articular process of C3 and on the right onto the articular processes of C1 or C2. The right hand pulls on the towel to fix C3, while the patient attempts to turn his head to the left, supported by the left hand, which also pulls on the end of the towel.

Unstable painful joints. For patients with structural instabilities, passive mobilization of the unstable joints is not the first choice. Priorities are rather mobilization of adjacent hypomobile joints and muscle control.

From a clinical point of view, grade II mobilizations might still be an option to reduce sensitivity of the hypermobile segments.[11] The Maitland concept defines grade II mobilizations as oscillating movements with a large amplitude without moving into resistance. These mobilizations do not aim to increase passive range of motion but rather to positively influence pain perception by offering non-nociceptive joint input.[62]

Thus, for example, a patient with mid-cervical instability could be treated in the supine position by unilateral posteroanterior mobilization (Fig. 6-12).

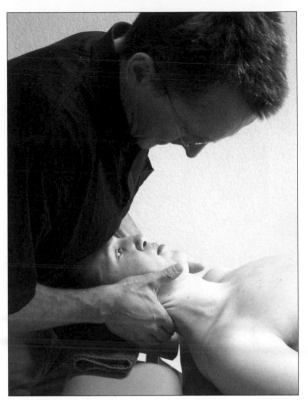

FIGURE 6-12 ■ Grade II unilateral posteroanterior mobilization in supine.

Treating neural structures

Instability of a mobile segment might cause nerve root irritations.[63] In this case dysfunction of neurodynamics is a secondary problem. Clinically, one will often find that neurodynamic signs will improve automatically with increased stability of the unstable segment. Therefore it is not surprising that upper limb neurodynamic test 1 (ULNT1) will show an increased elbow extension after activation of the deep cervical flexor muscles.

Detailed instructions, techniques and management of neural mobilization are described in Butler[64] and in Hall and Elvey.[65]

A commonly applied technique to improve sensitivity and mobility of the nervous system is the side-glide technique. Vicenzino et al.[66] demonstrated how this technique decreased local sensitivity at the lateral epicondyle and increased grip strength in patients with lateral epicondylitis. No changes in temperature

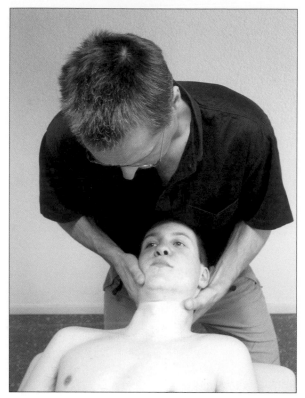

FIGURE 6-13 ■ Cervical side-glide towards the left.

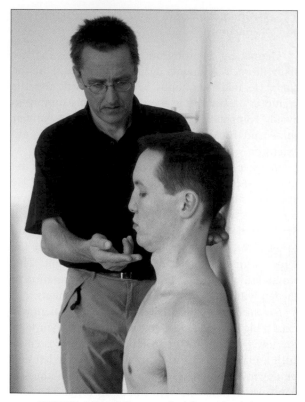

FIGURE 6-14 ■ Deep cervical flexors in sitting.

sensitivity were observed. Since the technique also changed sympathetic activity, the authors hypothesized that the side-glide technique activates the dorsal periaqueductal grey, thereby causing hypoalgesia.

Cowell and Philipps[67] and Hall et al.[68] also observed an effect of neural mobilization on cervicobrachial pain syndromes. They also used cervical side-glide techniques (Fig. 6-13).

Improving muscular stability

Basic exercise. Exercises for muscle stability are based on the graded cervical flexion test. All exercises are designed to focus on deep cervical flexor activity and should be performed with low-intensity muscle force. To gain control over muscle coordination the exercises should be performed 2–3 times a day, 10 repetitions of 10 seconds holding time.

The exercise is performed in exactly the same way as the test for the deep cervical flexors. Additionally, an exercise in sitting position should be performed

(Fig. 6-14). Initially, it will be easier for the patient to perform the exercise with the back leaning against a wall or a door, as far back against the wall as possible. His hands rest on his lap and the back of his head leans gently against the wall. Patients with a thoracic kyphosis who cannot adopt this position are allowed to move their buttocks slightly away from the wall.

The tummy is drawn in, the shoulder blades are positioned in slight retraction and gentle elevation or depression, depending on the habitual position of the individual patient. If the nervous system is highly mechanosensitive, shoulder depression should not be performed since this might cause an additional irritation of the nervous system. The final movement that is added is a gentle nod of the head. It is important that the head maintains contact with the wall and slides upwards against the wall. The advantages of performing the exercise in this position are:

■ The patient can perform the exercise throughout the day wherever he is.

- It is a functional position.
- Sliding against the wall provides sensory feedback.
- The wall prevents retraction.

Once the patient is comfortable with the wall exercise, he should learn to continue the activity without the feedback of the wall. He should imagine 'growing tall' while doing the exercise.

The patient is then asked to correct his posture throughout the day whenever he thinks of it. Reminders could be red traffic lights or the sound of the telephone ringing; whenever he sees or hears his cues, he should then perform a single 10-second hold of the exercise. The progression of this exercise depends on the normal daily life activities of the patient and the treatment goals. A young footballer, for example, who has problems when heading the ball will need an exercise progression for his deep cervical flexors that is designed to withstand the load of a ball on his head.

A mountain biker with problems on downhilling might rather need strength and endurance of his neck extensors. Those patients who do not put any specific load on their necks in their day-to-day lives should focus on functional muscle stability.

The following exercise examples do not require specific equipment to allow the patient to exercise where and whenever he thinks of it. Naturally, the therapist is free to adapt the exercises for his purposes and supplement with any equipment felt to be required like elastic exercise bands, pulleys, etc.

Focus on deep cervical flexors. Initially, the patient performs the basic exercise in supine. Then, he attempts to decrease the pressure of his occiput on the bed while the pressure of his cervical lordosis is maintained. The back of the head should then be gradually raised about 0.5 cm. Since this exercise is very difficult in supine, one might try to perform the movement in half-sitting or with a tilted headrest first (Fig. 6-15). At home, the patient may want to try to sit in a semi-reclined long-sitting position on the floor with his trunk against an ironing board, which is placed against his bed.

To lift the head off the bed, activity of the superficial flexor muscles like the sternocleidomastoid muscle is needed. It is essential that the therapist constantly

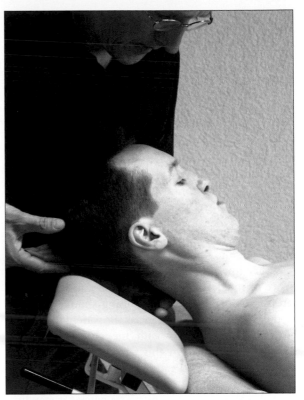

FIGURE 6-15 ■ Lifting off in semi-reclined position.

checks whether the patient continues to have control over the cervical lordosis. (He is not allowed to push the chin forward.)

Progression of the exercise requires performance on a flat surface or to move the chin towards the sternum. It is also important to change the starting position more towards extension. This is achieved by placing a small pillow underneath the thoracic spine and thereby positioning the craniocervical region into slight extension. Now the patient is asked to perform an upper cervical flexion ('head on neck') before lifting his head off the bed.

The final stage of the exercise programme could be to perform the movement in a supine position, with the head hanging over the end of the bed. Only those patients who need to perform high-load activities in their daily life will need to train at this level.

The football player mentioned above was also asked to do specific ball exercises: he was positioned standing 1 metre from a wall, facing the wall. With his forehead, he held a football against the wall. Progression of this exercise included decreased base (standing on one leg) or fast movements with hand weights.

Focus on extensor muscles. After the patient has learned the basic exercise, he is now positioned prone. He draws in his tummy, positions the shoulder blades in retraction and slight depression and lifts his forehead off the bed with his chin tucked in. Since the muscles in the back of the neck are much stronger than the ventral muscles, this exercise can usually be performed in a flat position straight away.

To increase the intensity of this exercise, a light weight, e.g. 1 kg, may be placed on the back of the head: otherwise, the patient should be standing, not only lifting the forehead but also extending the neck. It is very important to carefully observe the maintenance of the deep cervical extension and the cervical lordosis. For example, no bending should occur. A further progression can be to ask the patient to support himself on his elbows with the chin towards the sternum. Starting from this flexed position, he now performs a controlled extension.

Exercises in standing that involve arm movements have also shown good results. The patient is standing with his trunk bent to 60° by hip flexion. In both hands he holds 1 kg weights. First, the patient needs to position his head correctly; then he starts to quickly move his arms into flexion and/or abduction while he carefully tries not to lose the position of his neck. Again, exercises with a ball against the wall might be indicated.

Focus on functional stability. The exercise routine depends on the test position in which the patient failed to maintain the position of head and neck. The test that was failed is turned into the exercise.[42] Two cases will explain this procedure:

Example 1: The patient shows a hinging of cervical segments to extension on bilateral arm elevation. This patient should begin his training by performing the exercise against the wall. He positions his fingers in his cervical lordosis to feel and control the pressure he builds up on correct performance of the exercise (Fig. 6-16). The other arm is moved into elevation. Increased speed of the arm movement or hand weights will progress this exercise. Once this exercise is learned, the

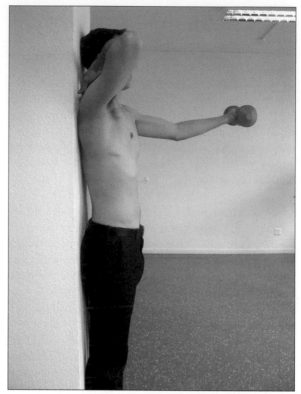

FIGURE 6-16 ■ Focusing on functional positions.

training can be continued in a free-standing position.

Example 2: The patient 2 is a physiotherapist who suffered a whiplash injury 3 years ago with continued cervical symptoms ('my neck gets very tired and feels like snapping'). The symptoms increase during the course of the day, so that he commonly needs a brace in the afternoons around 3 pm. His symptoms depend on his work posture: the more manual therapy he does (in a position of slight forward-bending), the worse his symptoms become. The physical examination shows a hinging in the cervical spine on lumbar forward-bending. If he pretends to perform a manual therapy mobilization, his head moves into protraction in the rhythm of his movements. This patient was supplied with exercises focusing on extensor muscles; furthermore, lumbar flexion was performed in sitting and standing with control of craniocervical stability. The patient was also asked to do controlled cervical flexion and extension while sitting with his elbows positioned on a bed. In the end, he practised posteroanterior mobilization techniques on a ball while maintaining craniocervical stability.

Contributing factors

Further to the treatment of neuromusculoskeletal dysfunctions, potential contributing factors should also be approached. These include biopsychosocial aspects[54,55] and ergonomic factors as well as an analysis of daily life activities.

Repetitive activities in a non-physiological position or compensatory movement patterns might maintain symptoms or lead to further episodes of symptoms.

Some examples will underline these thoughts:
Example 1: The first patient shows a slight instability of the C4–C5 segment on extension. Additionally, his cervicothoracic junction is hypomobile. Although he religiously performed his stabilization and mobilization exercises, he was never symptom-free and suffered frequent relapses. An analysis of his daily life activities showed that his symptoms occurred whenever he rode his mountain bike. He generally preferred flat surfaces but the low position of the handlebar and the hypomobility of his cervicothoracic junction forced his hypermobile cervical segments into extension. It was recommended to change the height of his handlebars to achieve a more upright posture.
Example 2: The second patient is a woman with mild insufficiency of the right alar ligaments whose hair was parted on the right side so her hair covered her left eye. She thus had a tendency to hold her head in slight lateroflexion to the right and habitually performed quick left rotations of her head to reposition her hair. This frequently caused new episodes of symptoms. After the third painful episode in a year, she accepted that she needed to change her hairstyle.
Example 3: The third patient suffers from a hypermobility of the C2–C3 segment on rotation to the left and extension. Additionally, his neck is stiff on rotation and lateroflexion to the right. He is an architect who spends a number of hours a day on the telephone, which he habitually holds between his left shoulder and his left ear to keep his hands free to write. This causes frequent lateroflexion to the left and an increased activity of the left levator scapula muscle. Muscle shortening will cause movement restriction on rotation and lateroflexion to the right. The patient was

informed of the biomechanical background of his symptoms and he bought a headset for his phone. He never had a relapse since.

Finally, it is important to assess the posture and activities at the workplace. Good ergonomic advice might be even more beneficial than mobilization and stabilization treatment in some computer users.

Conclusions

Successful management of cervical instability problems includes consideration of all biopsychosocial aspects.[54,55]

During neuromusculoskeletal treatment, any signs and symptoms need to be evaluated for priority and relevance.

To avoid relapses, it is of enormous importance to include a workplace and daily life activity intervention.

CASE STUDY

A 45-year-old male patient had a main complaint of deep nagging (sometimes stabbing) intermittent unilateral pain in the mid/low cervical region slightly spreading into the right scapular area (Fig. 6-17). Symptom area 2 was a superficial intermittent feeling of heaviness in the lateral side of the arm spreading into his thumb.

The neck symptoms are increased by:

- looking over his right shoulder while reversing his car
- looking up for a longer period when he is rock climbing
- making quick uncontrolled movements during work or leisure periods.

The neck symptoms are decreased by:

- returning the head back to the neutral position
- holding his neck with his hands
- wearing a collar, sometimes, to relax his neck.

The symptoms in the arm seem to be independent of the symptoms in the neck. They do not necessarily come on when the neck symptoms increase; but when he has provoked his neck many times during the day, his arm symptoms usually come on. He is not able to

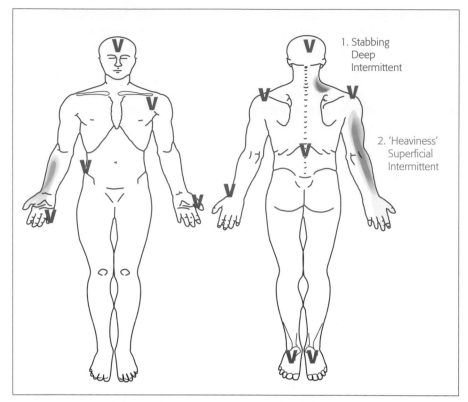

FIGURE 6-17 ■ Body chart case study.

relieve the arm symptoms with any particular positions or movements.

Generally, his sleep his undisturbed and, on waking, he feels rested and it is the best time of the day. At the end of the day, the symptoms are usually worse.

Reasoning

The localization of the neck symptoms would coincide with pain referral from C4–C5 and C5–C6 facet joint.[69] The pain has a typical intermittent peripheral nociceptive quality and is dependent upon stress to the cervical spine. The overall behaviour over 24 hours is atypical for a primary discogenic problem as he feels good in the morning.

The localization and quality of the arm symptoms would coincide with a more dermatomal distribution of C6 spinal nerve. As they seem to be independent from the neck symptoms, they are not a referred symptom from the same source. If the symptoms would have been primarily a lengthening dysfunction of the nervous system, it would have been expected that the patient describes arm movements or contralateral neck movements to increase the symptoms. If the problem would have been compression of a spinal nerve, it would have been expected that the patient would have had an increase of symptoms at night (due to the blood 'pressure gradient' from Sunderland[70] and an increase of symptoms with cervical movements which compress the nerve).

Special questions

- General health OK.
- No recent weight loss.
- The patient is able to work 100% as a mechanic in a factory (and gives the impression he is quite satisfied at his work).
- He is married with two children of 12 and 14 years of age.

- His hobbies are hiking and once/twice a week he goes rock climbing.
- He does not use any medication and he has never use cortisone.
- The standard X-rays of the cervical spine did not show any pathology.
- There are no associated symptoms like dizziness and there is no loss of strength.

Reasoning

From the medical point of view, there seem to be no red flags/contraindications and there are therefore no special precautions necessary. Furthermore, although there was no formal screening for psychosocial risk factors, there was no indication during the subjective interview of any obvious 'yellow flags' like, for instance, catastrophizing, fear-avoidance behaviour or any socioeconomic gain.

History

Six months ago the patient was involved in a car accident in which he was struck from behind. The next day his cervical symptoms appeared; they increased over the following week. On day 3 the arm symptoms slowly came on. He was diagnosed as a having a whiplash-associated disorder (WAD) type II and was initially managed with a collar and non-steroidal anti-inflammatory drugs (NSAIDs) for 4 weeks. After 2 weeks he was sent to physiotherapy where the first nine treatments over 5 weeks mainly consisted of hot packs and massage. This eased the symptoms only slightly. The subsequent nine treatments over 8 weeks focused on 'stretching' of muscles and electrotherapy with transcutaneous electrical nerve stimulation (TENS). The patient described that when only gentle stretches were applied, the symptoms decreased, whereas when end-of-range stretches were applied he usually felt worse. After these 4 months of treatment, he was not symptom-free, but he was told it just needed a bit more time. The patient returned to work 1 month after the accident. Concurrently, the patient is not satisfied with his condition and he even has the feeling that the symptoms are increasing without any cause.

The patient has no past history of cervical spine problems and/or trauma.

Reasoning

There is an adequate trauma to explain the patient's symptoms. The overall pattern would be indicative of a peripheral nociceptive/neurogenic problem. One main question, however, is why have the symptoms become chronic, as the patient does not show any classic risk factors for chronification of symptoms.[71]

When a problem is input-dominant, another question is: What is the primary source? If it would have been a stiff/hypomobile facet joint, then why did he not respond to end-of-range stretches?

The following indicators would lead to an initial hypothesis that one component could be an instability of the cervical spine:

- increase of symptoms with sustained looking up and with quick uncontrolled movements
- decrease of symptoms with holding the neck/collar
- good in the morning, increase end of day when the neck gets tired
- rear-end car accident
- delayed healing ('delayed instability'?)
- the response to the end-of-range stretches

The C5–C6 facet joint could be the primary source for area 1. And as the spinal nerve C6 exits through the intervertebral foramen of C5–C6, a possible instability of C5–C6 could cause a secondary irritation of this nerve.

As the condition was non-irritable and stable and there were no other special precautions, it was decided to perform the standard examination of the cervical spine, however without applying overpressure to the end positions (Box 6-1).

Reasoning

Analysis of the active movements. The cervical symptoms are being reproduced by rotation to the right and ipsilateral side-flexion. As rotation in the cervical spine below C2 is coupled with ipsilateral side-flexion, this would implicate the lower cervical spine to be its primary source. The symptoms are also reproduced with extension rather than flexion. These features would fit with translatory movements that 'close down' the intervertebral foramina on the right (= regular closing down pattern on the right).[72]

BOX 6-1
PHYSICAL EXAMINATION

PP	None
Inspection	Normal

Active movements

Flexion:	80° no symptoms
Extension:	70° area 1 (hinging in the mid-cervical spine)
Right rotation:	85° area 1
Left rotation:	95° no symptoms
Right side-flexion:	35° area 1
Left side-flexion:	10° no symptoms
Localized occiput – C2:	right rotation 5° no symptoms left rotation 35° no symptoms

Neurological examination

Sensation	normal
Reflexes	normal
Power	normal

Neurodynamic assessment: upper limb neural test 1
Left: lacking 10° of final elbow extension produces a pulling in the cubital fold
Right: lacking 40° of elbow extension reproducing the symptoms in the arm. With contralateral side-flexion these symptoms increase

PPIVMs	C0–C2	Right rotation 5° Extension slightly limited
	C2–C5	Normal
	C5–C6	Extension hypermobile Right side-flexion hypermobile

PAIVMs
Unilateral PA C4–C6 on the right slightly hypermobile
Unilateral PA C2 on the right slightly hypomobile, and when the neck was positioned in 10° of right rotation, there was no movement at all
Because of time constraints further testing, e.g. linear stress tests, were postponed

Rotation to the right is less than to the left, but with the side-flexion it's the other way around. Therefore, the movement restriction could be caused by a segmental restriction above C2. This is confirmed by the segmental rotation test in sitting.

Overall rotation to the left is 95° and the occiput part is 35°. This leaves approximately 60° for the rest of the cervical spine, which is normal. To the right, however, overall rotation is 85°, while the upper cervical contribution is only 5°. This means that the rest of

the cervical spine has to rotate 80°, which is excessive. This is confirmed by the hinging in the lower cervical spine that is visible with extension.

Therefore, the primary hypothesis is that the symptoms are being provoked by a low cervical hypermobility/instability in extension/right rotation, whereas there is a hypomobility in the upper cervical spine, which could contribute to the problem.

This is being confirmed by the PPIVMs.

This is further confirmed by the findings with the PAIVMs. The fact that the unilateral posteroanterior movement on C2 is more restricted when the head is in slight rotation to the right would implicate the C1–C2 joint.

The reproduction of the arm symptoms with the ULNT1 shows increased mechanosensitivity of the nervous system to mechanical stress, but as this could also be caused by excessive/abnormal segmental movement, this was initially thought to be a secondary phenomenon.

Treatment 1: initial management plan

The goal of the initial treatment was to increase the upper cervical rotation to the right without placing too much stress on the low cervical region. As the hypomobility is resistance-dominant, a grade IV mobilization is appropriate. One option could have been to mobilise with unilateral posteroanterior mobilizations on C2 on the right with the head in slight rotation towards the right. In this case, however, there was too much local tenderness. Therefore, it was decided to mobilize with upper cervical side-flexion towards the left.

Treatment 2 on day 4

Reassessment. The patient reported slight improvement with looking over his shoulder, but otherwise there was no change. On physical examination the right rotation and side-flexion provoked less symptoms, but otherwise the condition was unchanged.

Continuing/completion of the assessment. Linear stress testing showed instability of the C5–C6 segment (especially C6 versus C5 towards anterior provoked discomfort in the neck).

Assessment of the PPIVMs of the cervicothoracic region showed marked hypomobility in this region.

Furthermore, during these PPIVMs, the patient volunteered that he had the feeling that this was what his spine needed.

Treatment. Therefore treatment on day 4 consisted of mobilizations of both the upper cervical spine and of the cervicothoracic region. This included an automobilization of the cervicothoracic region.

Treatment 3 on day 8

The patient described a definite improvement of both the neck and the arm symptoms. On physical examination, side-flexion and rotation were symmetrical. His extension, however, was nearly unchanged. The ULNT had improved by 20° of elbow extension.

Continuing/completion of the assessment. Now the craniocervical flexion test was added. The patient showed marked substitution with the sternocleidomastoid muscle and was only able to perform correctly with a 2mm Hg pressure increase.

Treatment. The mobilization techniques were further progressed. The patient was instructed to perform the craniocervical flexion movement both in supine lying and in sitting against the wall on a 2 hourly basis.

Further treatment sessions

Treatments 4 and 5 were once per week, whereas treatments 6–9 were once every 2 weeks. From treatment 5 onwards passive mobilizations were no longer necessary and treatment mainly consisted of progression of the muscular exercises.

REFERENCES

1. Eisenstein S. Instability and low back pain a way out of the semantic maze. In: Szpalski M, Gunzburg R, Pope M, editors. Lumbar segmental instability. Philadelphia: Lippincott Williams and Wilkins; 1999. p. 39–51.
2. Mulholland R. Clinical definition of instability. In: Szpalski M, Gunzburg R, Pope M, editors. Lumbar segmental instability. Philadelphia: Lippincott Williams and Wilkins; 1999. p. 55–61.
3. Adams M. Biomehanics of the intervertebral disc, vertebra, and ligaments. In: Szpalski M, Gunzburg R, Pope M, editors. Lumbar segmental instability. Philadelphia: Lippincott Williams and Wilkins; 1999. p. 3–13.
4. Panjabi MM. The stabilizing system of the spine. Part I. Function, dysfunction, adaptation, and enhancement. J Spinal Disord 1992;5(4):383–9, discussion 397.
5. Zhu Q, Ouyang J, Lu W, et al. Traumatic instabilities of the cervical spine caused by high-speed axial compression in a human model. An in vitro biomechanical study. Spine 1999;24(5):440–4.
6. Siegmund GP, Myers BS, Davis MB, et al. Mechanical evidence of cervical facet capsule injury during whiplash: a cadaveric study using combined shear, compression, and extension loading. Spine 2001;26(19):2095–101.
7. Wilmink JT, Patijn J. MR imaging of alar ligament in whiplash-associated disorders: an observer study. Neuroradiology 2001; 43(10):859–63.
8. Lomoschitz F, Blackmore C, Mirza S, et al. Cervical spine injuries in patients 65 years old and older: epidemiologic analysis regarding the effects of age and injury mechanism on distribution, type, and stability of injuries. AJR Am J Roentgenol 2002;178:573–7.
9. Pope MH, Panjabi M. Biomechanical definitions of spinal instability. Spine 1985;10(3):255–6.
10. Panjabi MM, Lydon C, Vasavada A, et al. On the understanding of clinical instability. Spine 1994;19(23):2642–50.
11. Maitland G, Hengeveld E, Banks K, et al. Maitland's vertebral manipulation. 6th ed. Oxford: Butterworth-Heinemann; 2001.
12. Panjabi MM. The stabilizing system of the spine. Part II. Neutral zone and instability hypothesis. J Spinal Disord 1992;5(4):390–6, discussion 397.
13. Lee SW, Draper ER, Hughes SP. Instantaneous center of rotation and instability of the cervical spine. A clinical study. Spine 1997;22(6):641–7, discussion 647–8.
14. Kettler A, Hartwig E, Schultheiss M, et al. Mechanically simulated muscle forces strongly stabilize intact and injured upper cervical spine specimens. J Biomech 2002;35(3):339–46.
15. Pettman E. Stress tests of the craniovertebral joints. In: Boyling J, Palastanga N, editors. Grieve's modern manual therapy. 2nd ed. Edinburgh: Churchill Livingstone; 1994. p. 529–37.
16. Aspinall W. Clinical testing for craniovertebral hypermobility syndrome. J Orthop Sports Phys Ther 1990;12:47–54.
17. Sanchez Martin M. Occipital–cervical instability. Clin Orthop Relat Res 1992;283:63–73.
18. Pitkanen M, Manninen HI, Lindgrer KA, et al. Limited usefulness of traction-compression films in the radiographic diagnosis of lumbar spinal instability. Comparison with flexion-extension films. Spine 1997;22(2):193–7.
19. Cattrysse E, Swinkels RA, Oostendorp RA, et al. Upper cervical instability: are clinical tests reliable? Man Ther 1997;2(2):91–7.
20. McLain RF. Mechanoreceptor endings in human cervical facet joints. Spine 1994;19(5):495–501.
21. Mendel T, Wink CS, Zimny ML. Neural elements in human cervical intervertebral discs. Spine 1992;17(2):132–5.
22. Heikkila H, Astrom PG. Cervicocephalic kinesthetic sensibility in patients with whiplash injury. Scand J Rehabil Med 1996; 28(3):133–8.
23. Heikkila HV, Wenngren BI. Cervicocephalic kinesthetic sensibility, active range of cervical motion, and oculomotor function in patients with whiplash injury. Arch Phys Med Rehabil 1998;79(9):1089–94.

24. White A, Bernhardt M, Panjabi M. Clinical biomechanics and lumbar spinal instability. In: Szpalski M, Gunzburg R, Pope M, editors. Lumbar segmental instability. Philadelphia: Lippincott Williams and Wilkins; 1999. p. 15–25.

25. Wiesel SW, Rothman RH. Occipitoatlantal hypermobility. Spine 1979;4(3):187–91.

26. Delfini R, Dorizzi A, Facchinetti G, et al. Delayed post-traumatic cervical instability. Surg Neurol 1999;51(6):588–94, discussion 594-5.

27. McDermaid C. Vertebrobasilar incidents and spinal manipulative therapy of the cervical spine. In: Vernon H, editor. Craniocervical syndrome. London: Butterworth-Heinemann; 2001. p. 244–53.

28. Coman W. Dizziness related to ENT conditions. In: Grieve G, editor. Modern manual therapy of the vertebral column. Edinburgh: Churchill Livingstone; 1986. p. 28.

29. Endo K, Ichimaru K, Shimura H, et al. Cervical vertigo after hair shampoo treatment at a hairdressing salon: a case report. Spine 2000;25(5):632–4.

30. Bogduk N. Mechanisms and pain patterns of the upper cervical spine. In: Vernon H, editor. The cranio-cervical syndrome. Oxford: Butterworth-Heinemann; 2001. p. 110–16.

31. Spitzer WO, Skovron ML, Salmi LR, et al. Scientific monograph of the Quebec Task Force on Whiplash-Associated Disorders: redefining 'whiplash' and its management. Spine 1995;20(Suppl. 8):1S–73S.

32. Barnsley L, Lord S, Bogduk N. Whiplash injury. Pain 1994;58(3):283–307.

33. Jonsson H Jr, Bring G, Rauschning W, et al. Hidden cervical spine injuries in traffic accident victims with skull fractures. J Spinal Disord 1991;4(3):251–63.

34. Taylor JR, Twomey LT. Acute injuries to cervical joints. An autopsy study of neck sprain. Spine 1993;18(9):1115–22.

35. Foreman S, Croft A. Whiplash injuries. The cervical acceleration/deceleration syndrome. 2nd ed. Baltimore: Williams and Wilkins; 1995.

36. Herkowitz HN, Rothman RH. Subacute instability of the cervical spine. Spine 1984;9(4):348–57.

37. Twomey LT, Taylor JR. Age-related changes of the lumbar spine and spinal rehabilitation. Phys Rehabil Med 1991;2(3):153–69.

38. Dai L. Disc degeneration and cervical instability. Correlation of magnetic resonance imaging with radiography. Spine 1998; 23(16):1734–8.

39. Kirkaldy Willis W, Farfan H. Instability of the lumbar spine. Clin Orthop 1982;165:110–23.

40. Falla D. Unravelling the complexity of muscle impairement in chronic neck pain. Man Ther 2004;9:125–33.

41. Winters J, Peles J. Neck muscle activity and 3D kinematics during quasistatic and dynamic tracking movements. In: Winters J, Woolsley H, editors. Multiple muscle systems: biomechanics and movement organisation. New York: Springer; 1990. p. 461–80.

42. Sahrmann S. Diagnosis and treatment of movement impairment syndromes. St Louis: Mosby; 2002.

43. Maitland G, Hengeveld E, Banks K, et al. Maitland's vertebral manipulation. 7th ed. London: Elsevier Butterworth-Heinemann; 2005.

44. Jull G, Bogduk N, Marsland A. The accuracy of manual diagnosis for cervical zygapophysial joint pain syndromes. Med J Aust 1988;148(5):233–6.

45. Jull G, Treleaven J, Versace G. Manual examination: is pain provocation a major cue for spinal dysfunction? Aust J Physiother 1994;40(3):159–65.

46. Lord SM, Barnsley L, Wallis BJ, et al. Third occipital nerve headache: a prevalence study. J Neurol Neurosurg Psychiatry 1994;57(10):1187–90.

47. Hides JA, Stokes MJ, Saide M, et al. Evidence of lumbar multifidus muscle wasting ipsilateral to symptoms in patients with acute/subacute low back pain. Spine 1994;19(2):165–72.

48. Phillips DR, Twomey LT. A comparison of manual diagnosis with a diagnosis established by a uni-level lumbar spinal block procedure. Man Ther 1996;1(2):82–7.

49. Jull G, Zito G, Trott P, et al. Inter-examiner reliability to detect painful upper cervical joint dysfunction. Aust J Physiother 1997;43(2):125–9.

50. Jull G, Falla D, Treleaven J, et al. A therapeutic exercise approach for cervical disorders. In: Boyling J, Jull G, editors. Grieve's modern manual therapy. The vertebral column. Edinburgh: Elsevier Churchill Livingstone; 2004.

51. Butler D. Integrating pain awareness into physiotherapy – wise action for the future. In: Gifford L, editor. Topical issues in pain 1. Whiplash – Science and management. Falmouth: CNS Press; 1998. p. 1–23.

52. Gifford L. Schmerzphysiologie. In: Van der Berg F, editor. Angewandte Physiologie Teil 2: Organsysteme verstehen und beeinflussen. Stuttgart: Thieme; 2000. p. 467–518.

53. van den Berg F. Angewandte Physiologie Teil 1: Das Bindegewebe des Bewegungsapparates verstehen und beeinflussen. Stuttgart: Thieme; 1999.

54. Gifford L. Perspektiven zum biopsychosozialen Modell. Teil 1: Müssen einige Aspekte vielleicht doch akzeptiert werden? Manuelle Therapie 2002;6(3):139–45.

55. Gifford L. Perspektiven zum biopsychosozialen Modell. Teil 2: Einkaufskorb-Ansatz. Manuelle Therapie 2002;6(4): 197–206.

56. Svensson P, Graven-Nielsen T. Craniofacial muscle pain: review of mechanisms and clinical manifestations. J Orofac Pain 2001;15(2):117–45.

57. Sterling M, Jull G, Wright A. The effect of musculoskeletal pain on motor activity and control. J Pain 2001;2(3):135–45.

58. Hides JA, Richardson CA, Jull GA. Multifidus muscle recovery is not automatic after resolution of acute, first-episode low back pain. Spine 1996;21(23):2763–9.

59. Hides JA, Jull GA, Richardson CA. Long-term effects of specific stabilizing exercises for first-episode low back pain. Spine 2001;26(11):E243–8.

60. Stokes M, Young A. The contribution of reflex inhibition to arthrogenous muscle weakness. Clin Sci (Lond) 1984;67(1): 7–14.

61. Sterling M, Jull G, Wright A. Cervical mobilisation: concurrent effects on pain, sympathetic nervous system activity and motor activity. Man Ther 2001;6(2):72–81.

62. Melzack R. Gate control theory. On the evolution of pain concepts. Pain Forum 1996;5(2):128–38.

63. Rydevik B, Ollmarker K. Instability and sciatica. In: Szpalski M, Gunzburg R, Pope M, editors. Lumbar segmental instability. Philadelphia: Lippincott Williams and Wilkins; 1999. p. 75–84.

64. Butler D. The sensitive nervous system. Adelaide: Noigroup Publications; 2000.

65. Hall TM, Elvey RL. Nerve trunk pain: physical diagnosis and treatment. Man Ther 1999;4(2):63–73.

66. Vicenzino B, Collins D, Wright A. The initial effects of a cervical spine manipulative physiotherapy treatment on the pain and dysfunction of lateral epicondylalgia. Pain 1996;68(1):69–74.

67. Cowell IM, Phillips DR. Effectiveness of manipulative physiotherapy for the treatment of a neurogenic cervicobrachial pain syndrome: a single case study – experimental design. Man Ther 2002;7(1):31–8.

68. Hall T, Elvey R, Davies N, et al. Efficacy of manipulative physiotherapy for the treatment of cervicobrachial pain. In: Australia MPAA, ed. Tenth Biennial Conference of the MPAA, 1997; Melbourne.

69. Dwyer A, Aprill C, Bogduk N. Cervical zygapophyseal joint pain patterns. I: A study in normal volunteers. Spine 1990;15(6):453–7.

70. Sunderland S. Nerves and nerve injuries. London: Churchill Livingstone; 1978.

71. Scholten-Peeters GG, Bekkering GE, Verhagen AP, et al. Clinical practice guideline for the physiotherapy of patients with whiplash-associated disorders. Spine 2002;27(4):412–22.

72. Edwards B. Manual of combined movements. Melbourne: Churchill Livingstone; 1992.

7

HEADACHE AND THE CERVICAL SPINE

RAFAEL TORRES CUECO ■ GWENDOLEN JULL

Headaches are a very common disorder, with considerable social and economic impact. Epidemiological studies on European populations show an average headache prevalence of 51% over a period of 1 year, approximately 4% being chronic headaches.[1]

Headaches are classified as primary and secondary. Primary headaches are classified in four subgroups: migraine, tension-type headache, trigeminal autonomic cephalalgias and other primary headaches. Secondary headaches are caused by a recognizable disorder or pathology. One of the possible causes is a pathology or dysfunction of the cervical spine. This is the case for cervicogenic headaches.

The relationship between headaches and the cervical spine has been controversial. In the 1970s, neurologists considered that the cervical spine could in no way be responsible for a distinct headache type.[2] This reluctance to acknowledge the existence of a headache caused by a cervical spine disorder has been maintained until quite recently.[3–5] The reluctance can be partly justified by the fact that in those days there were no valid criteria for its diagnosis.

The term 'cervicogenic headache' was introduced in 1983 by the neurologist Sjaastad and colleagues.[6] The concept of cervicogenic headache (CEH) has been readily accepted by physical therapists, specialists of the musculoskeletal system and pain clinics' anaesthetists, who are more used to dealing with the phenomenon of somatic referred pain. In the same way that the lumbar zygapophyseal joints can be responsible for pain referred to the gluteal area and to the lower limbs, a dysfunction or pathology of the cervical spine can refer pain into the head.[7]

There are now sufficient clinical and experimental studies showing that different anatomical elements of the cervical spine, especially those innervated by the three first cervical nerves, can refer pain to the head and, therefore, clinically manifest as a headache.[8–13]

The varying interpretations of CEH pathophysiology have also hindered its acknowledgment, in addition to the significant terminological confusion.[14] Inaccurate terms have been used, such as cervical migraine, cervicocephalic syndrome, occipital neuralgia or spondylogenic headache. This terminological confusion, plus the fact that CEH is an entity shared by different health professionals each applying their own views, means that headaches can be inadequately diagnosed and their treatment is often unsuitable.

Despite the fact that the clinical diagnosis of CEH is still controversial, its pathophysiological mechanisms are currently among those best known and understood, and it is one of the few forms of headaches that can be diagnosed objectively, according to Bogduk.[7,11,15] The controversy around this entity, in the words of this author, is more ideological, sociological and political than scientific.[15] One of the reasons could be that the specialista to whom headache patients are referred to most often are neurologists and these specialists are not usually experts in neck assessment.[16]

The term CEH and its acknowledgment as a clinically distinguishable entity are based on the work of Sjaastad et al.[6] These authors, after a few preliminary studies,[12,17] established in 1990, the diagnostic criteria for CEH,[3] which were revised in 1998, when the Cervicogenic Headache International Study Group (CHISG) was founded.[18] The term CEH was accepted

240

in 1994 by the International Association for the Study of Pain (IASP).[19]

In 1988, the International Headache Society (IHS) recognized the cervical spine as a cause of headache,[20] but without accepting the term CEH. This changed under the 2004 IHS headache classification (ICHD-2). The term was finally accepted and the committee established new diagnostic criteria.[21] These criteria were further modified in the 2013 IHS classification (ICHD-3).[22]

An important aspect of CEH is its prevalence, so the collaboration of different health professionals is desirable. Following tension-type headaches and migraines, CEH is the most common type of headache. Recent population studies reveal that the prevalence of CEH in the general population is between 2.2% and 4.1%.[23,24] One-month prevalence of cervicogenic headache among adults has been estimated at 2.5%.[25] According to Sjaastad, we should question the accuracy of overly frequent diagnoses of migraines without aura and tension-type headaches because, in many cases, a possible cervical cause may be overlooked. Sjaastad and Bakketeig[26] suggest that, with a more accurate diagnosis, the incidence of CEH would approximate that of migraine without aura.

In patients with cervicalgia, the incidence of CEH appears to be high. Some studies suggest that it may be present in a third of the patients with cervical pain.[27] For these reasons, CEH is currently beginning to be considered as a fairly common form of chronic and recurrent headache.[16,28–32] The prevalence of CEH is not as high as migraine, although its incidence rises in certain types of patients, such as those who have suffered a whiplash injury and in subjects with symptomatic degenerative changes.

The differential diagnosis of CEH from other types of headaches is crucial because while there is evidence that manual therapy[31,33–36] and therapeutic exercise[31–37] are effective in the long term in CEH, there is no current evidence of good outcomes in migraine and tension-type headache.[38–40] Yet it is important to note that the relationship between headache and the cervical spine is more complex. Neck pain in patients with headache in no way implies its cervicogenic origin. Most primary headaches can refer pain to the cervical spine.[41–44] In fact, in patients with migraine, neck pain is more common than nausea.[44]

BACKGROUND

A history of the development of CEH is presented in Table 7-1. The first studies that related headaches to the cervical spine were derived from the works of Barré[45] in 1926 and Lieou.[46] Barré used the term 'posterior cervical sympathetic syndrome', since he believed that the headache was caused by the irritation of the cervical sympathetic nerve that runs along the vertebral artery. Unfortunately, these authors diverted the attention from other aetiological aspects of headache. The vertebral artery can trigger a headache, but an artery dissection is necessary for this to be possible. The stimulation of the sympathetic plexus that wraps around the vertebral artery only triggers a small contraction of the artery.[47] Bärtschi-Rochaix[10] also proposed a relationship between the vertebral artery and headaches and in 1949 coined the term 'cervical migraine'. His contribution in this field was initiated with the study of post-traumatic headaches, which was completed in 1968, establishing that headache was the result of degenerative changes in the spine

In 1949, Hunter and Mayfield[48] changed the perspective on cervicogenic headache by relating it to a disorder in the upper cervical roots. The one-sidedness of the pain was established as a typical characteristic of this headache. A number of patients were treated with avulsion of the greater occipital nerve, sectioning of the sensory root of C2 or intraspinal sectioning of the sensory roots of C2 and C3. The results were excellent in those cases in which a traumatic component was associated to the headaches.

In 1961, Kerr and Olafson[49] reported experimental evidence of an interconnection between the cranial and cervical sensory structures. They demonstrated

TABLE 7-1
Hypothesis of cervicogenic headache

Posterior cervical sympathetic syndrome	Barré 1926
Cervical migraine	Bärtschi-Rochaix 1949
Occipital neuralgia	Hunter and Mayfield 1949
Referred cervical pain	Kerr and Olafson 1961
Myodural bridge	Hack 1995
Cervicogenic headache	Sjaastad 1983 Bogduk 1984

the convergence between the cervical and trigeminal sensory units in the upper cervical cord (Fig. 7-1). Kerr[50] showed how stimulation of the dorsal root of C1 always triggered referred pain to the head, in particular to the supraorbital, frontal and vertex regions. Thereafter, for years, cervicogenic headaches were believed to be the result of the compression of the roots of the upper cervical levels and of the emerging nerves, mainly the medial branch of the posterior primary ramus of C2 or greater occipital nerve (Fig. 7-2). Subsequently, so-called 'occipital neuralgia' began to be a frequent diagnosis. Greater occipital nerve compression would justify the relationship between the cervical spine and headache.[51]

Occipital neuralgia in clinical practice is a rare entity.[52] It is caused by the involvement of the greater occipital nerve (or Arnold's nerve), the lesser occipital nerve or the third occipital nerve. These neuralgias may be due to irritation of these nerve trunks or of the spinal nerves from which they emerge due to a tumour, periarticular fibrosis, vascular malformations and, more commonly, due to direct traumatic causes.[8,15,53]

The neck-tongue syndrome[54–59] is a neuropathy that can be mistaken for a CEH. This syndrome is caused by compression of the ventral branch of the spinal nerve of C2 by direct irritation of the atlantoaxial joint. This typically occurs by an extremely ample rotational movement of the head and, sometimes, in hypermobile subjects. The symptoms are triggered by rapid rotation of the head and are characterized by the sudden onset of unilateral occipital pain that radiates to the ear and is associated with ipsilateral tongue hypoaesthesia. The latter symptom is explained by lingual nerve afferents reaching the second cervical nerve through the ansa cervicalis via the hypoglossal nerve[60] (Fig. 7-3).

In 1995, Hack et al.[61] found a bridge of connective tissue between the rectus posterior capitis minor and the dura mater (Fig. 7-4). This finding was later confirmed.[62–66] It has been suggested that this myodural bridge might be a headache-generating mechanism, as it transmits the tension generated by the suboccipital muscles to a sensitive structure such as the dura mater.[61,63,64,67–70] There is, however, no conclusive

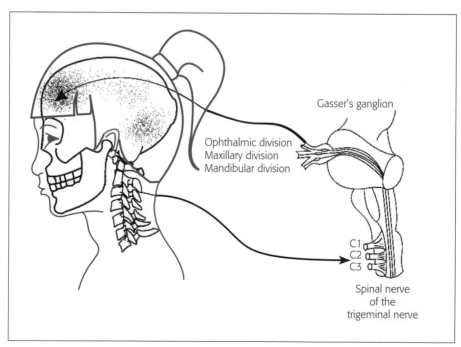

FIGURE 7-1 ■ Afferents of the first three cervical segments converging along with the afferents of the trigeminal nerve in the trigeminocervical nucleus.

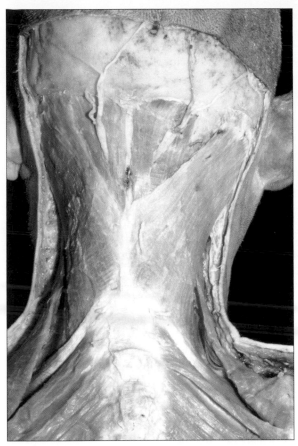

FIGURE 7-2 ■ Cervicogenic headache was considered for years to be a neuropathy due to entrapment of the greater occipital nerve.

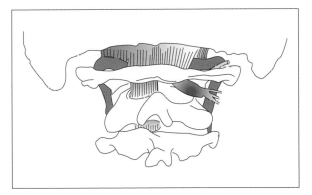

FIGURE 7-3 ■ The neck–tongue syndrome is caused by compression of the ventral branch of the spinal nerve C2 due to excessive amplitude movement of the atlantoaxial joint.

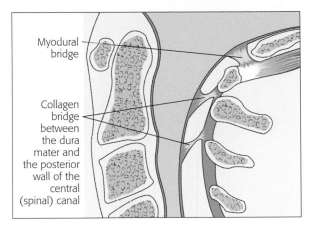

FIGURE 7-4 ■ The myodural bridge is a connective tissue structure that relates the posterior lesser rectus muscle of the head and the spinal dura.

evidence that this structure could suffer a mechanical dysfunction or that it may give rise to a headache.[71] Nevertheless, clinically, purported sensitivity of nerve tissue to the movement of upper cervical flexion has been found in up to 10% of a cohort with CEH.[72]

Today, thanks to the work of Kerr,[49,73,74] and, especially Bogduk et al.,[7,9,11,13,75–78] CEH is believed to relate to a pattern of referred pain caused by a dysfunction or disease of the cervical spine.

ANATOMICAL BASIS

As mentioned above, CEH is the clinical expression of a somatic referred pain from the cervical spine. The neuroanatomical basis of CEH is the common convergence in the pars caudalis of the trigeminocervical nucleus, the sensory afferents of the first three cervical nerves (C1, C2 and C3) and the trigeminal nerve afferents.[9–11,79–82] The trigeminocervical nucleus is a continuous column of grey matter formed by the caudal portion of spinal nucleus of the trigeminal nerve and the grey matter of the dorsal horns of the first three segments of the cervical spine. Therefore, any structure innervated by the spinal nerves C1–C3 can be a source of headache (Fig. 7-5, Table 7-2). The same mechanism explains how subjects with any type of headache may experience associated cervical pain.

The neuroanatomical basis of CEH is the common convergence in the trigeminocervical nucleus of the

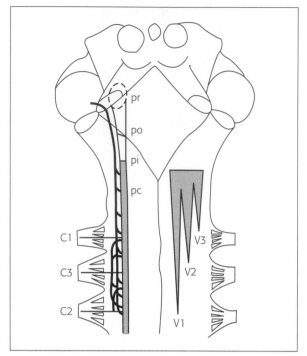

FIGURE 7-5 ■ The neuroanatomical basis of CEH is the common convergence in the pars caudalis of the trigeminocervical nucleus, of the sensory afferents of the first three cervical nerves (C1, C2 and C3) and trigeminal nerve afferents. The diagram shows the arrangement of the nuclei of the trigeminal nerve (pr, core; po, pars oralis; pi, pars interpolaris; pc, pars caudalis). On the right, the distribution in the trigeminocervical nucleus of the afferents of the three divisions of the trigeminal nerve is shown.

afferents of the first three cervical nerves (C1, C2 and C3) and of the trigeminal nerve afferents.

Bogduk[11] explains that convergence does not occur exclusively between cervical and trigeminal afferents, but between the nerves innervating the head and the cervical spine, since the innervation of the head does not depend solely on the trigeminal nerve. The cervical nerves are also involved. For example, the innervation of the occipital region to the coronal suture of the head depends on the greater occipital nerve, lesser occipital nerve and greater auricular nerve. CEH perceived in the frontal, temporal and orbital region is due to a phenomenon of convergence of the trigeminal and cervical afferents, whereas headaches perceived in the occipital region require the convergence between specific cervical levels and other cervical afferents. Thus, the referred pain from the cervical spine to the frontal or supraorbital region is a trigeminal referral, while pain in the occipital region is a cervicocervical referral.[7]

PATHOPHYSIOLOGY

First, it is important to note that the term CEH does not relate to a specific disease but encompasses a spectrum of typical disorders and pathologies of the cervical spine. CEH may originate from any cervical anatomical structure having nociceptive innervation, but mainly those belonging to the upper cervical spine.[83] Fredriksen and Sjaastad[10] consider that headaches may originate from the dorsal roots of C1 to C7, the intervertebral discs to the C7 level, the facet joints of C2–C3 to C6–C7, the trapezius and sternocleidomastoid muscles, the vertebral artery with its sympathetic plexus and, finally, the greater and lesser occipital peripheral nerves, the third occipital nerve and the greater auricular nerve. However, these possibilities are as yet theoretical, as the ability to produce headache in clinical and experimental studies has only been shown with regard to some of these structures.[11]

PAIN PATTERNS

One of the first experimental studies on referred craniocervical pain was carried out by Cyriax[84] in 1938, in a paper published under the title 'Rheumatic headache'. This author showed, for the first time, that the injection of hypertonic saline in the suboccipital muscles caused referred pain in the head. He found that the more cephalic the stimulated area, the more constant the pain referral to the head. Later research revealed that other neck muscles may also refer pain to the head such as the sternocleidomastoid, upper trapezius, splenius capitis, splenius cervicis, the suboccipital muscles, semispinalis capitis and semispinalis cervicis.[85–87]

More recent research has focused on the study of referred joint pain. Several studies have shown that C1–C2 lateral joints and C2–C3 facet joints and, to a lesser extent C3–C4, can be responsible for CEH. Facet pain patterns were first described by Dwyer et al.[88] The cervical segments C2–C3 to C6–C7 were stimulated

TABLE 7-2
Innervation of the structures of the upper cervical spine

	Innervation		
	C1	C2	C3
Joints	Atlanto-axial medial Atlanto-occipital	Atlantoaxial lateral	Facet joint C2–C3 Disc C2–C3
Ligaments	Transverse atlantoaxial Alar Tectorial membrane		
Muscles	Prevertebral Sternocleidomastoid Trapezius Suboccipital	Semispinalis Splenius	Multifidus Semispinalis
Dura mater	Of the upper cervical cord Of the posterior cranial fossa		
Arteries	Vertebral artery Internal carotid artery		

under fluoroscopic control, distending the joint capsule using contrast medium. Other experimental studies on referred pain from the craniovertebral joints have shown similar results.[89–93]

In trying to determine which articular segment is implicated in the pathogenesis of cervicogenic headache, some studies have used local anaesthetic joint blocks. Bovim et al.[94] conducted anaesthetic blocks of the spinal nerves C2–C5. Their study showed that headaches were reduced more frequently with the anaesthetic block of the nerve C2. No patient fully responded to the isolated blocks of nerves C3, C4 or C5.

Discs C2–C3 and C3–C4 have been suggested as a possible source of headache.[10,11,96,97] This claim was proven in studies that showed, in some patients, that headache may be reproduced by stimulation of C2–C3 intervertebral disc but not of lower discs.[97,98] Therefore, the disc may be responsible for a CEH, but Bogduk[11] warns that these studies are not conclusive because the result may merely be a false positive. Patients considered in this work may possibly present secondary hyperalgesia, so that a painful stimulus in

any structure within the same neurological segment may reproduce or aggravate pain. The phenomenon of pain, by itself, does not necessarily implicate the structure stimulated as a sole or primary source of pain.

The most reliable results come from clinical trials in which a complete remission of headache is obtained after selective anaesthesia of the atlanto-occipital and lateral atlantoaxial joints and facet joints C2–C3. Ehni and Benner[99] achieved complete remission of headache with a perianaesthetic block in patients with arthrosis of the lateral atlantoaxial joints. Aprill et al.[92] obtained complete relief of symptoms after anaesthetic infiltration of the lateral joints of C1–C2 in 21 of 31 patients suffering from headache and pain referred to the occipital region.

In patients with CEH associated with whiplash injury, Lord et al.[100] found that the most common source of pain was the C2–C3 joint, followed by C3–C4. However, pain was rarely referred to the head in joints located below C4–C5. Therefore, it can be conclude that segments most often referring pain to the frontal region and the head are C1–C2, C2–C3 and C0–C1 (Fig. 7-6).

Signs and symptoms associated with the neck

The most important aspects for the diagnosis of CEH are those signs and symptoms related to the cervical spine. The CHISG considered the following to be essential diagnostic criteria, in order of importance (most to least):

- Headache triggered by neck movements and /or sustained awkward postures (Ia1), or by applying an external pressure on the ipsilateral posterior region of the upper cervical or occipital region (Ia2).
- Reduced range of cervical mobility (Ib).
- Diffuse homolateral pain in the cervical spine, shoulder and arm (Ic).

In relation to the first criterion, what characterizes CEH and is considered important in diagnosis is that both its onset and its aggravation relate to sustained or awkward positions of the neck and performing neck movements.[6,12,13,17,32,130,134,140,141] Jull et al.,[31] in a study of 200 patients with CEH, showed how 60% of them reported that the headache was triggered by movements or postures of the cervical spine. This is a fact frequently recognized by the patients themselves. Sustained positions such as sitting with the cervical spine in flexion or end-range extension usually trigger a headache, as well as activities that require extensive and repetitive rotation of the cervical spine. Many patients have difficulty sleeping and are unable to find a comfortable neck position. Patients who 'struggle with their pillow' often wake with headache and neck stiffness. They themselves believe that uncomfortable or awkward neck positions during sleep are responsible for their headache.[6,12,32,130,140–143]

The onset of headache by pressure on certain points is another diagnostic criterion for CEH. The sensitivity to pressure around the mastoid area, C2 and different cervical muscles is well documented.[144–146] Palpation of the craniocervical joints with subsequent provocation of referred pain is a useful tool to confirm the cervical cause of the headache.

The second diagnostic criterion, reduction of the range of motion in the neck, will be discussed in the section on physical assessment of patients with CEH.

The third criterion of this group is the presence of a diffuse and non-radicular ipsilateral pain in the cervical spine, shoulder and arm – although, occasionally, it may be a radicular pain (Ic). Note that these symptoms are only indicative of the existence of a musculoskeletal dysfunction in the cervical spine. Their presence does not automatically imply that the patient has a cervicogenic headache.

Pain characteristics

The quality of pain can also help towards differential diagnosis. For example, during a migraine attack, the pain becomes pulsating and can be associated with sharp paroxysmal pains of short duration, which are interspersed within the headache and whose location is variable.[147] In tension-type headaches, patients describe the pain as oppressive, like having a 'tight band' or a weight around the head. The intense pressure behind the eye associated with ocular symptoms such as ptosis and tearing points to a diagnosis of chronic paroxysmal hemicrania or cluster headache[122,148] (Fig. 7-9). CEH pain, however, is a dull ache, similar to other somatic pain.

Pain intensity also has a diagnostic significance. CEH and tension-type headache pain is usually mild to moderate. Although it can sometimes be severe, it never reaches the level of unbearable pain, which is characteristic of chronic paroxysmal hemicrania or cluster headaches.[12,130] Unlike the pain of migraine, which can reach severe and disabling intensity if not treated, CEH pain fluctuates from mild to moderate. It is only severe in 20% of cases.[32]

The temporal pattern of headache is another important aspect of diagnosis (Table 7-10). The duration of cluster headaches is short, ranging between 15 and 60 minutes, with a frequency of attacks from one to three daily. Attacks often begin at night, waking the subject. It has active periods or phases – hence the name cluster headache or clusters – lasting between 2 and 8 weeks. These active phases usually occur every 1 or 2 years, often in spring and autumn. The clinical manifestations of chronic paroxysmal hemicrania are fairly similar to those of cluster headache. However, the attacks are much shorter, lasting between 10 and 20 minutes, but are much more frequent, reaching up to 15–20 attacks per day. Paroxysmal hemicrania tends to evolve to chronicity, although in some cases it is episodic.

Migraine is characterized by its episodic nature and limited duration of the attacks (4–72 hours), but they

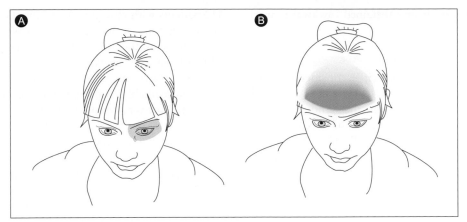

FIGURE 7-9 ■ Cluster headache and chronic paroxysmal hemicrania are characterized by severe pain behind the eye associated with ocular symptoms such as ptosis and tearing (A). In tension-type headaches, the patient described the pain as having a 'tight band' or a weight on the head (B).

TABLE 7-10		
The temporal pattern of headache		
	Duration of the attack	Frequency of attacks
Cervicogenic headache	Variable hours–days	
Cluster headache	15–60 minutes	1–3 days
Chronic paroxysmal hemicrania	10–20 m	15–20 days
Migraine	4–72 h	

usually last less than 24 hours. The temporal pattern of CEH is also episodic but, unlike migraine, it can be very variable (from a few hours to a few days) and always relates to a trigger activity or posture. There is practically no difference from the pain pattern of tension-type headaches. The history of the CEH is usually long, sometimes evolving over the years to chronic headache.[130]

Other non-essential elements that help in the differential diagnosis are the poor response of CEH to anti-migraine drugs (ergotamine and triptans) and no response to indometacin, as would be typical for paroxysmal hemicrania. Although a high percentage of patients with CEH take some sort of analgesic or anti-inflammatory drug, once the headache acquires a certain intensity, the use of these drugs barely offer relief.

The diagnostic criteria of CEH includes a number of associated symptoms such as nausea, vomiting, photophobia and phonophobia, but these (when present) are minor in nature. These symptoms, in greater intensities, are frequently associated with migraine, paroxysmal hemicrania and cluster headache. Nevertheless, they are not exclusive to these types of headache and can also accompany CEH. In addition, there are other features such as visual disturbances, dizziness, oedema in the periocular area, general irritability and poor concentration.[149] Although these symptoms are common to different types of headache, their severity may suggest a migraine or trigeminal autonomic cephalalgia rather than a muscleskeletal-type headache.

History of the onset

Headache is the most common pain we live with. However, less than 10% of the population with headaches seek medical care.[150] Therefore, patients suffering from CEH and other forms of headache, when they finally go to a doctor, report months or years' long histories.[17,32,102,130] A key aspect that can help differentiate the various forms of headache is the triggering factor. In the case of the CEH, the most common triggers are degenerative joint disease, neck injury from either a single event such as a motor vehicle crash (whiplash) or a sporting or recreational injury, or from the accumulation of repetitive minor trauma such as from sustained awkward work postures.

Post-traumatic cervicogenic headache

Although CEH is not, in principle, considered to be a post-traumatic headache, a history of a whiplash injury may be important from the standpoint of its pathogenesis.[83,129] Previous trauma, such as a whiplash injury, is common in patients with CEH[3,12,17,32,102,151,152] and is the most persistent symptom.[153] Headache, neck pain and limitation of cervical mobility are the symptoms of this clinical pattern.[152,154,155] In a prospective study by Drottning et al.[156] on the incidence of CEH following whiplash, headache was a very common symptom, particularly in the early stages. These authors found that 3% of patients who sought medical attention after whiplash injury had cervicogenic headache at 1 year post injury, and 25% of these had headache on more than 15 days a month.[156] At 6 years post injury, 35% of patients with cervicogenic headache at 1 year still had cervicogenic headaches.[157]

The International Association for the Study of Pain (IASP) recognizes that both whiplash and cervical degenerative disease may be directly responsible for CEH.[158] Lord et al.[100] conducted a study on 100 patients who had suffered whiplash, of whom 71 suffered from chronic headache. These authors demonstrated by anaesthetic blocks of the third occipital nerve, that in 27% of the 100 patients the source of headache was in the C2–C3 facet joint. They concluded that headache due to a disorder in the C2–C3 joint is a common situation in patients with chronic headache after whiplash. However, these researches, for safety reasons, did not perform anaesthetic blocks in C1–C2 lateral joints, so we do not know the real incidence of CEH arising from these joints. Another study of patients with chronic post-traumatic neck pain showed that in 54% of cases the pain came from the C2–C3 facet joints.[159] Therefore, whiplash can trigger cervicogenic headache.

However, the belief that headaches associated with whiplash are automatically CEH is mistaken. Cote el al.[160] showed that severe neck pain and headaches are more prevalent in individuals with a history of neck injury from a car collision, but a causal relationship between whiplash and chronic neck pain and headaches should not be inferred. Radanov et al.[161] studied 112 patients with chronic post-traumatic headache at an average time of over 2 years after whiplash. Using the criteria of the IHS-1 1998, headache following whiplash was tension-type in 37% of cases, migraine in 27%, cervicogenic in only 18%, while 18% of cases were unclassifiable. Although the diagnostic criteria used were not very sensitive or specific, whiplash can clearly be a trigger factor for any type of headache and not exclusively for CEH.

CEH commonly has an insidious onset. Patients often report a long history of headaches associated with cervical pain and stiffness. The frequency and intensity of headache progressively increase over the years and are often related to degenerative joint disease of the craniocervical spine.[162] According to Delfini et al.,[29] between 25% and 40% of patients with degenerative joint disease develop CEH. However, a more recent study suggests that, in elderly subjects, chronic musculoskeletal disorders could be the origin of cervicogenic headache or a comorbid associate of other headaches.[163]

Cervicogenic headache and central sensitization

An epidemiological study conducted by Hagen et al.[138] in 51,050 subjects showed that both subjects with migraine and those with non-migraine headaches are more likely to suffer associated musculoskeletal symptoms; those with musculoskeletal symptoms are four times more likely to suffer chronic headache and those with cervical symptoms are more likely to suffer headaches than those with musculoskeletal symptoms elsewhere in the body. There is thus a positive association between headache and musculoskeletal symptoms, for both genders, across age groups, and for all headache categories. There is also a strong association between cervical symptoms and headaches of any kind. These results might be explained in different ways: the relationship between headache and neck pain may not only be due to its cervicogenic nature, but simply due to the increased sensitization of the trigeminocervical nucleus. The other explanation, which does not exclude the above, is that headache is a common comorbid condition in patients with musculoskeletal pain, especially if it is chronic. Finally, many chronic headaches and much chronic musculoskeletal pain are associated with central sensitization.[164,165]

One of the issues readily raised is why some individuals with underlying chronic nociceptive sources develop CEH and other individuals with the same articular damage do not. Chua et al.[166] conducted a quantitative sensory testing study to systematically explore the differences in sensory pain processing in 17 CEH patients with underlying chronic cervical zygapophyseal joint pain compared to 10 patients with chronic cervical zygapophyseal joint pain but without CEH. The protocol comprised pressure pain threshold, thermal detection threshold, electrical pain threshold and measurement of the diffuse noxious inhibitory control. The main difference between patients with or without CEH was that the pressure hyperalgesia was clearly lateralized to the painful side of the head in the CEH patients and there was also cold and warm hyperaesthesia on this same side of the head and neck. These findings suggest that central sensitization is a pathophysiological mechanism in chronic cervical zygapophyseal joint pain patients with CEH.

Reliability of diagnostic criteria

Antonaci et al.[128] analysed the reliability of CHISG's diagnostic criteria. For this purpose, the criteria were grouped in seven points (Table 7-11). According to these authors, the diagnosis of CEH can be performed very reliably if the patient has five of the seven grouped criteria. The CEH diagnosis is *possible* when two criteria are met: unilateral headache and onset in the cervical region. CEH becomes *likely* when three of the following additional criteria are met: when triggered by neck movements or held positions or external pressure in the suboccipital or posterior cervical region; when there is a reduction in the cervical mobility; homolateral pain in the cervical spine, shoulder or arm; and a history of recent whiplash.

Possible CEH:
1. One-sidedness of headache.
2. Onset in the cervical region.

Probable CEH (at least 3 criteria):
1. Headache triggered by neck movements or held positions or external pressure on the suboccipital or posterior cervical region.
2. Reduction of cervical mobility.

TABLE 7-11
Grouped criteria

1. Unilateral headache without shifting sides
2. Signs and symptoms involving the neck (from most to least important):
   a. Headache caused by movements of the neck and/or maintained awkward postures and/or ipsilateral external pressure on the posterior region of the upper cervical spine or the occipital region
   b. Ipsilateral pain in the cervical spine, shoulder and arm being diffuse and non-radicular
   c. Reduced cervical mobility range
3. Episodes of pain, varying in duration or fluctuating to continuous pain
4. Moderate pain, not sharp or stabbing
5. Pain that starts in the cervical spine, which eventually expands to the oculo-fronto-temporal area, where the most intense pain is often located.
6. a. Anaesthetic blocks of the greater occipital nerve and/ or root of C2 or other appropriate blocks in the symptomatic side to remove the pain temporarily, provided that complete anaesthesia is obtained
   b. Whiplash relatively recently with respect to the onset
7. Varied symptoms related to the attack: symptoms and autonomic signs, nausea, vomiting, ipsilateral oedema and going towards the periocular area; vertigo; photophobia and phonophobia; blurred vision in the eye ipsilateral to pain

From Antonaci et al.[128]

3. Homolateral pain in the cervical spine, shoulder or arm.
4. History of recent whiplash.

From the diagnostic point of view, the two criteria that seem most important are the onset of pain in the cervical region with its subsequent propagation to the head, and the one-sidedness of pain. The temporal pattern and characteristics of pain also show a high specificity and sensitivity.

Vincent and Luna[167] performed similar work to confirm that the aspects that distinguish CEH from migraine and tension-type headaches are the location and radiation of pain, the temporal pattern and the onset of pain due to postures, movements or manual stimulation of the cervical spine. Van Suijlekom et al.[168] analysed the inter-observer reliability of CHISG diagnostic criteria for diagnosis of CH. They concluded that this was similar to that obtained in the diagnosis of migraine and tension-type headaches, using the IHS criteria.[171]

PHYSICAL EXAMINATION FOR CERVICOGENIC HEADACHE

The diagnostic criteria for CEH available today have been validated by several studies.[128,167–169] However, as pointed out by several authors, these criteria do not have sufficient specificity to differentiate CEH patients from migraine patients.[170] Physical impairments defined by both CHISG and IHS are few and non-specific. Physical examination of these patients is very often superficial, which would explain the difficulty of recognizing the involvement of the cervical spine in headache.[171]

Historical poor development of the physical examination for CEH promoted the role of anaesthetic blocks in determining the anatomical structure responsible for the headache.[172] However, anaesthetic blocks are not the solution to the problem of diagnosis. They are invasive techniques that should be performed under fluoroscopic guidance by a trained physician. Furthermore, there is an added difficulty, as blocks have to be performed at the time of the headache attack.[173] Other limitations include their low specificity and the difficulty in interpreting the results.[172,174,175] Therefore, a model of physical examination of the cervical spine is preferable that includes a thorough evaluation to identify the segment source of headache as well as the physical impairments in the cervical neuromuscular-articular system.

Sjaastad et al.[2] described a protocol of physical examination for CEH based on the analysis of five aspects: tenderness of the cervical musculature; sensitivity of nerves, tendons and occipital; facet joint tenderness; range of cervical mobility; and pinch and roll test. However, Jull and colleagues have always advocated a more extensive headache physical examination protocol, consistent with the examination used for a cervical musculoskeletal disorder.[31,43,72,102,162,176,177] In one study they investigated various aspects of musculoskeletal cervical function in persons with frequent intermittent headache (e.g. migraine, tension-type, cervicogenic headache), to determine if a group of physical impairments distinguished cervicogenic headache from other headache types.[43,177] The follow-

ing tests were conducted in 253 subjects (196 headache subjects and 57 non-headache control subjects): cervical range of motion, manual palpation to detect the presence or not of symptomatic cervical joint dysfunction, the craniocervical flexion test (CCFT), cervical flexor and extensor strength, cross-sectional area of the semispinalis capitis, longissimus capitis and upper trapezius at the C2 level using ultrasound imaging and the cervical joint position error test. The results of these studies show that the presence of a pattern of musculoskeletal dysfunction distinguished cervicogenic headache. Jointly, restricted movement, in association with palpable upper cervical joint dysfunction and impairment in the cervical neck flexor synergy (tested by the CCFT), had 100% sensitivity and 94% specificity to identify cervicogenic headache. This pattern of musculoskeletal impairment was not found in the migraine and tension-type headache patient groups, confirming that CEH is the headache which is secondary to cervical musculoskeletal dysfunction. This does not mean that other cervical physical impairments cannot present in patients with cervicogenic headache. Rather, the study showed that these three dysfunctions are the strongest associates of CEH. Other impairments may be found, but either they are not present in all those with CEH (e.g. not all patients with CEH have neural tissue mechanosensitivity) or they are not specific to CEH (e.g. muscle tenderness is also found in migraine and tension-type headaches).

Identifying physical findings that characterize CEH is not only important for diagnosis but also is necessary to inform a suitable and specific treatment programme. The following section reviews the physical impairments which may be associated with cervicogenic headache. The physical examination should identify comparable signs that are characteristically associated with cervicogenic headache. Before commencing the physical examination, the clinician must take into account the severity and irritability of the patient's clinical condition. Care must be taken in the examination of the patient with CEH, as central sensitization is present. Examination should be as painless as possible and not aim to provoke headache.

Head and neck posture

The forward head posture has been tenuously linked with CEH. Some studies have found an association,[140,178] while others have found no significant association between headache and posture.[72,173,179] Farmer et al.[180] recently analysed radiographs of posture and observed an association between a greater global cervical lordosis and increased likelihood of having CEH. However, they point out that this does not mean that posture is a cause of cervicogenic headache and if headache could be reduced by changing this measure.

In the clinic, the position of the head is analysed both in standing and sitting, especially when the patient reports that the headache appears or worsens in relation to postural positions. Measuring the position of the head can be done from a photograph of the patient, measuring the craniovertebral angle[180] (Fig. 7-10) Some measures can be obtained on a lateral radiograph: the lordosis can be measured using the Cobb method, but, depending on the upper end vertebra chosen, it can have a very different magnitude (Figs 7-11 and 7-12).

Joint dysfunction

Although any structure of the cervical spine is theoretically able to cause a headache, experimental[11] and clinical[72,162] studies, as well as clinical experience, show that the joints most commonly responsible are the three upper cervical segments (C0–C3). The clinical examination, while addressing the whole cervical region, should specifically target the craniocervical spine. This does not mean that the dysfunctions of the lower cervical or upper thoracic spine are unrelated to headache. In fact, they are sometimes involved in the symptoms.[94,181–183] More commonly, stiffness of the lower cervical and upper thoracic regions may impose abnormal stresses on the craniocervical spine and contribute indirectly to the headache syndrome.

Active mobility

Restricted range of active mobility is one of the diagnostic criteria for CEH. In this regard, various studies have been conducted to confirm the relationship between active cervical mobility and headache. Zwart[184] compared cervical mobility between subjects classified as cervicogenic headache, migraine, tension-type headache and a control group. The results confirmed that mobility was restricted in the CEH group and that

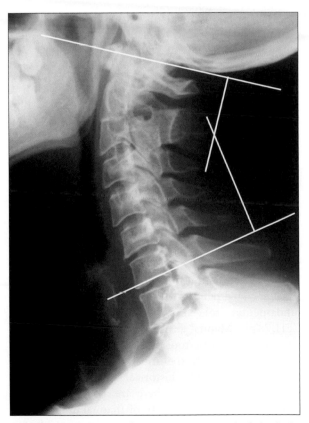

FIGURE 7-11 ■ In order to measure cervical lordosis, Cobb's angle can be measured from McGregor's line to C7.

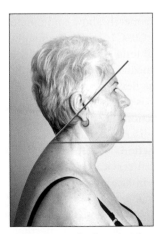

FIGURE 7-10 ■ Craniovertebral angle. The angle obtained is based on two lines: an oblique line connecting the tragus and the spinous process of C7 and another horizontal line at the level of C7.

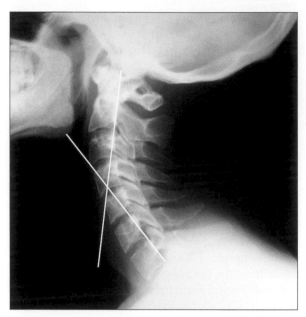

FIGURE 7-12 ■ Lordosis can be measured by drawing two lines: one from the posterior wall of C2, and the other one from the posterior wall of C7, measuring the angle formed when the lines cross one another.

this feature differentiated this subject group. There was no difference in mobility between the control group, tension-type headache and migraine groups. This important finding that reduced motion was a characteristic of CEH was confirmed in a similar study by Jull et al.[43] Other studies have also confirmed that reduced cervical mobility is a feature of CEH.[72,173] Asymmetries in rotation may occur especially in the case of CEH of C1–C2 origin.[185-187]

Manual segmental examination and other craniocervical clinical tests

Manual examination of joint mobility disorders and any associated pain provocation with the tests plays a fundamental role in the clinical diagnosis of CEH.[43,162,177] Manual examination is not only important as a diagnostic tool but also allows the physical therapist to design the most appropriate type of treatment.[188] Despite historical doubts about this examination method,[189] there are a number studies demonstrating the reliability of manual examination to detect symptomatic dysfunctions responsible for neck pain and headache[72,190-194] see also Chapter 4).

The segmental joint mobility tests, both physiological and accessory, are a qualitative assessment of the quantity and quality of movement of a particular spinal segment and also serve as pain provocation tests.[162] Thus, hypomobile or hypermobile joints can be distinguished and qualitative aspects of joint movement can be determined, such as tissue reaction to articular stress. Thus, these joint mobility tests are used as clinical tests to assess the joints responsible of the CEH. As such, this manual segmental examination is used to evaluate the joints C0–C1, C1–C2 and C2–C3 to identify the dysfunction and immediate source of headache as well as to evaluate the cervical and upper thoracic regions as possible areas contributing to the cervical disorder.

Other passive/assisted active tests of craniocervical regional mobility and associated pain provocation used in conjunction with assessment of active mobility include the craniocervical sagittal mobility test (Fig. 7-13) and craniocervical rotation in sitting (Fig. 7-14). The examination can be extended to include assessment of *combined movements* for the craniocervical spine, such as extension–rotation–ipsilateral bending (Fig. 7-15A), extension–rotation–contralateral bending (Fig. 7-15B) and flexion–rotation–ipsilateral bending (Fig. 7-15C). All tests can be sensitized with an added overpressure at the end of range of motion when necessary.

The different examination protocols for the C0–C1, C1–C2 and C2–C3 joints are discussed in Volume 1, Chapter 12. We merely show some pictures by way of examples for C0–C1 joints' segmental assessment, some analytical tests (Fig. 7-16) and the articular test for the anteromedial and posterolateral condylar glide (Fig. 7-17). The flexion–rotation test (FRT) described by Hall et al.[195] is an essential test in the assessment of C1–C2 dysfunction. The FRT (Fig. 7-18) has diagnostic validity to discriminate subjects with headache of C1–C2 dysfunction.[196,197] In asymptomatic subjects, the right and left cervical rotations reach between 43° and 44°, while in headache subjects, rotation was less than 30° or there was more than 10° asymmetry between the right and left cervical rotation. This test has a sensitivity of 90% and a specificity of 88% for differentiating subjects with cervicogenic headache due to C1–C2 joint dysfunction from control subjects.[195] Hall and colleagues have also shown a

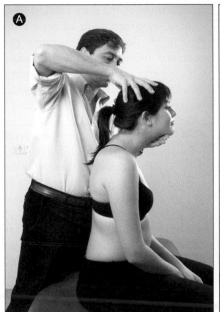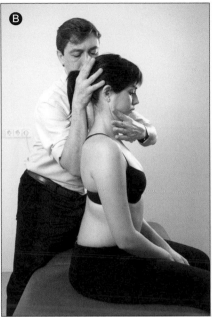

FIGURE 7-13 ■ Protraction (A) and retraction (B) movements to evaluate the sagittal craniocervical mobility.

relationship between the positivity of this test and the presence and severity of cervicogenic headache.[185]

Recently, Schneider et al.[194] developed a clinical decision guide for the diagnosis of cervical facet joint pain. They demonstrated that a cluster of tests was able to identify cervical zygapophyseal joint dysfunction with a high degree of specificity. The cluster includes the extension–rotation (ER) test (Fig. 7-19), unilateral posteroanterior accessory movements (Fig. 7-20) and the palpation for segmental tenderness (Fig. 7-21).[186] All tests have demonstrated moderate-to-excellent intra-rater and inter-rater reliability in patients with neck pain referred from zygapophyseal joints.[194]

Muscle tenderness

The presence of muscle tenderness has been researched in various forms of headache, including CEH.[86,87,109,131,144,146,198–205] Likewise, algometric studies have been conducted on different pericranial points and areas of muscle attachments. Bovim[146] compared pressure sensitivity in patients with CEH, migraine and tension-type headache. In this study, the sensitivity threshold to pressure was significantly lower in subjects with CEH. The most sensitive area corre-

sponded to the occipital region of the symptomatic side. The neuronal convergence explains the frequency with which certain muscles express tenderness in patients with CEH because the sternocleidomastoid muscles, upper trapezius, splenius capitis, splenius cervicis, semispinalis capitis and semispinalis cervicis, receive sensory innervation from the first three spinal nerves[87] (Fig. 7-22). This muscle sensitivity probably derives from a secondary hyperalgesia, perpetuated by a cervical nociceptive source and by a situation of central sensitization in the trigeminocervical system.[102]

Neuromuscular control

Painful joint dysfunction disrupts cervical and axioscapular neuromuscular function and poor neuromuscular control could contribute to the chronicity of joint dysfunction. The mobility of the craniocervical region and its complex biomechanics make it a vulnerable area that requires exquisite neuromuscular control. Muscles of the cervical spine, especially the suboccipital and deep flexor muscles, have a large number of proprioceptors and, along with the vestibular apparatus, vision and oculomotor muscles also have a major role in postural control.[206,207]

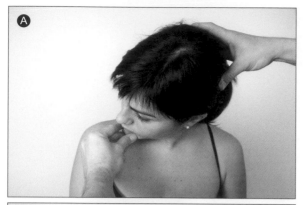

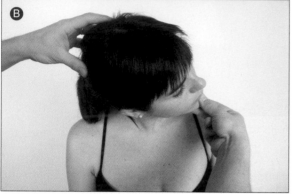

FIGURE 7-14 ■ (A, B) Craniocervical rotation assessment starting from a flexion of the lower cervical spine in the sitting position.

All muscles assist in control of movement and posture of the cervical spine and head, although there is some functional specificity. The powerful long muscles support the load of the head and are the major torque producers. The deep muscles contribute less to torque production but have a segment-stabilizing function.[208,209] There are also some differences in the response of these muscles to joint pain.

Evidence using the CCFT shows that persons with CEH present with weakness and an abnormal pattern of behaviour in the neck flexor synergy, where there is lesser activity in the deep flexor muscles, associated with increased activity of the superficial flexor muscles.[140,176,210–215] (Fig. 7-23). Atrophy of the extensors has also been demonstrated,[43] as has dysfunction in the axioscapular muscles – tightness in the levator scapulae and upper trapezius.[72] Patients with chronic cervical pathology also present with changes in the

muscle fibres of the deep cervical flexors: more specifically, a transformation of type I muscle fibres into type II[216,217] occurs. Degenerative changes have been observed using magnetic resonance imaging (MRI), with atrophy and fatty degeneration in the suboccipital muscles of patients with persistent moderate-to-severe whiplash-associated disorders.[218–220]

■ Individuals with CEH present with weakness and an abnormal pattern of behaviour in the neck flexor synergy, where there is lesser activity in the deep flexor muscles, associated with increased activity of the superficial flexor muscles.

Loss of endurance of the deep cervical spine flexor and extensor muscles is considered a specific dysfunction characteristic of patients with neck pain disorders, including cervicogenic headache. To determine the presence of this muscular deficit, specific tests are used, such as the craniocervical flexion test, active cervical extension and rotation in sitting tests, active upper cervical rotation in four point kneeling, etc. These are described in Chapter 13 of Volume 1 and Chapter 5 of Volume 2 (this volume).

Altered neuromuscular control is also expressed in excessive upper trapezius muscle activation. Nederhand et al.[221] studied subjects who had suffered whiplash and found increased activity of the trapezius manifested during various activities. This hyperactivity of the trapezius muscle fibres differentiated the group of subjects with whiplash from various control groups. An inability to relax the trapezius after performing certain activities was also observed. This study is consistent with the results obtained by Bansevicius and Saajstad,[222] which also showed enhanced activity of the upper trapezius. This increased activity is sometimes accompanied by changes in muscle extensibility in the trapezius muscle.[72,176,179]

Neural tissue mechanosensitivity

Several studies have attempted to establish a relationship between CEH and altered neural tissue mechanosensitivity at the craniocervical level. The innervation of the dura mater of the upper portion of the cord and the posterior cranial fossa[223,224] depends on the posterior plexus, formed by branches of the recurrent meningeal nerve of the craniocervical segments.

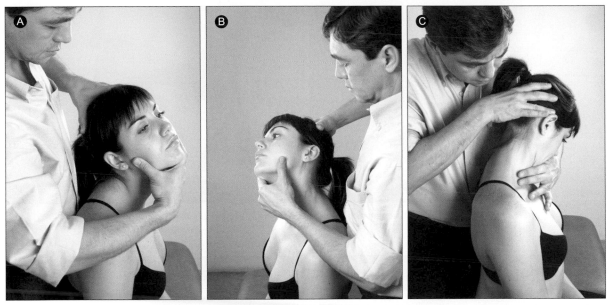

FIGURE 7-15 ■ Combined movements for the craniocervical spine: extension–rotation–ipsilateral bending (A), extension–rotation–contralateral bending (B) and flexion–rotation–ipsilateral bending (C).

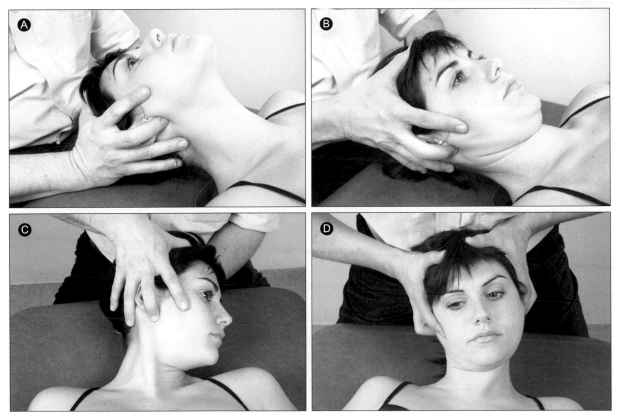

FIGURE 7-16 ■ (A–D) Analytical assessment of C0–C1 joints.

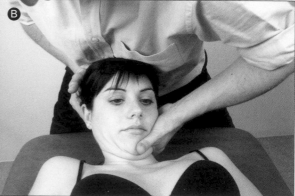
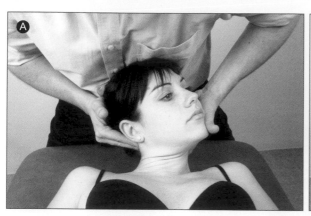

FIGURE 7-17 ■ (A, B) Articular test for the anteromedial and posterolateral condylar glide.

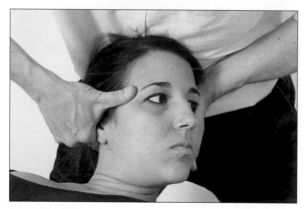

FIGURE 7-18 ■ Flexion–rotation test (FRT) adaptation from the author.

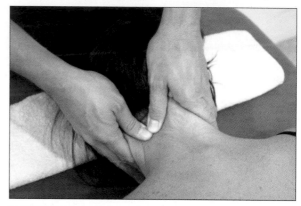

FIGURE 7-20 ■ Unilateral posteroanterior accessory mobility test.

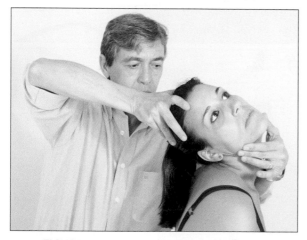

FIGURE 7-19 ■ Extension–rotation (ER) test.

Theoretically, an irritation of these structures could manifest as a headache. However, CEH is mainly a somatic referred pain rather than a neuropathic pain. In recent studies, symptoms of neural tissue mechanosensitivity have only been observed in a very small proportion of patients with CEH.[31,72] It is possible that this increased neural mechanosensitivity can be an expression of a more sensitized state.

An association may be established between neural tissue mechanosensitivity and CEH in cases of traumatic injury or compression of the greater occipital nerve, of the lesser occipital nerve or of the greater auricular nerve. However, this clinical entity has markedly different clinical characteristics from those of CEH and should be distinguished from CEH.[52,72,77]

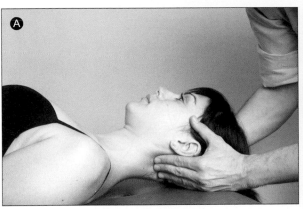
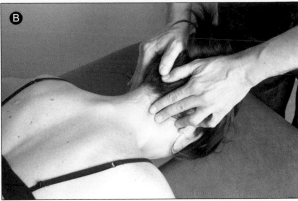

FIGURE 7-21 ■ Palpation for segmental tenderness over the articular pillars. Positions used for the palpation of the cervical spine: supine position (A) and prone position (B).

Assessment of neural tissue mechanosensitivity is performed with the upper cervical flexion test with the patient supine (Fig. 7-24). In this test, to provoke a greater sensitization of the neural tissue, craniocervical flexion is performed with, and then without, tension added to the neural system with the application of specific postures of the upper limb (e.g. ULNDT1) or lower limb (e.g. SLR) (Fig. 7-24). Alternately, to assess the greater occipital nerve mechanosensitivity, a variant of the slump test may be performed. In this variant, craniocervical flexion is performed and then a rotation and contralateral side-bending relative to the nerve evaluated is applied (Fig. 7-25). The greater occipital nerve may also be palpated at its emergence above the trapezius.

Kinaesthetic sensitivity

The assessment of alterations in cervical kinaesthetic perception has been researched in patients with CEH, without revealing any differences in these patients compared to those with migraine with aura and the control group.[72] The kinaesthetic sensitivity may be related to the severity of the disorder. For example, Sterling et al.[225] showed that patients with high levels of pain and disability indicative of more severe disorders showed kinaesthetic deficits, which were absent in subjects with lower pain levels. Other studies have shown deficits in postural control when symptoms of dizziness or unsteadiness are reported in association with the neck pain and headache.[226]

Pinch and roll test

This test is considered by some authors as a significant physical finding of CEH.[227,228] Bansevicius and Pareja[229,230] studied the validity of this sign in patients with CEH and its discriminative ability between CEH, tension-type headache and migraine without aura. They chose three skin areas: upper trapezius, angle of the jaw and supraorbital area. In patients with CEH, the difference in test sensitivity was significant between the side of the headache and the contralateral side. In addition, the test was positive more frequently in patients with CEH. Although this test has been suggested as useful for CEH diagnosis, it cannot determine the type of headache and is not specific for detecting dysfunction of the cervical spine.

TREATMENT

Treatment is designed according to the specific situation of the patient, prioritizing techniques according to the most relevant physical impairments. It is important to emphasize that the diagnosis of CEH should always be established by two conditions: the symptomatic diagnostic criteria are met and the patient has a specific pattern of cervical physical dysfunction. Therapeutic possibilities in CEH are many, including both conservative and surgical approaches. Conservative approaches include education, specific spinal mobilization and manipulation techniques, retraining the cervical and axioscapular musculature, the use of

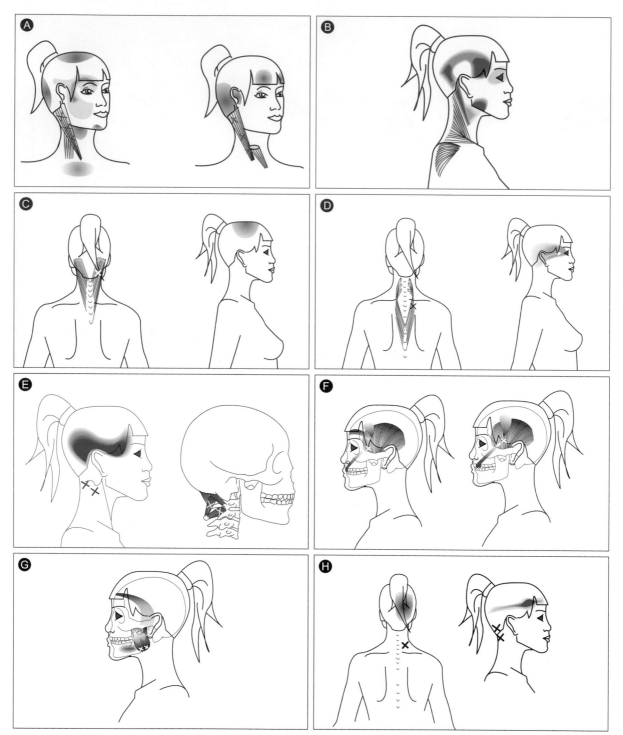

FIGURE 7-22 ■ Muscular pain referral patterns may be associated with headache: sternocleidomastoid (A), the upper trapezius (B), the splenius capitis (C), the splenium of the neck (D), the suboccipital muscles (E) the temporal muscle (F), superficial masseter and (G) the semispinalis capitis (H).

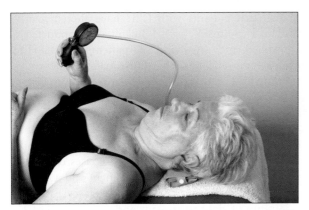

FIGURE 7-23 ■ Subjects with CEH show a pattern of weakness and abnormal recruitment of the deep flexor muscles, associated with increased activity of the superficial flexors.

functional active exercises, and management of somatosensory deficits when present.

Patients with neck pain and CEH may present simple or complex patterns. The majority have a noncomplex pattern and can be managed with education, manual therapy, therapeutic and functional exercises and, if necessary, sensorimotor control exercises. The occasional complex patient, often suffering a persistent whiplash-associated disorder, who presents with severe pain, multiple physical impairments, including dizziness, with signs of central sensitization, emotional distress and fear-avoidance behaviours, requires more complex management to address the multidimensionality of the problem. Many of these patients may benefit from treatment programmes for chronic pain that combine cognitive-behavioural, pain educational strategies, desensitization and gradual exposure. Such strategies for chronic pain management are discussed in Chapter 11.

Many patients with neck pain and with non-cervicogenic headache present in clinical practice. The question is if treatment in the form of cervical manual therapy and exercise should be offered to these patients. Both migraine and tension-type headaches are not caused by a cervical musculoskeletal dysfunction, so treatment targeting the cervical spine should not be a primary treatment. The treatment in these patients only makes sense when there are specific physical dysfunctions in the cervical spine, which, without bearing a relation to headaches, constitute a comorbid condition. In these cases the patient should know that

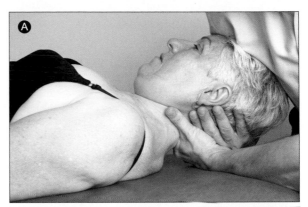

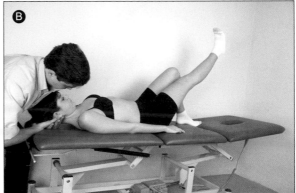

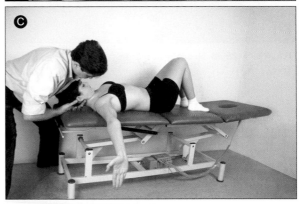

FIGURE 7-24 ■ Craniocervical flexion neurodynamic test – supine (A). Craniocervical flexion neurodynamic test associated with straight leg raise (B) and ULNDT1 (C)

our goal is not headache treatment, but the treatment of musculoskeletal disorders of the cervical spine.

Conservative treatment

Conservative treatment is currently considered the treatment of choice for CEH.[172] Analgesics and

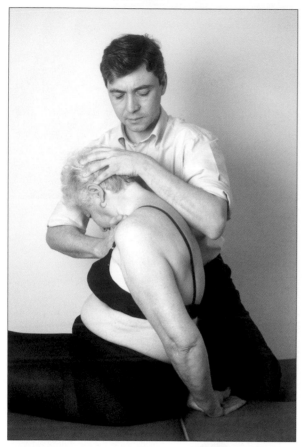

FIGURE 7-25 ■ Neurodynamic test of greater occipital nerve.

non-steroidal anti-inflammatory drugs (NSAIDs) are the pharmacological treatment commonly used for this type of headache.[231] However, as a monotherapy, only a partial, short-lasting pain relief is achieved, as occurs with other types of pain of musculoskeletal origin.[232–234] The use of pharmacological agents has been recommended in order to reduce painful symptoms and facilitate the patient's participation in the rehabilitation programme.[95]

Several controlled clinical studies have been conducted evaluating conservative treatment for CEH. Earlier trials principally evaluated manipulative therapy[33,235] and systematic reviews[233,236–238] concluded that manipulative procedures can be effective at short-term follow-ups. These early studies do not include any type of exercise for the neck muscles. It is now known that patients with CEH have altered neuro-muscular control.[72,140,179,239] Jull et al.[31] conducted a controlled study involving 200 patients with CEH to evaluate the effectiveness of manual therapy and a training programme directed towards the deep flexors and axioscapular stabilizers (lower trapezius and serratus anterior). The objective was to determine the efficacy of these two types of treatment alone and in combination. Patients were divided into four groups: manual therapy, muscle retraining exercises, combined manual therapy and exercise treatment and a control group. The treatment period lasted 6 weeks, with a minimum of eight treatments and a maximum of 12. Patients were monitored for 12 months. It was shown that both the manual therapy and exercise programme significantly reduced the frequency, intensity and duration of headaches. Exercise-based treatment showed the same effectiveness as manipulative treatment. There was no significant evidence of a greater effect when the two therapies were used simultaneously, but 10% more patients showed improvement in the group treated with a combination of the two types of treatment. This work demonstrates that both manual therapy and the exercises are effective therapeutic tools in the management of CEH and their effect is maintained long term. Also, for those patients in whom it is not advisable to perform manual therapy, a successful programme of specific exercises based on joint stabilization may be developed. A recent systematic review on the conservative physical therapy management of CEH shows that multimodal treatment that incorporates mobilization or manipulation of the cervical spine with training of the cervical and axioscapular muscles is the most effective therapeutic strategy for decreasing pain and disability, as well as for improving function.[240]

- Manual therapy and therapeutic exercises of motor control and strength and endurance training of the cervical and cervicoscapular muscles are effective in the treatment of CEH.
- It is advisable to use a combination of both therapeutic procedures.
- In those patients in whom it is not advisable to perform a manipulative treatment, a treatment based on specific therapeutic exercises can achieve the best results.

Joint dysfunction treatment

Addressing the CEH usually includes the treatment of joint dysfunction and re-education of the deep craniocervical and axioscapular muscles. The treatment programme will be designed according to the specific findings from the clinical examination of CEH patients.

The goals of manual therapy are to reduce pain and improve the cervical joint function associated with CEH. A variety of techniques can be used for the treatment of joint dysfunction: joint mobilization techniques applied rhythmically and in a gradual amplitude, craniocervical traction techniques, accessory movement techniques, mobilization with movement techniques, muscular energy techniques, functional techniques, high-velocity manipulation techniques, etc.[241]

The nature of articular treatment will depend on the type of joint dysfunction (hypomobile, hypermobile or unstable) presenting in the patient. When using mobilization techniques, slow progression is advised, beginning with soft tissue techniques (Fig. 7-26) and gentle passive stretching (Figs 7-27 and 7-28), manual cervical traction, progressive amplitude physiological movement techniques (Fig. 7-29), accessory movement techniques (Fig. 7-30), mobilization with movement techniques (Fig. 7-31A,B), functional techniques, and then, continuing, if required, with muscle energy techniques (Fig. 7-32) and high-velocity manipulative techniques (Fig. 7-33). In some cases if patients have tenderness of the cranial or cervical musculature, gentle pressure techniques can be performed on tender

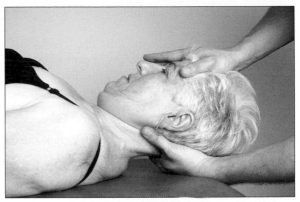

FIGURE 7-27 ■ Craniocervical extensors stretching technique.

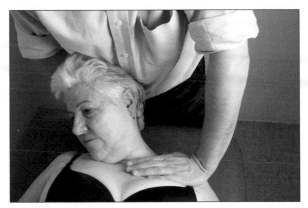

FIGURE 7-28 ■ Cervicoscapular muscle stretching technique

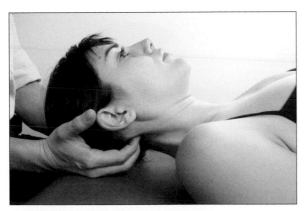

FIGURE 7-26 ■ Craniocervical inhibition technique.

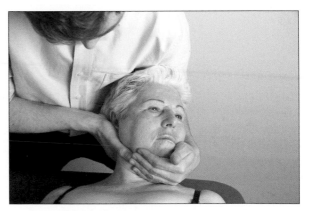

FIGURE 7-29 ■ C2 rotation articulatory technique.

points[71,242] (Fig. 7-34). The figures show some techniques by way of example.

In the treatment of patients with CEH, it is essential to consider irritability and severity of symptoms, and treatment should be adapted at all times to the clinical situation of the patient. It is imperative not to aggravate the patient's symptoms to avoid triggering a headache. In subjects with severe pain and an irritable condition, physiological and accessory movement techniques are recommended, without reaching the joint end-range. High-velocity techniques and mobilization techniques at the end-range will only be used when we are sure that this will not trigger the headache and only when deemed necessary. Manual therapy is especially effective when it is part of a multimodal rehabilitation programme, consisting of joint mobilization and manipulation techniques and specific exercises.[31,95,243,244]

The articular techniques applied in patients with CEH primarily address the craniocervical region, but one must not forget the influence of the lower cervical spine and upper thoracic spine in the biomechanics of the upper cervical segments. For details of the techniques used in the management of patients with CEH, the reader is referred to the section on assessment techniques and treatment of the craniocervical spine in Chapter 12 of Volume 1.

Craniocervical motor control exercises

Scientific evidence shows that it is not possible to recover the strength of the stabilizing muscles of the cervical spine through manual therapy alone. An appropriate programme of specific exercises is required, aimed at normalizing the behaviour and restoring the strength and endurance of the cervical musculature.[31,245,246]

A specific dysfunction in the deep flexors has been demonstrated in patients with CEH, as well as dysfunctions in the cervical extensors and axioscapular muscles. Jull et al.[31,162,247] have designed an exercise programme aimed at restoring these dysfunctions in patients with CEH. The initial exercises aim to train the tonic activation capacity of the deep muscles and thus improve their cervical spine-stabilizing role. The deep cervical flexor training is commenced in the supine position using a pressure feedback system

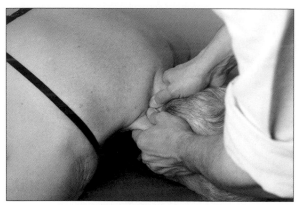

FIGURE 7-30 ■ Unilateral accessory intervertebral motion, posteroanterior.

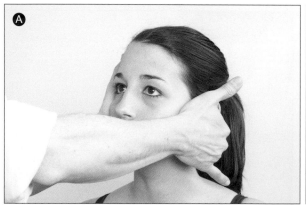
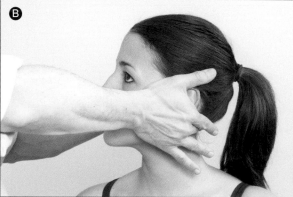

FIGURE 7-31 ■ (A, B) Mobilization with movement C1.

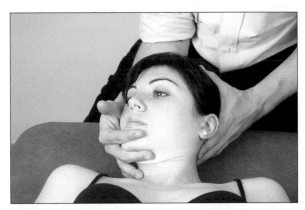

FIGURE 7-32 ■ C0–C1 posterolateral muscle energy technique.

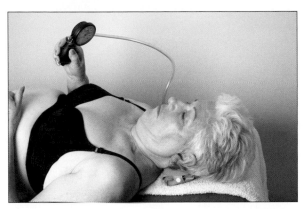

FIGURE 7-35 ■ Re-education of the deep cervical flexors with pressure biofeedback.

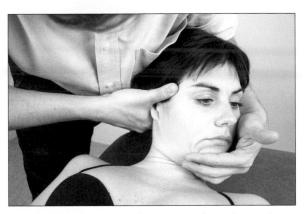

FIGURE 7-33 ■ High-velocity manipulation in rotation.

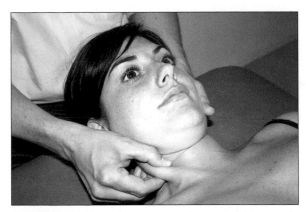

FIGURE 7-34 ■ Gentle pressure on the sternocleidomastoid muscle.

(Stabilizer) (Fig. 7-35). The patient trains until he can perform a correct craniocervical flexion action (with minimum activation of the superficial flexors) and has restored the tonic endurance capacity of the deep cervical flexors. Training of the extensor muscles is commenced in the four-point kneeling position and exercises are directed towards the suboccipital muscles (craniocervical extension and rotation exercises) and the deeper cervical extensors (cervical extension with the craniocervical region in a neutral position). The training programme for both the flexors and extensors is eventually progressed to address any strength and endurance deficits.

Other exercises are included, such as postural re-education exercises, cervicoscapular stabilizer exercises, self-mobilization of the craniocervical spine (Fig. 7-36), cervicocephalic kinaesthesia and sensorimotor functions retraining. These exercises are described in Chapters 5 and 8. In addition to the exercises, prescribing measures of postural ergonomics can help patients with CEH. As these individuals have difficulty sleeping because of the pain and often get up with painful neck stiffness, it may be advisable to sleep with a cervical roll using a rolled-up towel, wrapped with a net, as those used for applying plaster (Fig. 7-37).

To conclude, a comprehensive treatment protocol needs to be established for patients with CEH, which addresses different impairments present in these patients: education, treatment of joint dysfunction, neuromuscular control, retraining of the muscles of

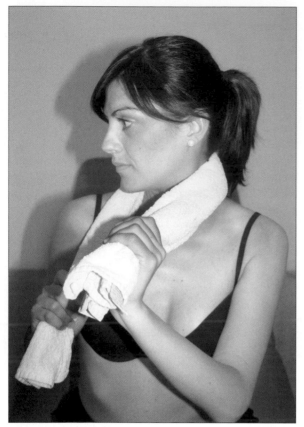

FIGURE 7-36 ■ Self-mobilization exercise for facet divergence.

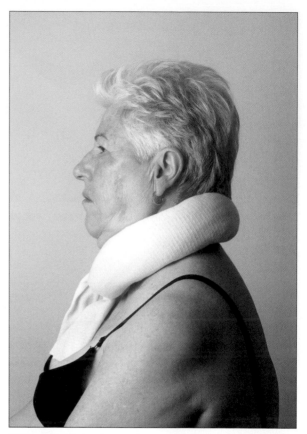

FIGURE 7-37 ■ Those subjects who have difficulty sleeping due to neck pain can be advised to sleep with a cervical roll.

the craniocervical, cervical and axioscapular regions, functional exercises and sports activities. The management of patients with complex and severe chronic headache and central sensitization requires a multidimensional approach (see Chapter 11).

Interventional and surgical techniques

Various interventional and surgical treatments for CEH have also been proposed with varying results. The use of epidural steroid injection is controversial both in its diagnostic and therapeutic aspect. While some authors consider it an effective treatment,[248] others advise against it because it is non-selective and has risks.[249] Anaesthetic blocks have been used both as a diagnostic method[13,94,249–251] and as a therapeutic procedure.[252–254] However, the short duration of effect limits its therapeutic use.[14,175] Infiltration around the

greater and lesser occipital nerve with corticosteroids has not always rendered good results.[175] Analgesic discography has also been carried out with a partial headache relief at 2 and 6 months.[255]

Articular injections of corticosteroids are effective, but their duration is limited (Fig. 7-38). In approximately 80% of patients, pain recurs before 20 days following treatment.[174,256] The only invasive treatment which has shown a longer duration of relief is percutaneous radiofrequency neurotomy of the facet joint responsible for the CEH.[172,257–262] However, some authors believe that its results are poor in the long term.[263,264] As Biondi[95] points out, anaesthetic procedures and neurolysis have the advantage of allowing earlier treatment based on manual therapy and physiotherapy with less discomfort to the patient. Different surgical procedures have also been described, such as

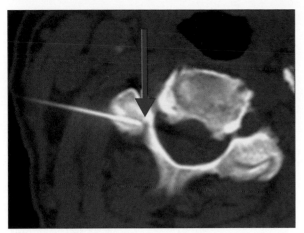

FIGURE 7-38 ■ Corticosteroid infiltrations in the facet joints are effective, but duration is limited. *(Picture courtesy of F. Aparisi.)*

radiofrequency nuchal plane devitalization (Blume intervention), microvascular decompression of roots and peripheral nerves and the discectomy and fusion of the craniocervical joints. Such techniques have been recommended in some cases when pain is refractory to any type of non-surgical treatment.[96,151,172,265-267]

CONCLUSION

Cervicogenic headache is beginning to be considered as a common type of headache. Progress leading to its recognition includes enhanced understanding of the anatomy of the trigeminal system and cervical pain patterns of the upper cervical spine, knowledge of the pathophysiological mechanisms and the establishment of diagnostic criteria which have proved to be worthy. These criteria allow a first diagnostic approach, which should be supplemented by an appropriate physical examination. Physical examination of the joint elements and neuromuscular control of the craniocervical spine identifies the physical impairments and, in many cases, the structure responsible for the headache.

Various conservative and invasive therapeutic approaches to CEH have been proposed. Conservative methods aimed at the functional improvement of the craniocervical spine through joint mobilization techniques, retraining of the stabilizing muscula-ture and treatment of sensorimotor deficits have shown good therapeutic efficacy and are now the treatment of choice. Such progress has allowed the development of therapeutic alternatives for a number of patients suffering from chronic and often debilitating headache.

REFERENCES

1. Stovner LJ, Zwart JA, Hagen K, et al. Epidemiology of headache in Europe. Eur J Neurol 2006;13(4):333–45.
2. Sjaastad O, Fredriksen TA, Petersen H, et al. Features indicative of cervical abnormality. A factor to be reckoned with in clinical headache work and research? Funct Neurol 2003;18(4): 195–203.
3. Sjaastad O, Fredriksen TA, Pfaffenrath V. Cervicogenic headache: diagnostic criteria. Headache 1990;30(11):725–6.
4. Leone M, D'Amico D, Grazzi L, et al. Cervicogenic headache: a critical review of the current diagnostic criteria. Pain 1998;78(1):1–5.
5. Sjaastad O, Fredriksen TA. Cervicogenic headache: criteria, classification and epidemiology. Clin Exp Rheumatol 2000;18(2 Suppl. 19):S3–6.
6. Sjaastad O, Saunte C, Hovdahl H, et al. 'Cervicogenic' headache. An hypothesis. Cephalalgia 1983;3(4):249–56.
7. Bogduk N. Mechanisms and pain patterns of the upper cervical spine. In: Vernon H, editor. The cranio-cervical syndrome. London: Butterworth-Heinemann; 2001. p. 110–16.
8. Bogduk N. The neck and headaches. Neurol Clin 2004;22(1): 151–71, vii.
9. Bogduk N. The anatomical basis for cervicogenic headache. J Manipulative Physiol Ther 1992;15(1):67–70.
10. Fredriksen TA, Sjaastad O. Cervicogenic headache: current concepts of pathogenesis related to anatomical structure. Clin Exp Rheumatol 2000;18(2 Suppl. 19):S16–18.
11. Bogduk N. Cervicogenic headache: anatomic basis and pathophysiologic mechanisms. Curr Pain Headache Rep 2001;5(4): 382–6.
12. Fredriksen TA, Hovdal H, Sjaastad O. 'Cervicogenic headache': clinical manifestation. Cephalalgia 1987;7(2):147–60.
13. Bogduk N, Marsland A. On the concept of third occipital headache. J Neurol Neurosurg Psychiatry 1986;49(7):775–80.
14. Pollmann W, Keidel M, Pfaffenrath V. Headache and the cervical spine: a critical review. Cephalalgia 1997;17(8): 801–16.
15. Bogduk N, McGuirk B. Management of acute and chronic neck pain. An evidence-based approach. Edinburgh: Elsevier; 2006.
16. Becker WJ. Cervicogenic headache: evidence that the neck is a pain generator. Headache 2010;50(4):699–705.
17. Pfaffenrath V, Dandekar R, Pollmann W. Cervicogenic headache – the clinical picture, radiological findings and hypotheses on its pathophysiology. Headache 1987;27(9):495–9.
18. Sjaastad O, Fredriksen TA, Pfaffenrath V, et al. Cervicogenic headache: diagnostic criteria. The Cervicogenic Headache International Study Group. Headache 1998;38(6):442–5.

19. Merskey H, Bogduk N. Classification of chronic pain. 2nd ed. Seattle: International Association for the Study of Pain (IASP) Press; 1994.

20. IHS. Classification and diagnostic criteria for headache disorders, cranial neuralgias and facial pain. Cephalalgia 1988; 8(Suppl. 7):1–96.

21. Headache Classification Committee of the International Headache Society (IHS). The International Classification of Headache Disorders, 3rd edition (beta version). Cephalalgia 2013; 33(9):629–808.

22. Headache Classification Committee of the International Headache Society. The International classification of headache disorders, 3rd edn (beta version). Cephalalgia 2013;33(9):629–808.

23. Sjaastad O, Bakketeig LS. Prevalence of cervicogenic headache: Vaga study of headache epidemiology. Acta Neurol Scand 2008;117(3):173–80.

24. Antonaci F, Sjaastad O. Cervicogenic headache: a real headache. Curr Neurol Neurosci Rep 2011;11(2):149–55.

25. Hogg-Johnson S, van der Velde G, Carroll LJ, et al. The burden and determinants of neck pain in the general population: results of the Bone and Joint Decade 2000-2010 Task Force on Neck Pain and Its Associated Disorders. J Manipulative Physiol Ther 2009;32(2 Suppl.):S46–60.

26. Sjaastad O, Bovim G. Cervicogenic headache. The differentiation from common migraine. An overview. Funct Neurol 1991;6(2):93–100.

27. Gore DR, Sepic SB, Gardner GM, et al. Neck pain: a long-term follow-up of 205 patients. Spine 1987;12(1):1–5.

28. Martelletti P. Proinflammatory pathways in cervicogenic headache. Clin Exp Rheumatol 2000;18(2 Suppl. 19):S33–8.

29. Delfini R, Salvati M, Passacantilli E, et al. Symptomatic cervicogenic headache. Clin Exp Rheumatol 2000;18(2 Suppl. 19):S29–32.

30. Nilsson N. The prevalence of cervicogenic headache in a random population sample of 20-59 year olds. Spine 1995; 20(17):1884–8.

31. Jull G, Trott P, Potter H, et al. A randomized controlled trial of exercise and manipulative therapy for cervicogenic headache. Spine 2002;27(17):1835–43, discussion 1843.

32. Jull G. Headaches associated with cervical spine – a clinical review. In: Grieve G, editor. Modern manual therapy of the vertebral column. Edinburgh: Churchill Livingstone; 1986. p. 322–9.

33. Nilsson N, Christensen HW, Hartvigsen J. The effect of spinal manipulation in the treatment of cervicogenic headache. J Manipulative Physiol Ther 1997;20(5):326–30.

34. Hall T, Chan HT, Christensen L, et al. Efficacy of a C1-C2 self-sustained natural apophyseal glide (SNAG) in the management of cervicogenic headache. J Orthop Sports Phys Ther 2007;37(3):100–7.

35. Haas M, Spegman A, Peterson D, et al. Dose response and efficacy of spinal manipulation for chronic cervicogenic headache: a pilot randomized controlled trial. Spine J 2010;10(2):117–28.

36. Chaibi A, Russell MB. Manual therapies for cervicogenic headache: a systematic review. J Headache Pain 2012;13(5):351–9.

37. Ylinen J, Nikander R, Nykanen M, et al. Effect of neck exercises on cervicogenic headache: a randomized controlled trial. J Rehabil Med 2010;42(4):344–9.

38. Astin JA, Ernst E. The effectiveness of spinal manipulation for the treatment of headache disorders: a systematic review of randomized clinical trials. Cephalalgia 2002;22(8):617–23.

39. Tuchin PJ, Pollard H, Bonello R. A randomized controlled trial of chiropractic spinal manipulative therapy for migraine. J Manipulative Physiol Ther 2000;23(2):91–5.

40. Nilsson N, Bove G. Evidence that tension-type headache and cervicogenic headache are distinct disorders. J Manipulative Physiol Ther 2000;23(4):288–9.

41. Fishbain DA, Cutler R, Cole B, et al. International Headache Society headache diagnostic patterns in pain facility patients. Clin J Pain 2001;17(1):78–93.

42. Leistad RB, Sand T, Westgaard RH, et al. Stress-induced pain and muscle activity in patients with migraine and tension-type headache. Cephalalgia 2006;26(1):64–73.

43. Jull G, Amiri M, Bullock-Saxton J, et al. Cervical musculoskeletal impairment in frequent intermittent headache. Part 1: Subjects with single headaches. Cephalalgia 2007;27(7): 793–802.

44. Calhoun AH, Ford S, Pruitt AP. Presence of neck pain may delay migraine treatment. Postgrad Med 2011;123(2):163–8.

45. Barré M. Sur un syndrome sympatique cervical posterieur et sa cause frequente: L'arthrite cervicale. Rev Neurol (Paris) 1926;33:1246–8.

46. Liéou YC. Syndrome sympathique cervical posterieur et arthrite cervicale chronique de la colonne vertébrale cervicale Etude clinique et radiologique. These de Strasbourg, 1928.

47. Bogduk N, Lambert GA, Duckworth JW. The anatomy and physiology of the vertebral nerve in relation to cervical migraine. Cephalalgia 1981;1:1–14.

48. Hunter C, Mayfield F. Role of the upper cervical roots in the production of pain in the head. Am J Surg 1949;48:743–51.

49. Kerr FW, Olafson RA. Trigeminal and cervical volleys. Convergence on single units in spinal gray at C1 and C2. Arch Neurol 1961;5:171–8.

50. Kerr RW. A mechanism to account for frontal headache in cases of posterior-fossa tumors. J Neurosurg 1961;18:605–9.

51. Knox DL, Mustonen E. Greater occipital neuralgia: an ocular pain syndrome with multiple etiologies. Trans Am Acad Ophthalmol Otolaryngol 1975;79(32):OP513–19.

52. Bogduk N. The anatomy of occipital neuralgia. Clin Exp Neurol 1981;17:167–84.

53. Cornely C, Fischer M, Ingianni G, et al. Greater occipital nerve neuralgia caused by pathological arterial contact: treatment by surgical decompression. Headache 2011;51(4):609–12.

54. Bogduk N. An anatomical basis for the neck-tongue syndrome. J Neurol Neurosurg Psychiatry 1981;44(3):202–8.

55. Bogduk N. Neck-tongue syndrome. Med J Aust 1980;2(1):4.

56. Bogduk N. C2 ganglion can be injured by compression between the posterior arch of the atlas and the lamina of C2. Spine 1999;24(3):308–9.

57. Lewis DW, Frank LM, Toor S. Familial neck-tongue syndrome. Headache 2003;43(2):132–4.

58. Borody C. Neck-tongue syndrome. J Manipulative Physiol Ther 2004;27(5):e8.

59. Queiroz LP. Unusual headache syndromes. Headache 2013;53(1):12–22.

60. Lance JW, Anthony M. Neck-tongue syndrome on sudden turning of the head. J Neurol Neurosurg Psychiatry 1980;43(2):97–101.

61. Hack GD, Koritzer RT, Robinson WL, et al. Anatomic relation between the rectus capitis posterior minor muscle and the dura mater. Spine 1995;20(23):2484–6.

62. Rutten HP, Szpak K, van Mameren H, et al. Anatomic relation between the rectus capitis posterior minor muscle and the dura mater. Spine 1997;22(8):924–6.

63. Mitchell BS, Humphreys BK, O'Sullivan E. Attachments of the ligamentum nuchae to cervical posterior spinal dura and the lateral part of the occipital bone. J Manipulative Physiol Ther 1998;21(3):145–8.

64. Dean NA, Mitchell BS. Anatomic relation between the nuchal ligament (ligamentum nuchae) and the spinal dura mater in the craniocervical region. Clin Anat 2002;15(3): 182–5.

65. Nash L, Nicholson H, Lee AS, et al. Configuration of the connective tissue in the posterior atlanto-occipital interspace: a sheet plastination and confocal microscopy study. Spine 2005;30(12):1359–66.

66. Kahkeshani K, Ward PJ. Connection between the spinal dura mater and suboccipital musculature: evidence for the myodural bridge and a route for its dissection – a review. Clin Anat 2012;25(4):415–22.

67. Alix ME, Bates DK. A proposed etiology of cervicogenic headache: the neurophysiologic basis and anatomic relationship between the dura mater and the rectus posterior capitis minor muscle. J Manipulative Physiol Ther 1999;22(8):534–9.

68. Hallgren RC, Hack GD, Lipton JA. Clinical implications of a cervical myodural bridge. AAO Journal 1997;30–5.

69. Hack GD, Hallgren RC. Chronic headache relief after section of suboccipital muscle dural connections: a case report. Headache 2004;44(1):84–9.

70. Enix DE, Scali F, Pontell ME. The cervical myodural bridge, a review of literature and clinical implications. J Can Chiropr Assoc 2014;58(2):184–92.

71. Torres-Cueco R. Cefalea cervicogénica. Criterios diagnósticos, exploración física y aproximación terapéutica. In: Padrós E, editor. Bases diagnósticas, terapéuticas y posturales del funcionalismo craneofacial. Madrid: Ripano; 2006. p. 736–58.

72. Zito G, Jull G, Story I. Clinical tests of musculoskeletal dysfunction in the diagnosis of cervicogenic headache. Man Ther 2006;11(2):118–29.

73. Kerr F. Central relationships of trigeminal and cervical primary afferents in the spinal cord and medulla. Brain Res 1972;43(2): 561–72.

74. Kerr F. The organization of primary afferents in the subnucleus caudalis of the trigeminal: a light and electron microscopic study of degeneration. Brain Res 1970;23(2):147–65.

75. Bogduk N. Anatomy and physiology of headache. Biomed Pharmacother 1995;49(10):435–45.

76. Bogduk N. Headaches and the cervical spine. Cephalalgia 1984;4(1):7–8.

77. Bogduk N. Cervical causes of headache and dizzinesss. In: Boyling JP, Palastanga N, editors. Grieve's modern manual therapy. The vertebral column. London: Churchill Livingstone; 2000. p. 317–31.

78. Bogduk N, Govind J. Cervicogenic headache: an assessment of the evidence on clinical diagnosis, invasive tests, and treatment. Lancet Neurol 2009;8(10):959–68.

79. Piovesan EJ, Kowacs PA, Tatsui CE, et al. Referred pain after painful stimulation of the greater occipital nerve in humans: evidence of convergence of cervical afferences on trigeminal nuclei. Cephalalgia 2001;21(2):107–9.

80. Bartsch T, Goadsby PJ. Increased responses in trigeminocervical nociceptive neurons to cervical input after stimulation of the dura mater. Brain 2003;126(Pt 8):1801–13.

81. Piovesan EJ, Kowacs PA, Oshinsky ML. Convergence of cervical and trigeminal sensory afferents. Curr Pain Headache Rep 2003;7(5):377–83.

82. Chua NH, Suijlekom HV, Wilder-Smith OH, et al. Understanding cervicogenic headache. Anesth Pain Med 2012;2(1):3–4.

83. Sjaastad O, Salvesen R, Jansen J, et al. Cervicogenic headache a critical view on pathogenesis. Funct Neurol 1998;13(1):71–4.

84. Cyriax J. Rheumatic headache. Br Med J 1938;2:1367–8.

85. Hoheisel U, Mense S, Simons DG, et al. Appearance of new receptive fields in rat dorsal horn neurons following noxious stimulation of skeletal muscle: a model for referral of muscle pain? Neurosci Lett 1993;153(1):9–12.

86. Davidoff RA. Trigger points and myofascial pain: toward understanding how they affect headaches. Cephalalgia 1998;18(7):436–48.

87. Borg-Stein J. Cervical myofascial pain and headache. Curr Pain Headache Rep 2002;6(4):324–30.

88. Dwyer A, Aprill C, Bogduk N. Cervical zygapophyseal joint pain patterns. I: A study in normal volunteers. Spine 1990;15(6):453–7.

89. Dreyfuss P, Michaelsen M, Fletcher D. Atlanto-occipital and lateral atlanto-axial joint pain patterns. Spine 1994;19(10): 1125–31.

90. Grenier F, Senegas J, Lavignolle B. Les nerfs rachidiens cervicaux et leur distribution La douleur cervicale. In: Senegas J, editor. Les cervicalgies La cervicarthrose et ses complications. Bordeaux: L'Unité de Pathologie Rachidienne CHR de Bordeaux; 1986. p. 39–62.

91. Fukui S, Ohseto K, Shiotani M, et al. Referred pain distribution of the cervical zygapophyseal joints and cervical dorsal rami. Pain 1996;68(1):79–83.

92. Aprill C, Axinn MJ, Bogduk N. Occipital headaches stemming from the lateral atlanto-axial (C1-2) joint. Cephalalgia 2002;22(1):15–22.

93. Cooper G, Bailey B, Bogduk N. Cervical zygapophysial joint pain maps. Pain Med 2007;8(4):344–53.

94. Bovim G, Berg R, Dale LG. Cervicogenic headache: anesthetic blockades of cervical nerves (C2-C5) and facet joint (C2/C3). Pain 1992;49(3):315–20.

95. Biondi DM. Cervicogenic headache: diagnostic evaluation and treatment strategies. Curr Pain Headache Rep 2001;5(4): 361–8.
96. Schofferman J, Garges K, Goldthwaite N, et al. Upper cervical anterior diskectomy and fusion improves discogenic cervical headaches. Spine 2002;27(20):2240–4.
97. Schellhas KP, Smith MD, Gundry CR, et al. Cervical discogenic pain. Prospective correlation of magnetic resonance imaging and discography in asymptomatic subjects and pain sufferers. Spine 1996;21(3):300–11, discussion 311-2.
98. Grubb SA, Kelly CK. Cervical discography: clinical implications from 12 years of experience. Spine 2000;25(11): 1382–9.
99. Ehni G, Benner B. Occipital neuralgia and the C1-2 arthrosis syndrome. J Neurosurg 1984;61(5):961–5.
100. Lord SM, Barnsley L, Wallis BJ, et al. Third occipital nerve headache: a prevalence study. J Neurol Neurosurg Psychiatry 1994;57(10):1187–90.
101. Ziegler DK, Hassanein RS, Couch JR. Headache syndromes suggested by statistical analysis of headache symptoms. Cephalalgia 1982;2(3):125–34.
102. Jull GA. Cervical headache: a review. In: Boyling JP, Palastanga N, editors. Grieve's modern manual therapy. The vertebral column. 2nd ed. London: Churchill Livingstone; 2000. p. 333–47.
103. Olesen J. Some clinical features of the acute migraine attack. An analysis of 750 patients. Headache 1978;18(5):268–71.
104. Saadah HA, Taylor FB. Sustained headache syndrome associated with tender occipital nerve zones. Headache 1987;27(4): 201–5.
105. Nelson CF. The tension headache, migraine headache continuum: a hypothesis. J Manipulative Physiol Ther 1994;17(3): 156–67.
106. Parker GB, Tupling H, Pryor DS. A controlled trial of cervical manipulation of migraine. Aust N Z J Med 1978;8(6):589–93.
107. Parker GB, Pryor DS, Tupling H. Why does migraine improve during a clinical trial? Further results from a trial of cervical manipulation for migraine. Aust N Z J Med 1980;10(2): 192–8.
108. Winston KR. Whiplash and its relationship to migraine. Headache 1987;27(8):452–7.
109. Sjaastad O, Bakketeig L. Tension-type headache: comparison with migraine without aura and cervicogenic headache. The Vaga study of headache epidemiology. Funct Neurol 2008;23(2):71–6.
110. Jensen R. Mechanisms of tension-type headache. Cephalalgia 2001;21(7):786–9.
111. Vandenheede M, Schoenen J. Central mechanisms in tension-type headaches. Curr Pain Headache Rep 2002;6(5):392–400.
112. Milanov I, Bogdanova D. Trigemino-cervical reflex in patients with headache. Cephalalgia 2003;23(1):35–8.
113. Jensen R. Peripheral and central mechanisms in tension-type headache: an update. Cephalalgia 2003;23(Suppl. 1):49–52.
114. Fernandez-de-las-Penas C, Schoenen J. Chronic tension-type headache: what is new? Curr Opin Neurol 2009;22(3): 254–61.
115. Saper JR. Chronic headache syndromes. Neurol Clin 1989;7(2):387–412.
116. Guerrero AL, Rojo E, Herrero S, et al. Characteristics of the first 1000 headaches in an outpatient headache clinic registry. Headache 2011;51(2):226–31.
117. Bhaskar S, Saeidi K, Borhani P, et al. Recent progress in migraine pathophysiology: role of cortical spreading depression and magnetic resonance imaging. Eur J Neurosci 2013;38(11):3540–51.
118. Hadjikhani N, Sanchez Del Rio M, Wu O, et al. Mechanisms of migraine aura revealed by functional MRI in human visual cortex. Proc Natl Acad Sci U S A 2001;98(8):4687–92.
119. Goadsby PJ, Charbit AR, Andreou AP, et al. Neurobiology of migraine. Neuroscience 2009;161(2):327–41.
120. Bahra A, Matharu MS, Buchel C, et al. Brainstem activation specific to migraine headache. Lancet 2001;357(9261): 1016–17.
121. Janig W. Relationship between pain and autonomic phenomena in headache and other pain conditions. Cephalalgia 2003;23(Suppl. 1):43–8.
122. Dodick DW, Capobianco DJ. Treatment and management of cluster headache. Curr Pain Headache Rep 2001;5(1): 83–91.
123. Goadsby PJ. Pathophysiology of cluster headache: a trigeminal autonomic cephalgia. Lancet Neurol 2002;1(4):251–7.
124. Leone M, Franzini A, Broggi G, et al. Hypothalamic deep brain stimulation for intractable chronic cluster headache: a 3-year follow-up. Neurol Sci 2003;24(Suppl. 2):S143–5.
125. May A, Leone M. Update on cluster headache. Curr Opin Neurol 2003;16(3):333–40.
126. Pringsheim T. Cluster headache: evidence for a disorder of circadian rhythm and hypothalamic function. Can J Neurol Sci 2002;29(1):33–40.
127. Vanelderen P, Lataster A, Levy R, et al. 8. Occipital neuralgia. Pain Pract 2010;10(2):137–44.
128. Antonaci F, Ghirmai S, Bono G, et al. Cervicogenic headache: evaluation of the original diagnostic criteria. Cephalalgia 2001;21(5):573–83.
129. Antonaci F, Fredriksen TA, Sjaastad O. Cervicogenic headache: clinical presentation, diagnostic criteria, and differential diagnosis. Curr Pain Headache Rep 2001;5(4):387–92.
130. Antonaci F, Bono G, Chimento P. Diagnosing cervicogenic headache. J Headache Pain 2006;7(3):145–8.
131. Jaeger B. Are 'cervicogenic' headaches due to myofascial pain and cervical spine dysfunction? Cephalalgia 1989;9(3):157–64.
132. Bono G, Antonaci F, Dario A, et al. Unilateral headaches and their relationship with cervicogenic headache. Clin Exp Rheumatol 2000;18(2 Suppl. 19):S11–15.
133. Sjaastad O, Bovim G, Stovner LJ. Laterality of pain and other migraine criteria in common migraine. A comparison with cervicogenic headache. Funct Neurol 1992;7(4):289–94.
134. Ehni G, Benner B. Occipital neuralgia and C1-C2 arthrosis. N Engl J Med 1984;310(2):127.
135. Wright EF. Referred craniofacial pain patterns in patients with temporomandibular disorder. J Am Dent Assoc 2000;131(9): 1307–15.

136. Fricton JR, Kroening R, Haley D, et al. Myofascial pain syndrome of the head and neck: a review of clinical characteristics of 164 patients. Oral Surg Oral Med Oral Pathol 1985; 60(6):615–23.

137. Kaniecki RG. Migraine and tension-type headache: an assessment of challenges in diagnosis. Neurology 2002;58(9 Suppl. 6):S15–20.

138. Hagen K, Einarsen C, Zwart JA, et al. The co-occurrence of headache and musculoskeletal symptoms amongst 51 050 adults in Norway. Eur J Neurol 2002;9(5):527–33.

139. Sjaastad O, Fredriksen TA, Sand T. The localization of the initial pain of attack. A comparison between classic migraine and cervicogenic headache. Funct Neurol 1989;4(1):73–8.

140. Watson DH, Trott PH. Cervical headache: an investigation of natural head posture and upper cervical flexor muscle performance. Cephalalgia 1993;13(4):272–84, discussion 232.

141. Petersen SM. Articular and muscular impairments in cervicogenic headache: a case report. J Orthop Sports Phys Ther 2003;33(1):21–30, discussion 30-2.

142. Sjaastad O, Fredriksen TA. Cervicogenic headache: the importance of sticking to the criteria. Funct Neurol 2002;17(1):35–6.

143. Gordon SJ, Trott P, Grimmer KA. Waking cervical pain and stiffness, headache, scapular or arm pain: gender and age effects. Aust J Physiother 2002;48(1):9–15.

144. Jensen R, Rasmussen BK, Pedersen B, et al. Cephalic muscle tenderness and pressure pain threshold in a general population. Pain 1992;48(2):197–203.

145. Jensen R, Rasmussen BK, Pedersen B, et al. Muscle tenderness and pressure pain thresholds in headache. A population study. Pain 1993;52(2):193–9.

146. Bovim G. Cervicogenic headache, migraine, and tension-type headache. Pressure-pain threshold measurements. Pain 1992;51(2):169–73.

147. Goadsby PJ. Recent advances in the diagnosis and management of migraine. BMJ 2006;332(7532):25–9.

148. Sjaastad O. Cluster headache and its variants. Headache 1988;28(10):667–8.

149. Bogduk N, Corrigan B, Kelly P, et al. Cervical headache. Med J Aust 1985;143(5):202, 206-7.

150. Spence J. Migraine and other causes of headache. Ann Emerg Med 1996;27(4):448–50.

151. Pikus HJ, Phillips JM. Characteristics of patients successfully treated for cervicogenic headache by surgical decompression of the second cervical root. Headache 1995;35(10):621–9.

152. Drottning M. Cervicogenic headache after whiplash injury. Curr Pain Headache Rep 2003;7(5):384–6.

153. Bogduk N, Aprill C. On the nature of neck pain, discography and cervical zygapophysial joint blocks. Pain 1993;54(2): 213–17.

154. Pearce JM. Whiplash injury: a reappraisal. J Neurol Neurosurg Psychiatry 1989;52(12):1329–31.

155. Antonaci F, Bulgheroni M, Ghirmai S, et al. 3D kinematic analysis and clinical evaluation of neck movements in patients with whiplash injury. Cephalalgia 2002;22(7):533–42.

156. Drottning M, Staff PH, Sjaastad O. Cervicogenic headache (CEH) after whiplash injury. Cephalalgia 2002;22(3):165–71.

157. Drottning M, Staff PH, Sjaastad O. Cervicogenic headache (CEH) six years after whiplash injury. Funct Neurol 2007;22(3):145–9.

158. Bono G, Antonaci F, Ghirmai S, et al. Whiplash injuries: clinical picture and diagnostic work-up. Clin Exp Rheumatol 2000;18(2 Suppl. 19):S23–8.

159. Barnsley L, Lord SM, Wallis BJ, et al. The prevalence of chronic cervical zygapophysial joint pain after whiplash. Spine 1995;20(1):20–5, discussion 26.

160. Cote P, Cassidy JD, Carroll L. Is a lifetime history of neck injury in a traffic collision associated with prevalent neck pain, headache and depressive symptomatology? Accid Anal Prev 2000;32(2):151–9.

161. Radanov BP, Di Stefano G, Augustiny KF. Symptomatic approach to posttraumatic headache and its possible implications for treatment. Eur Spine J 2001;10(5):403–7.

162. Jull G. Management of cervical headache. Man Ther 1997;2(4):182–90.

163. Uthaikhup S, Sterling M, Jull G. Cervical musculoskeletal impairment is common in elders with headache. Man Ther 2009;14(6):636–41.

164. de Tommaso M, Sardaro M, Vecchio E, et al. Central sensitisation phenomena in primary headaches: overview of a preventive therapeutic approach. CNS Neurol Disord Drug Targets 2008;7(6):524–35.

165. Staud R. Abnormal endogenous pain modulation is a shared characteristic of many chronic pain conditions. Expert Rev Neurother 2012;12(5):577–85.

166. Chua NH, van Suijlekom HA, Vissers KC, et al. Differences in sensory processing between chronic cervical zygapophysial joint pain patients with and without cervicogenic headache. Cephalalgia 2011;31(8):953–63.

167. Vincent MB, Luna RA. Cervicogenic headache: a comparison with migraine and tension-type headache. Cephalalgia 1999;19(Suppl. 25):11–16.

168. van Suijlekom JA, de Vet HC, van den Berg SG, et al. Interobserver reliability of diagnostic criteria for cervicogenic headache. Cephalalgia 1999;19(9):817–23.

169. Bono G, Antonaci F, Ghirmai S, et al. The clinical profile of cervicogenic headache as it emerges from a study based on the early diagnostic criteria (Sjaastad et al., 1990). Funct Neurol 1998;13(1):75–7.

170. Fishbain DA, Lewis J, Cole B, et al. Do the proposed cervicogenic headache diagnostic criteria demonstrate specificity in terms of separating cervicogenic headache from migraine? Curr Pain Headache Rep 2003;7(5):387–94.

171. Fredriksen TA, Sjaastad O. Cervicogenic headache (CEH): notes on some burning issues. Funct Neurol 2000;15(4):199–203.

172. Silverman SB. Cervicogenic headache: interventional, anesthetic, and ablative treatment. Curr Pain Headache Rep 2002;6(4):308–14.

173. Dumas JP, Arsenault AB, Boudreau G, et al. Physical impairments in cervicogenic headache: traumatic vs. nontraumatic onset. Cephalalgia 2001;21(9):884–93.

174. Bogduk N. The neck. Baillières Best Pract Res Clin Rheumatol 1999;13(2):261–85.

248. Reale C, Turkiewicz AM, Reale CA, et al. Epidural steroids as a pharmacological approach. Clin Exp Rheumatol 2000;18(2 Suppl. 19):S65–6.

249. van Suijlekom JA, Weber WE, van Kleef M. Cervicogenic headache: techniques of diagnostic nerve blocks. Clin Exp Rheumatol 2000;18(2 Suppl. 19):S39–44.

250. Bogduk N, Marsland A. The cervical zygapophysial joints as a source of neck pain. Spine 1988;13(6):610–17.

251. Gawel MJ, Rothbart PJ. Occipital nerve block in the management of headache and cervical pain. Cephalalgia 1992;12(1):9–13.

252. Feng FL, Schofferman J. Chronic neck pain and cervicogenic headaches. Curr Treat Options Neurol 2003;5(6):493–8.

253. Bogduk N. Role of anesthesiologic blockade in headache management. Curr Pain Headache Rep 2004;8(5):399–403.

254. Bogduk N. Distinguishing primary headache disorders from cervicogenic headache: clinical and therapeutic implications. Headache Currents 2005;2(2):27–36.

255. Blume HG. Cervicogenic headaches: radiofrequency neurotomy and the cervical disc and fusion. Clin Exp Rheumatol 2000;18(2 Suppl. 19):S53–8.

256. Barnsley L, Lord SM, Wallis BJ, et al. Lack of effect of intraarticular corticosteroids for chronic pain in the cervical zygapophyseal joints. N Engl J Med 1994;330(15):1047–50.

257. van Suijlekom HA, van Kleef M, Barendse GA, et al. Radiofrequency cervical zygapophyseal joint neurotomy for cervicogenic headache: a prospective study of 15 patients. Funct Neurol 1998;13(4):297–303.

258. Lord SM, Barnsley L, Bogduk N. Percutaneous radiofrequency neurotomy in the treatment of cervical zyga-

259. Lord SM, Barnsley L, Wallis BJ, et al. Percutaneous radiofrequency neurotomy for chronic cervical zygapophyseal-joint pain. N Engl J Med 1996;335(23):1721–6.

260. Martelletti P, van Suijlekom H. Cervicogenic headache: practical approaches to therapy. CNS Drugs 2004;18(12): 793–805.

261. van Suijlekom H, Van Zundert J, Narouze S, et al. 6. Cervicogenic headache. Pain Pract 2010;10(2):124–30.

262. Lee JB, Park JY, Park J, et al. Clinical efficacy of radiofrequency cervical zygapophyseal neurotomy in patients with chronic cervicogenic headache. J Korean Med Sci 2007;22(2): 326–9.

263. Stovner LJ, Kolstad F, Helde G. Radiofrequency denervation of facet joints C2-C6 in cervicogenic headache: a randomized, double-blind, sham-controlled study. Cephalalgia 2004;24(10): 821–30.

264. Mehnert MJ, Freedman MK. Update on the role of z-joint injection and radiofrequency neurotomy for cervicogenic headache. PM R 2013;5(3):221–7.

265. Bovim G, Fredriksen TA, Stolt-Nielsen A, et al. Neurolysis of the greater occipital nerve in cervicogenic headache. A follow up study. Headache 1992;32(4):175–9.

266. Biondi DM. Cervicogenic headache: a review of diagnostic and treatment strategies. J Am Osteopath Assoc 2005;105(4 Suppl. 2):16S–22S.

267. Fredriksen TA. Cervicogenic headache: invasive procedures. Cephalalgia 2008;28(Suppl. 1):39–40.

pophysial joint pain: a caution. Neurosurgery 1995;36(4): 732–9.

8

CLINICAL APPROACH TO DIZZINESS OF CERVICAL ORIGIN

RAFAEL TORRES CUECO ■ JULIA TRELEAVEN

Dizziness and various sensorimotor control impairments are commonly associated with pathology or dysfunction of the cervical spine. In fact, dizziness and unsteadiness are the most common symptoms associated with neck pain, especially after a whiplash injury.[1] The incidence of pseudo-vertiginous symptoms is very high in this type of patients, ranging between 40 and 85%.[1–6] Symptoms can be very varied in patients with neck pain, and may include dizziness, light-headedness, unsteadiness, nausea and blurred vision. They can be accompanied by several objective signs of sensorimotor control dysfunction such as altered cervical kinaesthetic sense,[1,7–12] altered neck motor control patterns,[13–15] altered standing balance[1,16–20] and altered oculomotor and neck coordination.[10,21–26] These sensorimotor proprioceptive disturbances in the cervical spine might be an important factor associated with chronicity in patients with neck pain.[12]

Terminology

The first difficulty faced by clinicians is the variety of terms used to refer to these pseudo-vertiginous sensations. Terms such as vertigo, dizziness, unsteadiness, light-headedness, giddiness, imbalance or instability hinder the interpretation of the patient's symptoms. The first step is, therefore, to clarify the terminology related to vertigo.[27]

Vertigo can be described as a false sensation of movement that the subject experiences in relation to the environment or vice versa. This type of true vertigo has its origin in the vestibular system and should be differentiated from dizziness or pseudo-vertigos of different aetiology.

Vestibular vertigo is classified as either *peripheral vertigo*, when the alteration occurs in the terminal organs of the vestibular system (utricle, saccule, semicircular canals and vestibular portion of the eighth cranial nerve), or *central vertigo*, when the alteration is located in the vestibular nuclei, cerebellum, perihypoglossal nucleus, and its different interconnecting tracts in the central nervous system (CNS).[28]

In 85% of people presenting with vertigo, the origin is peripheral, with the remaining 15% being central. Vertigo, when it has a labyrinthine aetiology, has a rotatory character, but it can be described in different ways; it is frequently accompanied by nausea, vomiting and sweating, but there is no loss of consciousness or falls.

Dizziness is a more ambiguous term that is described as a subjective sensation of unsteadiness with no objective loss of balance. The patient reports a feeling of unsteadiness, swaying or weakness, sometimes accompanied by nausea.[29] While the aetiology of vertigo is vestibular, the aetiology of dizziness is very diverse.[30] It can be a characteristic symptom of an alteration of the visual system, an alteration of the parietal and temporal lobes, the cerebellum, fatigue, stress, etc., as well as dysfunction or pathology of the cervical spine.

Imbalance is an objective loss of stability, with no perception of movement. It is usually the consequence of an alteration in the integration between sensory input and motor responses. This symptom appears while standing and walking, and is absent when sitting or lying down. Whereas vertigo can be of central or peripheral origin, severe imbalance in a younger patient usually indicates a central pathology.[27]

However, in elderly patients, it should be considered a normal response associated with age.

The first step of a subjective assessment is to differentiate between vertigo and dizziness and other pseudo-vertiginous complaints.

In order to define the symptoms associated with the cervical spine, in this chapter, the term cervicogenic dizziness and pseudo-vertiginous symptoms are used. These symptoms can improve with manual therapy, specific physical therapy exercises and retraining methods.

Cervicogenic dizziness can be experienced as a nearly constant symptom or as onset of very short duration.[5] These types of symptoms are more common in patients with more severe pain and are associated with poorer long-term prognosis in those with trauma. These pseudo-vertiginous symptoms can have a significant emotional impact and can be linked to anxiety, depression and fear-avoidance behaviours, which can have detrimental effects on the patient's professional, social and family life.[31]

Some patients with a persistent cervicogenic dizziness develop fear-avoidance behaviours and management should also address this if present.

CERVICAL SPINE AND DIZZINESS

The relationship between the cervical spine and the pseudo-vertiginous symptoms has, and still is, the source of controversy. While some authors reject the possible cervical aetiology of the symptoms,[32] others provide sufficient experimental and clinical evidence to support it.[5] However, the debate results more from the use of the term 'vertigo' than from the acknowledgement that patients with cervical pathology experience dizziness, unsteadiness, lightheadedness, etc.

The dizziness of cervical origin was first described in 1955 by Ryan and Cope,[33] who used the term 'cervical vertigo'. Cervicogenic dizziness (CD) has been defined by Furman and Cass[34] as 'a non-specific sensation of altered orientation in space and disequilibrium originating from abnormal afferent activity from the neck'.

As previously mentioned, this type of symptom is more frequent following cervical whiplash.[1] However, symptoms of dizziness or vertigo of traumatic origin cannot be exclusively attributed to the neck, since there are many other structures, such as the vestibule or brainstem, which can be the origin. In order to consider the existence of a cervicogenic dizziness, it is necessary to establish a time relationship between the dizziness and other cervical signs and symptoms. Therefore, the reduction of the dizziness should be associated with a neck pain improvement[3] and an adequate differential diagnosis is always obligatory.

Different hypotheses have attempted to explain the relationship between the cervical spine and dizziness.

Vascular hypothesis

The vascularization of the vestibular system depends on the labyrinthine artery, a branch of the anterior cerebellar artery, which, in turn, has its origin in the basilar artery. Vertigo is therefore one of the common symptoms of both vertebrobasilar insufficiency, and vertebral artery dissection.[35–38] One of the characteristics of this type of vertigo is that it rarely occurs in isolation, with no other neurological signs.[28,35,37] Although vascular aetiology is a factor that needs to be taken into account in subjects that suffer from vertigo, its importance has been overestimated, especially in elderly patients with arteriosclerosis. The nature and clinical expression of the pseudo-vertiginous symptoms of cervical spine origin do not correspond to the characteristics of central vertigo, such as the vertigo derived from a vertebrobasilar insufficiency. Therefore, the cervicogenic dizziness presents a different aetiology to the vascular aetiology.

Posterior cervical sympathetic syndrome

This syndrome, described by Barré[39] in 1926, and later by Lieou,[40] attempted to provide an aetiological reason for a complex clinical condition of neck pain, headaches and vertigo. These authors considered that these symptoms were caused by the irritation of the sympathetic plexus that surrounds the vertebral artery in its trajectory through the transverse foramina, as the consequence of articular degenerative changes.

However, this hypothesis has been rejected due to the observation that the stimulation of this sympathetic plexus only triggers a small contraction of the vertebral artery and thus only has a minimal effect on the regulation of the encephalic blood flow.[41,42]

Somatosensory hypothesis

This hypothesis suggests that the symptoms of CD are caused by the alteration of the afferent information proceeding from the articular and muscular proprioceptors of the cervical spine.[32,33] Currently, the cervical spine is considered to be an important proprioceptive organ that is involved in the control of head and eye movement control, balance and posture. This belief began with studies conducted by Magnus,[43] who proved that the tonic reflexes of the neck originate in receptors lodged in the craniocervical segments. The existence of abnormal input coming from the cervical spine caused discordance with the rest of the vestibular, visual and plantar information that converges into the central nervous system, disturbing the sensorimotor control system.[44–46] The pseudo-vertiginous sensations are the consequence of a conflict in the information gathered by the different postural sensory systems. This hypothesis currently offers the best explanation of the CD. In fact, experimental studies conducted in animals have demonstrated that the infiltration of different substances in the deep cervical muscles triggers alterations in balance, nystagmus and even ataxia.[47–50]

The pseudo-vertiginous sensations associated with cervicogenic dizziness are the consequence of a conflict with the information gathered by different postural sensory systems.

When conducted on normal subjects, the same type of study has demonstrated that the information coming from neck proprioceptors has a significant effect on sensorimotor control.[51,52] The infiltration of the cervical muscles with local anaesthetic substances can induce ataxia and dizziness in normal subjects.[51,53] Vibration of the neck muscles can also cause similar responses. The alteration of the afferent information of the deep cervical muscles and the cervical articular proprioceptors is considered the pathophysiological basis of CD.[2,32,46,51,54,55]

The alteration of the afferent information of the deep cervical muscles and the cervical articular proprioceptors is the pathophysiological basis of CD.

The articular or muscular dysfunctions of the cervical spine are, therefore, capable of producing dizziness, pseudo-vertiginous sensations, head and eye movement and balance control impairments. The severity of these symptoms is usually proportional to that of other cervical symptoms, such as pain or stiffness.[5,45,53,56] In order to have a better understanding of CD and associated symptoms, it is necessary to review how the sensorimotor control system works.

THE SENSORIMOTOR CONTROL SYSTEM

The sensorimotor control system is important for the control of head and eye movement control and postural stability. Maintenance of sensorimotor control is complex and requires the participation of a series of sensory organs known as postural sensors.

These sensory receptors are divided into exoreceptors and endoreceptors. The first group includes the peripheral vestibular system, the visual system and the plantar baroreceptors. Their role is to inform the CNS of the variations in position of the body in relation to the environment. However, the information obtained from the postural sensory receptors cannot be used if this system does not have complementary information regarding the reciprocal position of these postural exoreceptors. This information is crucial, since the changes of position recorded by the vestibular system, for instance, can indicate a movement of the entire body or only a movement of the head.

The reciprocal position of the exoreceptors is provided by the postural endoreceptors, which are composed of the oculomotor muscles and the proprioceptive sensors that are distributed over the body. The numerous sensors lodged in the cervical spine are especially relevant (Fig. 8-1). The vestibular system only gathers information regarding the change of position of the head, while the proprioceptive receptors of the neck inform of the position of the head in relation to the body. The postural endoreceptor is essential for sensorimotor control, although it has no direct relationship with the environment.

SENSORIMOTOR CONTROL SENSORY RECEPTORS

Exoreceptors

- Visual.
- Vestibular.
- Plantar baroreceptors.

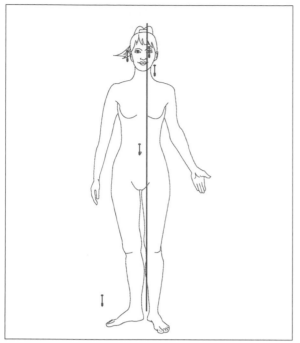

FIGURE 8-1 ■ The balance control uses information from postural exoreceptors (visual, vestibular and plantar baroreceptors) and from postural endoreceptors (oculomotor muscles and joint and muscle proprioceptors), including those hosted in the cervical spine.

Endoreceptors

- Oculomotor muscles.
- Articular and muscular proprioceptors:
  - cervical spine
  - foot and the ankle.

With respect to maintaining balance, for example, all of the information coming from the visual, vestibular and plantar exoreceptors as well as the prioprioceptive endoreceptors of the oculomotor muscles, the cervical spine, the paravertebral muscles and the muscles of the lower limbs is processed by the CNS in order to maintain the projection of the centre of gravity. In order to keep balance, the centre of gravity needs to fall within the support polygon. Balance is not a static function, as humans are constantly tilting around the tibiotalar joint, behaving like an inverted pendulum. This sensorimotor control system is extremely precise, in such a way that the projection of the centre of gravity is limited to an area of less than 1 cm², as evident in a posturograph (Fig. 8-2).

All of the information needed for sensorimotor control should be integrated in real time, as any minimal perturbation can cause imbalance. Thus, the quality of the regulation of the sensorimotor system not only depends on the correct functioning of the different sensors but also on the sensory integration of all the information obtained.

The quality of the regulation of the sensorimotor control system not only depends on the effective functioning of the different sensors but also on the sensory integration of all the information obtained.

If some of the information that reaches the CNS is not consistent, there is a conflict and the CNS must decide what information is correct. Otherwise, the subject may experience sensations of dizziness and unsteadiness.

However, the CNS has a great capacity to adapt, in such a manner that even when one or several sensory receptors provide inconsistent information, it is capable of adapting to this new situation in real time, and the subject will not have any symptoms of dizziness or imbalance. For instance, despite the gradual deterioration suffered by the vestibular system with ageing, elderly subjects can still maintain an acceptable level of balance thanks to the cooperation of vision and the proprioceptive system in balance control.[27]

The CNS has a great capacity to adapt, in such a manner that even when one or several sensors provide consistent information, it is capable of adapting to this new situation in real time, and the subject will not have any symptoms of dizziness or imbalance.

Until recently, the interest of clinicians, particularly of otoneurologists, has been primarily centred on the vestibular component for sensorimotor control, via tests specifically addressing vestibular function such as the vestibulo-ocular reflex, whose evaluation is carried out with electronystagmography or videonystagmography rather than specific tests of balance or head and eye movement control (Fig. 8-3). However, in sensorimotor control, the vestibular input is not the only or most important one and differential diagnosis of the signs and symptoms of altered sensorimotor control is important to direct appropriate management.

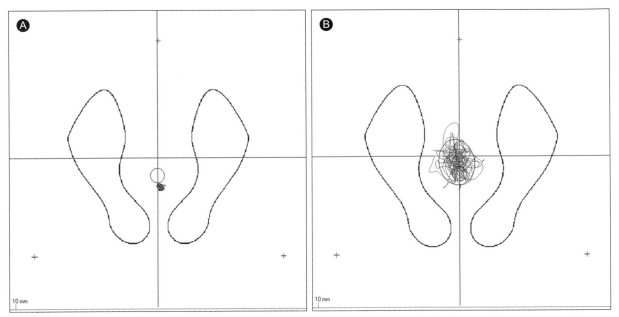

FIGURE 8-2 ■ The projection of the centre of gravity is not restricted to an area greater than 1 cm², as shown in the posturograph register (A). Posturograph register of a subject with a severe disruption of balance control (B).

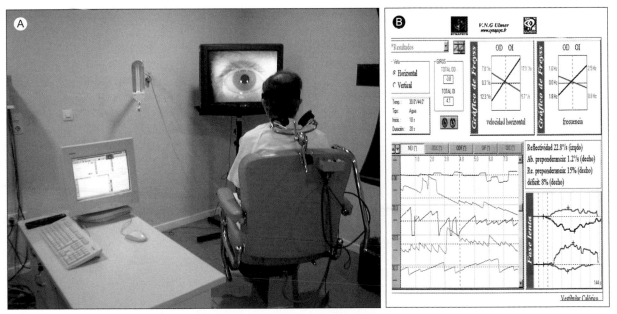

FIGURE 8-3 ■ Videonystagmography equipment (A) and results (B).

Postural sensory receptors

As previously mentioned, the postural exoreceptors are the vestibular system, the visual system and the plantar baroreceptors. Postural endoreceptors include the oculomotor muscles and the proprioceptive system, the cervical spine and the rest of the body.

Vestibular system

The vestibular system is an essential component for sensorimotor control, particularly in upright standing, thanks to the vestibular reflexes. The vestibular system is located in the inner ear and is formed by two functional units: (1) the utricle and saccule and (2) the semicircular canals. The cochlea participates in hearing and is not involved in balance control (Fig. 8-4).

The utricle and saccule are two chambers that have a specialized area known as the macula, where the ciliated sensory cells are located (Fig. 8-5). The ciliated sensory cells are covered by a gelatinous layer over which calcium carbonate crystals, known as otoliths, are deposited. These particles move during head movements due to the action of gravity. Thus, when the head is tilted in relation to the vertical line, the otoliths tend to glide laterally, and tilt the sensory ciliated cells, causing their depolarization (Fig. 8-6).

The utricular and saccular maculae are located on perpendicular planes between each other. This helps the vestibular system to determine the position of the head in the three planes of space. The utricle and saccule provide information on the position of the head in relation to the force of gravity and of the changes in the lineal acceleration in the coronal, sagittal and vertical directions. Sensory information from the utricle and saccule serves as an afferent input to the vestibulo-spinal reflex (VSR), which helps to maintain postural stability, and to the vestibulo-cervical reflex (VCR), which aids head movement control.

Three semicircular canals (horizontal, sagittal and coronal) are in contact with the utricle and each canal is situated at a right angle in relation to the others. These canals are filled with endolymphatic fluid, and on their edge they have a dilatation, the ampulla. This is where sensory ciliated cells are located (Fig. 8-7). The semicircular canals detect rotation in any direction, as well as the intensity of the change in the

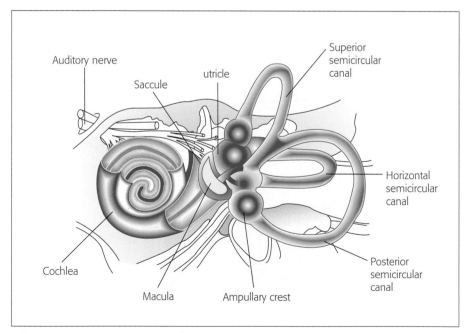

FIGURE 8-4 ■ The vestibular apparatus is located in the inner ear and consists of two functional units: (1) the utricle and saccule and (2) the semicircular canals.

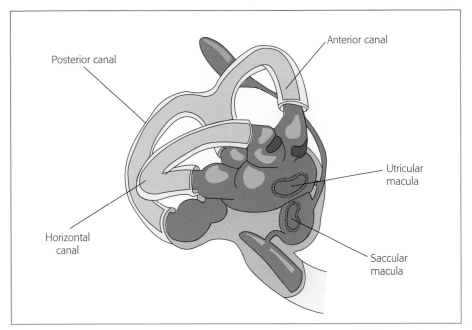

FIGURE 8-5 ■ The utricle and saccule are two chambers that have a specialized area called the macula, comprising the sensory hair cells.

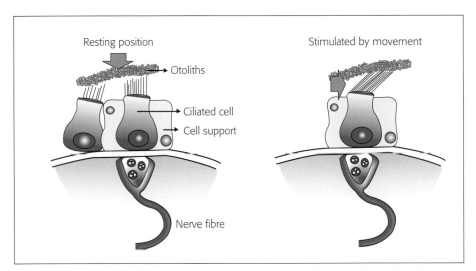

FIGURE 8-6 ■ The otoliths tend to slide during movement of the head and, in doing so, tilt the cilia of the sensory cells, causing depolarization.

rotation that is known as angular acceleration. The information from the semicircular canal provides the sensory input to the vestibulo-ocular reflex (VOR), which causes activation of the oculomotor muscles to stabilize gaze and the VCR to control head motion.

Visual system

It is necessary to use vision in order to precisely adjust the body's position in relation to the environment. The visual input is a powerful postural input: the precision of the human postural system with eyes open is,

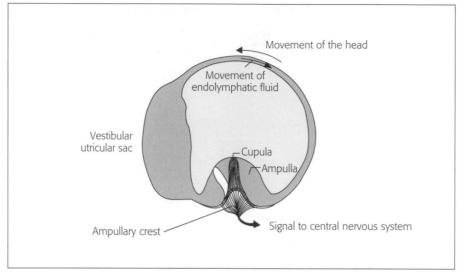

FIGURE 8-7 ■ The three semicircular canals (horizontal, sagittal and coronal) are filled with endolymph and, at the ends, have a dilation known as ampulla, where sensory hair cells are lodged.

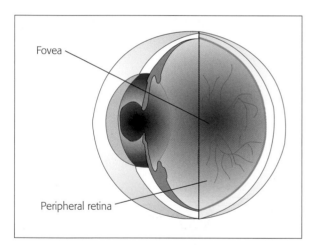

FIGURE 8-8 ■ Humans have two types of vision: foveal vision, recorded by the central part of the retina or fovea, which ensures the accuracy of sight, and peripheral vision, which depends on the peripheral portion of the retina.

in general, 250% higher than with eyes closed. There are two types of vision: first, *foveal vision*, which is registered by the central part of the retina or fovea, which has numerous cones and rods, and ensures precise vision; secondly, there is *peripheral vision*, which depends on the peripheral portion of the retina (Fig. 8-8). Both foveal and peripheral vision play a role in sensorimotor control. Vision allows subjects to

maintain balance with their eyes open, despite the vestibular system being completely destroyed.

Eye movements can be classified according to direction of both eyes in either convergence or divergence movements. In these vergence movements, both eyes move in opposite horizontal directions, allowing the eyes to capture near or far objects.

Eye movements are also classified as fixational, gaze-shifting or gaze-stabilizing movements.[57] Fixational movements involve very small eye movements such as microsaccades, drifts and microtremors. These small movements are aimed at constantly shifting the visual image minutely over the fovea.

Gaze-shifting movements are smooth pursuit and saccadic movements. Smooth pursuit eye movements allow the eyes to follow an object that is moving, and to perceive it in detail. Saccadic movements are rapid movements of the eyes that abruptly change the focus point. The velocity of pursuit eye movements is possible under 30° per second. Greater velocities tend to require catch-up saccades. Saccadic movements guide the fovea to an object initially positioned at an eccentric retinal location.

Gaze-stabilizing movements may include the VOR, the cervico-ocular reflex (COR) and the optokinetic reflex. The VOR stabilizes the images on the retina during head movement by producing an eye movement in the opposite direction to the head movement. The COR has a lesser role but also generates compensatory gaze shifts which oppose those produced by the rotation of the head. The optokinetic reflex (OKR) is a combination of saccadic and smooth pursuit eye movements. The OKR is produced when an individual follows a moving object with their eyes for a distance and then subsequently saccades in the opposite direction to reacquire a target.

Plantar baroreceptors

The sole of the foot contains a significant number of exoreceptors that are capable of recording minimal variations in pressure. The stimulation of these baroreceptors can significantly modify postural control. Furthermore, both the foot and the ankle have many proprioceptors implicated in the control of the line of gravity projection (Fig. 8-9).

The architecture of the foot provides a great versatility of movement that ensures its great capacity of adaptation. In some cases painful hyperpressure plantar areas can disturb baroreceptor input and modify postural control.

Cervical proprioceptive system

The main functional responsibility of the cervical spine is positioning the head in order to orientate the sensory organs, eyes, nose and ears, in multiple directions. It is crucial for the head to be stabilized in order to organize the posture of the rest of the body and maintain dynamic balance. As previously discussed, the head holds three types of systems that are fundamental for sensorimotor control: the vestibular system, which detects gravity and head accelerations; the visual system, which is capable of stabilizing the head and body in relation to the environment; and proprioceptive information from the cervical spine, which provides details of the head's position in relation to the trunk.

The vestibular system can only detect head movement in relation to the environment; therefore, the CNS also needs information regarding the head orientation in relation to the rest of the body, and this information is provided by the proprioceptors of the cervical spine. Proprioceptive information from the cervical spine also plays a decisive role in coordinating eye and head movements. The vestibular and visual information produces postural, head and eye movement corrections, but these responses are modified by afferent input from the neck.[32,58] The three first cervical spinal segments have the most influence on sensorimotor control. This region has a significant number of proprioceptive receptors, both in the muscle (muscle spindles and Golgi tendon organs), and the articular

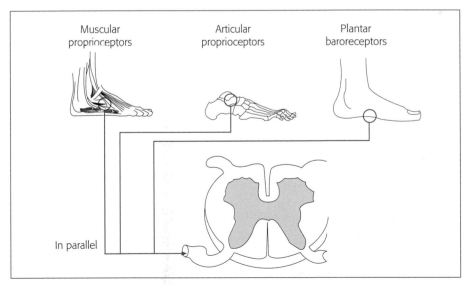

FIGURE 8-9 ■ The foot is an important exoreceptor because of the baroreceptors on the sole and endoreceptors with numerous joint proprioceptors.

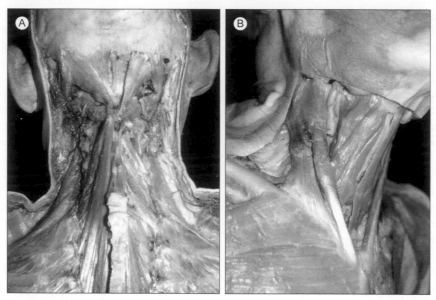

FIGURE 8-10 ■ Cervical proprioception involves the deep muscles (suboccipital muscles and deep cervical flexors) (A) and the superficial muscles (sternocleidomastoid and upper trapezius) (B).

capsules (Pacini's corpuscles and Ruffini's receptors).[59,60] This proprioceptive function involves not only the deep suboccipital and deep neck flexor muscles but also some superficial muscles such as the sternocleidomastoid and upper trapezius (Fig. 8-10). The first group of muscles is responsible for recording minimal variations in the position of the head, while the second group of muscles act as tensors, capable of linking the position of the head to the position of the vestibular and the visual systems.[61,62] There are connections between the lateral vestibular nucleus and the sternocleidomastoid muscle through the medial vestibular spinal tract. This link can be observed with the *vestibular evoked myogenic potential*.[63,64] Some authors believe that one of triggers of CD is an asymmetry of the cervical muscles activity or tone.[65] The dizziness is primarily triggered during the cervical rotation movements and it can be the consequence of muscular stretching. The stretching of a muscle which has an abnormal activity generates abnormal proprioceptive information that alters the performance of the sensorimotor control system. This type of cervicogenic dizziness is manifested, especially, when the subject moves the head after having maintained an eccentric position for a long time, and is perceived as a brief imbalance, which subsides when the subject identifies the stable reference point in the usual environment.[65]

All of this information from muscles and joints contributes to the construction of the kinaesthetic position and movement sense of the cervical spine.[66] In addition to these mechanoreceptors that are responsible for providing positional information to the CNS, the joints of the cervical spine have several connections with the trochlear, abducens, trigeminal and vestibular nuclei.[67–72] Thus, the cervical afferents not only modulate body posture but also stabilize the head in relation to the trunk through the cervical reflexes, interacting with the vestibular and visual reflexes that stabilize the head and eyes in space.[32,73,74]

Sensorimotor control is largely maintained by involuntary reflex control. Visual and vestibular systems are interrelated via the VOR, whose role is stabilizing the visual field.[75,76] During head movements the eye moves in relation to the head to guarantee that the image remains stable on the retina. If there is a retinal slip, the vision is blurred and the surroundings appear to move around. Then, the VOR is responsible for creating a compensatory eye movement in order to abolish the effect on vision of the head movement.

The input from the cervical spine is linked to the vestibular system by the VCR to stabilize the position of the head.[77] The VCR counters the movement sensed by the otoliths or semicircular canals, stabilizing the position of the head, mainly in the horizontal plane.[78,79]

The COR generates compensatory gaze shifts which oppose those produced by the rotation of the head and the cervico-collic reflex (CCR) stabilizes the head with respect to the trunk in response to stretching of the neck muscles.[73,77,78,80,81] The COR cooperates with the VOR, in keeping a good perception of visual field during movement.[77] The COR makes a small contribution to gaze stability in comparison with the VOR but can compensate for altered VOR. The CCR stabilizes the head on the body, avoiding an excess of cervical rotation. This reflex probably originates in the neuromuscular spindles of the deeper muscles of the neck.[73] The input from the cervical spine is related to the anti-gravitational extensor motor system via the tonic neck reflex (TNR), keeping a stable posture when the body is moving in relation to the head.[82]

Abnormal cervical afferent input can cause discordance with the rest of the vestibular, visual and plantar information that converges in the CNS, producing disturbances in the sensorimotor control system.[44-46] Therefore, sensorimotor control impairments such as altered neck motor control patterns, altered cervical kinaesthetic sense, altered oculomotor and neck coordination and standing balance can be the consequence of a conflict in the information gathered by the different postural sensory systems.

DIFFERENTIAL DIAGNOSIS OF CERVICOGENIC DIZZINESS

The diagnosis should establish a correlation between dizziness and the cervical spine, excluding a vestibular disorder and a neurovascular injury, using the subject's previous history, the clinical assessment of cervical musculoskeletal and relevant sensorimotor impairments and the use of vestibular functional tests.[3] At present, the primary criteria for CD is that it must be concluded that a subject suffers from CD only when the other pathologies have been ruled out.[83]

The diagnosis of the CD should establish a correlation between dizziness and the cervical spine,

excluding a vestibular disorder and a neurovascular injury, using the subject's previous history, the clinical assessment and the use of vestibular function tests.

The differential diagnosis of vertigo of neurovascular dysfunction is described in Chapter 10. It is only necessary here to highlight that vertebrobasilar insufficiency is an uncommon entity, and the majority of pseudo-vertiginous symptoms relevant to the cervical spine are not caused by this pathology.

VESTIBULAR VERTIGO

Among the causes of vestibular vertigo, we can highlight Meniere's disease, otosclerosis, immune labyrinth disorders, labyrinth infections, vestibular neuronitis, ototoxic drugs, labyrinth injuries, acoustic neuromas and benign paroxysmal positional vertigo (BPPV).[84]

Central vertigo can be secondary to vascular disorders, such as vertebrobasilar insufficiency, or dissection, cerebellar infarction, malformations at the base of the skull, such as Chiari syndrome, and CNS tumours.

Characteristics of peripheral vertigo

Vestibular vertigo is characterized by a sensation of movement experienced by the subject in relation to the environment or vice versa and it is frequently of a rotatory nature. The onset is sudden: it lasts minutes, hours or days, and is accompanied by vegetative manifestations and hearing symptoms. Peripheral vertigo can be differentiated from central vertigo, given that the former often has a shorter duration (disappears after a while), with the exception of vestibular neuritis and Meniere's disease; it can be accompanied by hearing loss and/or tinnitus, and there are no neurological signs.[85] Table 8-1 outlines the differences between central and peripheral vertigo.

Benign paroxysmal positional vertigo

The most common peripheral vestibular vertigo is benign paroxysmal positional vertigo (BPPV). It is characterized by a sudden onset of rotational vertigo that typically lasts between 10 and 30 seconds. It can be triggered by rolling over in bed and tilting the head back. It is characterized by its short duration, rapid fatigue, and disappearance when the position that provoked it is maintained and/or changed and the appearance each time such a position is adopted. It can cease spontaneously or after otolith repositioning manoeuvres, and it sometimes reappears after a while.[86] Table 8-2 outlines the differences between cervicogenic dizziness and some peripheral and central causes of vertigo.

The aetiology of this entity seems to be the traumatic, infectious, degenerative or idiopathic detachment of the otoliths of the utricular macula and their deposit in a semicircular canal.[86–89] There are two possibilities with regard to the location: cupulolithiasis, if the otoliths remain attached to the cupula of the ampullary crest,[90,91] and canalolithiasis, if the otoliths fall into a semicircular canal where they are free-floating.[92,93]

In the majority of cases, the otolithic debris is located in the posterior semicircular canal (Fig. 8-11).[94] The vertigo is triggered when the patient extends or rotates the head; the otoliths are displaced into the posterior semicircular canal and generate an abnormal stimulus. This stimulation triggers vertigo that can be accompanied by nausea and vomiting.

The diagnosis of the BPPV is based on the Dix–Hallpike manoeuvre, which reproduces the vertigo and triggers nystagmus, with a latency of 2 seconds and a duration of 10–20 seconds. This diagnostic test is mainly for the posterior semicircular canal. The BPPV of the horizontal canal is diagnosed by the supine roll test or Pagnini–McClure manoeuvre.[95]

Dix–Hallpike manoeuvre

The Dix–Hallpike manoeuvre is performed with the patient sitting on the examination table with the legs extended. The patient's head is then rotated to the affected ear 45°. The clinician helps the patient to lie down backwards quickly with the head held in approximately 20° of extension. The manoeuvre is positive when the patient experiences vertigo associated with

TABLE 8-1 Diagnostic differences between central and peripheral vertigo		
	Peripheral BPPV	Central
Findings in the Dix–Hallpike test		
Latency of nystagmus symptoms	2–40 s	None
Severity of the vertigo	Severe	Moderate
Duration of the nystagmus	< 1 min	> 1 min
Fatigability	Yes	No
Habituation	Yes	No
Other findings		
Postural instability	Walking is possible, unidirection instability	Falls when walking, severe instability
Loss of hearing and tinnitus	They may be present	Normally not present
Other neurological symptoms	Absent	Normally present

From Swartz and Longwell.[99]

TABLE 8-2 Differences between cervical pseudo-vertigo and the rest of vertiginous phenomena				
	Frequent symptoms	Frequency	Duration	Trigger factors
Benign paroxysmal positional vertigo	Vertigo	Episodic	Seconds	Changes in the position of the head
Cervicogenic pseudo-vertigo	Dizziness, imbalance	Episodic	Minutes–hours	Related to positions or movements of the head
Labyrinthine concussion	Vertigo, imbalance	Episodic	Hours–days	Increases with movement
Central vestibular dysfunction	Dizziness, imbalance	More constant	Days–weeks	Can be seen in combination with pathologies of the inner ear

From Wrisley et al.[3]

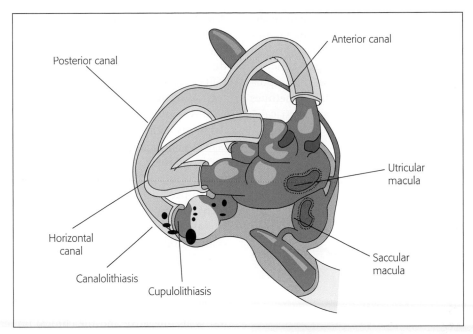

FIGURE 8-11 ■ The aetiology of BPPV seems to be the shedding of otoliths of utricular and saccular maculae and their deposit at sites further down the canal.

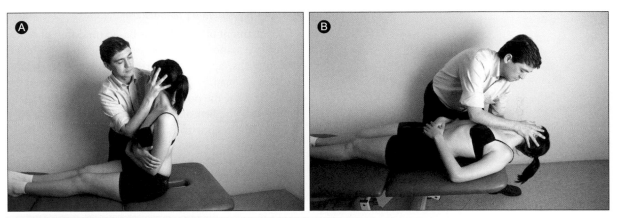

FIGURE 8-12 ■ (A, B) The Dix–Hallpike manoeuvre.

nystagmus. The nystagmus appears within the first 45 seconds after a characteristic 5–10 second period of latency[96] and then dissipates when this position is held (Fig. 8-12).

Supine roll test or Pagnini–McClure manoeuvre

To identify a BPPV of the lateral canal the supine roll test or Pagnini–McClure manoeuvre is used.[97] In this manoeuvre, the patient is lying down with the head resting on the bed with a cervical flexion of about 30°. The therapist turns the head by about 90° to each side while supine. During this manoeuvre, if the horizontal nystagmus is towards the ground, it is named geotropic nystagmus and if is towards the ceiling is an apogeotropic nystagmus. In the geotropic type of horizontal canal BPPV (HC-BPPV) the induced nystagmus is stronger when the head is turned toward the affected ear. In contrast, in the apogeotropic HC-BPPV the nystagmus is stronger when the head turns to the healthy ear. The presence of a geotropic nystagmus indicates that the patients has canalolithiasis and an ageotropic indicates a cupulolithiasis (Fig. 8-13).

To obtain a good therapeutic response, it is important to determine the affected side, which is sometimes difficult as the responses can be rather symmetrical.[98]

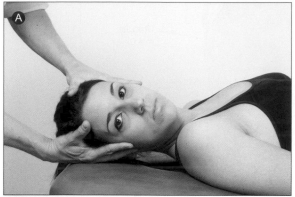

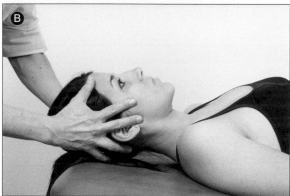

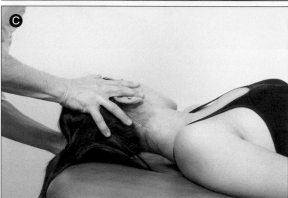

FIGURE 8-13 ■ (A–C) The supine roll test or Pagnini–McClure manoeuvre.

A nystagmus in the horizontal canal has different characteristics to a nystagmus in the posterior canal: the latency is shorter (0–3 s), the intensity is greater, the duration may be longer than 1 minute and the fatigability is less than that observed in the positional nystagmus of the posterior canal.[105]

It is always recommended to carry out a differential diagnosis with vestibular vertigo. The first assessment is neck active range of motion. If the characteristics of vertigo point to a BPPV, the Dix–Hallpike manoeuvre is performed. If the patient cannot tolerate this test due to neck pain or limitation of the range of movement, it can be performed with the patient in the lateral decubitus position, with their head facing the ceiling. Consequently, the cervical spine is maintained in a 45° rotation, by lowering the head of the examining table. If the test is positive, an Epley or Semont manoeuvre is performed. If Dix–Hallpike's manoeuvre is negative, the supine roll test is performed. If this test is also negative and the clinical presentation corresponds to a vestibular vertigo, the patient should be referred to an otoneurologist.

Otolith repositioning manoeuvres

The treatment of the BPPV is based on different repositioning manoeuvres, whose purpose is to mobilize the otoliths, applying a series of movements to the patient's head.[99] The repositioning manoeuvres described for the posterior canal are the Epley manoeuvre and the Semont manoeuvre. The treatment of BPPV in the horizontal canal, with the geotropic variant, can be carried out with the so-called barbecue technique or the Gufoni manoeuvre. A modified Sermont manoeuvre and the Gufoni method are proposed for the ageotropic variant.

Epley manoeuvre

The manoeuvre starts with the patient long sitting on the bed with their head turned 45° towards the affected ear. The clinician helps the patient to lie down backwards quickly with the neck in extension, maintaining the head rotation. In this way, the particles move from the cupula to the centre of the semicircular canal. Then, the therapist assists the patient to turn the head 45° towards the affected ear. The patient turns on the examining table until she reaches the lateral decubitus position, so that the nose is pointing to the floor. Then, the patient moves her knees towards the chest and returns to the sitting position. Finally, she returns the head to the neutral position. The holding time in each of these positions is approximately between 30 seconds and 1 minute (Fig. 8-14).

This manoeuvre is contraindicated in cases of carotid artery stenosis, an unstable coronary pathology and a serious cervical pathology, such as a myelopathy, cervical instability or rheumatoid arthritis.[100]

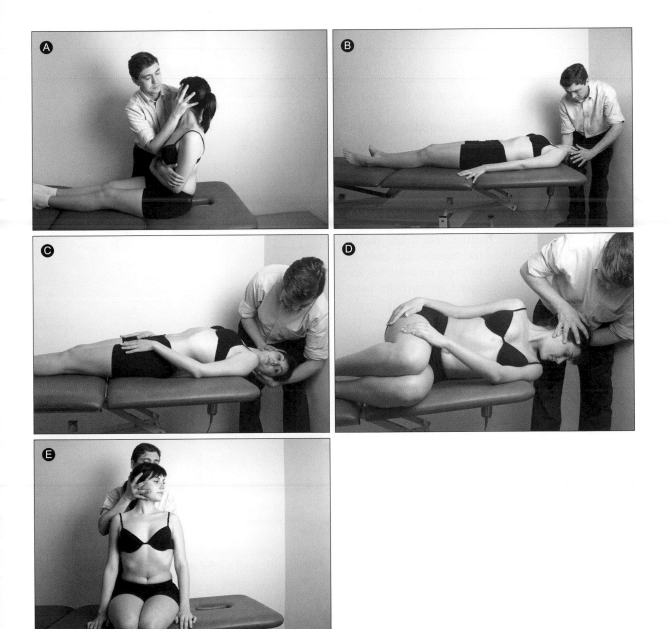

FIGURE 8-14 ■ (A–E) The Epley manoeuvre.

A Cochrane systematic review confirmed that Epley's manoeuvre is a safe and effective treatment of BPPV.[101] A single repositioning manoeuvre is effective in 75% of cases, and two manoeuvres are effective in 97% of cases.[102] The Epley manoeuvre is the only recommended method of treating BPPV of the posterior semicircular canal, with an A evidence level according to the American Academy of Neurology.[103]

Semont manoeuvre

This manoeuvre involves the rapid mobilization of the patient from one lateral decubitus position to another.[104] The patient is sitting on the bed with the head turned 45% towards the unaffected side. The therapist takes the patient rapidly to the lateral decubitus of the affected side, and this position is held for at least 1 minute. Then, the patient is taken quickly to the lateral decubitus of the other side and this position is held for 3 minutes with the head facing the floor (Fig. 8-15). Finally, the patient is slowly brought back to an upright seated position. The debris should then fall into the utricle of the semicircular canal. In order to stabilize the result of these manoeuvres, the patient is advised to not extend or turn the head. However, these measures seem unnecessary.[105–107] The recurrence of vertigo after the repositioning manoeuvres is not very frequent and does not reach 15% per year.[108]

Patients can be taught to practice the Semont manoeuvre at home as they are able to achieve canalith repositioning. The manoeuvre that is usually recommended is a variation of the Epley manoeuvre.[109] It is also possible to teach Brandt–Daroff's exercises.[86]

Brandt–Daroff exercises

These exercises can be easily learned by patients and are applicable for any canal. The Brandt–Daroff exercises are performed in a similar fashion to the Semont manoeuvre. Patients sit on the edge of the examining table, turn their head 45% to one side and quickly lie down on the other side, with their head facing the ceiling. Then, they wait in this position either until the vertigo disappears, or until at least 30 seconds have passed. Finally, patients return to the sitting position, wait another 30 seconds and perform the same exercise on the other side (Fig. 8-16).

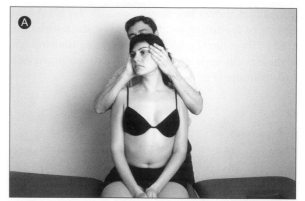

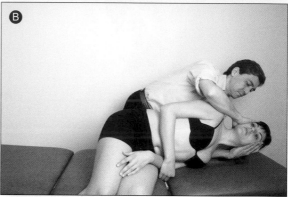

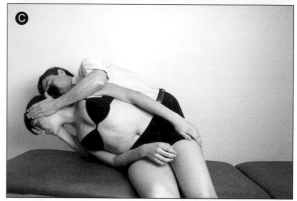

FIGURE 8-15 ■ (A–C) The Semont manoeuvre.

Horizontal canal BPPV repositioning

Lateral canal BPPV is often unresponsive to canalith repositioning designed to treat posterior canal BPPV. The most commonly used treatment is the Lempert manoeuvre or barbecue roll manoeuvre.[110] The patient starts in the supine position with the head fully rotated

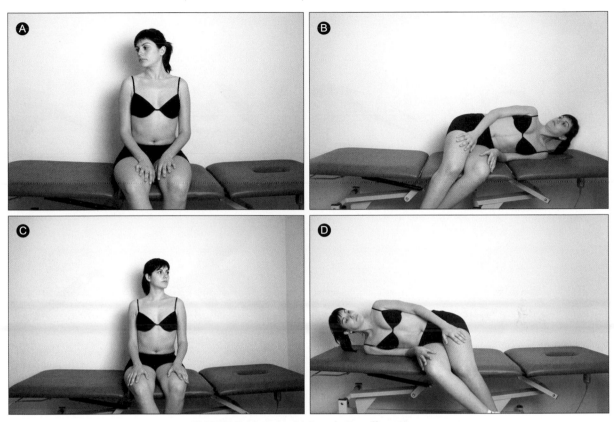

FIGURE 8-16 ■ (A–D) Brandt–Daroff exercises.

to the affected ear; the head is then turned quickly 90° towards the unaffected side and, sequentially, a series of 90° turns towards the unaffected side are undertaken until the patient has turned 360° and is back to the affected ear-down position. From there, the patient is turned to the face-up position and then brought up to the sitting position (Fig. 8-17). This manoeuvre was originally only outlined for the variant with geotropic nystagmus, but it can also be used for the treatment of apogeotropic form.

Another treatment for this canal is the Gufoni manoeuvre.[111] The patient quickly moves from the sitting position to the lateral decubitus of the unaffected side, then turns the head 45° (facing the floor) and sits up again.

Other common vestibular vertigos

Meniere disease or *endolymphatic hydrops* is a disorder of the inner ear that can cause episodes of vertigo and hearing loss. The symptoms of Meniere disease are variable but the most common are severe attacks of spontaneous rotational vertigo, that last anywhere between 20 minutes to several hours, tinnitus and hearing loss.

Labyrinthitis and *vestibular neuronitis* are characterized by vertigo episodes of longer duration, which can be aggravated with changes in position in any direction, and can force the patient to stay in bed for several days.[89]

CLINICAL ASSESSMENT OF CERVICOGENIC DIZZINESS AND SENSORIMOTOR CONTROL IMPAIRMENTS

The assessment of CD is complex, since there is no single specific and conclusive diagnostic test. In the assessment it is necessary to consider the subjective

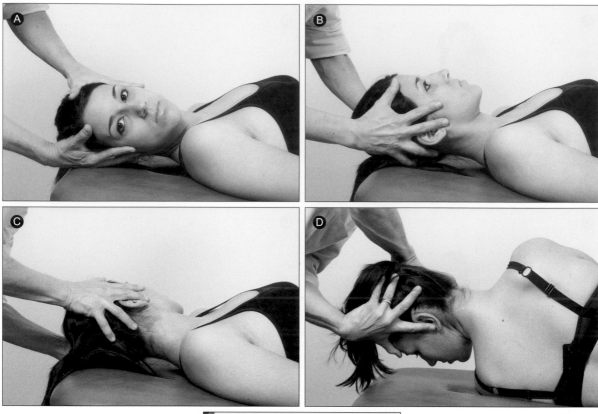

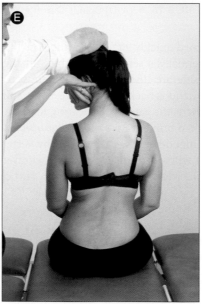

FIGURE 8-17 ■ (A–E) The barbecue roll manoeuvre.

examination in conjunction with findings of cervical musculoskeletal and sensorimotor dysfunction.

Subjective assessment

Clinical features and patient history can be indicative of cervicogenic dizziness. First, there should be a time relationship between the onset of the CD and other neck symptoms. However, it should be pointed out that is not uncommon for subjects with vestibular vertigo to report neck symptoms, since they can develop neck stiffness trying to reduce head movements in order avoid a vertiginous crisis; thus, a primary vestibular pathology creating a secondary neck problem.

Cervicogenic dizziness is a frequent complaint following a whiplash injury and it tends to be more severe in subjects with persistent symptoms.[112] It should be noted that whiplash injury can be also associated with traumatic vestibular pathology, including BPPV, due to the labyrinthine concussion. A whiplash injury is considered to be a direct cause of BPPV, especially when head trauma is associated.[113] A whiplash injury can also be linked to a concussion of the brainstem or an injury of the cervical arteries that can be expressed as a central vertigo.[28,32,114,115]

If, after trauma, vertigo is accompanied by an acute and severe unilateral headache, it is possible that the cause is a cervical artery dissection. In these cases, neurological signs and symptoms usually appear, such as alterations of vision, motor incoordination or alteration of gait.[28,35,38] It is thus essential to perform an adequate neurological examination to assist differential diagnosis when this is suspected.[116]

Possible aetiologies of post-traumatic dizziness:

- cervicogenic dizziness
- benign paroxysmal positional vertigo
- labyrinthine concussion
- brainstem concussion
- cervical artery dissection.

A patient with CD reports a subjective sensation of imbalance, and not the rotatory vertigo characteristic of vestibular vertigo.[1] The symptoms of CD can be described as unsteadiness or subjective imbalance and can be associated with subjective visual sensations like blurred vision and focusing difficulties.[117]

The frequency of symptoms, the temporal relationship with neck pain, its duration and trigger factors can also help to distinguish cervical dizziness from the other types of vertiginous sensations. CD is episodic and lasts minutes or hours.

The trigger factors of CD are all those activities that are associated with movements or positions of the head. Frequently, the dizziness sensation appears with the first movement of the head, after it has been held in a sustained rotation position for some time.

The cervicogenic dizziness is a subjective unsteadiness sensation and not the rotatory vertigo that is characteristic of vestibular vertigo.

Physical assessment

Signs of cervical musculoskeletal dysfunction such as joint dysfunction, altered neuromotor control and range of motion should be demonstrated in patients with CD.[118,119]

Furthermore, a series of tests relating to cervical sensorimotor control have also been developed in order to support the cervical aetiology of dizziness. These include the cervical nystagmus test, cervical joint position and movement sense tests, oculomotricity tests (e.g. smooth-pursuit neck torsion test) and posturological examination, both clinical and with the aid of a posturography platform. Many of these tests have been described by Jull et al.[119] Treleaven et al.[1,22,26] It is suggested that no one test alone can diagnose CD, but that clinical reasoning of the findings in a cluster of tests, associated with the patient's subjective reports and cervical musculoskeletal impairments, is most useful for differential diagnosis of CD.

Nystagmus test with cervical rotation

The therapist observes the appearance of nystagmus while the patient turns the body, keeping the head stable[120–122] (Fig. 8-18). In theory, a CD can be identified using this test, as the cervical proprioceptors are stimulated without stimulating the vestibular system.

Oosterveld et al.[123] showed that 64% of 262 patients with cervical pain who attended an Otorhinolaryngology Department after a cervical whiplash had nystagmus with this manoeuvre. However, the nystagmus that appears with this type of test is not always specific of CD. It has been demonstrated that up to 50% of

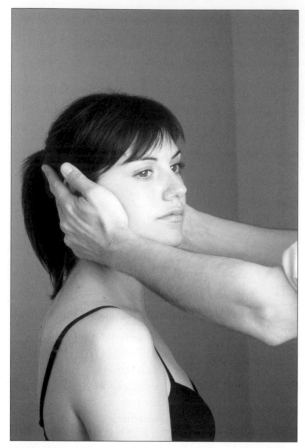

FIGURE 8-18 ■ The nystagmus test with cervical rotation: the patient rotates the trunk while the therapist stabilizes the head.

the subjects with no pathology of the cervical spine showed nystagmus with this test,[122,124] likely due to manifestation of a normal COR.[3] Recently however, L'Heureux-Lebeau et al.[125] demonstrated differences in this nystagmus test with cervical rotation held for 30 seconds each in (a) left torsion, (b) neutral, (c) right torsion and (d) neutral with 52% of patients with CD exhibiting a positive test (nystagmus > 2° in any one of the four positions as measured by videonystagography) compared to 8% in patients with diagnosed BPPV. Thus, it is thought this might be useful, particularly when in association with other findings suggestive of CD.

Cervicocephalic kinaesthesia

Different tests have been developed in order to support the cervical spine aetiology of the dizziness

based on the assessment of the cervicocephalic kinaesthesia or propioception. One of these is the *joint position error* (JPE) test developed by Revel et al.[126] It measures the patient's ability to find the natural head posture after having performed a head movement with the eyes closed. This alteration of the cervical kinaesthesia reflects abnormal afferent input from neck joint and muscle proprioceptors or an alteration of CNS processing of this information. Subjects who have persistent neck pain or have suffered a cervical whiplash and refer a CD have demonstrated lower accuracy than normal subjects in this test.[1,4,6,8,10,126,127]

To assess the joint position error, the subject is seated 90 cm away from the wall with eyes closed and with the cervical spine in the neutral natural head position. A laser pointer is placed on the head of the patient, and it projects onto a blackboard or a piece of paper. The therapist first asks the patient to concentrate on their neutral resting position. Patients then carry out a specific movement to their comfortable range and then are asked to return to this neutral position with their eyes closed. The patient's head is repositioned back to the original starting position and repeated. The difference between neutral and end point is measured in centimetres after each movement. The average of three relatively consistent attempts should be measured (Fig. 8-19). The movements should be performed slowly, as by performing them in such a way that the cervical proprioception is more involved than the vestibular system. The accuracy is measured in centimetres, which can be converted into degrees and can be used as an outcome measure (Fig. 8-20).

The JPE test using the laser has been validated against more sophisticated equipment and thus can be considered a suitable clinical measure.[128] Furthermore, according to this study, an error less than 3° is considered to be normal, between 3° and 4.5° acceptable and the test is considered positive when the error is more than 4.5°.[126] The same test can be used to improve proprioceptive kinaesthetic control in subjects suffering from cervicogenic dizziness.[129]

Chen and Treleaven[130] have recently developed a modified JPE test (*JPE torsion test*) in which the subject, instead of rotating the cervical spine, rotates the trunk while the therapist gently keeps the head steady. In this case the laser pointer is attached to the chest. In the

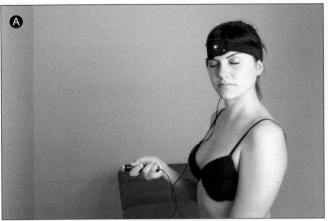 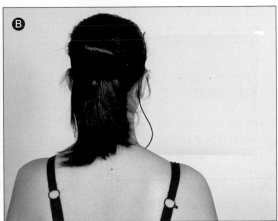

FIGURE 8-19 ■ The cervicocephalic kinaesthesia test. The patient starts in the neutral head position, which is projected by the laser beam. She then closes her eyes and performs each of these movements: right cervical rotation, left cervical rotation and extension (A). After each movement, she attempts to come back to the neutral position as accurately as possible (B).

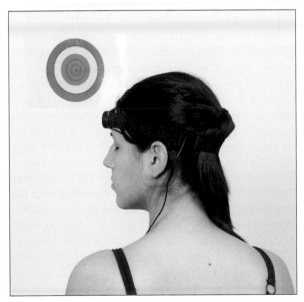

FIGURE 8-20 ■ The JPE can be measured in degrees. An error less than 3° is considered to be normal, between 3° and 4.5° is acceptable and the test is positive when the error is more than 4.5°

conventional JPE test, the movement of the head during the test can also stimulate the vestibular system. In the JPE torsion test, the trunk rotation produces a relative neck rotation, stimulating the cervical neck afferents, but it has no effect on the vestibular system. In Chen and Treleaven's study, the patients with neck pain had significantly greater errors in one of the conventional JPE tests and in almost all the JPE torsion tests when compared to an asymptomatic control group. This suggests that the JPE torsion test may be a more appropriate test than the conventional JPE when trying to differentiate altered cervical afferent information from vestibular dysfunction in people with chronic neck pain with dizziness. Nevertheless, this hypothesis needs further exploration.

Kristjansson et al.,[9] using Revel's test, have shown that kinaesthetic errors can help to distinguish asymptomatic subjects from those with neck symptoms, both insidious and secondary to whiplash. However, the results obtained from other works show limited evidence of kinaesthetic alterations in subjects with non-traumatic cervical pain.[131] JPE deficits appear to be more prevalent in subjects with post-traumatic neck pain[9] and, especially, in those that report more severe symptoms, dizziness and higher levels of disability.[1,8,12,132] Furthermore, in a recent paper, L'Heureux-Lebeau et al.[125] also concluded this to be a helpful test to differentiate CD from BPPV, where JPE of 4.5° in at least one direction of movement is considered abnormal.

Rod and frame test

Cervical spine abnormal proprioceptive afferences can also cause an alteration in verticality perception which requires external information from vision to be integrated with vestibular information and cervical spine proprioception. It has been suggested that altered proprioceptive afferent input originating from the cervical region can disturb the perception of the vertical orientation.[133]

The perception of verticality can be measured quantitatively with the rod and frame test. This test is currently carried out with computer software that generates a luminescent vertical rod surrounded by a square frame on the screen.[134] The rod and the frame can rotate independently one from each other. The subject is required to position an offset rod into the vertical position using a joystick (Fig. 8-21).

Grod and Diakow[135] have shown that the rod and frame test was impaired in subjects with neck pain. Bagust et al.[136] compared 71 patients with neck pain with 17 asymptomatic control subjects and showed that symptomatic subjects were significantly less accurate in the perception of verticality compared to asymptomatic controls. Similarly, Uthaikhup et al.[133] have shown that elderly patients with neck pain have greater difficulty in perceiving verticality in comparison to those without neck pain. However, there is large variability even in asymptomatic control subjects and this test can also be impaired in those with brain injury

or vestibular pathology, so this may not be as useful as other tests of cervical proprioception for differential diagnosis of CD.[133,135–137]

Oculomotor control tests

As detailed above, the COR complements the VOR in helping to maintain gaze stability, especially during low-frequency slow head movements. Oculomotor dysfunctions are very common between whiplash-associated disorder (WAD) in patients and they are thought to be related to disturbances of cervical or vestibular afferents or a deficit in the CNS integration sensorimotor control information. Oculomotor disorders deserve more attention as they may be involved in many symptoms reported by patients that are scarcely paid any attention to due to their subjective nature. Patients often report some visual and oculomotor disturbances in idiopathic neck pain or after a whiplash injury, such as blurred vision, visual fatigue, and some of these patients have been described as diplopia to near vision, altered oculomotor divergence, unilateral or bilateral deficit of the internal rectum muscle, nausea or dizziness after convergence test, etc.[24,117,138] Oculomotor dysfunctions may be hidden causes of disability following whiplash injury and may indicate a poor prognosis.[139,140] One oculomotor test thought to be a specific test to the presence of a CD is the smooth-pursuit neck torsion (SPNT) test.[141]

Smooth-pursuit neck torsion test. This test compares the ability to follow a moving target smoothly with the eyes, with the head and neck in the neutral position versus a torsioned position (Fig. 8-22). A decrease in the ability to follow smoothly in the torsion positions is indicative of cervical afferent involvement in eye movement control. Supporting the cervical afferent cause is that these changes during neck torsion are not seen in those with brain injury or peripheral vestibular pathology.[141,142] There are currently many studies that show alterations of SPNT in subjects that have suffered a cervical whiplash,[1,21–23,141] idiopathic neck pain and CD.[138,140] Originally developed by Tjell and Rosenhall,[141] it has a good sensitivity (72%) and specificity (91%) as a diagnostic test for a cervical whiplash injury.[21,141] Subjects with post-traumatic neck pain, especially those complaining of dizziness, have higher deficits in the test than subjects with non-traumatic

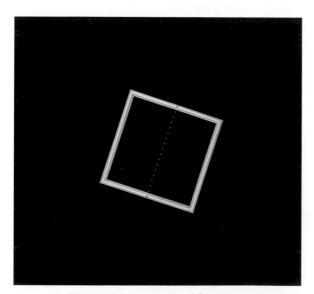

FIGURE 8-21 ■ Rod and frame test.

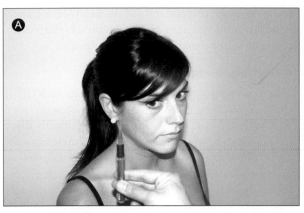
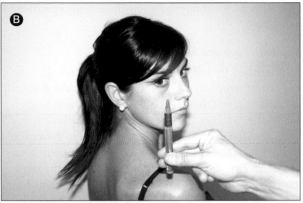

FIGURE 8-22 ■ The smooth-pursuit neck torsion (SPNT) test: head in neutral position (A) and trunk rotation (B).

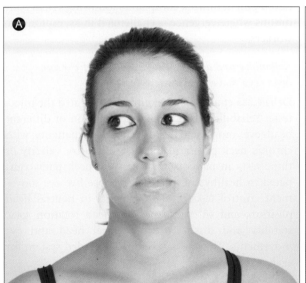
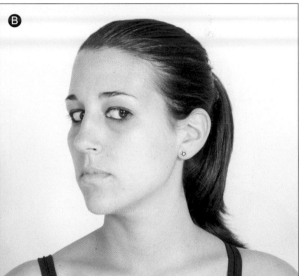

FIGURE 8-23 ■ (A, B) The eye mobility test.

neck pain.[10,21,22,138,141,143,144] Electro-oculography can be used in order to conduct research studies and objectively records the eye movements,[22,23,143] although recent work suggests that it may be possible to detect these differences visually.[145] In this study, visual assessment of fast eye movements between two targets for 10 seconds in the neutral position and then repeated when the neck was torsioned to the left and right 45° were performed[145] (Fig. 8-23). More work is needed to examine this further using the original methodology of the SPNT.

Gaze stability test

The gaze stability test is assessed as described by Jull et al.,[119] by asking patients to keep their eyes fixed on a point and perform cervical movements of rotation and flexion–extension (Fig. 8-24). The test is positive if patients are unable to keep their eyes fixed, cannot move their head smoothly or in a suitable range of motion (approximately 40°) or if visual symptoms or dizziness appear.[82] Patients with neck pain have demonstrated impairments in this task (26, 145), although again this test in isolation is not a specific test for

CD and can be abnormal in in those with vestibular pathology.

Sequential eye and head movements

As described by Jull et al.[119] and Treleaven et al.,[26] the test is performed in the following manner: the patient is asked to move their eyes 30° to the right and to then rotate the head in the same direction while keeping their gaze fixed. The patient is then asked to move the eyes back to the starting position, keeping their head fixed and afterwards the head moves back to the starting position (Fig. 8-25). The same test is performed to the left and into flexion and extension.[26,119] Inability to move the eyes independently of the head is considered abnormal and was seen in those with whiplash compared to asymptomatic control individuals.[26]

Ocular vergence tests

When carrying out assessments of patients with CD, it can be interesting to evaluate if oculomotor vergence is impaired. Again, while this is not specifically diagnostic, it can be useful to help guide tailored management. Some of the convergence tests are described in Figures 8-26 and 8-27. It should be noted that, currently, there is limited research in this area, with only one study to date that has demonstrated altered vergence in people with neck pain.[146] The majority of research in this area has been concerned with the development of neck complaints following visual conditions where vergence is challenged in asymptomatic workers.[147]

Reliability and discriminative validity of clinical head–eye movement control tests

Della Casa et al.[145] have recently investigated the intertester reliability of the visual observation of different head–eye movement control tests in patients with chronic neck pain and the discriminative validity of these tests in patients with chronic neck pain compared to healthy controls. They chose five eye movement control tests: eye movements in neutral head position, and 45° right and left head rotation, gaze stability and dissociated sequential head and eye movements. They also developed a graded system for each test.

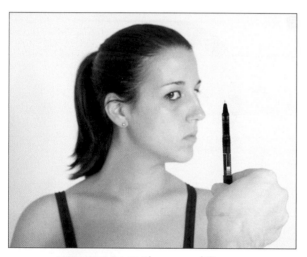

FIGURE 8-24 ■ The gaze stability test.

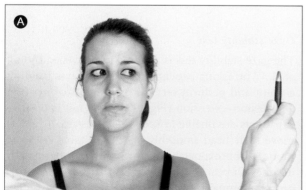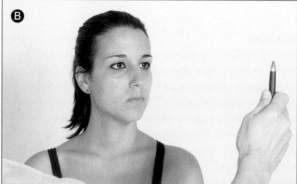

FIGURE 8-25 ■ (A, B) Sequential eye and head movements.

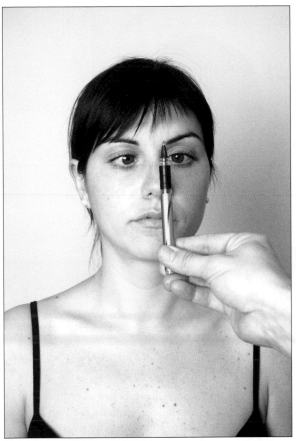

FIGURE 8-26 ■ *Convergence test:* the subject looks at the tip of a pen as it gets closer from a distance of 20 cm to the base of the nose. This shows if the one eye is unable to converge during the test and it goes in divergence.

TABLE 8-3	
Rating scale of eye movements in neutral head position	
Rating	**Definition**
0 = negative	Smooth, precise, fast eye movements, fast change of gaze direction, head remains stable
1 = moderately positive	Slightly irregular eye movements. Short stops before changing gaze direction. Head slightly unstable
2 = strongly positive	Eye movements clearly slower or irregular. Prolonged maintenance of gaze direction before changing direction. Obvious head movement. Test cannot be performed

From Della Casa et al.[145] with author's permission.

TABLE 8-4	
Rating scale of gaze stability	
Rating	**Definition**
0 = negative	Gaze stable. Smooth, well-coordinated, precise and fast movement of the head, fluent change of head movement direction
1 = moderately positive	Gaze stable. Slightly irregular head movement
2 = strongly positive	Gaze repeatedly unstable. Head movement slow and irregular

From Della Casa et al.[145] with author's permission.

In the eye movement in neutral head position test, subjects were required to hold their head in the neutral position while moving their eyes sideways from one marker to the other as fast as possible for 10 seconds (Table 8-3).

In the gaze stability test, subjects were asked to hold a stable gaze while moving their head from left to right as far and as fast as possible for 10 seconds (Table 8-4).

In the sequential head and eye movements test, subjects moved their eyes to the right or to the left with the head remaining still and then they rotated the head in the same direction with gaze remaining fixed. All these movements were to be repeated for 10 seconds. For the eye movements in neck rotation test, the subjects held a 45° relative right or left rotation and moved the gaze as fast as possible for 10 seconds (Table 8-5).

It was shown that visual assessment by physiotherapists of head–eye movement control tests is reliable. Two or more positive tests out of five can be interpreted as impaired head–eye movement control. This tests battery was able to discriminate between patients with chronic neck pain and controls and thus could also be useful for the differential diagnosis of CD. However, future refinement of the tests in accordance with previous research findings and comparison to more sophisticated assessment as well as comparison to other pathologies such as peripheral vestibular pathology is warranted.

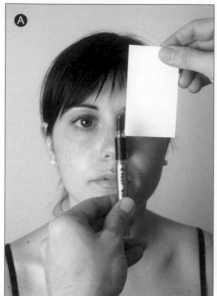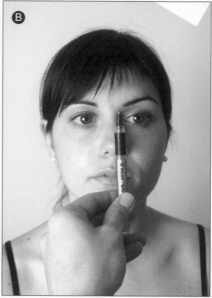

FIGURE 8-27 ■ (A, B) The cover test is useful when the previous tests are normal and detects the presence of ocular deviation. A pen is placed 20 cm away from the patient's eyes; each eye is covered alternatively with the hand or a card. Every time one of the eyes is uncovered, it should stay fixed. If the uncovered eye performs a return movement, there is a convergence deficit. It should be emphasized that there is not necessarily a relation between convergence deficits and cervicogenic dizziness.

TABLE 8-5	
Rating scale of sequential head and eye movements	
Rating	**Definition**
0 = negative	Clear, regular, smooth, dissociated movements of head and eyes
1 = moderately positive	Slightly decelerated eye movements, occasional associated eye–head movements, head unstable
2 = strongly positive	Clearly decelerated, irregular and often associated eye–head movements, test not feasible

From Della Casa et al.[145] with author's permission.

Standing balance assessment

In the evaluation of sensorimotor impairments in patients with CD, it is important to do postural balance assessment to direct management. However, this type of examination is not exclusively designed for patients with CD and has little discriminative value in CD on its own. Nevertheless, the results may help to confirm or refute CD as the diagnosis. Some clinical tests can be used such as the Romberg, tandem, the step and the Fukuda–Unterberger test.[148] Generally, altered balance in people with neck pain is associated with altered anterior posterior sway, especially when vision is altered.

Romberg test. It helps to observe changes in posture and in the amplitude of the postural body sway with feet together and eyes closed for 30 seconds. This test is usually performed with the patient's index fingers pointing forward (Fig. 8-28). The Romberg test can also be performed by eliminating the plantar afferences, placing a foam mat under the feet (Fig. 8-29). Patients with vestibular pathology demonstrate greater deficits in this test when compared to those with CD.

Recent work suggests that it may be possible to use a test of comfortable stance (rather than narrow stance) eyes closed,[142] performed with the head torsioned to either side to observe if there is an increase in postural body sway in these positions compared to the neutral position,[149] to detect altered balance of a cervical nature. However, it is not known whether

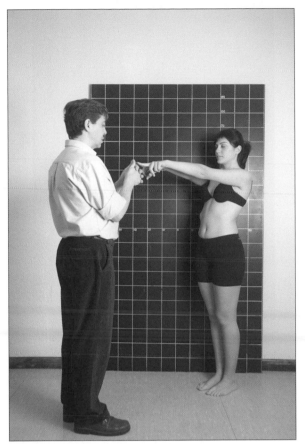

FIGURE 8-28 ■ Postural Romberg test. Changes are observed in the position and amplitude of the postural oscillations when the patient closes her eyes for about 30 seconds.

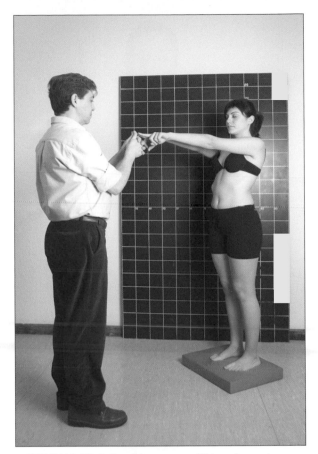

FIGURE 8-29 ■ Romberg test modifying plantar input.

these subtle changes can be detected without sophisticated equipment.

Tandem test. Patients are asked to stand with their feet in tandem for 30 seconds while keeping their eyes closed (Fig. 8-30). Treleaven et al.[18] and Field et al.[150] have shown that patients with neck pain, in particular those with whiplash-associated disorders, especially if they reported instability or dizziness, often presented a positive tandem test: i.e. failed to maintain the position for 30 seconds.

Fukuda–Unterberger test. Fukuda showed that the asymmetries of the postural tone can be detected during dynamic activities. The test, also known as the

stepping test, involves asking the patient to step in place without moving, with eyes closed. In normal circumstances, the patient should not travel less than 1 m forward or turn more than 45° in 50 steps.[151–155]

A series of conditions must be met in order for this test to be valid: the lack of a sound or light source that may orientate the patient; the patient's hip should be flexed 45°; the rhythm of the steps should be 1.2–1.4 Hz; and the subject should keep the eyes looking forward before closing them and be barefoot (Fig. 8-31).

The test is repeated while observing the influence of the nuchal reflex (Fig. 8-32). The rotation of the cervical spine increases the tone of the extensor muscles of the lower limb of the same side. In this way, if a subject performs this test with the head turned to the right, due to the increase in tone of the right extensor muscles, she will tend to move to the left

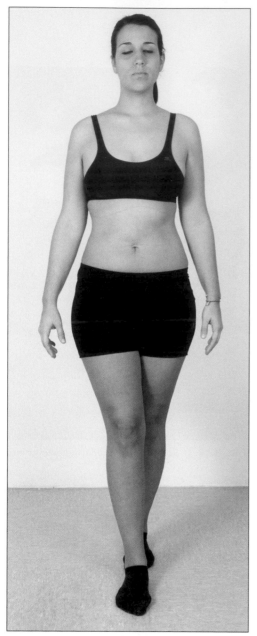

FIGURE 8-30 ■ The tandem test.

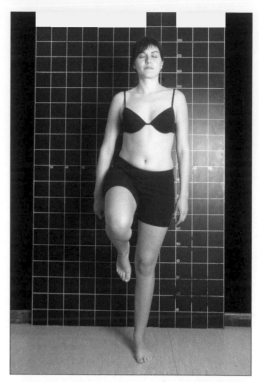

FIGURE 8-31 ■ The Fukuda–Unterberger test.

well as its sensitivity and specificity for vestibular pathology.[20,156,157]

Functional balance

Functional balance measures include the step test, tandem walk and walking with head turns and up and down.[20,158,159] The step test measures the number of times one foot is completely placed onto and off a 10 cm block within 15 seconds and has been shown to be impaired in subjects with neck pain.[20] Walking with large range, slow, head turns and movements in the sagittal plane can also be impaired in those with neck pain.[20,132,136]

Posturography

Posturography records postural body sway on a computerized dynamometric platform. Posturography makes it possible to quantify postural oscillations and, depending on the conditions in which the test is carried out, to observe the relative contribution of

(Fig. 8-33). The normal direction is when the patient turns to the opposite direction to the neck rotation.[154] However, an abnormal response is not necessarily associated with CD and more research is required to determine the relevance in CD assessment as

each sensory system (vestibular, visual and proprioceptive) to postural (Fig. 8-34).

Although posturography does not diagnose the aetiology of the balance dysfunction, it helps to

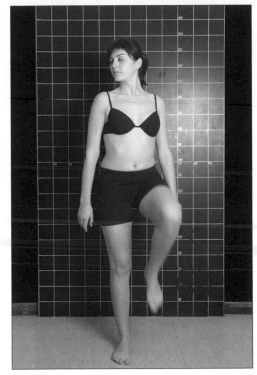

FIGURE 8-32 ■ The Fukuda–Unterberger test to analyse the influence of nuchal reflex. However, this test is not specific for CD

quantify the postural control deficits in patients with CD.[160,161] It is currently considered to be a useful tool in the analysis of postural control impairments in subjects with CD, especially in those that have suffered cervical whiplash.[18,20,23,24,54,149,150,162–177]

Posturographic examination is composed of a series of tests where conflictive situations are created for the postural system, by modifying different information from the sensory systems (visual, vestibular and proprioceptive).

The various posturographic tests attempt to subject the patients to certain conditions (eyes open, eyes closed, standing on one foot, standing on both feet, etc.) which determine the information from the visual, vestibular and proprioceptive sensory systems to establish the displacement of the centre of pressure (CoP).

The CoP represents the result from the forces of inertia of the body and the forces to restore the balance of the postural control system. When a subject maintains a stable position, her CoP approximately represents the projection of her centre of gravity. Based on the ground reaction vector and its application points, these systems calculate the CoP and its displacement based on time.[173,174] Records obtained represent the displacements in the anteroposterior (AP) axis and medial-lateral (ML) axis of the CoP, as well as the forces exerted. The registration time for the test has been studied and currently it is considered that optimum reliability is achieved with a duration of 20–30 seconds.[175,176]

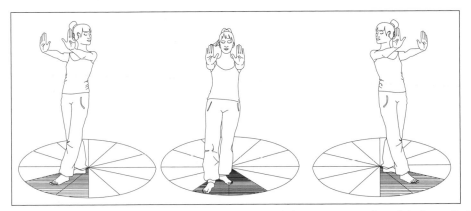

FIGURE 8-33 ■ The rotation of the cervical spine increases the tone of the extensor muscles of the lower limb on the same side.

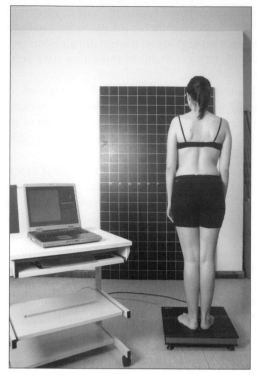

FIGURE 8-34 ■ Satel posturographic platform.

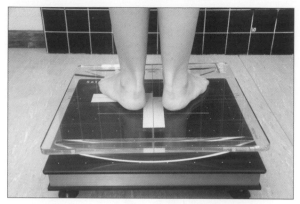

FIGURE 8-35 ■ A plane that increases oscillations in the coronal plane was placed on the posturographic platform.

Posturographic tests can take different sequences and integrate different conditions. The interest of these different sequences is to investigate the postural interactions between the different postural data. The subject usually starts in the position of maximum stability with eyes open (EO) on a stable platform (SP); the complexity of the situation gradually increases, influencing the different mechanisms involved in balance control – eyes closed (EC), unstable platform (US).

The visual input is eliminated with eyes closed or altered with optokinetic stimulation. Afterwards, the test can be performed on a dynamic posturography platform or by placing a moving plate on the platform, which causes oscillations in the sagittal and coronal planes (Fig. 8-35). This somatosensory input can also be modified with a foam pad placed on the platform. It is also tested with eyes open and eyes closed. The possible influence of the cervical spine can be assessed if the tests are carried out with neck torsion to the left or right.[149]

Different tests can be performed, depending on the type of available platform. Here are some examples:

1. SP with EO: this allows for maximum stability, since the patient uses all the postural sensory information (visual, vestibular and proprioceptive).
2. SP with EC: balance is obtained with the vestibular and proprioceptive system.
3. SP with EO and optokinetic stimulation: the optokinetic stimulation creates a visual conflict that should be compensated by the vestibular and proprioceptive system.
4. UP with EO and imbalance in the sagittal or coronal plane: in this situation, a proprioceptive conflict is created, since the body sways cause platform movement in these planes, and this needs to be compensated by the visual, vestibular systems and also neck proprioception (Fig. 8-36).
5. UP with EC and imbalance in the sagittal or coronal plane: in this case, the proprioceptive conflict created by the movement of the platform in these planes, with the elimination of the visual input, should be compensated with the vestibular system.

In order to make this test more sensitive in subjects with CD all these tests can be performed with the neck in different positions, such as right and left torsion or neck extension.[149a–d] For example: SP with EO and the cervical spine in extension, right or left neck torsion:

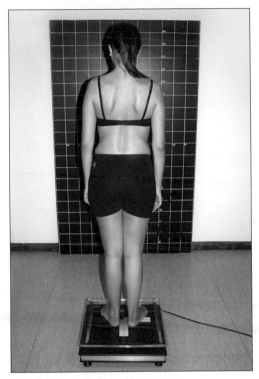

FIGURE 8-36 ■ Posturographic examination on an unstable platform in the sagittal plane.

there is a conflict with the cervical afferent information and mainly with the extension of the head, there is also a disturbance in the vestibular information, that can be compensated with visual and other somatosensory body information[7] UP with EC: somatosensory body information should compensate the conflict between the vestibular system, visual and cervical afferent information.

Posturographic analysis. A considerable amount of information is provided by a posturographic computerized system analysis. We will only point out some data that may facilitate the analysis of the signal obtained with the stabilometric platform.

There are different parameters to describe the complexity of the CoP pattern. There is little standardization in data collection protocols and methods used to analyse the fluctuations of the CoP.[180] Studies to establish the reliability of the variables of CoP[181,182]

have been conducted. The variables that have shown good reliability in the assessment of postural control are the range of CoP (mm), mean velocity variable (MVLO), root mean square (RMS) and mean frequency (MFRQ).[181–185]

However, it now seems that these parameters measuring displacement length, area and velocity of CoP are not sufficient to analyse the complexity of the signal obtained and thus determine changes in postural control. A decrease in body sway is not always indicative of a good postural control strategy. In fact this decrease may be indicative of excessive rigidity in patients who are subjectively unstable.[186] Indeed, some patients have what has been termed 'postural blindness'. These patients show lower CoP displacement with eyes closed than with eyes open, showing a coefficient of Romberg below normal (2.88).[187] This postural blindness has been interpreted as a manifestation of a failure of integration of visual information in subjects with postural control deficits but can also be the result of a hypervigilance strategy, common in patients who feel themselves unstable and are afraid of falling when closing their eyes.

Therefore, one of the approaches to the analysis of the CoP signal is the wavelet analysis, decomposing it into multiple independent frequency bands with fast Fourier transforms (FFTs). This type of signal analysis is thought to be reliable to identify specific postural control changes related to altered proprioceptive input from the neck.[188]

CoP oscillations can be represented linearly (stabilogram), vectographically (statokinesiogram) or spectral based on the frequency spectrum analysis. Today, normative values are published using standardized platforms. One of them is *Normes 85 of the Association Posture et Equilibre*[189] described by Gagey. The difficulty is that the construction of these platforms must meet very specific protocols.[190] Statokinesiograms describe the different successive positions of the CoP in relation to a reference, located on the geometric centre of the support polygon. The statokinesiogram is drawn on a diagram and helps determine the mean position in the sagittal and coronal planes, from which the values of surface and length are calculated. The surface is the confidence ellipse area, expressed in square millimetres, and it contains the successive positions of the CoP. The surface

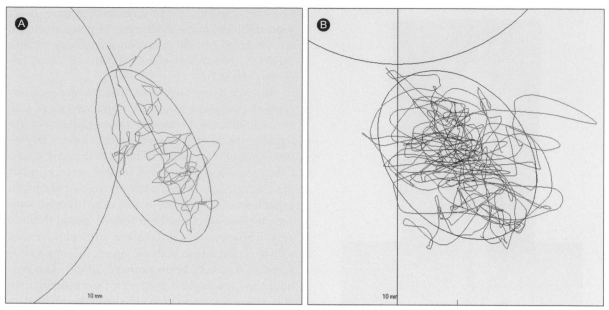

FIGURE 8-37 ■ The statokinesogram allows us to quantify the surface and length. (A) The subject shows a small area and a very small length. (B) The surface is slightly larger and with a considerably greater length.

evaluates the efficiency of the postural system in order to maintain the centre of gravity in its average balance position.

Surface	Mean (upper and lower limit)
Eyes open	91 (39–210)
Eyes closed	225 (79–638)

The length expresses the path that runs through the CoP during the test (Fig. 8-37).

Romberg's quotient is the product, expressed in percentage of the surface with eyes open in relation to the surface with eyes closed. In this way, it is possible to analyse the participation of the visual input in orthostatic balance. Normally, the surface increases around 250%, with normal values of Romberg's quotient being 2.88 (between 1.12 and 6).[77]

Similar to Romberg's quotient, the relevance of the plantar afferent information in postural control can be calculated with the plantar quotient. This can be obtained from the relationship between the surface recorded when performing the test on foam and that obtained on a stable platform. Evidently, there are no normative values due to the different thickness and density of the foam used.

The stabilogram records the coordinates of the successive positions of the centre of pressure in relation to time, and two graphs are obtained: one graph for the forward–backward (Y) movements and another graph for the right–left (X) movements. The mean X and mean Y values are obtained by calculating the oscillations obtained with the stabilogram (Fig. 8-38).[189] The mean Y corresponds to the average of the different positions of the CoP in the forward–backward direction.

The FFT decomposes postural sway data into different frequency bands. In this way, the different frequency bands are postulated to correspond to the different types of sensorimotor regulation channels. Distinct CoP signal frequency bandwidths have been identified, ranging from moderate to ultralow.[188] The slower frequencies correspond to the visual[191–193] and vestibular regulation channels,[194] while the low frequencies are related to cerebellar regulation[195,196] and the faster frequencies belong to the spinal reflex regulation and muscle activity.[195,197,198] It has been hypothesized that these high frequencies involve greater use of the proprioceptive control mechanisms[188,199–201] (Fig. 8-39). Four frequency bands often studied are:

■ Ultralow (0–0.10 Hz) corresponds to the slow visual circuits.

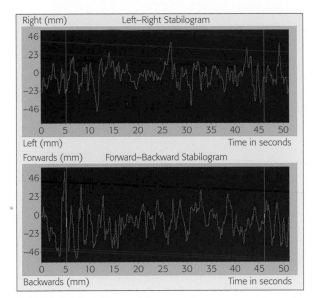

FIGURE 8-38 ■ The stabilogram allows two graphs to be obtained: one for forward–backward movements (Y) and another for right–left movements (X).

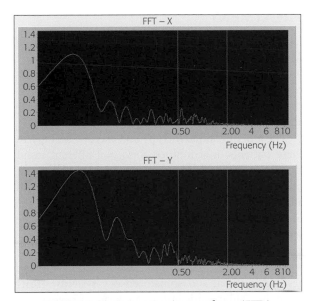

FIGURE 8-39 ■ Fast Fourier transforms (FFTs).

- Very low (0.10–0.39 Hz) corresponds to vestibular system activity.
- Low (0.39–1.56 Hz) corresponds to the cerebellar regulations.
- Moderate (1.56–6.25 Hz) represent the spinal reflex regulation and myotatic activity.

The vestibular and somatosensory system stabilize posture more efficiently at higher frequencies of body sway, while visual and vestibular system are more effective at lower frequencies.[202] At present, more research is needed in order to characterize posturographic reports in patients with neck pain as well as in those with cervicogenic dizziness. The studies that have specifically analysed frequency bandwidths suggest that subjects who have suffered cervical whiplash tend to use low frequencies.[177,178,203] Similarly, Quek et al.[177] found significant increase in the very low frequencies and a decrease in the moderate frequencies in older patients with neck pain. These results suggest that people with neck pain may have a reduced ability to recruit the muscular proprioception system and so they are more dependent on the vestibular system. Likewise, Röijezon et al.[203] studied the differences between subjects with a WAD and chronic non-specific neck pain. They found an increased magnitude of the slow sway component in WAD subjects, but not in chronic non-specific neck pain patients. They observed a correlation between the magnitude of the slow component in WAD and more severe balance disturbances, more severe sensory symptoms and a poorer physical functioning. This increased magnitude of the slow sway component in WAD patients may be a characteristic of altered cervical proprioceptive information or an altered integration of this information in the CNS.

Sensorial organization test

This test consists of the analysis of the relative contribution of somatosensory, visual and vestibular receptors to the patient's equilibrium. The objective of the test is to detect the sensory system responsible for the altered balance (Box 8-1).

There are platforms that offer many other interesting tools to assess the balance using a visual biofeedback.

Balance surface. The balance surface is the area that a subject can cover with the projection of her centre of gravity, without losing balance. To obtain this value, the subject is positioned on the platform and watches on the computer screen the status of the projection of her centre of gravity. Then, pivoting around her ankles, she tries to cover the largest possible area, without

BOX 8-1
SENSORIAL ORGANIZATION TEST

PATTERN OF SOMATOSENSORY AND VESTIBULAR DYSFUNCTION (SOMATOSENSORY INDEX)

This index tells us about the effect of cancelled visual input on balance. The standard platform eyes closed (SP–EC) test provides abnormally low values compared with the standard platform eyes open (SP–EO) test. The somatosensory stimuli are inadequate and are unable to compensate for the situation when the visual input on a stable platform disappears.

PATTERN OF VISUAL–VESTIBULAR DYSFUNCTION (VISUAL INDEX)

In this case, the tests altering sensory performed with eyes open provide poor results. For example, the unstable platform eyes open (UP–EO) test shows low values compared to SP–EO. Visual stimuli are inadequate and are unable to compensate for the alteration of somatosensory input.

PATTERN OF VESTIBULAR DYSFUNCTION (VESTIBULAR INDEX)

The test run with UPEC compared to the position of maximum stability or SP–EO offers abnormally low values. The vestibular information is unable to compensate for the situation caused by the *elimination* of the visual input and the change in somatosensory input.

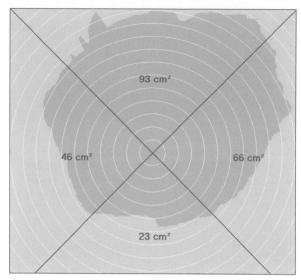

FIGURE 8-40 ■ Quantifying balance surface.

losing balance. With this information one can establish the limits of a subject's stability and the areas where her balance control is deficient (Fig. 8-40).

Summary

In summary, diagnosis of CD should be based on clinical reasoning following consideration of the patient's subjective reports and history in combination with results from the physical examination that should include a cervical musculoskeletal assessment as well as tests for sensorimotor control. Table 8-6 is a list of tests for sensorimotor control. It should be pointed out that a combination of tests is more important than any single test alone in the diagnosis of CD. They should also be used in conjunction with subjective assessment and other musculoskeletal findings.

Other tests of vestibular function may also be required, as directed by the examination findings (Table 8-7).

TREATMENT

Over the last few years, different strategies have been developed to manage CD and sensorimotor control impairments. These treatment methods can include manual therapy, therapeutic exercise, neck kinaesthetic retraining, oculo-cervical coordination, balance and tailored sensorimotor control exercises.

The aim of manual therapy and exercise therapy, in these patients, is to reduce abnormal afferent input from joints and muscles in order to normalize the neck proprioceptive sensitivity.[5,23] The treatment should adapt to specific articular and muscular impairments of the patient.[23,204] However, the CD can alter the sensory integration of the different sensorimotor control systems. It is therefore often necessary to use specific exercises that improve the integration of the vestibular, visual and somatosensory systems. Treatment directed towards improving head and eye movement control, proprioception and balance can be tailored according to the examination findings. Different vestibular rehabilitation exercises can also be incorporated as treatment strategy in CD.[205,206] Exercises that create conflictive situations between the different types of information in order to aid their integration are also useful.[23,119]

TABLE 8-6

Sensorimotor physical assessment tests relevant for cervicogenic dizziness (CD)

Indicated	Condition	Specificity of the test in differential diagnosis of CD[a]
Nystagmus related to neck rotation	Nystagmus test with cervical rotation	+
	Nystagmus test with cervical rotation held for 30 s (nystagmus greater than 2°/s)	+++
Cervicocephalic kinaesthesia	Joint position error test > 4.5° in any direction	+++
	Joint position error test in neck torsion	+++
	Rod and frame test	+
Oculomotor control tests	Smooth-pursuit neck torsion test	+++
	Gaze stability test	++
	Sequential eye and head movements	++
	Ocular vergence tests	+
Standing balance assessment	Postural Romberg test	+
	Tandem test	++
	Posturography	+
	Posturography – neck torsion	+++
Functional and dynamic tests	Fukuda–Unterberger test	+
	Walking with large slow head movements	++
	Step test	+

[a]High (+++), moderate (++), low (+).

Manual therapy

As stated by Jull et al.,[119] the treatment of patients with CD should not only address the somatosensory and proprioceptive impairments but also the joints and other structures implicated in the dysfunctional afferent barrage.

Reid and Rivett,[205] in 2005, performed a systematic review of the efficiency of the manual therapy in the treatment of the CD and suggested positive results, with a significant improvement of the signs and symptoms of CD after manual treatment.

Other studies have combined manual therapy with other treatments, such as electrotherapy, muscle relaxation exercises, biofeedback, and a neck collar.[45,207]

More recently, studies have been conducted into the long-term effectiveness of manual therapy on CD. Malmstrom et al.[118] studied the effect of different strategies in 22 patients with CD, and monitored them over a follow-up period of 2 years. This study was intended to report physical findings that could be linked to neck pain and dizziness and the long-term

effect of treatment of 22 patients. Treatment consisted of soft tissue techniques, local manual therapy, stabilization technique for neck, trunk and shoulders and body awareness and some home training programmes. In this study they found that cervical mobility recorded normal or even larger than expected values but mobility of the cervicothoracic spine was reduced. The authors hypothesized that the combination of a mobile/hypermobile cervical spine with a concomitant hypomobile cervicothoracic region as well as poor stability and postural imbalance could put stress on the neck, thus creating an abnormal proprioceptive inflow. They also found that these patients showed sensitivity to muscle palpation, and in relation to the zygapophysial joints, as well as poor postural balance and poor dynamic stability. In this study, treatment based on these findings reduced neck pain as well as dizziness over the long term but some patients also needed a maintenance strategy.[118]

Reid et al.[208] conducted a double-blind randomized controlled clinical trial to study the effectiveness of the

TABLE 8-7
Test indicated in the differential diagnosis of vestibular vertigo

Test	Indicated	Positive findings	Differential diagnosis
Hallpike–Dix	Vertigo with neck extension, rolling in bed, lasting a few seconds to minutes	Vertigo and nystagmus	Posterior canal BPPV
Pagnini–McClure	Vertigo and nystagmus with rolling in bed	Vertigo and horizontal nystagmus	Horizontal canal BPPV
VBI tests	Vertigo sustained head positions extension and rotation	Vertigo and nystagmus or other neurological symptoms after sustained neck extension, rotation	VBI
Cranial nerve testing	Neurological symptoms. Vertigo, vertigo associated with trauma	Positive cranial nerve test	VBI, VAD, central vestibular
Dynamic visual acuity	Vertigo	Loss of three or more lines of visual acuity relative to static visual acuity	Peripheral vestibular
Head impulse test	Vertigo with rapid movement to one direction	Vertigo and nystagmus or saccadic eye movement	Peripheral vestibular
Head thrust test	Vertigo with head movement	Vertigo and nystagmus or saccadic eye movement	Peripheral vestibular
Spontaneous nystagmus	Vertigo with spontaneous nystagmus	Nystagmus in sitting position. Nystagmus not altered by changes in body positions	Acute peripheral vestibular brainstem or cerebellar disorder
Gaze nystagmus	Vertigo with eye movements	Nystagmus only present for certain directions of gaze	Brainstem or cerebellar disorder. Normal variant. Ocular muscle fatigue. Congenital nystagmus
Head shaking nystagmus test	Vertigo with rapid head movements	Saccadic eye movements and inability to fixate gaze.	Peripheral vestibular. Central vestibular
Smooth pursuit neutral	Vertigo with eye movement	Saccadic catch- up movements with eye follow task in neutral neck position	Central vestibular
Saccades	Vertigo with eye movement	Decreased speed, latency and accuracy	Central vestibular
Limb coordination tests	Balance deficits, vertigo	Dysmetria or dysrythmia	Central vestibular

BPPV, benign paroxysmal positional vertigo; VAD, vertebral artery dissection; VBI, vertebrobasilar isuficiency.

sustained natural apophyseal glides (SNAGs) technique in the treatment of CD. The SNAG treatment had an immediate clinical effect and, statistically, it had a significant sustained effect in reducing dizziness, cervical pain and disability caused by cervical dysfunction. These researchers have since[209–211] conducted further randomized controlled clinical trials in people with CD.[213–215] In one study they compared the effect of two manual therapy interventions (4–6 treatments) in 86 patients with chronic CD: self-SNAG exercises

versus passive joint mobilization (PJM) with range of motion (ROM) exercises, or a placebo.[209,210] Both SNAGs and PJMs provided comparable immediate and sustained (12 weeks) reductions in intensity and frequency of chronic cervicogenic dizziness. While SNAG treatment improved cervical ROM, and the effects were maintained for 12 weeks after treatment, the effect of PJM on this impairment was not as good. Neither SNAGs nor PJMs have meaningful effect on joint repositioning accuracy or balance in people with cervicogenic dizziness.[209] Reid et al.[211] followed these patients to study long-term outcomes. At 12 months, both manual therapy groups had less dizziness frequency and higher global perceived effect compared to placebo, whereas there were no between-group differences in dizziness intensity, pain intensity or head repositioning accuracy. These studies have provided evidence that manual therapy has long-term beneficial effects for the treatment of chronic cervicogenic dizziness. It is also important to address specific patient complaints, adapting the intervention to each individual clinical situation, and to initially avoid an excessively intensive treatment. The results, however, suggest that it may be important to include treatment directed towards different sensorimotor control impairments to further improve treatment outcomes.

Therapeutic exercise

Subjects with CD may show cervical and axioscapular neuromuscular altered function.[212–221] Pain and fatigue of the cervical muscles are also capable of altering sensorimotor control. Recovering a normal pattern of neck muscle activation can help to reduce pain and normalize cervical proprioception, thus improving the postural control.[204] The motor control exercises of the craniocervical flexor muscles, the deep extensor and axioscapular muscles can be an important part of the treatment.

It has also been suggested that patients with CD have difficulty relaxing the cervical muscles: therefore, an abnormal relaxation time could be a factor involved in the CD.[222] This proprioceptive disturbance and nociceptive input from the neck is more evident when the patients are hypervigilant, when they are afraid of suffering dizziness or feelings of unsteadiness. The treatment of patients with CD should thus include neck and scapular muscle stabilizers retraining[23] and, perhaps, cervical kinematic training and muscle relaxation in those patients with hypervigilance.

Cervicocephalic kinaesthesia

The same test (JPE) used in the evaluation of the cervicocephalic kinaesthesia can be used as a retraining method. The therapist may ask the patient to reach the starting position, beginning with the natural head position and, after closing the eyes and performing

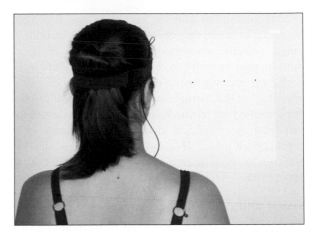

FIGURE 8-41 ■ Re-education of cervicocephalic kinaesthesia.

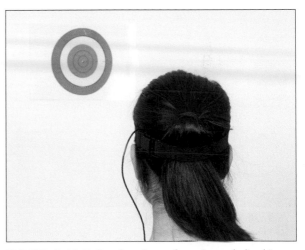

FIGURE 8-42 ■ Re-education of cervicocephalic kinaesthesia with a target.

movements in one direction – flexion, extension, right and left rotation – then opening their eyes to get feedback on their performance. The patient can then attempt to find different points in range with their closed eyes (Figs 8-41 and 8-42).

Retraining cervical movement sense with virtual reality

Recently, Sarig-Bahat et al.[223–226] have developed a virtual reality system to assess cervical kinematics that can be used as a retraining method in patients with neck pain. This system has proven to be a valid and reliable assessment tool for neck pain and it is also beneficial in improving cervical kinematics, including range, velocity, smoothness and accuracy of neck motion, pain intensity, neck disability in subjects with neck pain and improving exercise compliance.[227] The advantage of this virtual reality system is that it can be implemented for telemedicine and remote assessment and training of cervical kinematics in patients with chronic neck pain[227] (Fig. 8-43). Nevertheless, similar exercises using a laser and target for feedback also appear to be effective.

Visual and oculo-cervical exercises

The COR complements the VOR in maintaining the visual stability during the slow cephalic movements, and therefore oculo-cervical coordination exercises may help in the treatment of the CD.

Revel et al.[7] have shown that a rehabilitation programme based on oculo-cervical coordination exercises and neck proprioception is not only capable of improving the cervicocephalic kinaesthesia but also can improve cervical mobility, pain and the perceived disability.

Eye mobility exercises

In order to facilitate the retraining of the patient, eye mobility exercises without moving the head are a good starting point. The patient follows different drawings of varying eye movement complexity with the eyes at an adequate distance (Fig. 8-44). The eye mobility exercises can be performed with the neck torsioned 45° to the right and to the left. These and the following exercises should be performed while sitting down initially, standing on a stable platform, and then on an unstable platform or on a foam surface.

Oculomotor convergence exercises

Oculomotor control can be improved with specific exercises to improve eye convergence (Fig. 8-45), such as near-point convergence training.

Slow visual pursuit exercises

These exercises involve the same procedure as the smooth-pursuit neck torsion test. The patient, with the head in the neutral position, without moving it, follows a moving target with her eyes in different directions. The therapist observes the patient's ability

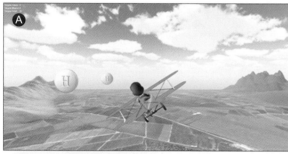

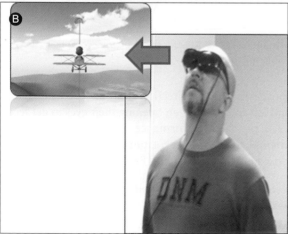

FIGURE 8-43 ■ Virtual reality exercises. The participant is required to follow the moving target as quickly (A) and as accurately (B) as possible.

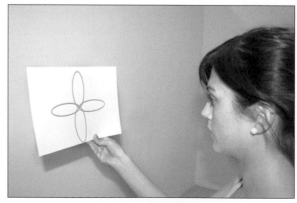

FIGURE 8-44 ■ Ocular motility exercises following different visual targets.

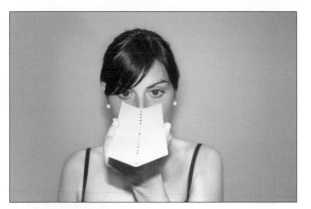

FIGURE 8-45 ■ Eye convergence training.

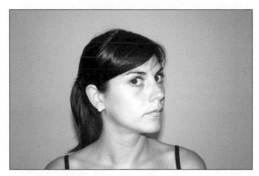

FIGURE 8-47 ■ Gaze stability exercises.

from one hand to the other while following the trajectory of the ball with the eyes.

Gaze stability exercises

The patient should keep the eyes fixed on a point and perform neck movements of rotation and flexion–extension that become wider and faster each time (Fig. 8-47). The progression can be asking the patient to look at a point, close the eyes and turn the head, always maintaining the orientation of the eyes towards the initial point. The patient opens the eyes to check that she is still looking at the initial point. Progressively, the visual reference point is located in different positions that are more end range. This exercise can also be performed by altering the plantar input if the patient is standing on a foam mat (Fig. 8-48). The difficulty of this exercise increases if the patient is asked to fix the eyes on a card with white and black vertical lines or if the focus point is several words rather than a single spot.

Cervico-ocular dissociation exercises

The patient is asked to perform dissociated movements of the head and the target (e.g. head moves in one direction, then eyes, then head back to starting position, then eyes, or while the head turns in one direction, the target moves in the opposite direction) (Fig. 8-49).

Balance control exercises

After identifying the sensory deficit responsible for balance impairment through postural tests and posturography, we can design exercises that stimulate the system that is more deficient. The deficit of a postural

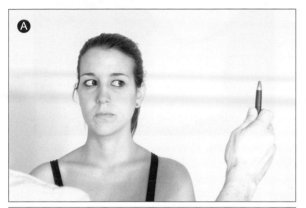

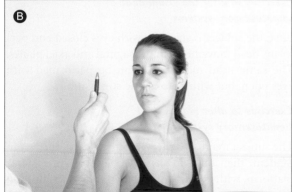

FIGURE 8-46 ■ (A, B) Slow visual pursuit exercises.

to follow the target and whether there are saccadic eye movements or symptoms such as dizziness or unsteadiness are reproduced. Then, with a trunk rotation of 45°, the subject performs the same eye pursuit movement (Fig. 8-46). The patient can also throw a ball

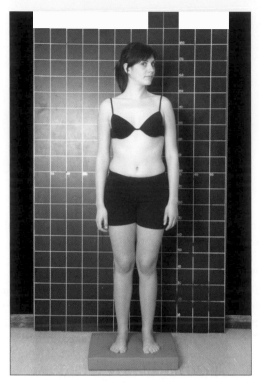

FIGURE 8-48 ■ Gaze stability exercise: altering the plantar input.

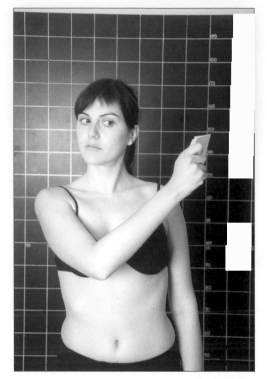

FIGURE 8-49 ■ Cervico-ocular dissociation exercises.

system tends to be compensated by the other systems and, therefore, balance retraining attempts to eliminate or alter the information of the systems on which the individual depends so that she is forced to train the dysfunctional system.

Standing balance training is incorporated as a re-education of different postural strategies. Balance retraining attempts to eliminate or alter the information of the systems on which the individual is more dependent on, creating conflictive situations in order to favour their integration.[23] In this way, different vestibular rehabilitation exercises can be incorporated as a treatment strategy in CD.[228,229] It has been shown that with a vestibular rehabilitation programme, dizziness can be reduced and there is an improvement in balance control.[228] This retraining can be achieved with the aid of the posturography platform or without it. The advantage of using the platform is that it allows us to quantify precisely the improvement of the patient in the postural control.

Exercises to alter the visual and somatosensory systems

First, the subject is standing with eyes closed and performs head movements in the sagittal and axial planes. The same head movements can be performed with eyes open, but with optokinetic stimulation.

Exercises to alter plantar and somatosensory systems

The subject maintains the balance first with the feet in tandem, then on a foam surface or on an unstable platform, with eyes open, and then moves the head in the sagittal and axial planes (Fig. 8-50).

Regarding the unstable platform, it is important for its base to have a wide radius of curvature that does not allow postural oscillations to be greater than 4–5°, which correspond to the amplitudes controlled by the standing postural system. Beyond these amplitudes, the stimulation of the semicircular canals plays a more important role.[154]

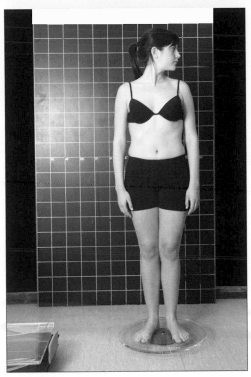

FIGURE 8-50 ■ Exercises with altered plantar and somato-sensory input.

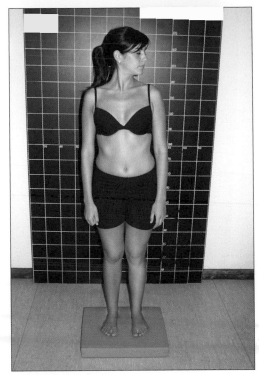

FIGURE 8-51 ■ Exercises with altered plantar, somatosensory and visual input.

Exercises to alter plantar, somatosensory and visual systems

The subject keeps balance on a foam surface or an unstable platform, with eyes closed or with an optokinetic stimulation, and then moves the head in the sagittal and axial planes (Fig. 8-51).

Balance training

The patient performs rocking body movements using their ankles. Initially, the patient only rocks in one direction (forward–back, right–left) and then makes the shape of a circle, all this on a stable surface. Later on, the same exercise can be performed on a foam surface (Fig. 8-52). The patient also performs rotation and flexion–extension movements of the cervical spine, standing on a foam surface or an unstable platform. Some exercises can also be performed while walking, with open eyes and then closed eyes, on a foam mat.

In addition to these balance control exercises, oculo-cervical coordination and head coordination exercises can be added (Fig. 8-53).

Walking and turning

The patient is asked to walk in one direction, to turn quickly 180° and to walk in the opposite direction.

Walking and oculo-cervical control

The patient is asked to walk, first with the head in the neutral position, looking to one side and then the other or up and down. The patient looks straight ahead and turns the head from one side and to the other or up and down.

Modern posturography platforms have several retraining programmes adapted to the patient's sensory deficit.

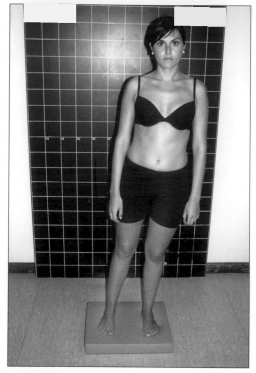

FIGURE 8-52 ■ Exercises balancing on foam.

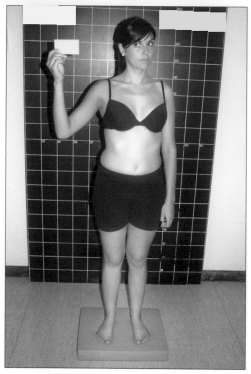

FIGURE 8-53 ■ Balance control on foam and oculo-cervical dissociation.

Stabilization

The patient observes the projection of her centre of gravity as a small point moving on a computer screen, and has to stay inside an area that becomes smaller. This test records the ability to maintain the projection of the centre of gravity on a reduced surface area (Fig. 8-54). The visual image can be eliminated and replaced by a sound that appears each time the centre of gravity is out of the target.

Load

On the computer screen a target appears, and the patient directs the projection of the centre of gravity towards it and maintains it for a few seconds. This target appears on different sections of the screen (Fig. 8-55). The progression in the difficulty of the test lies in the fact that the targets appear further away from the initial position of the projection of the centre of gravity of the subject.

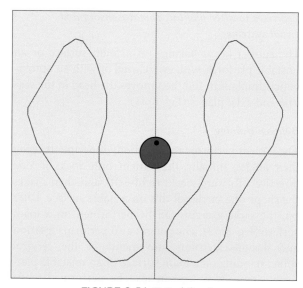

FIGURE 8-54 ■ Stabilization.

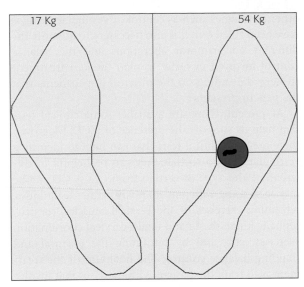

FIGURE 8-55 ■ Loading.

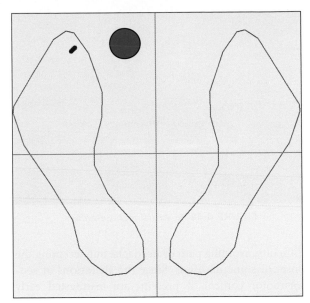

FIGURE 8-57 ■ Postural control.

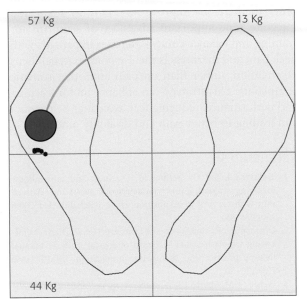

FIGURE 8-56 ■ Load transfer.

Load transfer

In this exercise, targets appear on the screen and they move in an arch of 90°. The patient has to reach them by moving her centre of gravity projection (Fig. 8-56). The exercise is carried out in different quadrants on the screen area. The exercise makes it possible to train the dynamic transfer of the load and to control support. This exercise is developed in different quadrants of the screen. This exercise allows for the retraining of the dynamic transference of the load.

Postural control

Once the subject controls stability, the load and the transfer of support begins to train balance control in relation to situations involving random destabilization that are similar to those faced in everyday life. Targets begin to appear quickly on the screen and in different random locations, and the patient must reach them (Fig. 8-57). The quick appearance of the targets makes it possible to train the ability to anticipate with regard to postural control.

Virtual reality exercises

Posturography platforms have several virtual reality retraining programmes that can create visuo-vestibular perception conflicts in a 3D environment. In this programme, for example, the plane must reach several targets in a moving environment that creates an optokinetic effect (Fig. 8-58).

Summary

All the sensorimotor retraining exercises should be performed several times a day, with progressive

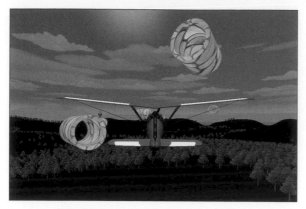

FIGURE 8-58 ■ Virtual reality exercises.

difficulty, avoiding pain or headache but accepting the onset of some dizziness. Since the alterations of sensorimotor control, if present, are manifested early after a car accident,[6,12] these exercises should be undertaken as soon as possible but avoiding an increase in the pain severity. The basic principle of the treatment of sensorimotor disorders is to help the patient to adapt to situations that trigger dizziness or pseudo-vertiginous symptoms.[31,230–232] Therefore, it is important for the patient to perform these exercises daily at home in several sessions of short duration. The difficulty of the exercises will increase progressively and will depend on the degree of severity, the initial symptoms and the age of the patient. As the clinical situation improves, it is advisable to begin physical activities that may cause stress on the sensorimotor control system such as dancing, biking or tennis.

> The basic principle of the treatment of sensorimotor disorders is to help the patient to adapt to situations that trigger dizziness or pseudo-vertiginous symptoms.

CONCLUSION

Cervicogenic dizziness is characterized by a subjective sensation of unsteadiness and instability and it is usually associated with neck pain, cervical musculoskeletal and sensorimotor impairments in eye–neck coordination, cervical kinaesthetic sense, neck motor control patterns and standing balance. The diagnosis of CD is based on the existing relationship between dizziness and sensorimotor impairments and the presence of cervical musculoskeletal dysfunction, once

other aetiologies such as central or vestibular vertigos have been ruled out. It is also necessary to quantify the different sensorimotor alterations and the balance control involved in order to plan the best treatment strategy depending on the physical impairments that the patient presents.

At present, there are available some clinical tests that help us support the presence of a CD. Moreover, there are also clinical tests that can help to identify a vestibular vertigo so that they can be helpful to differentiate this type of vertigo from CD. A CD can be managed using different manual therapy techniques, retraining exercises of the cervical muscles, cervico-cephalic kinaesthesia and oculo-cervical coordination exercises, etc., and by retraining the postural and standing balance control. The final aim of the treatment is to train the patient with exercises that involve graduated exposure to different alterations of the afferent input of the sensorimotor control system, in order to therefore improve its ability to adapt and integrate. One important advantage of sensorimotor training and balance control exercises in patients with neck pain and dizziness is the use of an external focus of attention, rather than on pain and other somatic complaints. This strategy can enhance motor learning and performance, reducing fear avoidance behaviours and leading to better pain and disability outcomes.

REFERENCES

1. Treleaven J, Jull G, Sterling M. Dizziness and unsteadiness following whiplash injury: characteristic features and relationship with cervical joint position error. J Rehabil Med 2003; 35(1):36–43.
2. Oostendorp R, Van Europen A, van Erp J, et al. Dizziness following whiplash injury: a neuro-otological study in manual therapy practice and therapeutic implication. JMMT 1999; 7(3):123–30.
3. Wrisley DM, Sparto PJ, Whitney SL, et al. Cervicogenic dizziness: a review of diagnosis and treatment. J Orthop Sports Phys Ther 2000;30(12):755–66.
4. Heikkila H, Johansson M, Wenngren BI. Effects of acupuncture, cervical manipulation and NSAID therapy on dizziness and impaired head repositioning of suspected cervical origin: a pilot study. Man Ther 2000;5(3):151–7.
5. Reid SA, Rivett DA. Manual therapy treatment of cervicogenic dizziness: a systematic review. Man Ther 2005;10(1):4–13.
6. Sterling M, Jull G, Vicenzino B, et al. Characterization of acute whiplash-associated disorders. Spine 2004;29(2):182–8.
7. Revel M, Minguet M, Gregoy P, et al. Changes in cervico-cephalic kinesthesia after a proprioceptive rehabilitation

program in patients with neck pain: a randomized controlled study. Arch Phys Med Rehabil 1994;75(8):895–9.

8. Heikkila H, Astrom PG. Cervicocephalic kinesthetic sensibility in patients with whiplash injury. Scand J Rehabil Med 1996; 28(3):133–8.

9. Kristjansson E, Dall'Alba P, Jull G. A study of five cervico-cephalic relocation tests in three different subject groups. Clin Rehabil 2003;17(7):768–74.

10. Heikkila HV, Wenngren BI. Cervicocephalic kinesthetic sensi-bility, active range of cervical motion, and oculomotor func-tion in patients with whiplash injury. Arch Phys Med Rehabil 1998;79(9):1089–94.

11. Kristjansson E, Hardardottir L, Asmundardottir M, et al. A new clinical test for cervicocephalic kinesthetic sensibility: 'the fly'. Arch Phys Med Rehabil 2004;85(3): 490–5.

12. Sterling M, Jull G, Vicenzino B, et al. Development of motor system dysfunction following whiplash injury. Pain 2003; 103(1–2):65–73.

13. Woodhouse A, Vasseljen O. Altered motor control patterns in whiplash and chronic neck pain. BMC Musculoskelet Disord 2008;9:90.

14. Sjolander P, Michaelson P, Jaric S, et al. Sensorimotor distur-bances in chronic neck pain – range of motion, peak velocity, smoothness of movement, and repositioning acuity. Man Ther 2008;13(2):122–31.

15. Woodhouse A, Stavdahl O, Vasseljen O. Irregular head move-ment patterns in whiplash patients during a trajectory task. Exp Brain Res 2010;201(2):261–70.

16. Michaelson P, Michaelson M, Jaric S, et al. Vertical posture and head stability in patients with chronic neck pain. J Rehabil Med 2003;35(5):229–35.

17. Sjostrom H, Allum JH, Carpenter MG, et al. Trunk sway meas-ures of postural stability during clinical balance tests in patients with chronic whiplash injury symptoms. Spine 2003;28(15): 1725–34.

18. Treleaven J, Jull G, Lowchoy N. Standing balance in persistent whiplash: a comparison between subjects with and without dizziness. J Rehabil Med 2005;37(4):224–9.

19. Stapley PJ, Beretta MV, Dalla Toffola E, et al. Neck muscle fatigue and postural control in patients with whiplash injury. Clin Neurophysiol 2006;117(3):610–22.

20. Stokell R, Yu A, Williams K, et al. Dynamic and functional balance tasks in subjects with persistent whiplash: a pilot trial. Man Ther 2011;16(4):394–8.

21. Tjell C, Tenenbaum A, Sandström S. Smooth pursuit neck torsion test – a specific test for whiplash associated disorders? J Whiplash Relat Disorders 2003;1:9–24.

22. Treleaven J, Jull G, LowChoy N. Smooth pursuit neck torsion test in whiplash-associated disorders: relationship to self-reports of neck pain and disability, dizziness and anxiety. J Rehabil Med 2005;37(4):219–23.

23. Treleaven J, Jull G, LowChoy N. The relationship of cervical joint position error to balance and eye movement disturbances in persistent whiplash. Man Ther 2006;11(2): 99–106.

24. Storaci R, Manelli A, Schiavone N, et al. Whiplash injury and oculomotor dysfunctions: clinical-posturographic correla-tions. Eur Spine J 2006;15(12):1811–16.

25. Grip H, Jull G, Treleaven J. Head eye co-ordination using simultaneous measurement of eye in head and head in space movements: potential for use in subjects with a whiplash injury. J Clin Monit Comput 2009;23(1): 31–40.

26. Treleaven J, Jull G, Grip H. Head eye co-ordination and gaze stability in subjects with persistent whiplash associated disor-ders. Man Ther 2011;16(3):252–7.

27. Ramírez R. Tratamiento de los trastornos del equilibrio. Infor-macion Terapeutica del Sistema Nacional de Salud 2002; 26(2):44–7.

28. Furman JM, Whitney SL. Central causes of dizziness. Phys Ther 2000;80(2):179–87.

29. Meadows J, Magee D. An overview of dizziness and vertigo for the orthopaedic manual therapist. In: Boyling J, Palastanga N, editors. Grieve's modern manual therapy. The vertebral column. 2nd ed. London: Churchill Livingstone; 1994. p. 381–9.

30. Neuhauser H, Lempert T. Vertigo and dizziness related to migraine: a diagnostic challenge. Cephalalgia 2004;24(2): 83–91.

31. Yardley L, Luxon L. Treating dizziness with vestibular rehabili-tation. BMJ 1994;308(6939):1252–3.

32. Brandt T, Bronstein AM. Cervical vertigo. J Neurol Neurosurg Psychiatry 2001;71(1):8–12.

33. Ryan GM, Cope S. Cervical vertigo. Lancet 1955; 269(6905):1355–8.

34. Furman J, Cass S. Balance disorders: a case-study approach. Philadelphia: F.A. Davis; 1996.

35. Grad A, Baloh RW. Vertigo of vascular origin. Clinical and electronystagmographic features in 84 cases. Arch Neurol 1989;46(3):281–4.

36. Husni EA, Bell HS, Storer J. Mechanical occlusion of the ver-tebral artery. A new clinical concept. JAMA 1966;196(6): 475–8.

37. Schellinger PD, Schwab S, Krieger D, et al. Masking of verte-bral artery dissection by severe trauma to the cervical spine. Spine 2001;26(3):314–19.

38. Bonkowsky V, Steinbach S, Arnold W. Vertigo and cranial nerve palsy caused by different forms of spontaneous dissections of internal and vertebral arteries. Eur Arch Otorhinolaryngol 2002;259(7):365–8.

39. Barré M. Sur un syndrome sympathique cervical postérieur et sa cause frequente: L'arthrite cervicale. Rev Neurol (Paris) 1926;33:1246–8.

40. Lieou YC. Syndrome sympathique cervical posterieur et arthrite cervicale chronique de la colonne vertébrale cervicale Etude clinique et radiologique. These de Strasbourg, 1928.

41. Bogduk N, Lambert GA, Duckworth JW. The anatomy and physiology of the vertebral nerve in relation to cervical migraine. Cephalalgia 1981;1(1):11–24.

42. Bogduk N. Cervical causes of headache and dizziness. In: Boyling JP, Palastanga N, editors. Grieve's modern manual

therapy. The vertebral column. 2nd ed. London: Churchill Livingstone; 1994. p. 317–31.

43. Magnus R. Some results of studies in the physiology of posture. Cameron prize lectures. Lancet 1926;211:531–6.

44. Brandt T. Cervical vertigo – reality or fiction? Audiol Neurootol 1996;1(4):187–96.

45. Bracher ES, Almeida CI, Almeida RR, et al. A combined approach for the treatment of cervical vertigo. J Manipulative Physiol Ther 2000;23(2):96–100.

46. Borg-Stein J, Rauch S, Krabak B. Evaluation and management of cervicogenic dizziness. Clin Rev Phys Rehabil Med 2001; 13(4):255–64.

47. Igarashi M, Alford BR, Watanabe T, et al. Role of neck proprioceptors for the maintenance of dynamic bodily equilibrium in the squirrel monkey. Laryngoscope 1969;79(10):1713–27.

48. Igarashi M, Miyata H, Alford BR, et al. Nystagmus after experimental cervical lesions. Laryngoscope 1972;82(9):1609–21.

49. Biemond A, De Jong JM. On cervical nystagmus and related disorders. Brain 1969;92(2):437–58.

50. Hinoki M, Hine S, Okada S, et al. Optic organ and cervical proprioceptors in maintenance of body equilibrium. Acta Otolaryngol Suppl 1975;330:169–84.

51. de Jong PT, de Jong JM, Cohen B, et al. Ataxia and nystagmus induced by injection of local anesthetics in the Neck. Ann Neurol 1977;1(3):240–6.

52. Heikkilä H. Cervical vertigo. In: Boyling J, Jull G, editors. Grieve's modern manual therapy. 3rd ed. London: Elsevier Churchill Livingstone; 2004. p. 233–42.

53. Wyke B. Cervical articular contribution to posture and gait: their relation to senile disequilibrium. Age Ageing 1979;8(4): 251–8.

54. Karlberg M, Persson L, Magnusson M. Impaired postural control in patients with cervico-brachial pain. Acta Otolaryngol Suppl 1995;520(Pt 2):440–2.

55. Brandt T, Orberk E, Weber R, et al. Pathogenesis of cervical artery dissections: association with connective tissue abnormalities. Neurology 2001;57(1):24–30.

56. Froehling DA, Silverstein MD, Mohr DN, et al. The rational clinical examination. Does this dizzy patient have a serious form of vertigo? JAMA 1994;271(5):385–8.

57. Thiagarajan P, Ciuffreda KJ. Versional eye tracking in mild traumatic brain injury (mTBI): effects of oculomotor training (OMT). Brain Inj 2014;28(7):930–43.

58. Thurrell A, Bertholon P, Bronstein AM. Reorientation of a visually evoked postural response during passive whole body rotation. Exp Brain Res 2000;133(2):229–32.

59. Kulkarni V, Chandy MJ, Babu KS. Quantitative study of muscle spindles in suboccipital muscles of human foetuses. Neurol India 2001;49(4):355–9.

60. Boyd-Clark LC, Briggs CA, Galea MP. Muscle spindle distribution, morphology, and density in longus colli and multifidus muscles of the cervical spine. Spine 2002;27(7):694–701.

61. Toupet M. [Convergence of visual and neck proprioceptives on the vestibulo-ocular reflex arc and the 'vestibulo-cerebellum' (author's transl)]. Ann Otolaryngol Chir Cervicofac 1982;99(3):119–28.

62. Biguer B, Donaldson IM, Hein A, et al. Neck muscle vibration modifies the representation of visual motion and direction in man. Brain 1988;111(Pt 6):1405–24.

63. Zhou G, Cox LC. Vestibular evoked myogenic potentials: history and overview. Am J Audiol 2004;13(2):135–43.

64. Pérez-Guillem V, González-García E, García-Piñero A, et al. Potencial vestibular miogénico evocado: un aporte al conocimiento de la fisiología y patología vestibular. Patrones cuantitativos en la población normal. Acta Otorrinolaringol Esp 2005;56:349–53.

65. Boquet J. Asimetrías tónicas en la nuca y desequilibrios propioceptivos. In: Gagey P, Weber B, editors. Posturología. Regulación y alteraciones en la bipedestación. Barcelona: Masson; 2001.

66. Dutia MB. The muscles and joints of the neck: their specialisation and role in head movement. Prog Neurobiol 1991; 37(2):165–78.

67. Bartsch T, Goadsby PJ. Increased responses in trigeminocervical nociceptive neurons to cervical input after stimulation of the dura mater. Brain 2003;126(Pt 8):1801–13.

68. Metherate RS, da Costa DC, Herron P, et al. A thalamic terminus of the lateral cervical nucleus: the lateral division of the posterior nuclear group. J Neurophysiol 1986;56(6): 1498–520.

69. Schwabe A, Drepper J, Maschke M, et al. The role of the human cerebellum in short- and long-term habituation of postural responses. Gait Posture 2004;19(1):16–23.

70. McLain RF. Mechanoreceptor endings in human cervical facet joints. Spine 1994;19(5):495–501.

71. Yoganandan N, Knowles SA, Maiman DJ, et al. Anatomic study of the morphology of human cervical facet joint. Spine 2003;28(20):2317–23.

72. Wyke B. Neurology of the cervical spinal joints. Physiotherapy 1979;65(3):72–6.

73. Peterson BW, Goldberg J, Bilotto G, et al. Cervicocollic reflex: its dynamic properties and interaction with vestibular reflexes. J Neurophysiol 1985;54(1):90–109.

74. Kanaya T, Gresty MA, Bronstein AM, et al. Control of the head in response to tilt of the body in normal and labyrinthine-defective human subjects. J Physiol 1995;489(Pt 3):895–910.

75. Brandt T. Modelling brain function: the vestibulo-ocular reflex. Curr Opin Neurol 2001;14(1):1–4.

76. Raphan T, Cohen B. The vestibulo-ocular reflex in three dimensions. Exp Brain Res 2002;145(1):1–27.

77. Peterson BW, Choi H, Hain T, et al. Dynamic and kinematic strategies for head movement control. Ann N Y Acad Sci 2001; 942:381–93.

78. Dutia M, Price R. Interaction between the vestibulo-collic reflex and the cervico-collic stretch reflex in the cescerebrate cat. J Physiol 1987;387:19–30.

79. Gdowski GT, McCrea RA. Integration of vestibular and head movement signals in the vestibular nuclei during whole-body rotation. J Neurophysiol 1999;82(1):436–49.

80. Jurgens R, Mergner T. Interaction between cervico-ocular and vestibulo-ocular reflexes in normal adults. Exp Brain Res 1989;77(2):381–90.

81. Schubert MC, Das V, Tusa RJ, et al. Cervico-ocular reflex in normal subjects and patients with unilateral vestibular hypofunction. Otol Neurotol 2004;25(1):65–71.

82. Kristjansson E, Treleaven J. Sensorimotor function and dizziness in neck pain: implications for assessment and management. J Orthop Sports Phys Ther 2009;39(5):364–77.

83. Bruzzone MG, Grisoli M, De Simone T, et al. Neuroradiological features of vertigo. Neurol Sci 2004;25(Suppl. 1):S20–3.

84. Ramirez R. Trastornos del equilibrio. Un abordaje multidisciplinario. Madrid: McGraw-Hill Interamericana; 2003.

85. Alpini D, Caputo D, Pugnetti L, et al. Vertigo and multiple sclerosis: aspects of differential diagnosis. Neurol Sci 2001;22(Suppl. 2):S84–7.

86. Solomon D. Benign paroxysmal positional vertigo. Curr Treat Options Neurol 2000;2(5):417–28.

87. Epley JM. Positional vertigo related to semicircular canalithiasis. Otolaryngol Head Neck Surg 1995;112(1):154–61.

88. Brandt T. Steddin S. Current view of the mechanism of benign paroxysmal positioning vertigo: cupulolithiasis or canalolithiasis? J Vestib Res 1993;3(4):373–82.

89. Parnes LS, Agrawal SK, Atlas J. Diagnosis and management of benign paroxysmal positional vertigo (BPPV). CMAJ 2003;169(7):681–93.

90. Schuknecht HF. Cupulolithiasis. Arch Otolaryngol 1969;90(6):765–78.

91. Schuknecht HF, Ruby RR. Cupulolithiasis. Adv Otorhinolaryngol 1973;20:434–43.

92. Hall SF, Ruby RR, McClure JA. The mechanics of benign paroxysmal vertigo. J Otolaryngol 1979;8(2):151–8.

93. Parnes LS, McClure JA. Free-floating endolymph particles: a new operative finding during posterior semicircular canal occlusion. Laryngoscope 1992;102(9):988–92.

94. Honrubia V, Baloh RW, Harris MR, et al. Paroxysmal positional vertigo syndrome. Am J Otol 1999;20(4):465–70.

95. Vannucchi P, Giannoni B, Pagnini P. Treatment of horizontal semicircular canal benign paroxysmal positional vertigo. J Vestib Res 1997;7(1):1–6.

96. Dix MR, Hallpike CS. The pathology, symptomatology and diagnosis of certain common disorders of the vestibular system. Proc R Soc Med 1952;45(6):341–54.

97. McClure JA. Horizontal canal BPV. J Otolaryngol 1985;14(1):30–5.

98. Lee SH, Kim JS. Benign paroxysmal positional vertigo. J Clin Neurol 2010;6(2):51–63.

99. Swartz R, Longwell P. Treatment of vertigo. Am Fam Physician 2005;71(6):1115–22.

100. Humphriss RL, Baguley DM, Sparkes V, et al. Contraindications to the Dix-Hallpike manoeuvre: a multidisciplinary review. Int J Audiol 2003;42(3):166–73.

101. Hilton M, Pinder D. The Epley (canalith repositioning) manoeuvre for benign paroxysmal positional vertigo. Cochrane Database Syst Rev 2002;(1):CD003162.

102. White J. Bening paroxysmal position vertigo: how to diagnose and quickly treat it. Cleve Clin J Med 2004;71(9):722–8.

103. Fife TD, Iverson DJ, Lempert T, et al. Practice parameter: therapies for benign paroxysmal positional vertigo (an evidence-based review): report of the Quality Standards Subcommittee of the American Academy of Neurology. Neurology 2008;70(22):2067–74.

104. Semont A, Freyss G, Vitte E. Curing the BPPV with a liberatory maneuver. Adv Otorhinolaryngol 1988;42:290–3.

105. Lopez-Escamez JA, et al. Multiple positional nystagmus suggests multiple canal involvement in benign paroxysmal vertigo. Acta Otolaryngol 2005;125(9):954–61.

106. Massoud EA, Ireland DJ. Post-treatment instructions in the nonsurgical management of benign paroxysmal positional vertigo. J Otolaryngol 1996;25(2):121–5.

107. De Stefano A, Dispenza F, Citraro L, et al. Are postural restrictions necessary for management of posterior canal benign paroxysmal positional vertigo? Ann Otol Rhinol Laryngol 2011;120(7):460–4.

108. Nunez RA, Cass SP, Furman JM. Short- and long-term outcomes of canalith repositioning for benign paroxysmal positional vertigo. Otolaryngol Head Neck Surg 2000;122(5):647–52.

109. Radtke A, von Brevern M, Tiel-Wilck K, et al. Self-treatment of benign paroxysmal positional vertigo: Semont maneuver vs Epley procedure. Neurology 2004;63(1):150–2.

110. Lempert T, Tiel-Wilck K. A positional maneuver for treatment of horizontal-canal benign positional vertigo. Laryngoscope 1996;106(4):476–8.

111. Casani AP, Nacci A, Dallan I, et al. Horizontal semicircular canal benign paroxysmal positional vertigo: effectiveness of two different methods of treatment. Audiol Neurootol 2011;16(3):175–84.

112. Treleaven J. Dizziness, unsteadiness, visual disturbances, and postural control: implications for the transition to chronic symptoms after a whiplash trauma. Spine 2011;36(25 Suppl.):S211–17.

113. Dispenza F, De Stefano A, Mathur N, et al. Benign paroxysmal positional vertigo following whiplash injury: a myth or a reality? Am J Otolaryngol 2011;32(5):376–80.

114. Gresty MA, Bronstein AM, Brandt T, et al. Neurology of otolith function. Peripheral and central disorders. Brain 1992;115(Pt 3):647–73.

115. Lempert T, Gresty MA, Bronstein AM. Benign positional vertigo: recognition and treatment. BMJ 1995;311(7003):489–91.

116. Thomas LC. Cervical arterial dissection: an overview and implications for manipulative therapy practice. Man Ther 2016;21:2–9.

117. Treleaven J, Takasaki H. Characteristics of visual disturbances reported by subjects with neck pain. Man Ther 2014;19(3):203–7.

118. Malmstrom EM, Karlberg M, Melander A, et al. Cervicogenic dizziness – musculoskeletal findings before and after treatment and long-term outcome. Disabil Rehabil 2007;29(15):1193–205.

119. Jull G, Sterling S, Falla D, et al. Whiplash, headache, and neck pain: research-based directions for physical therapies. Philadelphia: Churchill Livingstone Elsevier; 2008.

nociceptive processing mechanisms may underlie neck pain, depending on whether or not it is of traumatic onset, and this could be one reason for apparently better responses to physical treatments in patients with non-traumatic neck pain.[49,50] It also suggests that neck pain classification systems will need to take these findings into account and that a single classification system for all neck pain may not be optimal. These proposals require further investigation.

Mechanical hyperalgesia locally over the cervical spine seems to be common to both chronic whiplash and idiopathic neck pain and probably indicates an ongoing peripheral nociceptive source of pain.[41,51] In addition to its presence in the chronic stages of neck pain conditions, local mechanical hyperalgesia has also been shown to occur following acute whiplash injury, irrespective of symptom intensity and disability levels reported by the patient.[28,30] However, the local mechanical hyperalgesia resolved within several weeks in those who recovered or reported continuing milder symptoms but persisted unchanged in whiplash patients reporting persistent symptoms of a moderate/severe nature at 6 months post injury.[28]

In contrast, the phenomena of widespread sensory hypersensitivity may be unique to WAD. Scott et al.[41] showed chronic WAD subjects to have a more complex presentation involving lowered pain thresholds for pressure, heat and cold stimuli in areas remote to the cervical spine which were not present in idiopathic neck pain subjects. The reasons for these differences between the conditions are not clear but it has been demonstrated that conditions with more severe and widespread pain show greater degrees of sensory hypersensitivity.[52] Patients with WAD generally report higher levels of pain and disability[41] and, at least clinically, tend to have more widespread pain. The findings of Scott and colleagues[41] added to the previous body of knowledge demonstrating WAD to be a condition involving more complex changes in the neurobiological processing of pain most likely occurring within the central nervous system.

It is important to note that the widespread sensory hypersensitivity that is a consistent feature of chronic WAD has been shown to be present soon after injury, at least in those whiplash-injured people with poor functional recovery.[53,54] Most importantly, sensory features of cold hyperalgesia appear to be prognostic

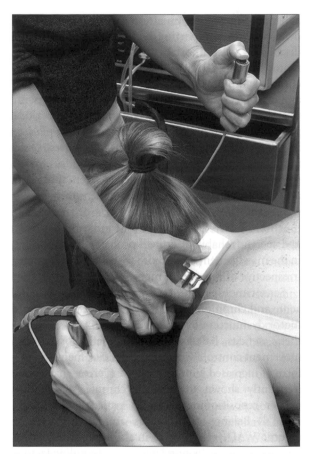

FIGURE 9-2 ■ Measurement of cold pain thresholds over the cervical spine in the laboratory setting. The thermode is preset to 30°C and increased at 1°C /second until the participant first feels pain.

indicators for poor recovery at long-term follow-ups of 6 months and 2 years post injury (Figs 9-2 and 9-3).[34,55–57] It is essential that physiotherapists are alert to features of a patient's clinical presentation that may indicate a propensity for the development of chronic symptoms and, for this reason, assessment of sensory function will be important.

PSYCHOLOGICAL FACTORS INVOLVED IN WHIPLASH-ASSOCIATED DISORDERS

As with any painful musculoskeletal condition, relationships between psychological factors and health outcomes have been well documented and this is no

81. Schubert MC, Das V, Tusa RJ, et al. Cervico-ocular reflex in normal subjects and patients with unilateral vestibular hypofunction. Otol Neurotol 2004;25(1):65–71.

82. Kristjansson E, Treleaven J. Sensorimotor function and dizziness in neck pain: implications for assessment and management. J Orthop Sports Phys Ther 2009;39(5):364–77.

83. Bruzzone MG, Grisoli M, De Simone T, et al. Neuroradiological features of vertigo. Neurol Sci 2004;25(Suppl. 1):S20–3.

84. Ramirez R. Trastornos del equilibrio. Un abordaje multidisciplinario. Madrid: McGraw-Hill Interamericana; 2003.

85. Alpini D, Caputo D, Pugnetti L, et al. Vertigo and multiple sclerosis: aspects of differential diagnosis. Neurol Sci 2001;22(Suppl. 2):S84–7.

86. Solomon D. Benign paroxysmal positional vertigo. Curr Treat Options Neurol 2000;2(5):417–28.

87. Epley JM. Positional vertigo related to semicircular canalithiasis. Otolaryngol Head Neck Surg 1995;112(1):154–61.

88. Brandt T. Steddin S. Current view of the mechanism of benign paroxysmal positioning vertigo: cupulolithiasis or canalolithiasis? J Vestib Res 1993;3(4):373–82.

89. Parnes LS, Agrawal SK, Atlas J. Diagnosis and management of benign paroxysmal positional vertigo (BPPV). CMAJ 2003;169(7):681–93.

90. Schuknecht HF. Cupulolithiasis. Arch Otolaryngol 1969;90(6):765–78.

91. Schuknecht HF, Ruby RR. Cupulolithiasis. Adv Otorhinolaryngol 1973;20:434–43.

92. Hall SF, Ruby RR, McClure JA. The mechanics of benign paroxysmal vertigo. J Otolaryngol 1979;8(2):151–8.

93. Parnes LS, McClure JA. Free-floating endolymph particles: a new operative finding during posterior semicircular canal occlusion. Laryngoscope 1992;102(9):988–92.

94. Honrubia V, Baloh RW, Harris MR, et al. Paroxysmal positional vertigo syndrome. Am J Otol 1999;20(4):465–70.

95. Vannucchi P, Giannoni B, Pagnini P. Treatment of horizontal semicircular canal benign paroxysmal positional vertigo. J Vestib Res 1997;7(1):1–6.

96. Dix MR, Hallpike CS. The pathology, symptomatology and diagnosis of certain common disorders of the vestibular system. Proc R Soc Med 1952;45(6):341–54.

97. McClure JA. Horizontal canal BPV. J Otolaryngol 1985;14(1):30–5.

98. Lee SH, Kim JS. Benign paroxysmal positional vertigo. J Clin Neurol 2010;6(2):51–63.

99. Swartz R, Longwell P. Treatment of vertigo. Am Fam Physician 2005;71(6):1115–22.

100. Humphriss RL, Baguley DM, Sparkes V, et al. Contraindications to the Dix-Hallpike manoeuvre: a multidisciplinary review. Int J Audiol 2003;42(3):166–73.

101. Hilton M, Pinder D. The Epley (canalith repositioning) manoeuvre for benign paroxysmal positional vertigo. Cochrane Database Syst Rev 2002;(1):CD003162.

102. White J. Bening paroxysmal position vertigo: how to diagnose and quickly treat it. Cleve Clin J Med 2004;71(9):722–8.

103. Fife TD, Iverson DJ, Lempert T, et al. Practice parameter: therapies for benign paroxysmal positional vertigo (an evidence-based review): report of the Quality Standards Subcommittee of the American Academy of Neurology. Neurology 2008;70(22):2067–74.

104. Semont A, Freyss G, Vitte E. Curing the BPPV with a liberatory maneuver. Adv Otorhinolaryngol 1988;42:290–3.

105. Lopez-Escamez JA, et al. Multiple positional nystagmus suggests multiple canal involvement in benign paroxysmal vertigo. Acta Otolaryngol 2005;125(9):954–61.

106. Massoud EA, Ireland DJ. Post-treatment instructions in the nonsurgical management of benign paroxysmal positional vertigo. J Otolaryngol 1996;25(2):121–5.

107. De Stefano A, Dispenza F, Citraro L, et al. Are postural restrictions necessary for management of posterior canal benign paroxysmal positional vertigo? Ann Otol Rhinol Laryngol 2011;120(7):460–4.

108. Nunez RA, Cass SP, Furman JM. Short- and long-term outcomes of canalith repositioning for benign paroxysmal positional vertigo. Otolaryngol Head Neck Surg 2000;122(5):647–52.

109. Radtke A, von Brevern M, Tiel-Wilck K, et al. Self-treatment of benign paroxysmal positional vertigo: Semont maneuver vs Epley procedure. Neurology 2004;63(1):150–2.

110. Lempert T, Tiel-Wilck K. A positional maneuver for treatment of horizontal-canal benign positional vertigo. Laryngoscope 1996;106(4):476–8.

111. Casani AP, Nacci A, Dallan I, et al. Horizontal semicircular canal benign paroxysmal positional vertigo: effectiveness of two different methods of treatment. Audiol Neurootol 2011;16(3):175–84.

112. Treleaven J. Dizziness, unsteadiness, visual disturbances, and postural control: implications for the transition to chronic symptoms after a whiplash trauma. Spine 2011;36(25 Suppl.):S211–17.

113. Dispenza F, De Stefano A, Mathur N, et al. Benign paroxysmal positional vertigo following whiplash injury: a myth or a reality? Am J Otolaryngol 2011;32(5):376–80.

114. Gresty MA, Bronstein AM, Brandt T, et al. Neurology of otolith function. Peripheral and central disorders. Brain 1992;115(Pt 3):647–73.

115. Lempert T, Gresty MA, Bronstein AM. Benign positional vertigo: recognition and treatment. BMJ 1995;311(7003):489–91.

116. Thomas LC. Cervical arterial dissection: an overview and implications for manipulative therapy practice. Man Ther 2016;21:2–9.

117. Treleaven J, Takasaki H. Characteristics of visual disturbances reported by subjects with neck pain. Man Ther 2014;19(3):203–7.

118. Malmstrom EM, Karlberg M, Melander A, et al. Cervicogenic dizziness – musculoskeletal findings before and after treatment and long-term outcome. Disabil Rehabil 2007;29(15):1193–205.

119. Jull G, Sterling S, Falla D, et al. Whiplash, headache, and neck pain: research-based directions for physical therapies. Philadelphia: Churchill Livingstone Elsevier; 2008.

120. Phillipszoon AJ, Bos JH. Neck torsion nystagmus. Pract Otorhinolaryngol (Basel) 1963;25:339–44.

121. Fitzgerald DC. Persistent dizziness following head trauma and perilymphatic fistula. Arch Phys Med Rehabil 1995; 76(11):1017–20.

122. Norre ME. Cervical vertigo. Diagnostic and semiological problem with special emphasis upon 'cervical nystagmus'. Acta Otorhinolaryngol Belg 1987;41(3):436–52.

123. Oosterveld WJ, Kortschot HW, Kingma GG, et al. Electronystagmographic findings following cervical whiplash injuries. Acta Otolaryngol 1991;111(2):201–5.

124. Calseyde P, Ampe W, Depondt M. E.N.G. and the cervical syndrome neck torsion nystagmus. Adv Otorhinolaryngol 1977;22:119–24.

125. L'Heureux-Lebeau B, Godbout A, Berbiche D, et al. Evaluation of paraclinical tests in the diagnosis of cervicogenic dizziness. Otol Neurotol 2014;35(10):1858–65.

126. Revel M, Andre-Deshays C, Minguet M. Cervicocephalic kinesthetic sensibility in patients with cervical pain. Arch Phys Med Rehabil 1991;72(5):288–91.

127. Loudon JK, Ruhl M, Field E. Ability to reproduce head position after whiplash injury. Spine 1997;22(8):865–8.

128. Roren A, Mayoux-Benhamou MA, Fayad F, et al. Comparison of visual and ultrasound based techniques to measure head repositioning in healthy and neck-pain subjects. Man Ther 2009;14(3):270–7.

129. Jull G, Falla D, Treleaven J, et al. Retraining cervical joint position sense: the effect of two exercise regimes. J Orthop Res 2007;25(3):404–12.

130. Chen X, Treleaven J. The effect of neck torsion on joint position error in subjects with chronic neck pain. Man Ther 2013;18(6):562–7.

131. Rix GD, Bagust J. Cervicocephalic kinesthetic sensibility in patients with chronic, nontraumatic cervical spine pain. Arch Phys Med Rehabil 2001;82(7):911–19.

132. Armstrong BS, McNair PJ, Williams M. Head and neck position sense in whiplash patients and healthy individuals and the effect of the cranio-cervical flexion action. Clin Biomech (Bristol, Avon) 2005;20(7):675–84.

133. Uthaikhup S, Jull G, Sungkarat S, et al. The influence of neck pain on sensorimotor function in the elderly. Arch Gerontol Geriatr 2012;55(3):667–72.

134. Bagust J. Assessment of verticality perception by a rod-and-frame test: preliminary observations on the use of a computer monitor and video eye glasses. Arch Phys Med Rehabil 2005;86(5):1062–4.

135. Grod JP, Diakow PR. Effect of neck pain on verticality perception: a cohort study. Arch Phys Med Rehabil 2002;83(3): 412–15.

136. Bagust J, Rix GD, Hurst HC. Use of a computer rod and frame (CRAF) test to assess errors in the perception of visual vertical in a clinical setting. A pilot study. Clin Chiro 2005;8(3): 134–9.

137. Humphreys BK. Cervical outcome measures: testing for postural stability and balance. J Manipulative Physiol Ther 2008;31(7):540–6.

138. Hildingsson C, Wenngren BI, Bring G, et al. Oculomotor problems after cervical spine injury. Acta Orthop Scand 1989; 60(5):513–16.

139. Hildingsson C, Toolanen G. Outcome after soft-tissue injury of the cervical spine. A prospective study of 93 car-accident victims. Acta Orthop Scand 1990;61(4):357–9.

140. Hildingsson C, Wenngren BI, Toolanen G. Eye motility dysfunction after soft-tissue injury of the cervical spine. A controlled, prospective study of 38 patients. Acta Orthop Scand 1993;64(2):129–32.

141. Tjell C, Rosenhall U. Smooth pursuit neck torsion test: a specific test for cervical dizziness. Am J Otol 1998;19(1):76–81.

142. Treleaven J, LowChoy N, Darnell R, et al. Comparison of sensorimotor disturbance between subjects with persistent whiplash-associated disorder and subjects with vestibular pathology associated with acoustic neuroma. Arch Phys Med Rehabil 2008;89(3):522–30.

143. Prushansky T, Dvir Z, Pevzner E, et al. Electro-oculographic measures in patients with chronic whiplash and healthy subjects: a comparative study. J Neurol Neurosurg Psychiatry 2004;75(11):1642–4.

144. Kelders WP, Kleinrensink GJ, van der Geest JN, et al. The cervico-ocular reflex is increased in whiplash injury patients. J Neurotrauma 2005;22(1):133–7.

145. Della Casa E, Affolter Helbling J, Meichtry A, et al. Head-eye movement control tests in patients with chronic neck pain; inter-observer reliability and discriminative validity. BMC Musculoskelet Disord 2014;15:16.

146. Brown S. Effect of whiplash injury on accommodation. Clin Experiment Ophthalmol 2003;31(5):424–9.

147. Richter HO. Neck pain brought into focus. Work 2014;47(3): 413–18.

148. Hill K, Bernhardt J, McGann A, et al. A new test of dynamic standing balance for stroke patients: reliability, validity and comparison with healthy elderly. Physiotherapy Canada 1996;48.

149. Yu LJ, Stokell R, Treleaven J. The effect of neck torsion on postural stability in subjects with persistent whiplash. Man Ther 2011;16(4):339–43.

149a. Alund M, Larsson SE, Ledin T, et al. Dynamic posturography in cervical vertigo. Acta Otolaryngol Suppl 1991;481:601–2.

149b. Roth V, Kohen-Raz R. Posturographic characteristics of whiplash patients. En: Proceedings of the XXth Regular Meeting of The Barany Society 1998; Wuerzburg, Germany, 11–17 September 1998.

149c. Nacci A, Ferrazzi M, Berrettini S, et al. Vestibular and stabilometric findings in whiplash injury and minor head trauma. Acta Otorhinolaryngol Ital 2011;31(6):378–89.

149d. Yu LJ, Stokell R, Treleaven J. The effect of neck torsion on postural stability in subjects with persistent whiplash. Man Ther 2011;16(4):339–43.

150. Field S, Treleaven J, Jull G. Standing balance: a comparison between idiopathic and whiplash-induced neck pain. Man Ther 2008;13(3):183–91.

151. Fukuda T. The stepping test: two phases of the labyrinthine reflex. Acta Otolaryngol 1959;50(2):95–108.

152. Gagey PM, Bizzo G, Debruille O. [Are the parameters of the Fukuda's stepping test valid?]. Agressologie 1983;24(7):331–6.

153. Weber B, Gagey PM, Noto R. [Does repetition change the performance of Fukuda's test?]. Agressologie 1984;25(12): 1311–14.

154. Gagey P, Weber B. Posturología. Regulación y alteraciones de la bipedestación. Barcelona: Masson; 2001.

155. Choy NL, Johnson N, Treleaven J, et al. Balance, mobility and gaze stability deficits remain following surgical removal of vestibular schwannoma (acoustic neuroma): an observational study. Aust J Physiother 2006;52(3):211–16.

156. Alpini D, Ciavarro GL, Zinnato C, et al. Evaluation of head-to-trunk control in whiplash patients using digital CranioCorpoGraphy during a stepping test. Gait Posture 2005;22(4): 308–16.

157. Cohen HS, Sangi-Haghpeykar H, Ricci NA, et al. Utility of stepping, walking, and head impulses for screening patients for vestibular impairments. Otolaryngol Head Neck Surg 2014;151(1):131–6.

158. Bohannon RW, Larkin PA, Cook AC, et al. Decrease in timed balance test scores with aging. Phys Ther 1984;64(7): 1067–70.

159. Hill K, Bernhardt J, McGann A, et al. A new test of dynamic standing balance for stroke patients: reliability, validity and comparison with healthy elderly. Physiotherapy Canada 1996;48:257–62.

160. Norre ME, Forrez G, Stevens A, et al. Cervical vertigo diagnosed by posturography? Preliminary report. Acta Otorhinolaryngol Belg 1987;41(4):574–81.

161. Norre ME. Head extension effect in static posturography. Ann Otol Rhinol Laryngol 1995;104(7):570–3.

162. Alund M, Larsson SE, Ledin T, et al. Dynamic posturography in cervical vertigo. Acta Otolaryngol Suppl 1991;481:601–2.

163. Alund M, Ledin T, Odkvist L, et al. Dynamic posturography among patients with common neck disorders. A study of 15 cases with suspected cervical vertigo. J Vestib Res 1993;3(4): 383–9.

164. Chester JB Jr. Whiplash, postural control, and the inner ear. Spine 1991;16(7):716–20.

165. Karlberg M, Johansson R, Magnusson M, et al. Dizziness of suspected cervical origin distinguished by posturographic assessment of human postural dynamics. J Vestib Res 1996;6(1):37–47.

166. Karlberg M, Magnusson M, Malmstrom EM, et al. Postural and symptomatic improvement after physiotherapy in patients with dizziness of suspected cervical origin. Arch Phys Med Rehabil 1996;77(9):874–82.

167. Rubin AM, Woolley SM, Dailey VM, et al. Postural stability following mild head or whiplash injuries. Am J Otol 1995;16(2):216–21.

168. Mallinson AI, Longridge NS. Dizziness from whiplash and head injury: differences between whiplash and head injury. Am J Otol 1998;19(6):814–18.

169. Allum JH, Shepard NT. An overview of the clinical use of dynamic posturography in the differential diagnosis of balance disorders. J Vestib Res 1999;9(4):223–52.

170. Kogler A, Lindfors J, Odkvist LM, et al. Postural stability using different neck positions in normal subjects and patients with neck trauma. Acta Otolaryngol 2000;120(2):151–5.

171. Allum JH, Bloem BR, Carpenter MG, et al. Differential diagnosis of proprioceptive and vestibular deficits using dynamic support-surface posturography. Gait Posture 2001;14(3): 217–26.

172. Madeleine P, Prietzel H, Svarrer H, et al. Quantitative posturography in altered sensory conditions: a way to assess balance instability in patients with chronic whiplash injury. Arch Phys Med Rehabil 2004;85(3):432–8.

173. Gil-Agudo A, Baydal-Bertomeu J, Fernández-Bravo C, et al. Determinación de parámetros cinéticos en las pruebas de equilibrio y marcha de pacientes con latigazo cervical. Rehabilitación 2006;40(3):141–9.

174. Michaelson P, Michaelson M, Jaric S, et al. Vertical posture and head stability in patients with chronic neck pain. J Rehabil Med 2003;35(5):229–35.

175. Dehner C, Heym B, Maier D, et al. Postural control deficit in acute QTF grade II whiplash injuries. Gait Posture 2008; 28(1):113–19.

176. Bianco A, Pomara F, Petrucci M, et al. Postural stability in subjects with whiplash injury symptoms: results of a pilot study. Acta Otolaryngol 2014;134(9):947–51.

177. Quek J, Brauer SG, Clark R, et al. New insights into neck-pain-related postural control using measures of signal frequency and complexity in older adults. Gait Posture 2014;39(4): 1069–73.

178. Roth V, Kohen-Raz R. Posturographic characteristics of whiplash patients. In: Proceedings of the XXth regular meeting of the Barany Society, 1998; Würzburg, Germany, 11–17 September 1998.

180. Doyle RJ, Hsiao-Wecksler ET, Ragan BG, et al. Generalizability of center of pressure measures of quiet standing. Gait Posture 2007;25(2):166–71.

181. Raymakers JA, Samson MM, Verhaar HJ. The assessment of body sway and the choice of the stability parameter(s). Gait Posture 2005;21(1):48–58.

182. Lin D, Seol H, Nussbaum MA, et al. Reliability of COP-based postural sway measures and age-related differences. Gait Posture 2008;28(2):337–42.

183. Lafond D, Corriveau H, Hebert R, et al. Intrasession reliability of center of pressure measures of postural steadiness in healthy elderly people. Arch Phys Med Rehabil 2004;85(6):896–901.

184. Centomo H, Termoz N, Savoie S, et al. Postural control following a self-initiated reaching task in type 2 diabetic patients and age-matched controls. Gait Posture 2007;25(4): 509–14.

185. Cornilleau-Peres V, Shabana N, Droulez J, et al. Measurement of the visual contribution to postural steadiness from the COP movement: methodology and reliability. Gait Posture 2005;22(2):96–106.

186. Carpenter MG, Frank JS, Silcher CP, et al. The influence of postural threat on the control of upright stance. Exp Brain Res 2001;138(2):210–18.

187. Gagey PM, Toupet M. Orthostatic postural control in vestibular neuritis: a stabilometric analysis. Ann Otol Rhinol Laryngol 1991;100(12):971–5.

188. Liang Z, Clark R, Bryant A, et al. Neck musculature fatigue affects specific frequency bands of postural dynamics during quiet standing. Gait Posture 2014;39(1):397–403.

189. APF. Normes 85. Paris: Association Francaise de Posturologie; 1985.

190. Bizzo G, Guillet N, Patat A, et al. Specifications for building a vertical force platform designed for clinical stabilometry. Med Biol Eng Comput 1985;23(5):474–6.

191. Chagdes JR, Rietdyk S, Haddad JM, et al. Multiple timescales in postural dynamics associated with vision and a secondary task are revealed by wavelet analysis. Exp Brain Res 2009; 197(3):297–310.

192. Friedrich M, Grein HJ, Wicher C, et al. Influence of pathologic and simulated visual dysfunctions on the postural system. Exp Brain Res 2008;186(2):305–14.

193. Patel M, Fransson PA, Johansson R, et al. Foam posturography: standing on foam is not equivalent to standing with decreased rapidly adapting mechanoreceptive sensation. Exp Brain Res 2011;208(4):519–27.

194. Oppenheim U, Kohen-Raz R, Alex D, et al. Postural characteristics of diabetic neuropathy. Diabetes Care 1999;22(2): 328–32.

195. Paillard T, Costes-Salon C, Lafont C, et al. Are there differences in postural regulation according to the level of competition in judoists? Br J Sports Med 2002;36(4):304–5.

196. Kapoula Z, Matheron E, Demule E, et al. Postural control during the Stroop test in dyslexic and non dyslexic teenagers. PLoS ONE 2011;6(4):e19272.

197. Golomer E, Dupui P, Sereni P, et al. The contribution of vision in dynamic spontaneous sways of male classical dancers according to student or professional level. J Physiol (Paris) 1999;93(3):233–7.

198. Lacour M, Bernard-Demanze L, Dumitrescu M. Posture control, aging, and attention resources: models and posture-analysis methods. Neurophysiol Clin 2008;38(6):411–21.

199. Golomer E, Dupui P, Bessou P. Spectral frequency analysis of dynamic balance in healthy and injured athletes. Arch Int Physiol Biochim Biophys 1994;102(3):225–9.

200. Golomer E, Dupui P. Spectral analysis of adult dancers' sways: sex and interaction vision-proprioception. Int J Neurosci 2000;105(1–4):15–26.

201. Nagy E, Toth K, Janositz G, et al. Postural control in athletes participating in an ironman triathlon. Eur J Appl Physiol 2004;92(4–5):407–13.

202. Ghilardi P, Casani A, Fattori B, et al. Static posturography and whiplash. In: Alpini D, Brugnoni G, Cesarani A, editors. Whiplash injuries. 2nd ed. Milan: Springer; 2014. p. 171–84.

203. Röijezon U, Björklund M, Djupsjöbacka M. The slow and fast components of postural sway in chronic neck pain. Man Ther 2011;16(3):273–8.

204. Persson L, Karlberg M, Magnusson M. Effects of different treatments on postural performance in patients with cervical root compression. A randomized prospective study assessing

205. Reid SA, Rivett DA. Manual therapy treatment of cervicogenic dizziness: a systematic review. Man Ther 2005;10(1): 4–13.

206. Treleaven J. Sensorimotor disturbances in neck disorders affecting postural stability, head and eye movement control – Part 2: case studies. Man Ther 2008;13(3):266–75.

207. Wing LW, Hargrave-Wilson W. Cervical vertigo. Aust N Z J Surg 1974;44(3):275–7.

208. Reid SA, Rivett DA, Katekar MG, et al. Sustained natural apophyseal glides (SNAGs) are an effective treatment for cervicogenic dizziness. Man Ther 2008;13(4):357–66.

209. Reid SA, Callister R, Katekar MG, et al. Effects of cervical spine manual therapy on range of motion, head repositioning, and balance in participants with cervicogenic dizziness: a randomized controlled trial. Arch Phys Med Rehabil 2014;95(9): 1603–12.

210. Reid SA, Rivett DA, Katekar MG, et al. Comparison of Mulligan sustained natural apophyseal glides and Maitland mobilizations for treatment of cervicogenic dizziness: a randomized controlled trial. Phys Ther 2014;94(4):466–76.

211. Reid SA, Callister R, Snodgrass SJ, et al. Manual therapy for cervicogenic dizziness: long-term outcomes of a randomised trial. Man Ther 2015;20(1):148–56.

212. Watson DH, Trott PH. Cervical headache: an investigation of natural head posture and upper cervical flexor muscle performance. Cephalalgia 1993;13(4):272–84, discussion 232.

213. Jull G, Barrett C, Magee R, et al. Further clinical clarification of the muscle dysfunction in cervical headache. Cephalalgia 1999;19(3):179–85.

214. Falla D, Jull G, Rainoldi A, et al. Neck flexor muscle fatigue is side specific in patients with unilateral neck pain. Eur J Pain 2004;8(1):71–7.

215. Falla D, Jull G, Edwards S, et al. Neuromuscular efficiency of the sternocleidomastoid and anterior scalene muscles in patients with chronic neck pain. Disabil Rehabil 2004;26(12): 712–17.

216. Falla D, Jull G, Hodges PW. Feedforward activity of the cervical flexor muscles during voluntary arm movements is delayed in chronic neck pain. Exp Brain Res 2004;157(1): 43–8.

217. Falla D, Bilenkij G, Jull G. Patients with chronic neck pain demonstrate altered patterns of muscle activation during performance of a functional upper limb task. Spine 2004;29(13): 1436–40.

218. Falla D. Unravelling the complexity of muscle impairment in chronic neck pain. Man Ther 2004;9(3):125–33.

219. Falla DL, Jull GA, Hodges PW. Patients with neck pain demonstrate reduced electromyographic activity of the deep cervical flexor muscles during performance of the craniocervical flexion test. Spine 2004;29(19):2108–14.

220. Nederhand MJ, Hermens HJ, IJZerman MJ, et al. Chronic neck pain disability due to an acute whiplash injury. Pain 2003;102(1–2):63–71.

221. Falla D, Rainoldi A, Merletti R, et al. Myoelectric manifestations of sternocleidomastoid and anterior scalene muscle fatigue in chronic neck pain patients. Clin Neurophysiol 2003;114(3):488–95.

222. Elert J, Kendall SA, Larsson B, et al. Chronic pain and difficulty in relaxing postural muscles in patients with fibromyalgia and chronic whiplash associated disorders. J Rheumatol 2001;28(6):1361–8.

223. Sarig-Bahat H, Weiss PL, Laufer Y. Cervical motion assessment using virtual reality. Spine 2009;34(10):1018–24.

224. Sarig-Bahat H, Weiss PL, Laufer Y. Neck pain assessment in a virtual environment. Spine 2010;35(4):E105–12.

225. Sarig Bahat H, Weiss PL, Laufer Y. The effect of neck pain on cervical kinematics, as assessed in a virtual environment. Arch Phys Med Rehabil 2010;91(12):1884–90.

226. Sarig Bahat H, Chen X, Reznik D, et al. Interactive cervical motion kinematics: sensitivity, specificity and clinically significant values for identifying kinematic impairments in patients with chronic neck pain. Man Ther 2015;20(2):295–302.

227. Sarig Bahat H, Takasaki H, Chen X, et al. Cervical kinematic training with and without interactive VR training for chronic neck pain – a randomized clinical trial. Man Ther 2015;20(1):68–78.

228. Hansson EE, Mansson NO, Hakansson A. Effects of specific rehabilitation for dizziness among patients in primary health care. A randomized controlled trial. Clin Rehabil 2004;18(5):558–65.

229. Schneider KJ, Meeuwisse WH, Nettel-Aguirre A, et al. Cervicovestibular rehabilitation in sport-related concussion: a randomised controlled trial. Br J Sports Med 2014;48(17):1294–8.

230. Shepard NT, Telian SA, Smith-Wheelock M, et al. Vestibular and balance rehabilitation therapy. Ann Otol Rhinol Laryngol 1993;102(3 Pt 1):198–205.

231. Yardley L, Beech S, Zander L, et al. A randomized controlled trial of exercise therapy for dizziness and vertigo in primary care. Br J Gen Pract 1998;48(429):1136–40.

232. Cohen HS, Kimball KT. Increased independence and decreased vertigo after vestibular rehabilitation. Otolaryngol Head Neck Surg 2003;128(1):60–70.

9

PHYSICAL AND PSYCHOLOGICAL FACTORS INVOLVED IN WHIPLASH: IMPLICATIONS FOR PHYSIOTHERAPY ASSESSMENT AND MANAGEMENT

MICHELE STERLING

INTRODUCTION

Whiplash-associated disorders (WAD) are a common, disabling and costly condition. While the figures vary depending on the cohort studied, most international data indicate that up to 50% of people will not fully recover.[1] The symptoms of those who do not fully recover may range from milder levels of neck pain and associated disability to moderate/severe pain and disability that have significant effects on the person's everyday life.[1,2] The associated cost secondary to whiplash injury, including medical care, disability and lost work productivity, as well as personal costs, is substantial.[3,4]

Most treatments evaluated, to date, for the acute stages of the whiplash injury are yet to demonstrate efficacy in terms of decreasing the incidence of those who develop persistent symptoms.[5–7] This is not to suggest that little has been learnt from these randomized controlled trials. Indeed it is apparent that maintenance of activity and sensible advice is superior to rest and prescription of a collar for most whiplash-injured individuals.[8] However, even in the presence of such a treatment approach, significant numbers of patients develop persistent symptoms. One reason for this may be due to the non-specific nature of the treatments that have been investigated which appear to view WAD as a homogeneous condition with little consideration to potential mechanisms involved. It would appear that WAD is a more complex condition than previously assumed. In recent years, investigations have begun to provide insight of the characteristics of the whiplash condition – both physical and

psychological – that allows speculation of potential underling mechanisms.

This chapter outlines the whiplash injury, possible structures involved and classification before discussing the burgeoning knowledge of the physical and psychological manifestations of the condition and the implications for clinical physiotherapy practice.

THE WHIPLASH INJURY

Symptoms following whiplash injury can be diverse in nature. The predominant symptom is neck pain that typically occurs in the posterior region of the neck but can also radiate to the head, shoulder and arm, thoracic, interscapular and lumbar regions.[9] Symptoms such as headache, dizziness/loss of balance, visual disturbances, paraesthesia, anaesthesia, weakness and cognitive disturbances such as concentration and memory difficulties are also common.[9–11] The onset of symptoms may occur immediately or, in many patients, may be delayed for up to 12–15 hours.[12]

The mechanism of whiplash injury has not been fully elucidated but it is generally accepted that it involves a complex buckling of the cervical spine with concomitant flexion and extension occurring simultaneously at different segmental levels.[13] Bioengineering studies where cadavers were subjected to simulated rear-end crashes have demonstrated perturbations in segmental movement, including intersegmental hyperextension in the lower cervical spine, S-curve formation and differential acceleration of the upper cervical spine.[14,15] Secondary thoracic spine movement also occurs, including superiorly directed acceleration and extension/rotation of the upper thoracic spine, which has been referred to as thoracic ramping.[15] Documented spinal kinematics in response to whiplash injury have mainly focused on the most commonly reported accident, the rear-end collision. It should be noted that other collision directions, including front-end and side-impact collisions, do frequently occur. There is some evidence to suggest that muscle activation may affect head and neck responses to a greater extent in these collision directions when compared to a rear impact, thus having some protective capacity on soft tissues.[15,16]

It is conceivable that virtually any cervical spine structure may be injured following whiplash injury. The quest to identify structures injured following a whiplash collision, in vivo, is complicated by the insensitivity of current imaging technology to identify these more subtle lesions.[17] Nevertheless, when evidence is taken together from bioengineering studies, identifying the possibility for lesions to occur,[18] and cadaveric studies, where clear lesions are demonstrated in non-survivors of a motor vehicle crash (MVC), there is reasonable argument for the presence of pathoanatomical lesions in at least some of the injured people.[19] Damaged structures may include, amongst others, zygapophyseal joints, intervertebral discs, synovial folds, vertebral bodies and nerve tissue (including dorsal root ganglia, spinal cord or brainstem).[19]

Clinical studies provide some support for the findings of potential structural lesions from both bioengineering and cadaveric studies. Lord et al.[20] linked zygapophyseal arthropathy with chronic WAD by achieving substantial pain relief in some patients with persistent pain following a whiplash injury using placebo-controlled zygapophyseal joint blocks. Smith and colleagues have also shown decreases in psychological distress and quantitative sensory measures of pain and hyperalgesia following radiofrequency neurotomy of zygapophyseal joints in patients with chronic WAD.[21,22]

CLASSIFICATION OF WHIPLASH INJURY AND RECOVERY PATHWAYS

The Quebec Task Force (QTF) classification of whiplash injuries (Table 9-1)[23] was put forward in 1995 and it remains the classification method still currently used

TABLE 9-1

The Quebec Task Force (QTF) classification of whiplash-associated disorders

QTF classification grade	Clinical presentation
0	No complaint about neck pain No physical signs
I	Neck complaint of pain, stiffness or tenderness only No physical signs
II	Neck complaint Musculoskeletal signs, including: ■ decreased range of movement ■ point tenderness
III	Neck complaint Musculoskeletal signs Neurological signs, including: ■ decreased or absent deep tendon reflexes ■ muscle weakness ■ sensory deficits
IV	Neck complaint and fracture or dislocation

From Spitzer et al.[23]

throughout the world. While the QTF system is rather simplistic and based only on signs and symptoms, it allows practitioners and other stakeholders involved in the management of patients with WAD to have a common language about the condition. Most patients fall into the WAD II classification, although health outcomes for this group can be diverse and this has been outlined as one problem with the QTF system.[24] Modifications to the QTF system have been proposed but have generally been more complicated[24] and, for this reason, are not easily taken up by all stakeholders involved in the management of WAD.

Cohort studies have demonstrated that recovery, if it occurs, takes place within the first 2–3 months following the injury, with a plateau of the condition following this time point.[2,25] Even in those with poor overall recovery, there appears to be an initial decrease in symptoms to some extent in this early post-injury period. Recently, three distinct clinical recovery pathways following whiplash injury were identified using trajectory modelling analysis[2]:

1. A pathway of good recovery where initial levels of pain-related disability were mild to moderate and recovery was good, with 45% or people predicted to follow this pathway.
2. A pathway of initial moderate/severe pain-related disability with some recovery but with disability levels remaining moderate at 12 months, with 39% of injured people predicted to follow this pathway.
3. A pathway of initial severe pain-related disability and some recovery to moderate/severe disability, with 16% of individuals predicted to follow this pathway.

Physical characteristics of the whiplash condition

Whereas it is probably important that a specific structural lesion can be identified in whiplash- injured individuals, it has been argued that the identification of the pathoanatomical source of symptoms provides little basis for appropriate management of musculoskeletal pain, and emphasis should instead be placed on treatment approaches directed towards mechanisms and processes underlying the painful condition.[26,27] These authors were, in this case, referring to neuropathic pain conditions, but a similar approach to other musculoskeletal conditions is necessary. With respect to whiplash-associated disorders, it is emerging that a variety of physical and psychological impairments characterize the condition.

Movement, motor and sensorimotor dysfunction

The most commonly identified motor deficit in WAD is that of movement loss or decreased cervical range of movement.[28,29] Most prospective studies have shown that all whiplash-injured individuals have a loss of cervical active range of movement from soon after injury.[30,31] Kasch et al.[30] reported that restoration of movement loss had occurred in all individuals by 3 months post injury, irrespective of recovery or non-recovery. However, if whiplash subjects are classified more precisely, it can be seen that those with persistent moderate/severe levels of pain and disability (measured with NDI) continue to display active movement loss at 3 months post injury. In contrast, participants who had recovered or reported lesser (but still significant) pain and disability showed restoration of movement loss[28] similar to that seen by Kasch and colleagues (Fig. 9-1). This demonstrates the importance of differentiating individuals with whiplash based on pain and disability levels.

Altered patterns of muscle recruitment in both the cervical spine and shoulder girdle regions have been clearly shown to be a feature of chronic WAD.[32,33] Longitudinal data demonstrate that these changes are

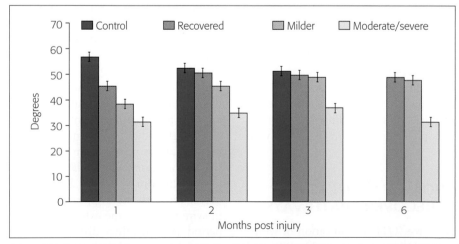

FIGURE 9-1 ■ Mean (SEM) for whiplash groups (recovered, mild pain and disability, moderate/severe pain and disability) and controls at < 1 month, 2, 3 and 6 months post injury for active extension.

apparent from very soon after injury,[28,33] with greater deficits in those reporting higher levels of pain and disability.[28] It is important to note that the disturbed motor patterns persist, not only in those with ongoing chronic symptoms but also in those with milder pain and disability and those who report full recovery with this phenomena occurring at significant time periods post injury – 3 months and 2 years.[28,34] These persisting deficits in muscle control may leave recovered individuals more vulnerable to future episodes of neck pain, but this proposal has not yet been substantiated.[34] Nevertheless, these findings demonstrate the significant effect whiplash injury has on the motor function of the cervical spine and indicate that early and specific rehabilitation will probably be important in the management of all those with a whiplash injury, irrespective of reported symptoms.

Sensorimotor dysfunction is also a feature of both acute and chronic WAD. Investigation of this sensorimotor dysfunction has focused on three areas: kinaesthetic deficits, balance disturbance and loss of eye movement control. Kinaesthetic deficits, mainly in the form of increased joint repositioning errors, have been frequently shown to exist in chronic WAD, with greater repositioning errors in patients with dizziness.[10,35] Balance disturbances are also evident in chronic WAD (again worse in those reporting dizziness) and seem to be unrelated to confounding factors such as medication type, anxiety or compensation status.[36] The smooth pursuit neck torsion test has been used as a measure of neck-influenced eye movement control.[37] In this test, eye movement control is measured with the head in a neutral position and then compared to eye movement with the trunk rotated beneath the head (neck torsion).[37] Patients with WAD show disturbed eye movement control in the neck torsioned position that is not apparent in patients with vestibular disorders or central nervous system disorders.[37] Chronic whiplash-injured patients with dizziness again show greater loss of eye movement control.[38]

It is apparent that sensorimotor dysfunction will be an important issue for consideration in the assessment and treatment of whiplash injury. It would appear that while all those with chronic WAD show deficits to a certain extent, those patients reporting dizziness and/or unsteadiness show greater deficits, indicating that emphasis may need to be placed on these factors in the management of dizzy whiplash-injured individuals. Only the measure of joint repositioning error has been investigated in the acute stage of whiplash injury, where it has been shown that greater errors are present within a few weeks of injury, particularly in those with moderate/severe levels of pain and disability.[28]

The mechanisms underlying sensorimotor disturbances in WAD are not entirely clear, although most clinicians subscribe to the proposal that it is due to the disordered afferent input from damaged cervical spine articular and/or muscular structures.[10,39] However, other factors are yet to be ruled out, such as the effect of inflammatory mediators on muscle spindle activity, effects of pain on central nervous system function, vestibular dysfunction and potential effects of medication and anxiety.

Evidence for central hyperexcitability in whiplash

Whereas motor dysfunction has been shown to be a consistent feature of WAD, such dysfunctions are also present in those with idiopathic neck pain: i.e. neck pain of a non-traumatic nature.[32,33,40] In contrast, sensory hypersensitivity (central hyperexcitability) may be a feature that differentiates the two neck pain conditions and could help to explain the higher levels of pain and disability so often reported by patients with WAD.[41]

Consistent evidence from numerous cohorts demonstrates the presence of sensory hypersensitivity (or decreased pain thresholds) to a variety of stimuli in WAD. Two recent systematic reviews have concluded that there is moderate evidence that the sensory presentation of widespread sensory hypersensitivity at sites both local and remote to the injured area found in chronic WAD indicates the presence of augmented nociceptive processing or sensitization within the central nervous system.[42,43] Later findings would support this, with clear evidence of spinal cord hyperexcitability,[44] as well as impaired descending inhibitory mechanisms.[45] Whereas there are some reports of similar findings indicative of central sensitization in non-traumatic neck pain when compared to healthy controls,[46] direct comparisons of non-traumatic neck pain and WAD have shown more pronounced sensory disturbances in the latter traumatic neck pain group.[41,47,48] These findings suggest different nociceptive processing mechanisms may underlie neck pain, depending on whether or not it is of traumatic onset, and this could be one reason for apparently better responses to physical treatments in patients with non-traumatic neck pain.[49,50] It also suggests that neck pain classification systems will need to take these findings into account and that a single classification system for all neck pain may not be optimal. These proposals require further investigation.

Mechanical hyperalgesia locally over the cervical spine seems to be common to both chronic whiplash and idiopathic neck pain and probably indicates an ongoing peripheral nociceptive source of pain.[41,51] In addition to its presence in the chronic stages of neck pain conditions, local mechanical hyperalgesia has also been shown to occur following acute whiplash injury, irrespective of symptom intensity and disability levels reported by the patient.[28,30] However, the local mechanical hyperalgesia resolved within several weeks in those who recovered or reported continuing milder symptoms but persisted unchanged in whiplash patients reporting persistent symptoms of a moderate/severe nature at 6 months post injury.[28]

In contrast, the phenomena of widespread sensory hypersensitivity may be unique to WAD. Scott et al.[41] showed chronic WAD subjects to have a more complex presentation involving lowered pain thresholds for pressure, heat and cold stimuli in areas remote to the cervical spine which were not present in idiopathic neck pain subjects. The reasons for these differences between the conditions are not clear but it has been demonstrated that conditions with more severe and widespread pain show greater degrees of sensory hypersensitivity.[52] Patients with WAD generally report higher levels of pain and disability[41] and, at least clinically, tend to have more widespread pain. The findings of Scott and colleagues[41] added to the previous body of knowledge demonstrating WAD to be a condition involving more complex changes in the neurobiological processing of pain most likely occurring within the central nervous system.

It is important to note that the widespread sensory hypersensitivity that is a consistent feature of chronic WAD has been shown to be present soon after injury, at least in those whiplash-injured people with poor functional recovery.[53,54] Most importantly, sensory features of cold hyperalgesia appear to be prognostic

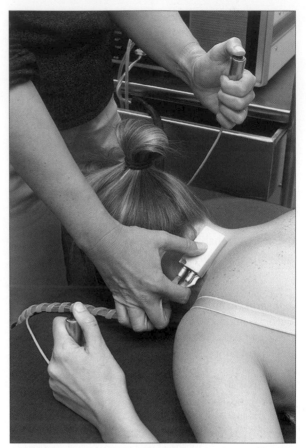

FIGURE 9-2 ■ Measurement of cold pain thresholds over the cervical spine in the laboratory setting. The thermode is preset to 30°C and increased at 1°C /second until the participant first feels pain.

indicators for poor recovery at long-term follow-ups of 6 months and 2 years post injury (Figs 9-2 and 9-3).[34,55–57] It is essential that physiotherapists are alert to features of a patient's clinical presentation that may indicate a propensity for the development of chronic symptoms and, for this reason, assessment of sensory function will be important.

PSYCHOLOGICAL FACTORS INVOLVED IN WHIPLASH-ASSOCIATED DISORDERS

As with any painful musculoskeletal condition, relationships between psychological factors and health outcomes have been well documented and this is no

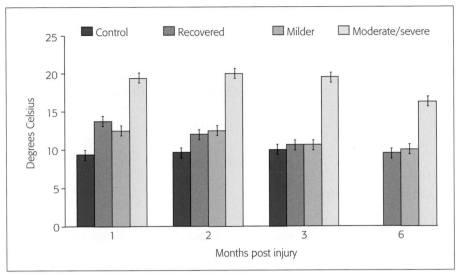

FIGURE 9-3 ■ Cold pain thresholds (measured over the cervical spine) in controls (1–3 months) and three whiplash groups (recovered, NDI < 8; milder symptoms, NDI 10–28; and moderate/severe symptoms, NDI > 30) at 1, 2, 3 and 6 months post injury.[54] The whiplash group with persistent moderate/severe symptoms demonstrates cold hyperalgesia from within 1 month of injury that does not resolve.

different for whiplash. It is generally considered that psychological factors do not by themselves alone fully explain poor recovery following the injury but that they are likely to interact with other processes and play a role in the persistence of symptoms. In the case of whiplash injury, some factors including post-traumatic stress symptoms,[57,58] pain catastrophizing[59] and negative expectations of recovery[60] have shown prognostic capacity in some studies. Other psychological factors include depression[59,61] and fear of movement,[62,63] and have conflicting evidence for prognosis, with some studies showing an association with poor recovery and others finding no association.

WAD is initiated by a traumatic event, usually an MVC. Post-traumatic stress disorder (PTSD) is a common psychological sequela following MVCs,[6] yet it is only recently that it has been investigated in WAD. The effect of the distress surrounding the crash itself, as opposed to or in addition to distress about neck pain, may have a significant influence on outcome. Recent data indicate that PTSD symptoms are not uncommon in individuals who have sustained whiplash injuries following an MVC.[58,65,66] The early presence of post-traumatic stress symptoms has been shown to be associated with poor functional recovery

from the injury.[55,57,58] A significant proportion (10–25%) of whiplash-injured individuals also meet the diagnostic criteria for PTSD, in addition to the cardinal signs of neck pain,[58,67,68] and this co-morbidity of pain and PTSD may contribute to poor recovery following the injury.

The development of pain/disability and PTSD symptoms seems to be related, and research has begun to focus on the potential shared neurobiological pathways between PTSD and pain.[69,70] In regard to research of WAD, in addition to PTSD symptoms predicting pain-related disability following injury, the reverse relationship also exists where, initially, higher pain levels predict later PTSD symptoms.[56] In this study cold hyperalgesia also predicted both pain-related disability as well as PTSD symptoms.[56] Further exploration of the relationship between pain-related disability and PTSD symptoms has been conducted in experimental studies. Interventions aimed at improving PTSD symptoms had been shown to also have effects on decreasing pain and disability. In a preliminary randomized controlled trial, Dunne et al.[71] showed that trauma-focused cognitive behavioural therapy (CBT), an evidence-based treatment for PTSD,[72] resulted in clinically relevant changes in pain and disability in addition to expected decreases in PTSD symptoms and PTSD diagnosis in patients with chronic WAD. In a later study, also in chronic WAD, it was shown that a trauma-cue exposure resulted in greater cold and mechanical hyperalgesia measured at sites over the cervical spine.[73]

Thus data is accumulating that demonstrates close relationships between the pain, disability and PTSD symptoms following whiplash injury.

THE PREDICTION OF OUTCOME FOLLOWING WHIPLASH INJURY

With up to 50% of those sustaining a whiplash injury reporting ongoing pain and disability, it is important to be able to clinically identify both those at risk of poor recovery as well as those who will recover well. This may assist in targeting ever-shrinking health resources to those in most in need of them. The most consistent risk factors for poor recovery are, initially, higher levels of reported pain and, initially, higher levels of disability.[1,74] A recent meta-analysis indicated that initial pain scores of greater than 5.5/10 on a visual analogue scale (VAS) and scores of greater than 29% on the Neck Disability Index (NDI) are useful cut-offs cores for clinical use.[74] In view of the consistency of these two factors to predict poor functional recovery, they should be mandatory in the assessment of patients with acute WAD.[75]

Other factors have also been identified that show prognostic capacity in various studies. These include psychological factors of initial moderate post-traumatic stress symptoms, pain catastrophizing and symptoms of depressed mood.[1,57,59] Additionally, lower expectations of recovery have been shown to predict poor recovery.[60,76]

Cold hyperalgesia has been shown to predict disability and mental health outcomes at 12 months post injury[34,56] and decreased cold pain tolerance measured with the cold pressor test predicted ongoing disability.[53] A recent systematic review concluded that there is moderate evidence available to support cold hyperalgesia as an adverse prognostic indicator.[77] Other sensory measures such as lowered pressure pain thresholds (mechanical hyperalgesia) show inconsistent prognostic capacity. Walton et al.[78] showed that decreased pressure pain thresholds over a distal site in the leg predicted neck pain-related disability at 3 months post injury but other studies have shown that this factor is not an independent predictor of later disability.[34] The exact mechanisms underlying the hyperalgesic responses are not clearly understood but are generally acknowledged to reflect augmented nociceptive processing in the central nervous system or central hyperexcitability.[42,79]

Some factors commonly assessed by physiotherapists do not show prognostic capacity and these include measures of motor and sensorimotor function such as the craniocervical flexion test, joint repositioning errors and balance loss.[80] Decreased range of neck movement is inconsistent, in that some studies have found it to be predictive and others have not.[74] This is not to say that these factors should not be considered in the clinical assessment of patients with WAD, but they should not be used to gauge prognosis. Other factors commonly considered to predict outcome such as those associated with compensation processes and accident-related factors are not robust prognostic indicators.[81] Few demographic or social factors such as income and educational levels demonstrate consistent prognostic capacity, although age demonstrates inconsistent predictive capacity.[74]

Most prognostic studies of WAD have been phase 1 or exploratory studies, with few confirmatory or validation studies conducted.[82] Validation studies are important in order to confirm the prognostic capacity of identified factors in a new and independent cohort. A recent study undertook validation of a set of prognostic indicators that included initial disability, cold hyperalgesia, age and post-traumatic stress symptoms. The results indicated that the predictive set showed good accuracy to discriminate patients with moderate/severe disability from patients with full recovery or residual milder symptoms at 12 months post injury.[57] These results are clinically useful as physiotherapists usually aim to broadly identify patients likely to report persistent moderate/severe symptoms.

Based on data of previous cohort studies, a clinical prediction rule to identify both chronic moderate/severe disability and full recovery at 12 months post injury was recently developed. The results indicated that an initial NDI score of $\geq$ 40%, age $\geq$ 35 years and a score of $\geq$ 6 on the hyperarousal subscale of the Post-traumatic Stress Diagnostic Scale[83] could predict

TABLE 9-2

Prognostic indicators of poor functional recovery following whiplash injury based on findings of systematic reviews

Factors showing consistent evidence for being prognostic indicators for poor recovery	Factors showing consistent evidence of not being prognostic indicators	Factors with inconsistent evidence
■ Initial pain levels: > 5.5/10 ■ Initial disability levels: NDI > 29% ■ Symptoms of post-traumatic stress ■ Negative expectations of recovery ■ High pain catastrophizing ■ Cold hyperalgesia	■ Accident-related features (e.g. collision awareness, position in vehicle, speed of accident) ■ Findings on imaging ■ Motor dysfunction	■ Older age ■ Female gender ■ Neck range of movement ■ Compensation-related factors

patients with moderate/severe disability at 12 months with fair sensitivity, good specificity and a positive predictive value of 72%.[84] It is also important to predict patients who will recover well, as these patients will likely require less intensive intervention. Initial NDI scores of ≤ 32% and age ≤ 35 years predicted full recovery at 12 months post injury, with a positive predictive value of 71%.[84] A third medium-risk group could either recover or develop chronic pain and disability (> 32% on the NDI score and >3 on the hyperarousal subscale).The hyperarousal subscale comprises five items that evaluate the frequency of symptoms: having trouble falling asleep; feelings of irritability; difficulty concentrating; being overly alert; and being easily startled.[85]

Table 9-2 summarizes consistent prognostic indicators for poor functional recovery, factors with consistent evidence of not being associated with poor recovery and factors with inconsistent evidence.

IMPLICATIONS FOR PHYSIOTHERAPY ASSESSMENT OF WHIPLASH

The clinical assessment of the patient with whiplash injury should attempt to reflect the physical and psychological processes shown to be involved in the condition. It is clear that a precise and thorough assessment of the whiplash-injured patient will be required and this will be particularly important in the acute stage of injury in order to identify risk factors for chronicity that may be targeted for treatment.

The patient assessment will need to include an adequate history, such as previous history of neck pain and headache, as well as the possible mechanism of injury. Although accident-related features have not been shown to be consistent prognostic indicators of outcome,[86] they have shown some predictive capacity in certain studies.[87] Since pain and disability levels have been repeatedly shown to be a consistent indicator of prolonged recovery,[74] it is essential that validated tools to measure these constructs are used in the initial assessment. The patient should be screened for the presence of any 'red flag' condition (WAD IV – fracture/dislocation) as well psychosocial 'yellow flags'. With respect to whiplash , the psychological factor of post-traumatic stress appears to be involved in the transition from the acute to chronic stages of the condition and clinicians may want to include a measure of post-traumatic stress symptoms (e.g. Impact of Events Scale) in their assessment of the whiplash-injured patient.[75]

As outlined previously in this chapter, the identification of sensory hypersensitivity in patients with WAD is important for two reasons: first, because of the association of sensory hypersensitivity with poor or delayed recovery[56,57] and, secondly, because care should be taken with physical interventions to avoid further provocation of central hyperexcitability and symptom exacerbation. Information is gained in the patient interview and history that may alert the clinician to the presence of sensory hypersensitivity. Whiplash-injured patients with sensory hypersensitivity invariably also report higher levels of pain and disability,[54] emphasizing the importance of obtaining a measure of these factors. Additional clues to the presence of sensory hypersensitivity may include the following: high irritability of the condition[88]; the presence of mechanical and thermal allodynia (e.g. pain when the shirt sleeve or bed clothes touch the skin or intolerance of cold); and difficulty sleeping due to the pain. Additionally, the presence of non-painful symptoms such as paraesthesia or anaesthesia should be recorded.

It has been shown that taking into account both painful and non-painful symptoms can improve the accuracy of a neuropathic pain diagnosis made from the subjective reports of the patient,[89] but whether this can be extrapolated to the whiplash condition is not clear.

Physical examination will provide further indication of the presence or not of sensory hypersensitivity. Hyperalgesic or even allodynic responses to manual examination of the cervical spine are common in whiplash patients and likely reflect central hyperexcitability. The use of pressure algometry in the clinical situation is becoming more common and will probably be a useful tool in the assessment of whiplash. Of course, clinical neurological examination (sensation loss, muscle power, reflexes) will be necessary where indicated, since some patients will be classifiable as WAD III (neurological deficit). However, these appear to be the minority of the whiplash-injured patients, with the majority showing marked sensory disturbance but without conduction loss (WAD II), thus reflecting the heterogeneous nature of this classification group.[24]

The presence of cold hyperalgesia and sympathetic disturbances seems to be important in the outcome following whiplash injury.[77] The clinical assessment of cold pain threshold is difficult with the currently available laboratory equipment being expensive and thus not feasible for clinical use. A recent study demonstrated that a VAS of pain > 5/10 with application of ice to the cervical spine correlates well with laboratory measures of cold hyperalgesia and may be useful in clinical practice.[90]

Physiotherapists routinely assess cervical range of movement and this will remain a mainstay of assessment due to the prognostic capacity of this measure. Assessment will also need to include muscle recruitment patterns of the cervical and shoulder girdle regions. Furthermore, the assessment of sensorimotor dysfunction is relatively simple to undertake in the clinical situation and will be particularly important in whiplash- injured patients who report dizziness associated with their neck pain. Readers are referred to Jull et al.[91] for a detailed account of how to undertake these assessments.

In the presence of high levels of pain and disability and sensory hypersensitivity, the examination of the whiplash-injured patient may need to be curtailed, at least in the first instance. For reasons outlined earlier, it is important that symptoms and hyperalgesic responses are not exacerbated in this patient group.

IMPLICATIONS FOR PHYSIOTHERAPY MANAGEMENT

Currently available guidelines for the management of acute WAD promote reassurance to the patient, the maintenance of activity levels, neck exercises and simple analgesics.[75] However, the emerging multifactor nature of WAD suggests that while the current guidelines may benefit some whiplash patients with a less complex presentation, they are likely to be inadequate for the management of those with a complex condition that includes both marked physical dysfunction and psychological distress.

It is not clear at present if physiotherapy interventions have the capacity to modulate sensory hypersensitivity. Spinal manual therapy exerts a hypoalgesic effect for mechanical hyperalgesia[92] but it is not known if similar effects occur for cold hyperaglesia. Results from a preliminary randomized controlled trial of physiotherapy (exercise and manual therapy) for chronic whiplash indicate that the presence of cold and mechanical hyperalgesia mitigates against an effective reduction in pain and disability levels seen in those without these features,[93] although this finding was not replicated in a later larger study.[50] These patients may require pharmacological intervention to achieve adequate pain relief.

This is not to suggest that physiotherapy, including exercise and manual therapy, is not indicated for those with neck pain from whiplash injury. A combined specific exercise and manual therapy approach has demonstrated efficacy in the management of cervicogenic headache (idiopathic neck pain).[49] This treatment approach has been shown to decrease pain and disability in patients with chronic whiplash without the presence of mechanical and cold hyperalgesia.[93] A more general graded exercise programme has also shown some effectiveness in this patient group.[94] However, a recent study demonstrated no greater effect with an intensive 12-week exercise programme compared to a single session with a physiotherapist providing information and exercise advice.[50] Additional processes such as psychological factors and central hyperexcitability may require specific targeting in addition to exercise, and approaches along these lines are currently being tested.

CONCLUSION

The physiotherapist plays an important role in the assessment and management of individuals with whiplash injuries. It is now recognized that WAD is a complex heterogeneous condition involving varying degrees of physical (motor, sensorimotor and sensory) disturbances as well as psychological distress. Clinicians should make every attempt to precisely examine the patient and this will need to include assessment of physical and psychological factors in addition to reported levels of pain and disability. This data, together with sound clinical reasoning skills, lays the foundation for the early identification of those at risk of poor recovery and the institution of tailored and appropriate interventions for all whiplash-injured patients in order to provide an optimal chance of recovery.

REFERENCES

1. Carroll L, Holm L, Hogg-Johnson S, et al. Course and prognostic factors for neck pain in whiplash-associated disorders (WAD). Results of the Bone and Joint Decade 2000–2010 Task Force on Neck Pain and Its Associated Disorders. Spine 2008;33(42):583–92.
2. Sterling M, Hendrikz J, Kenardy J. Developmental trajectories of pain/disability and PTSD symptoms following whiplash injury. Pain 2010;150(1):22–8.
3. Crouch R, Whitewick R, Clancy M, et al. Whiplash associated disorder: incidence and natural history over the first month for patients presenting to a UK emergency department. Emerg Med J 2006;23(2):114–18.
4. MAIC. Annual report 2011-2012. Brisbane; 2012.
5. Jull G, Kenardy J, Hendrikz J, et al. Management of acute whiplash: a randomized controlled trial of multidisciplinary stratified treatments. Pain 2013;154:1798–806.
6. Lamb S, Gates S, Williams M, et al. Emergency department treatments and physiotherapy for acute whiplash: a pragmatic, two-step, randomised controlled trial. Lancet 2013;381(9866): 546–56.
7. Teasell R, McClure J, Walton D, et al. A research synthesis of therapeutic interventions for whiplash-associated disorder (WAD): part 2 – interventions for acute WAD. Pain Res Manag 2010;15(5):295–304.
8. Scholten-Peeters G, Bekkering G, Verhagen A, et al. Clinical practice guideline for the physiotherapy of patients with whiplash associated disorders. Spine 2002;27(4): 412–22.
9. Barnsley L, Lord S, Bogduk N. The pathophysiology of whiplash. Spine State of the Art Reviews 1998;12(2):209 42.
10. Treleaven J, Jull G, Sterling M. Dizziness and unsteadiness following whiplash injury – characteristic features and relationship with cervical joint position error. J Rehabil Med 2003;35(1):36–43.
11. Radanov B, Sturzenegger M. Predicting recovery from common whiplash. Eur Neurol 1996;36:48–51.
12. Provinciali L, Baroni M. Clinical approaches to whiplash injuries: a review. Crit Rev Phys Rehabil Med 1999;11:339–68.
13. Davis C. Injury threshold: whiplash associated disorders. J Manipulative Physiol Ther 2000;23(6):420–7.
14. Cusick J, Pintar F, Yoganandan N. Whiplash syndrome: kinematic factors influencing pain patterns. Spine 2001;26(11): 1252–8.
15. Stemper B, Yoganandan N, Rao R, et al. Influence of thoracic ramping on whiplash kinematics. Clin Biomech (Bristol, Avon) 2005;20:1019–28.
16. Brolin K, Halldin P, Leijonhufvud I. The effect of muscle activation on neck response. Traffic Inj Prev 2005;6: 67–76.
17. Uhrenholt L, Grunnet-Nilsson N, Hartvigsen J. Cervical spine lesions after road traffic accidents. a systematic review. Spine 2002;27(17):1934–41.
18. Yoganandan N, Pintar F, Cusick J. Biomechanical analyses of whiplash injuries using an experimental model. Accid Anal Prev 2002;34:663–71.
19. Curatolo M, Bogduk N, Ivancic P, et al. The role of tissue damage in whiplash associated disorders. Spine 2011;36(25S): S309–15.
20. Lord S, Barnsley L, Wallis B, et al. Chronic cervical zygapophysial joint pain after whiplash: a placebo-controlled prevalence study … including commentary by Derby R Jr. Spine 1996; 21(15):1737–45.
21. Smith A, Jull G, Schneider G, et al. Cervical radiofrequency neurotomy reduces psychological distress and pain catastrophization, but not post-traumatic stress in individuals with chronic WAD. Pain Res Manag 2013;18(2):e13.
22. Smith A, Jull G, Schneider G, et al. Cervical radiofrequency neurotomy reduces Central hyperexcitability and improves neck movement in individuals with chronic whiplash. Pain Med 2014;15(1):128–41.
23. Spitzer W, Skovron M, Salmi L, et al. Scientific Monograph of Quebec Task Force on Whiplash associated Disorders: redefining "Whiplash" and its management. Spine 1995;20(8S): 1–73.
24. Sterling M. A proposed new classification system for whiplash associate disorders – implications for assessment and management. Man Ther 2004;9(2):60–70.
25. Kamper S, Rebbeck T, Maher C, et al. Course and prognostic factors of whiplash: a systematic review and meta-analysis. Pain 2008;138(3):617–29.
26. Woolf C, Bennett G, Doherty M, et al. Towards a mechanism-based classification of pain. Pain 1998;77:227–9.

27. Jensen T, Baron R. Translation of symptoms and signs into mechanisms in neuropathic pain. Pain 2003;102(2):1–8.
28. Sterling M, Jull G, Vizenzino B, et al. Development of motor system dysfunction following whiplash injury. Pain 2003;103:65–73.
29. Dall'Alba P, Sterling M, Trealeven J, et al. Cervical range of motion discriminates between asymptomatic and whiplash subjects. Spine 2001;26(19):2090–4.
30. Kasch H, Flemming W, Jensen T. Handicap after acute whiplash injury. Neurology 2001;56:1637–43.
31. Sterling M, Jull G, Vicenzino B, et al. Characterisation of acute whiplash associated disorders. Spine 2004;29(2):182–8.
32. Jull G, Kristjansson E, Dall'Alba P. Impairment in the cervical flexors: a comparison of whiplash and insidious onset neck pain patients. Man Ther 2004;9(2):89–94.
33. Nederhand M, Hermens H, Ijzerman M, et al. Cervical muscle dysfunction in chronic whiplash associated disorder grade 2. The relevance of trauma. Spine 2002;27(10):1056–61.
34. Sterling M, Jull G, Kenardy J. Physical and psychological predictors of outcome following whiplash injury predictive capacity at long term follow-up. Pain 2006;122:102–8.
35. Heikkilä H, Wenngren B. Cervicocephalic kinesthetic sensibility, active range of cervical motion and oculomotor function in patients with whiplash injury. Arch Phys Med Rehabil 1998;79:1089–94.
36. Treleaven J, Jull G, LowChoy N. Standing balance in persistent whiplash: a comparison between subjects with and without dizziness. J Rehabil Med 2005;37:224–9.
37. Tjell C, Rosenhall U. Smooth pursuit neck torsion test: A specific test for cervical dizziness. Am J Otol 1998;19:76–81.
38. Treleaven J, Jull G, LowChoy N. Smooth pursuit neck torsion test in whiplash-associated disorders: relationship to self-reports of neck pain and disability, dizziness and anxiety. J Rehabil Med 2005;37:219–23.
39. Revel M. Cervicocephalic kinesthetic sensibility in patients with cervical pain. Arch Phys Med Rehabil 1991;72:288–91.
40. Tjell C, Rosenhall U. Smooth pursuit neck torsion test – a specific test for WAD. Journal of Whiplash and Related Disorders 2002;1(2):9–24.
41. Scott D, Jull G, Sterling M. Widespread sensory hypersensitivity is a feature of chronic whiplash-associated disorder but not chronic idiopathic neck pain. Clin J Pain 2005;21(2):175–81.
42. Stone A, Vicenzino B, Lim E, et al. Measures of central hyperexcitability in chronic whiplash associated disorder – a systematic review and meta-analysis. Man Ther 2012;18(2):111–17.
43. Van Oosterwijck J, Nijs J, Meeus M, et al. Evidence for central sensitization in chronic whiplash: a systematic literature review. Eur J Pain 2013;17:299–312.
44. Lim E, Sterling M, Stone A, et al. Central hyperexcitability as measured with nociceptive flexor reflex threshold in chronic musculoskeletal pain: a systematic review. Pain 2011;152(8):1811–20.
45. Ng T, Pedler A, Vicenzino B, et al. Less efficacious conditioned pain modulation and sensory hypersensitivity in chronic whiplash-associated disorders in Singapore. Clin J Pain 2014;30(5):436–42.
46. Johnston V, Jimmieson N, Jull G, et al. Quantitative sensory measures distinguish office workers with varying levels of neck pain and disability. Pain 2008;137:257–65.
47. Chien A, Eliav E, Sterling M. Sensory hypoaesthesia is a feature of chronic whiplash but not chronic idiopathic neck pain. Man Ther 2010;15(1):48–53.
48. Elliott J, Jull G, Sterling M, et al. Fatty infiltrate in the cervical extensor muscles is not a feature of chronic insidious onset neck pain. Clin Radiol 2008;63(6):681–7.
49. Jull G, Trott P, Potter H, et al. A randomised controlled trial of physiotherapy management for cervicogenic headache. Spine 2002;27(17):1835–43.
50. Michaleff Z, Maher C, Lin C, et al. Comprehensive physiotherapy exercise program or advice alone for chronic whiplash (PROMISE): a pragmatic randomised controlled trial (ACTRN12609000825257). Lancet 2014;384(9938):133–41.
51. Chien A, Eliav E, Sterling M. Sensory function in chronic whiplash associated disorders. In: 11th World Congress on Pain 2005; Sydney.
52. Carli G, Suman A, Biasi G, et al. Reactivity to superficial and deep stimuli in patients with chronic musculoskeletal pain. Pain 2002;100:259–69.
53. Kasch H, Qerama E, Bach F, et al. Reduced cold pressor pain tolerance in non-recovered whiplash patients: a 1 year prospective study. Eur J Pain 2005;9(5):561–9.
54. Sterling M, Jull G, Vicenzino B, et al. Sensory hypersensitivity occurs soon after whiplash injury and is associated with poor recovery. Pain 2003;104:509–17.
55. Sterling M, Jull G, Vicenzino B, et al. Physical and psychological factors predict outcome following whiplash injury. Pain 2005;114:141–8.
56. Sterling M, Hendrikz J, Kenardy J. Similar factors predict disability and PTSD trajectories following whiplash injury. Pain 2011;152(6):1272–8.
57. Sterling M, Hendrikz J, Kenardy J, et al. Assessment and validation of prognostic models for poor functional recovery 12 months after whiplash injury: a multicentre inception cohort study. Pain 2012;153(8):1727–34.
58. Buitenhuis J, DeJong J, Jaspers J, et al. Relationship between posttraumatic stress disorder symptoms and the course of whiplash complaints. J Psychosom Res 2006;61(3):681–9.
59. Walton D, Pretty J, MacDermid J, et al. Risk factors for persistent problems following whiplash injury: results of a systematic review and meta-analysis. J Orthop Sports Phys Ther 2009;39(5):334–50.
60. Holm L, Carroll L, Cassidy D, et al. Expectations for recovery important in the prognosis of whiplash injuries. PLoS Med 2008;5(5):e105.
61. Carroll L, Liu Y, Holm L, et al. Pain-related emotions in early stages of recovery in whiplash-associated disorders: their presence, intensity and association with pain recovery. Psychosom Med 2011;73(8):708–15.
62. Pedler A, Sterling M. Assessing fear-avoidance beliefs in patients with whiplash associated disorders: a comparison of 2 measures. Clin J Pain 2011;27(6):502–7.

63. Williamson E, Williams M, Gates S, et al. A systematic review of psychological factors and the development of late whiplash syndrome. Pain 2008;135:20–30.

64. Deleted in proofs.

65. Sterling M, Kenardy J, Jull G, et al. The development of psychological changes following whiplash injury. Pain 2003;106(3):481–9.

66. Sullivan M, Thibault P, Simmonds M, et al. Pain, perceived injustice and the persistence of post-traumatic stress symptoms during the course of rehabilitation for whiplash injuries. Pain 2009;145(3):325–31.

67. Mayou R, Bryant B. Psychiatry of whiplash neck injury. Br J Psychiatry 2002;180:441–8.

68. Jaspers J. Whiplash and post-traumatic stress disorder. Disabil Rehabil 1998;20:397–404.

69. Asmundson G, Coons M, Taylor S, et al. PTSD and the expereince of pain: research and clinical implications. Can J Psychiatry 2002;47(10):930–7.

70. McLean S, Clauw D, Abelson J, et al. The development of persistent pain and psychological morbidity after motor vehicle collision: integrating the potential role of stress response systems into a biopsychosocial model. Psychosom Med 2005; 67:783–90.

71. Dunne R, Kenardy J, Sterling M. A randomised controlled trial of cognitive behavioural therapy for the treatment of PTSD in the context of chronic whiplash. Clin J Pain 2012;28(9):755–65.

72. NHMRC. Australian guidelines for the treatment of adults with ASD and PTSD; 2007.

73. Dunne-Proctor R, Kenardy J, Sterling M. The impact of Post-traumatic Stress Disorder on physiological arousal, disability and sensory pain thresholds in patients with chronic whiplash. Clin J Pain 2016;32(8):645–53.

74. Walton D, Macdermid J, Giorgianni A, et al. Risk factors for persistent problems following acute whiplash injury: update of a systematic review and meta-analysis. J Orthop Sports Phys Ther 2013;43(2):31–43.

75. MAA. Guidelines for the management of whiplash associated disorders. Sydney: Motor Accident Authority (NSW); <www.maa.nsw.gov.au> 2014.

76. Carroll L, Holm L, Ferrari R, et al. Recovery in whiplash-associated disorders: do you get what you expect. J Rheumatol 2009;36:1063–70.

77. Goldsmith R, Wright C, Bell S, et al. Cold hyperalgesia as a prognostic factor in whiplash associated disorders: a systematic review. Man Ther 2012;17(5):402–10.

78. Walton D, McDermid J, Teasell R, et al. Pressure pain threshold testing demonstrates predictive ability in people with acute whiplash. J Orthop Sports Phys Ther 2011;41(9):658–65.

79. Curatolo M, Arendt-Nielsen L, Petersen-Felix S. Evidence, mechanisms and clinical implications of central hypersensitivity in chronic pain after whiplash injury. Clin J Pain 2004;20(6): 469–76.

80. Daenen L, Nijs J, Raadsen B, et al. Cervical motor dysfunction and its predictive value for long-term recovery in patients with acute whiplash-associated disorders: a systematic review. Man Ther 2013;45(2):113–22.

81. Spearing N, Connelly L, Gargett S, et al. Systematic review: Does compensation have a negative effect on health after whiplash? Pain 2012;153:1274–82.

82. Sterling M, Carroll L, Kasch H, et al. Prognosis after whiplash injury: Where to from here? Discussion Paper 3. Spine 2011;36(25S):s330–4.

83. Foa E, Cashman L, Jaycox L, et al. The validation of a self-report measure of posttraumatic stress disorder: the posttraumatic diagnostic scale. Psychol Asses 1997;9(4):445–51.

84. Ritchie C, Hendrikz J, Kenardy J, et al. Development and validation of a screening tool to identify both chronicity and recovery following whiplash injury. Pain 2013;154:2198–206.

85. Foa E Posttraumatic stress diagnostic scale: manual. Minneapolis: NCS Pearson; 1995.

86. Scholten-Peeters G, Verhagen A, Bekkering G, et al. Prognostic factors of whiplash-associated disorders: a systematic review of prospective cohort studies. Pain 2003;104(1–2):303–22.

87. Sturzenegger M, Radanov B, Stefano GD. The effect of accident mechanisms and initial findings on the long-term course of whiplash injury. J Neurol 1995;242:443–9.

88. Zusman M. Mechanisms of musculoskeletal physiotherapy. Phys Ther Rev 2004;9:39–49.

89. Bouhissera D, Attal N. Novel strategies for neuropathic pain. In: Villannueva L, Dickensen A, Ollat H, editors. The pain system in normal and pathological states. Seattle: IASP Press; 2004. p. 299–310.

90. Maxwell S, Sterling M. An investigation of the use of a numeric pain rating scale with ice application to the neck to determine cold hyperalgesia. Man Ther 2012;18(2):172–4.

91. Jull G, Falla D, Treleaven J, et al. A therapeutic exercise approach for cervical disorders. In: Jull G, Boyling J, editors. Grieve's modern manual therapy. 3rd ed. Edinburgh: Churchill Livingstone; 2005.

92. Vicenzino B, Collins D, Benson H, et al. An investigation of the interrelationship between manipulative therapy-induced hypoalgesia and sympathoexcitation. J Manipulative Physiol Ther 1998;21(7):448–53.

93. Jull G, Sterling M, Kenardy J, et al. Does the presence of sensory hypersensitivity influence outcomes of physical rehabilitation for chronic whiplash? – A preliminary RCT. Pain 2007;129(2): 28–34.

94. Stewart M, Maher C, Refshauge K, et al. Randomized controlled trial of exercise for chronic whiplash-associated disorders. Pain 2007;128(1–2):59–68.

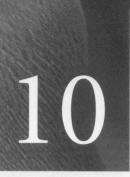

10

CERVICAL MANIPULATION AND NEUROVASCULAR ACCIDENTS

RAFAEL TORRES CUECO ■ LUCY THOMAS

━━━━━━━━━━━━━━━━━━━━━━━━━━━━━━━━━━━

Manipulative therapy of the cervical spine, and in particular high-velocity manipulative techniques, may on rare occasions lead to serious complications involving the extracranial cervical arteries: that is, the vertebrobasilar system and, less commonly, the internal carotid artery.[1-4] Although the internal carotid arteries provide the majority (80%) of the blood supply, the vertebral and basilar arteries provide 20% of the total cerebral flow[5,6] and, therefore, their compromise can cause ischaemia of the brainstem and the cerebellar structures, causing serious long-term effects and, in some cases, death.[7,8] Cervical arterial dissection leading to cerebrovascular ischaemia or stroke is in fact the most serious side effect that can occur subsequent to cervical spine manipulation.[4,9] Injuries to the cervical arteries are not only the consequence of a cervical manipulation but also of minor mechanical trauma to the neck, and can even appear spontaneously, with no obvious injury of the vertebrobasilar system when performing rotation or cervical extension techniques.[10-13] The problem lies in the fact that some of the most frequent symptoms of cervical arterial injury are similar to those of a cervical musculoskeletal pathology, such as cervical pain and headaches. These are also the most common early symptoms of vertebral or carotid arterial dissection.[14] Whereas such neurovascular complications are not common, the potential serious long-term sequelae have led this topic to be widely reviewed in recent years.

PREVALENCE

While it is considered a highly uncommon complication, the reported incidence of cervical arterial injury following neck manipulation varies widely in the different studies published.[15-19] Haldeman et al.[12] considered that the risk of arterial dissection after cervical manipulation is significantly low, with 1 in 5.85 million manipulations. However, the risk has more usually been estimated higher, reaching 1 in 400,000 and 1 in 1.5 million manipulations.[3,15,17,20-23]

In the last 20 years, the literature has shown an increase in the frequency of vertebral artery injuries as a consequence of manipulation.[16,24,25] It has been suggested that the incidence of serious complications is underestimated, since in many cases, such complications are not reported to the public authorities.[4,26] This has been confirmed by confidential information obtained from lawsuits in Australia[27] and by a study conducted by Rivett and Reid,[28] in which 1 in 163,371 manipulations resulted in a cerebrovascular incident. It is also possible that a number of cases go unrecognized and heal spontaneously.[10,26] However, in general, the incidence is low but warrants much better education of practitioners who provide manipulative therapy to the cervical spine.[2]

Although cerebrovascular incidents are considered a highly infrequent complication, the consequences for both patient and practitioner can be devastating.[20,29] This type of procedure is not entirely free of risks, and hence the importance of this topic.

344

Cerebrovascular incidents are the most serious side effects following a vertebral manipulation. Although cerebrovascular incidents are considered a highly uncommon complication, manipulative procedures are not free of risks.

ANATOMY OF THE CERVICAL ARTERIES

Although the vertebral artery is the artery more frequently injured after a manipulative procedure,[12] the internal carotid artery can also suffer the same type of injuries[9,30] (Fig. 10-1).

Vertebral artery

The vertebral artery runs vertically from the subclavian artery towards the cervical spine, and is divided into four areas or segments relative to particular anatomical relationships.[31,32] These four regions are known as pretransverse segment (V1), transverse segment (V2), atlantoaxial segment (V3) and intracranial segment (V4) (Fig. 10-2).

The pretransverse segment (V1) is located between the longus colli and the anterior scalenus, in close proximity to the stellate ganglion, and is located in front of the transverse process of C7, where it enters inside the transverse foramen of C6. Although the artery usually accesses the cervical spine at this level, it can also enter through the transverse foramen of higher levels, even as far as C3.[31]

The transverse segment (V2) is composed of the entire part that passes up through the transverse foramina of the cervical vertebrae until it emerges at C2. In this trajectory, it is accompanied by vessels and a sympathetic plexus. At each level, it is located in front of the spinal nerves upon emergence through the intervertebral foramen. The artery is coated with connective tissue that adheres to the soft tissue around it. Thus, the external layer of the artery, the adventitia, is attached, directly or indirectly, into the periosteum of the transverse foramen and the muscular fascia,[33] while remaining secure inside the foramen.

The atlantoaxial segment (V3) is the part of the artery that runs from its exit at the transverse foramen of C2 to its entry through the occipital foramen.[31] In this segment, the artery changes from a vertical orientation to a horizontal orientation, describing two curves: one that goes forwards and outwards, from the transverse foramen of C2 to the transverse foramen of C1; and another that goes backwards and inwards, from the foramen of C1 to the posterior part of the occipital foramen (Fig. 10-3). This arterial segment is

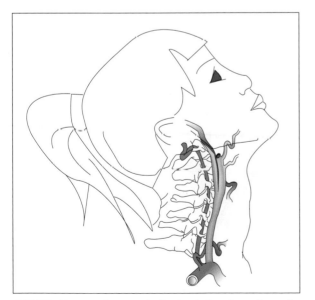

FIGURE 10-1 ■ The encephalic circulation depends on the vertebral and internal carotid arteries.

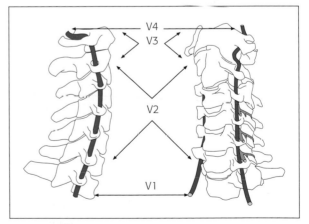

FIGURE 10-2 ■ The vertebral artery is divided into four segments, each one with particular anatomical relationships: pretransverse segment (V1), transverse segment (V2), atlantoaxial segment (V3) and intracranial segment (V4).

in contact with the posterior cervical muscles and crosses the atlanto-occipital membrane. At the level of C1, the vertebral artery rests on its posterior arch, in a canal, and is supported by a ligamentous ring, the retroglenoid ligament, before crossing the atlanto-occipital membrane and the dura mater to enter the skull[33–37] (Fig. 10-4). On occasions, this ligament may be ossified, forming a bony bridge (posterior ponticle) that may be complete or incomplete[38,39] (Fig. 10-5). In this segment the artery is more susceptible to suffer an injury due to the significant tensile and shearing forces as a consequence of the high degree of mobility, especially in rotation, of this region of the cervical spine[40–43] (Fig. 10-6).

The intracranial segment (V4) pierces the dura mater 10–15 mm from the midline, and is located anterolaterally to both sides; it is joined to its counterpart to form the basilar artery, which subsequently feeds into the circle of Willis. It is worth noting that there are wide individual variations in the anatomy of the vertebrobasilar system, and this suggests that its vulnerability varies also from one individual to another.[36,44,45] The basilar artery has numerous brainstem branches, the cerebellar arteries (anterior, from which a labyrinthine artery emerges; posteroinferior cerebellar; superior cerebellar), and the posterior cerebral artery.

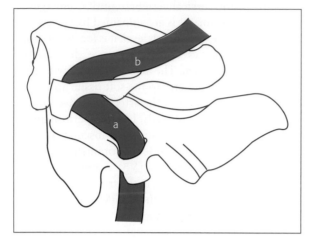

FIGURE 10-3 ■ In the V3 segment, the vertebral artery goes from a vertical orientation to a horizontal orientation, describing two curves: (a) one that goes forwards and outwards, from the transverse foramen of C2 to the transverse foramen in C1; and (b) that goes backwards and inwards, from the foramen of C1 to the posterior part of the occipital foramen.

Internal carotid artery

The internal carotid artery branches off from the common carotid artery around the level of C3 and is

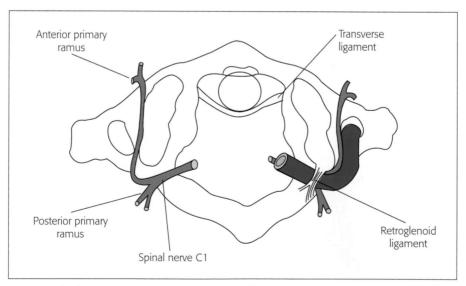

FIGURE 10-4 ■ The vertebral artery rests on the posterior arch of C1, forming a channel, in which the retroglenoid ligament stabilizes it.

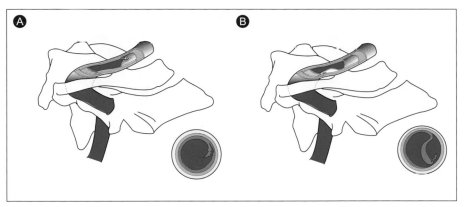

FIGURE 10-10 ■ Rupture of the tunica intima (A) and arterial dissection (B).

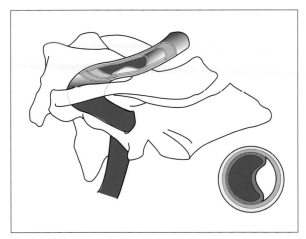

FIGURE 10-11 ■ Rupture of the tunica media and arterial dissection as a consequence of the intramural bleeding of the vasa vasorum.

trigger a vasospasm. The dissection of the arterial walls can extend along the artery.[2,80,102,103]

Alterations of the local circulation, as a consequence of the dissection, associated with the exposure of the subendothelial tissue of the artery, can promote platelet aggregation and the formation of thrombus that can be embolized and block the circulation distally.[98,99,104] (Fig. 10-12). The arterial dissection can, therefore, lead to a temporary ischaemia or permanent cerebral or brainstem ischaemia: for example, lateral medullary or Wallenberg syndrome. Nevertheless, in some cases, cerebral ischaemia does not occur thanks to the ability of the collateral circulation to provide adequate perfusion to the brainstem.[45,105]

When there is a dissection of the cervical arteries, if spontaneous, in 88% of cases there is a complete clinical recovery.[106] Mortality during the first month is only 2%, and 1% within the next 10 years.[107] However, in a review of accidents after manipulation conducted by Di Fabio, the mortality reached 18% of cases.[108] In general, though, the majority of patients who suffer arterial dissection have a good outcome with no or low levels of disability.[2,90]

Vasospasm is the other theoretical mechanism responsible for ischaemia. Vertebrobasilar ischaemia has been described, even with fatal results, after a manipulation, in which the angiography, Doppler ultrasound or an autopsy has not been able to find evidence of a minimal vascular injury.[2,90,109–112] It was proposed, therefore, that in these cases the mechanism responsible for the neurological after-effects could be a temporary arterial spasm.[92,110,113–116] Improvements in imaging capabilities in recent years have made these instances less common, as more subtle radiographic features can now be more readily identified. It is known that vasospasms are one of the most important causes of mortality after a serious vascular trauma.[117] These vasospasms have also been observed in vertebral arteries after a cervical trauma.[92,118,119] Cases of temporary ischaemia due to vasospasms in the internal carotid artery have likewise been described, without an injury or vascular pathology.[120] This type of vasospasm seems to occur as a response to strong vasoconstrictive substances released by blood elements, and by the wall of the vessels, secondary to the trauma of the arterial wall.[53] Even so, the role played by vasospasms in the

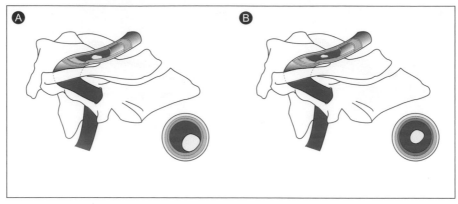

FIGURE 10-12 ■ Formation of thrombus (A) and embolization (B).

injury of the cervical artery due to a minimal trauma is currently mere speculation and it is considered unlikely that such vasospasm would be sufficient to cause permanent ischaemia.[80,97]

RISK FACTORS

Injuries of the cervical arteries can occur as the consequence of cervical manipulation or a non-traumatic event. The problem faced by therapists is identifying those subjects in a risk situation. In the last few years, several reviews have been conducted with the purpose of identifying the risk factors associated with cervical manipulation.[2,4,12,40,41,108,121–126]

One of the difficulties in understanding the risk factors is that these complications are relatively infrequent. As highlighted by Haldeman et al.,[124] in large hospitals in the United States and Canada, there are no more than three cases of dissection of the vertebral artery per year and, therefore, many of the statements regarding this entity are only the result of the extrapolation or generalization of the observations obtained from a small number of patients, case series or expert opinions.[2]

The risk factors for a cerebrovascular incident can be classified as those related to the patient and those related to the manipulative technique.

Risk factors related to the patient

The proposed risk factors related to the patient include anatomical anomalies of the vertebral arteries, previ-ous traumas of the cervical arteries, anomalies in the components of the arterial walls, age, sex, cardiovascular factors such as hypertension, oral contraceptives, smoking and migraines.

Anatomical anomalies of the vertebral arteries

There is wide anatomical variability in the cervical arteries, and this implies that their vulnerability may differ widely from one individual to another.[36,44,45] Different anatomical anomalies, such as hypoplasia, or anomalies in their origin and path, may favour their injury during a manipulative treatment.[36,80]

Hypoplasia of the vertebral arteries. Asymmetry of the vertebral arteries has been proposed as a factor that favours the appearance of vertebrobasilar complications in the cervical manipulation.[127] This asymmetry is very common, and is present between 7.5 and 13.7% of the population.[38] The left vertebral artery is, in general, thicker than the right one.[45,128] We should consider that, although the lumen of the vertebral artery is reduced with cervical rotation and, consequently, blood flow may decrease, cerebral perfusion is usually maintained due to connection with the circle of Willis. This is the case because in order to reduce the cerebral perfusion, a significant reduction of the flow of the cervical arteries is necessary on the one hand, and on the other hand, the collateral circulation also needs to be insufficient to maintain adequate perfusion. However, when one of the arteries is noticeably hypoplastic, the cerebral perfusion can be critically reduced during the rotation of the cervical spine.

Anomalies in the origin and path of the cervical arteries.

The anomalies in the origin and path of the cervical arteries are varied, but one of the most serious anomalies is the lack of connection between the arteries of the circle of Willis.

In regards to adverse events that occur after a manipulation, an abnormal origin of the postero-inferior cerebellar artery has been described. This artery usually emerges from the vertebral artery in its intracranial segment, and therefore it cannot be injured by a trauma. However, on occasions, it can emerge from the vertebral artery before entering the foramen magnum and, therefore, cervical trauma could injure it directly.[129]

Dissection of the vertebral artery has also been described in cases where the artery has an anomalous access to the cervical spine through the transverse foramen of C3 instead of C6.[130]

Previous traumas of the cervical arteries

One of the causes for the dissection of the cervical arteries is serious cervical trauma.[131–133] This traumatic aetiology was thought by some to make up for 24–59% of all dissections,[131,134] most often due not to vertebral manipulation but to motor vehicle accidents.[135] However, more recently, cervical arterial dissection is thought to be more commonly associated with minor or trivial trauma.[26,90,136,137] Dissection can also occur spontaneously, though often this is in association with trivial event involving some strain of the neck.[26,30] Some authors consider that there should be a distinction between a traumatic and a spontaneous cervical artery dissection, since there are significant differences between the type of injuries and the residual after-effects.[138] Thus, in traumatic dissections, aneurysms are more frequent, they progress to arterial occlusion more frequently and the residual neurological deficits are greater. In contrast, in patients with a spontaneous dissection, recovery is more common. Often, in serious traumas of the cervical spine, the dissection of the vertebral artery can be masked by other serious tissue injuries.[139] Therefore, there is a need for an adequate physical assessment that includes a neurological examination of every patient that has suffered a cervical trauma.

- In serious traumas of the cervical spine, the dissection of the vertebral artery can be masked by other serious injuries.
- In patients that have suffered a cervical trauma, it is necessary to perform an adequate physical examination that includes a neurological exploration.

Dissection of the cervical arteries can also be the result of a minimal indirect trauma to the head or neck or a trivial movement, such as the extension position of the cervical spine during a dental procedure[140] or when coughing[30,141] or sneezing, maintaining the cervical spine in rotation,[49] having one's hair washed at a beauty salon,[142–145] doing yoga,[103,146] or other sporting activities[26,136,137,147] or painting the ceiling.[103] Furthermore, it is known that the rupture of the tunica intima is a common cause of spontaneous dissection of a cervical artery, when performing a physiological movement of the cervical spine, such as extension and rotation, and without any known trauma,[13,18,104,148] although more recently some authors have described the tunica media and outer layers of the arterial wall to be primarily affected in spontaneous dissection.

On occasions, a cerebrovascular adverse event occurs after manipulation despite the patient receiving several previous manipulations without incident.[12,97] This situation is not infrequent and is suggested by post mortem studies in which recent and old thrombus were found, potentially related to spontaneous dissections or previous manipulations.[27,149] This finding shows how a spontaneous arterial injury, or one due to manipulation, can remain subclinical, and may heal spontaneously, yet the risk of extending an existing injury and causing serious vertebrobasilar complications when performing the manipulation is very high.

A spontaneous arterial injury or one due to manipulation can remain subclinical, and the risk of serious vertebrobasilar complications following manipulation is very high.

Abnormalities in the structural components of the arterial walls

One of the factors that appears to be involved in the dissection of the cervical arteries after a manipulation is the existence of an underlying arteriopathy[10,150] or genetic anomalies of the structural elements of the arterial walls, such as collagen and elastin.[10,90]

Histological studies[151,152] of the vertebral artery show the existence of structural defects in the inner elastic layer in subjects that have had a dissecting aneurysm. This layer, belonging to the tunica intima, is composed primarily of elastic fibres and is considered the most resistant of the arterial walls. The study by Sato[152] also showed that the defects of the inner elastic layer are associated with a thinning of the tunica intima. These two associated alterations reduce the resistance of the arterial wall and are located at a point preceding the entrance of the vertebral artery in the dura mater, and this coincides with the C1–C2 sector, where the injuries of the vertebral artery are more frequent.

A family history that includes an arterial dissection or arteriopathy could be useful to identify possible patients at risk.[153,154] Pathologies that can predispose subjects to the dissection of the cervical arteries include fibromuscular dysplasia,[155–157] Ehlers–Danlos syndrome type IV[158–160] and Marfan syndrome.[161–163] Schievink[164] suggested that 20% of patients with dissection of the cervical arteries suffer from some alteration of the connective tissue, and this is supported by other authors, but this may not be an established hereditary tissue disorder, demonstrated, for example, by skeletal, ocular or skin abnormalities, or facial dysmorphisms.[165] In addition, the systemic hyperlaxity is thought to be a risk factor,[97] due to its possible relationship with a benign variant of Ehlers–Danlos syndrome. However, other studies have failed to find convincing evidence of connective tissue disorders in patients with dissection[136] or any genetic association.[90]

Some authors have suggested that an anomaly in the metabolism of homocysteine, such as hyperhomocysteinemia, can increase the risk of an arterial injury, since it causes structural fragility of the arterial walls,[72,166] but this has not been confirmed by more recent studies although it may be important in some groups.[167]

Furthermore, other risk factors have been identified, such as age, gender, hypertension, oral contraceptives and migraines.

Regarding age, it is commonly considered that the risks for a vertebrobasilar injury are higher in elderly subjects, due to the degeneration of the cervical spine, arteriosclerosis and atherosclerotic changes. However, it appears that arteriosclerosis and atherosclerosis may be protective for dissection[90] and dissection of the cervical arteries is actually a more frequent cause of cerebrovascular incidents in young adults aged ≤ 45 years old.[10,168] It is known, for instance, that cerebrovascular injuries in sport, most commonly undertaken by younger people, are due primarily to the dissection of the vertebral or carotid arteries.[136,169] With regards to the published cases of adverse events after a manipulation, the majority of victims are young adults between the ages of 30 and 45 years old.[108,121] However, it has been said that this higher occurrence of accidents in this age group may just reflect the characteristics of patients that seek manipulative treatment more often.[124,170]

Other risk factors, such as gender,[10] and cardiovascular factors such as hypertension,[171,172] use of oral contraceptives[40,173] and smoking,[174] cannot be validated with enough evidence.[90]

Migraine is a risk factor for cerebrovascular incident in young adults, and some authors link it to adverse events subsequent to cervical manipulation.[149,175] However, it has not been currently demonstrated that these events occur more frequently in these subjects[40]; even so, it is not recommended to manipulate the cervical spine of a subject with a migraine crisis.[170]

It has been said that there may be seasonal risk factors for dissection,[168,176,177] suggesting a transient environmental factor may be to blame. Schievink et al.[177] examined a group of 200 patients and observed that there was an extremely high occurrence of dissections of the vertebral artery in the month of October; 58% more patients suffered the dissection during autumn compared with the rest of the year. Some authors[42,178] have presented cases of dissection of the vertebral artery in subjects that had suffered a respiratory infection, and the number of cases of arterial dissection also increased in the seasons in which respiratory infections were more frequent. It is possible that pro-inflammatory mechanisms associated with infection may make the artery more fragile and vulnerable to trauma.[90,141]

Risk factors related to manipulation

Mann and Refshauge[27] analysed the different aspects that characterized high-velocity manipulation techniques, such as strength, velocity, amplitude, direction and their relationship with vascular accidents. Symons et al.[88] have studied the forces supported by the vertebral artery during a manipulation, demonstrating that their magnitude is considerably lower than that necessary to cause its disruption.[179]

Commonly, it is considered that the force and amplitude of the impulse, more than the velocity, are the parameters responsible for the injury of the vertebral artery. In fact, it is considered by some authors that the velocity of the manipulation minimizes the risks of tissue injury. However, others suggest this premise may not be relevant in arteries, due to their viscoelastic nature.[27] It might be expected a manoeuvre performed at high speed is more likely to cause an arterial injury than one performed at a slower speed.[180] Before performing a high-velocity manipulation, it is advisable to use manoeuvres that increase arterial viscoelasticity, such as muscular stretching or physiological mobilization techniques.

Amplitude of the manipulation is one of the parameters considered to be directly related to the injury of the cervical arteries. The fact that the majority of the dissections occur in the atlantoaxial segment seems to be related to the high mobility of the vertebral artery.[42,60,114,181] However, the amplitude of movement induced by manipulation is considered to be much smaller than that induced by mobilization techniques and therefore to have less effect on the vertebral artery.[86,182]

There is a relationship between adverse events caused by manipulation and the direction of the manipulative thrust. It has been demonstrated that manipulative techniques in rotation seem to be associated with a higher risk of cerebrovascular incidents.[22,104,108,183,184] One of the reasons which may explain this is the fact that cervical rotation is thought to alter the blood flow in the contralateral vertebral artery. Nevertheless, this theory is currently controversial. Whereas different studies, both experimental and with specimens,[59,65,185] as well as those using different techniques, such as arteriography,[62,186] Doppler ultrasound[70,75,187–190] and angiography with magnetic resonance,[191–194] show that rotation can diminish the flow

of the vertebral artery of the opposite side to the rotation, other studies do not find significant haemodynamic changes.[36,195–197] Other clinicians have shown increases in flow in neck rotation in the contralateral vertebral artery, leading to the suggestion that measurement of blood flow may be highly variable between individuals and therefore not particularly useful for determination of the risk of an adverse event from neck manipulation.[76]

Mitchell et al.,[189,198] using transcranial Doppler ultrasound, analysed the V4 portion of the vertebral artery in young asymptomatic subjects to determine if the movements of the cervical spine are capable of reducing the perfusion within the posterior fossa. Their study showed that maximum rotation of the cervical spine can reduce perfusion in both vertebral arteries, although more significantly on the side opposite to the rotation. It is evident that these alterations in perfusion are more likely in older subjects, in whom the vascular pathology is more prevalent.[108] These findings give some justification, according to the authors, to the practice of the functional test of the vertebral artery in rotation, particularly in older patients. In another work, conducted by Sakaguchi et al.,[190] 1108 patients received an ultrasound of the vertebral artery. Many of the patients showed a change in the velocity of the flow during rotation. Among these patients, 12.3% had symptoms during cervical rotation, possibly related to vertebrobasilar insufficiency (VBI), such as vertigo and blurred vision, suggesting compression in the vertebral artery. One subject from this group then underwent an angiography of the posterior cerebral artery and a single-photon emission computed tomography (SPECT) during cervical rotation to confirm this. The first evidence of compression occurring during a submaximal cervical rotation showed an obvious arterial compression between C1–C2, and the second one, a pronounced decrease in the perfusion of the occipital cortex, the cerebellum and the brainstem.

Arnold et al.[199] showed, with Doppler ultrasound, the effect of different positions used as functional tests of the vertebral artery in 21 subjects, 6 with possible VBI, and they observed a pronounced decrease in the arterial flow in the position of maximum rotation.

In contrast, however, there are other works that did not show changes in arterial perfusion during rotation.

Thiel et al.[196] compared 30 asymptomatic subjects to 12 subjects with symptoms that could be attributed to a VBI and which were triggered by the manoeuvre of combined neck extension plus rotation. Their results showed that the different positions of the head and neck had little effect on the flow of the vertebral artery. They used this work to question the validity of the manoeuvres employed in pre-manipulative tests, although the results were not entirely reliable, as the authors themselves were not sure of whether the symptoms corresponded to a VBI or another pathology. Cote et al.[195] submitted the results of Thiel's study to a statistical analysis, and they reached the same conclusion – the extension–rotation test is not a valid manoeuvre to rule out a VBI – and advised against its use. In support of this, some authors reported studies which showed marked reduction or occlusion of blood flow in the vertebral artery in contralateral rotation yet no signs or symptoms of VBI were experienced by participants.[196,200] Similarly, ultrasound studies of individuals who tested positive on pre-manipulative positional tests have shown normal blood flow.[200]

Thomas et al.[76,193] used magnetic resonance angiography to measure blood flow simultaneously in all four cervical arteries during various pre-manipulative positions and found while blood flow in some vessels was decreased in some rotation positions, it tended to be compensated for by the other arteries and total blood flow to the brain was maintained.

It is important to note that most of the blood flow studies have examined effects of head position, but few have examined the effect of the manipulative thrust. However, Licht et al. have observed, with Doppler ultrasound, that the velocity of the vertebral artery flow is not significantly modified immediately after a high-velocity manipulation, neither in asymptomatic subjects,[201] nor in those whose pre-manipulative tests were positive.[202] This finding was also confirmed in a more recent ultrasound[203] and magnetic resonance study.[204]

A study conducted by Zaina et al.[197] showed that, in normal subjects, rotation, including maximum rotation, did not cause significant changes in the perfusion of the vertebral artery. Three years earlier, this group of researchers had developed a reliable method based on the measurement of two parameters: the peak velocity of the flow in C1–C2 in the position of maximum rotation of the cervical spine and the percentage of volume of the flow in C5–C6.[36] Zaina et al.,[197] in their last work, demonstrated – although only clearly in the left vertebral artery – that there was a reduction of the velocity in C1–C2 when moving from a maximum rotation to the neutral position. This finding justifies that, during the pre-manipulative tests, clinicians evaluate the appearance of a response for a few seconds after moving from a maximum rotation position to the neutral position. Yet, since this study was exclusively conducted in normal subjects, its conclusions cannot be extrapolated to subjects with VBI. The only studies which have been conducted on symptomatic individuals and that have shown marked changes in blood flow in the vertebral arteries on head rotation have used elderly patients with severe cardiovascular disease.[194,205]

These striking discrepancies can be explained by methodological differences, such as the parameter used to quantify the arterial flow, what movement or combination of movements were analysed, if the subjects that were studied were symptomatic or asymptomatic, the type of ultrasound scanner used, if the study was conducted with the subject in the supine position or sitting down, and the experience of the researcher with this type of study.[197] Despite these findings, it is important to appreciate there are some individuals in whom blood flow is affected by head position and it is these people in whom care must be taken with manual techniques.

Although the results are conflicting regarding the decreased perfusion during the cervical rotation, it is evident that, as this is the movement with the highest degree of amplitude in the craniocervical spine and potentially biomechanical strain, it can generate a significant amount of stretching over the vertebral artery. This elongation can reach 3–5% of the neutral length with a contralateral rotation.[88,179]

In this craniocervical region, the tension over the artery can be at its greatest, since those areas where the ends are relatively fixed, as is the case between the transverse foramen of C1 and C2, a large amplitude rotation to the opposite side may induce a stretching of the vertebral artery in this section.[206] Haynes et al.[38,207] have suggested that the decrease in the flow of the vertebral artery during the rotation movement is not due to a elongation of the arterial lumen induced by such stretching, but mostly to a focal compression of the lumen where it exits the transverse foramen of C2. This theory had been proposed by Dumas et al.[192] using angiography with MRI. While this author considered that, starting with 35° of rotation between C1 and C2, there was stretching of the artery and disturbance of blood flow, Haynes[38] argues that at least 45° are necessary for this stretching to occur. The stress undergone by the vertebral artery during rotation can increase even more with the extension of the cervical spine, since the artery is also relatively fixed between the point where the artery penetrates the dura mater[208] and the groove of the posterior arch of the atlas (Fig. 10-13). It is important to recall that the movements of extension and rotation are coupled in the craniocervical spine[58] and, therefore, rotation of this region is able to induce a significant amount of extension, which may generate significant tension in the suboccipital portion of the vertebral artery. However more recent studies have suggested that this may not be the case in typical manipulative positions.[76,179,182]

Nevertheless, some authors consider that a healthy vertebral artery can tolerate this stretching without suffering an injury.[76,179,193] The maximum degree of stretching tolerated by the vertebral arteries during the manipulation only reaches 46%,[38] a lower percentage than that of 139% and 162% necessary to cause their failure.[88]

The risk factors related to the manipulation are:

- Excessive force.
- Excessive velocity.
- Traction.
- Excessive rotation and extension.

The coupled ipsilateral side-bending movement, which necessarily occurs, would seem to limit the stretching of the vertebral artery during the contralateral rotation movement.[58,192] Side-bending is the movement that generates the least amount of tension on the artery.[209,210]

Therefore, it should be assumed that, in the absence of new evidence, the range of rotation should be limited with an initial side-bending, as long as it does not exceed 45°, and thus avoiding any extension component.

In regards to the carotid artery, the manipulation proposed to pose greater risk is that which involves cervical extension associated with a contralateral side-bending or rotation[47,81,82,211] (Fig. 10-14).

In conclusion, the most important risk factors for an arterial injury due to manipulation are a previous trauma of the cervical spine that includes a subclinical injury of a cervical artery, and disorders or altered states that involve a fragility of the arterial walls.[90,212] The development of an arterial dissection does not seem so dependent on the forces applied during the manipulation, but on a situation of arterial vulnerability of

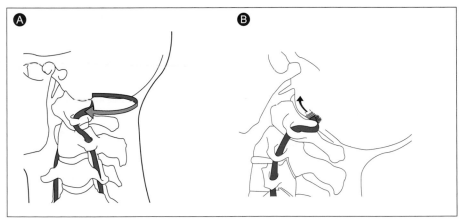

FIGURE 10-13 ■ The two movements that can favour an overstretching of the vertebral artery are rotation (A) and extension (B).

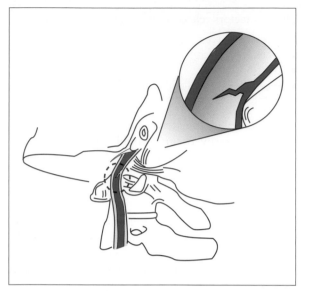

FIGURE 10-14 ■ The manipulation that has more potential risks of injury of the carotid artery is one that involves extension associated with a contralateral inclination or a rotation.

the patient, as a consequence of a trauma or previous pathology.[26,29,90,212] Therefore, cerebrovascular incidents following neck manipulation most likely occur due to an aggravation of a previous injury, or a premorbid condition such as a vascular pathology,[2,3,12] genetic susceptibility[10,14,212] or an alteration of the connective tissue.[29,87,89,90,136,156,165,179]

Evidence suggests that a healthy vertebral artery is not at risk if the manipulative technique is performed correctly.[179] However, an artery with structural fragility may be at risk with almost any movement. In these patients at risk, a manipulation of the craniocervical spine in rotation is potentially dangerous.[38,40,213] Therefore, before applying any type of manipulative technique, it is advisable to assess in traumatic cases if the patient's symptomatology may be related to a vascular injury and also to rule out, if possible, an arteriopathy or pathology that may weaken the artery walls.

The most important risk factors for an arterial injury due to manipulation are:

- Previous trauma of the cervical spine that includes a subclinical injury of the cervical artery.
- Disorders or altered states that involve fragility of the arterial walls, such as a vascular pathology, genetic susceptibility or connective tissue disorders.

CLINICAL HISTORY OF NEUROVASCULAR INCIDENTS AND MANIPULATION

The most important risk factors, as described earlier, are the presence of an injury of the cervical arteries and/or previous ischaemic episodes, and this makes it absolutely mandatory for every therapist using these manipulative techniques to identify these situations. When the patient's history suggests the possibility of symptoms or temporary ischaemia, no treatment should be initiated, and the patient should be referred for an exhaustive neurological examination.

Signs and symptoms of a neurovascular injury

The signs and symptoms that may indicate a neurovascular injury are varied, including facial paraesthesia, lip anaesthesia, diplopia, blurred vision, nausea, vomiting, instability, ataxia, dysarthria, drop attacks and nystagmus.

The majority of therapists fail to recognize that the earliest and most common sign of dissection of a cervical artery is a headache, plus or minus cervical pain.[14,214,215] Some cases have been published in which the only symptom was acute cervical pain.[216,217] Nichols et al.[218] demonstrated experimentally that the vertebral artery can cause headaches. These authors inserted an inflatable ball in the vertebral and basilar arteries of healthy subjects and saw that, when they inflated the ball and the walls of the artery were stretched, the subject referred pain on the forehead, cheek, occipital area, posterior part of the neck and even the trapezius. Also, Munari et al.[219] have demonstrated that the carotid artery, during a percutaneous angioplasty, may refer cervical and facial pain and headaches. However, the location of pain in itself is not a reliable indicator of dissection.[137]

The earliest and most common sign of the dissection of a cervical artery is a headache, which may or may not be associated with cervical pain.

The presence of a sudden and intense headache usually precedes the signs of ischaemia.[164,215] In some

cases pain may be the only symptom.[216,220] Advances in angiography with MRI have shown that many patients who were previously diagnosed with headaches or post-manipulation vertigo actually had an undiagnosed dissection of the tunica intima.[206] The clinical relevance of this fact cannot be underestimated, as the description of the nature of this headache provided by the patient is usually the only diagnostic clue. Beletsky et al.,[134] in a study conducted with 116 subjects that had suffered a dissection of the vertebral or internal carotid artery, observed that the most frequent symptoms were headaches and cervical pain, which affected 74% of individuals. Headaches and cervical pain are not only the most frequent symptoms but also often the only ones in an injury of the cervical artery.[206,216,217]

The main characteristics of a headache caused by the dissection of a cervical artery are its sudden onset, its high severity and its difference from any other headache suffered before.[215]

Characteristics of a headache caused by the dissection of a cervical artery:

- Sudden onset.
- High severity.
- Different from any other headache suffered before.
- Occurs after an intense physical activity or a forced and rapid movement or position.

Caution should be taken, especially in subjects who report an acute onset of cervical pain and headache after practicing a sport, an intense physical activity, or a forced and rapid head movement or position.[18,29,215,221] Silbert et al.[221] studied the characteristics of a headache caused by the dissection of the internal carotid and vertebral arteries in 161 patients, and showed that the headache was unilateral and always on the same side as the dissection, and it could have a continuous and pulsating nature. Headaches caused by dissection of the internal carotid or vertebral artery are different in that the former may be more intense in the frontotemporal region and the latter in the occipital region.

The clinical problem is that the initial symptoms of an arterial dissection may be similar to musculoskeletal symptoms and, therefore, some of these patients may request a manipulative treatment.[11,124,221,222] Different published cases may indicate that the symptoms reported by the patients who suffered a cerebrovascular incident during a manipulation were the reason why the patients sought therapeutic treatment, but were symptoms of arterial dissection.[206,215,223] Therefore, the clinical problem that may lead to a diagnostic error is that cervical pain caused by arterial pathology may coexist with a history of mechanical cervical pain.

The clinical problem is that the initial symptoms of an arterial dissection may be similar to musculoskeletal symptoms.

Other common symptoms of dissection of the vertebral artery and the resulting lateral spinal cord syndrome are vertigo, dysphagia, dysarthria, diplopia, drop attacks, ataxia, nystagmus, nausea, vomiting, paraesthesia, Horner syndrome and pulsating tinnitus.[10,214,224]

Visual symptoms are also common: early studies suggested they may occur in up to 86% of subjects with a dissection of the vertebral artery.[186,225–227] More recent estimates suggest around 50% of patients with posterior circulation stroke will report some visual deficit.[8] These visual symptoms include diplopia, blurred vision, nystagmus, loss of the corneal reflex and alteration of the visual field. When the VBI affects the visual cortex, it can be manifested by a ipsilateral hemianopia or quadrantanopia, depending on the extent of the condition.[226] The patient can also experience hallucinations in the visual field, such as sparkling or flashing lights. The diplopia may be due to involvement of cranial nerves III, IV or VI.

The most common auditory symptoms include hypoacusis or partial loss of hearing[225,228,229] and tinnitus.[139,230,231] If the patient reports the sudden appearance of pulsating tinnitus and if, in addition, this is associated with headaches and neck pain, manipulation should be avoided, since it may be a sign of a dissecting aneurysm of the vertebral or internal carotid artery.[232–234]

The presence of facial and ipsilateral perioral paraesthesiae are common and well-known symptoms of VBI and internal carotid artery dissection; they are especially prevalent in Wallenberg syndrome.[186,227,235,236] They are usually associated with hypoaesthesia and facial and ipsilateral perioral anaesthesia. The mechanism behind these paraesthesiae seems to be a condition of the trigeminothalamic bundle of the thalamus.

Painless dysphonia is a common symptom of Wallenberg syndrome.[237] This dysphonia, manifested with a characteristic hoarse voice, may be due to the paresis of a vocal cord, since the control of the vocal muscles occurs in the vagal nucleus.

Dizziness and vertigo are frequent symptoms of VBI.[8,186,227] Classically, vertigo has been considered the cardinal symptom of VBI, yet it does not occur in every patient. Husni et al.[186] demonstrated that, in patients with VBI, only 40% suffer from vertigo, while 100% suffer dizziness. Although some recent literature has shown vertigo may be present as an isolated symptom in VBI,[8,238] it rarely appears in isolation, without other neurological signs.[225] It should be noted that the most frequent type of vertigo that appears isolated is benign paroxysmal positional vertigo.[239–241] The nystagmus that accompanies a vestibular pathology, unlike VBI, is fatigable, and both vertigo and dizziness are also common features associated with craniocervical spine pain.[242,243] Therefore, it is important to perform a correct differential diagnosis of the vertiginous symptoms, since many cases of manipulative treatment with fatal results have been described in this type of patient.[170]

Drop attacks, a sudden leg weakness or collapse without loss of consciousness is one of the classic manifestations of vertebrobasilar ischaemia, yet it is not the most common.[244]

The dissection of the internal carotid artery may lead to Horner syndrome, with its classic symptoms of ptosis, miosis and facial anhidrosis; other symptoms of carotid dissection may include facial flushing,[18,72] vertigo, headaches, alterations of the visual field, nausea, vomiting and paralysis of the cranial nerves X, XI and XII.[245] If a patient has signs or symptoms of temporary ischaemia of the internal carotid artery, a complete neurological examination should be performed, since a complete cerebrovascular event may occur after a few episodes of ischaemia.

SYMPTOMS OF DISSECTION OF THE VERTEBRAL ARTERY

- Visual symptoms: diplopia, blurry vision, nystagmus, paralysis of cranial nerve VI, loss of the corneal reflex and alteration of the visual field.
- Auditory symptoms: hypoacusis and pulsatile tinnitus.
- Painless dysphonia and dysarthria.
- Nausea.

- Paraesthesiae and/or facial and ipsilateral perioral anaesthesia.
- Dizziness and vertigo.
- Drop attacks.

SYMPTOMS OF DISSECTION OF THE INTERNAL CAROTID ARTERY

- Horner syndrome.
- Vertigo.
- Headaches.
- Alterations of the visual field.
- Nausea and vomiting.
- Paralysis of cranial nerves X, XI and XII.
- Limb weakness and paraesthesia.

On some occasions, the dissection of the cervical artery is accompanied by symptoms referred to the cervical spine and the upper limb, simulating a cervical radiculopathy. The vertebral artery in the transverse foramen is close to the anterior spinal roots. The increase in diameter of the artery, due to an intramural haematoma or a dissecting aneurysm, may cause a radiculopathy by compressing the nerve root.[246–248] This usually affects the lower cervical nerve roots.

Onset of symptoms

The symptoms of an arterial dissection are manifested, in most cases, almost immediately or within the first 24–48 hours,[60,170] but in some cases they can be delayed up to 2 months, which is enough time to prevent the patient from establishing a relationship between a traumatic event and the symptoms, and this has important diagnostic and therapeutic consequences.[134] A few authors have stated that the most delayed manifestation of the symptoms after a vertebrobasilar ischaemia is 5 years.[135] However, one of the clinical problems is that the decrease in arterial flow can be asymptomatic, as the collateral circulation may maintain an adequate posterior cranial perfusion.[149]

A cerebrovascular incident after a manipulation may initially manifest itself with isolated local signs and symptoms, but as it develops it may become apparent with completely different symptomatic clinical pictures, such as Wallenberg syndrome, and cerebromedullospinal disconnection syndrome, as well as other brainstem, cerebellar or thalamic syndromes.

Wallenberg syndrome

This syndrome, also known as lateral medullary syndrome, occurs due to the obstruction of the postero-inferior cerebellar artery.[11,129,237,249] It is the most common cerebrovascular event after a manipulation, since the obstruction takes places in this location, due to the propagation of a thrombus caused by an injury of the third section (V3) of the vertebral artery. This syndrome is also known as lateral medullary syndrome, since the posteroinferior cerebellar artery irrigates the lateral portion of the medulla oblongata. The signs and symptoms are due to the destruction of the nuclei and the tracts located in the dorsolateral medulla oblongata. The following structures are usually affected: the inferior cerebellar peduncle, which causes ataxia and hypotonia on the side of the injury; the descending spinal tract and the nucleus of cranial nerve V, which cause the loss of thermal and ipsilateral painful sensitivity on the face, and loss of the corneal reflex; the lateral ascending spinothalamic, which causes the loss of thermal and painful sensitivity on the trunk and the ipsilateral limbs; the descending sympathetic tract, which leads to Horner syndrome; the inferior vestibular nucleus, which causes nystagmus, vertigo and nausea; and the ambiguous nucleus of the glossopharyngeal and the vagus nerve, which are manifested with hoarse voice and dysphagia.

Cerebromedullospinal disconnection syndrome

This syndrome, also known as 'locked-in syndrome', is caused by the obstruction of the basilar artery and ischaemia of the pons.[250] The subject maintains consciousness, but loses all voluntary movements, except vertical ocular and convergence movements. This occurs in 5% of the dissections of the vertebral artery.[60,97,114,170] Izquierdo-Casas et al.[251] presented a case of a locked-in syndrome after a cervical manipulation in which a blood thrombus was embolized as the consequence of a dissection of the V2 segment of the vertebral artery (Fig. 10-15). These are rare but devastating outcomes of a cervical manipulation and it is important that clinicians take all possible steps to avoid such an adverse outcome.

MANIPULATIVE EXAMINATION

The presence of signs or symptoms of neurovascular compromise completely contraindicates any type of manipulative technique. It is therefore necessary to identify beforehand those subjects that are potentially

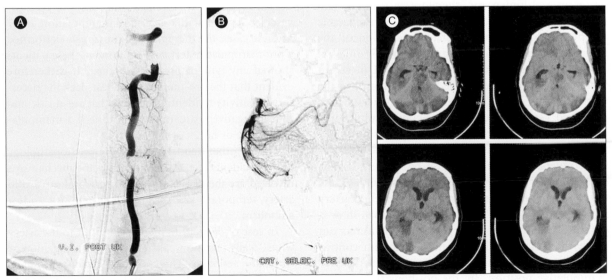

FIGURE 10-15 ■ Entrapment syndrome after a cervical manipulation. (A) Arteriography of the left vertebral artery compatible with a dissection of the V2 segment. (B) Filling defect of the basilar artery caused by the presence of an intraluminal blood clot. (C) Computed tomography in which the areas of ischaemia can be seen in the protuberance of both cerebellar hemispheres and in the area of the right posterior cerebral artery. *(Images courtesy of Dr Izquierdo-Casas.)*

at risk, and to this end a series of functional or positional tests of the vertebral artery have been described.

Functional tests of the vertebral artery

Classically, it has been stated that a functional test of the vertebral artery performed before the manipulation would allow us to rule out a VBI. Since the first description of a test of the vertebral artery, by De Kleyn and Nieuwenhuyse[54] in 1927, different tests have been described, but they are mere variations of a position of rotation and neck extension. While some authors place the cervical spine in rotation and extension directly, others recommend doing it in sequences and progressively, starting from a cervical position of less stress to more stress. These tests have been, for decades, a standard procedure for those who use manipulative techniques in the cervical spine, with the belief that a negative test allows for the application of a manipulative technique without risk.

The functional tests of the vertebral artery are no more than screening tests and, therefore, should theoretically have high sensitivity to help identify subjects at risk of adverse events following cervical manipulation. They are based on the premise that the positions of rotation, or rotation and extension, common therapeutic positions, are capable of reducing the vertebral arterial lumen and, therefore, in subjects with prior stenosis, induce the appearance of ischaemic symptoms due to the insufficient perfusion of the brainstem neural structures and the posterior fossa. However, as described, studies conducted in recent years regarding changes in the haemodynamics of the vertebral artery during pre-manipulative tests have produced very diverse and conflicting results. Some of these studies show a decrease in perfusion of the vertebral artery in the position of the tests,[75,188,189,199,201] while others, on the contrary, do not present significant changes.[36,195–197,252] Thus, the sensitivity of the tests to identify an obstruction of the vertebral artery is controversial. Yet, from these works that show a decrease in perfusion, a few practical conclusions can be reached, such as the fact that maximum contralateral rotation, and the tension applied in the pre-manipulative position, are the positions that tend to reduce the flow of the vertebral artery more intensely than even the rotation and extension or De Kleyn's test.[199] It is important to note that these functional

tests can be completely negative in some subjects with a severe alteration of the arterial perfusion. There are also cases of subjects that do not experience any type of symptom during the pre-manipulative tests yet have a complete atresia (absence) of a vertebral artery,[253] or with a complete occlusion of the artery during a movement of cervical rotation, as shown with angiography.[28,254]

- The pre-manipulative tests cannot detect patients that are predisposed to suffer a dissection of the vertebral artery.
- Even in case of a previous arterial dissection or complete obstruction of the artery, the pre-manipulative tests may produce false negatives, since the contralateral artery can maintain sufficient vascular perfusion.

The predictive value of the pre-manipulative tests has thus been questioned by several authors. who show that these tests are unable to identify patients that are predisposed to suffer a vertebral artery dissection.[20,40,195,202,252,254] Similarly, there have been cases of cerebrovascular incidents in subjects whose pre-manipulative tests were negative.[28,112] This fact was even more evident after the review conducted by Haldeman et al.[124] of 64 forensic court cases of cerebrovascular accidents after a cervical manipulation. In 27 of these cases, the therapist had previously performed a pre-manipulative test, and yet none of these patients showed any type of positive response. It is therefore evident that the pre-manipulative tests lack the necessary sensitivity to identify subjects that are at risk, and thus a negative test cannot determine if a manipulation is safe or not.

On the other hand, regarding the physiopathology of the accidents after a manipulation, the mechanisms involved are the dissection of the vertebral or carotid artery, temporary vasospasm and thrombosis and/or embolism.

In case of dissection, there is an insult to the artery whose walls may be weakened due to a congenital or traumatic aetiology. Therefore, a test that supposedly analyses the arterial susceptibility will be limited to provide any useful clinical information regarding the potential risk or injury. In a pathological situation such as this one, the test would actually put the patient at risk.[255] Regarding a temporary vasospasm, a pre-manipulative test cannot foresee this either. In addition, the functional tests also do not have any ability to test the effect of the manipulative thrust. In case of a previous arterial dissection, the pre-manipulative tests may produce false negatives, since the contralateral artery can maintain enough vascular perfusion, even with a complete obstruction of the artery.[206] Furthermore, this is the most serious risk situation, in which the pre-manipulative test can have catastrophic results.

The other mechanism related to adverse events after neck manipulation is a blood thrombus caused by a previous endothelial injury. It is possible that a manipulative manoeuvre performed in a pathological situation such as this could favour the embolization of the blood clot and a resulting cerebrovascular incident.[255]

The pre-manipulative tests cannot identify other types of arterial stenosis that may contraindicate a manipulation, such as an atherosclerosis or hypoplasia, due to the compensating mechanisms of the perfusion that have been already described.

Another issue with the pre-manipulative tests is the frequent false positives that can appear if the differential diagnosis of vertigo is not sufficiently made. The provocation manoeuvres of the vertebral artery are similar to the tests, such as the Dix–Hallpike test, used in the diagnosis of one of the most frequent forms of peripheral vertigo, benign paroxysmal positional vertigo (BPPV). Also, the stimulation of the articular proprioceptive and cervical muscular receptors during the pre-manipulative tests can similarly trigger cervicogenic dizziness that has nothing to do with the vascular pathology. These findings have recently led some authors to consider abandoning the use of pre-manipulative tests because of their low specificity and sensitivity.[202,255]

Nevertheless, and taking into account that the tests of the vertebral artery do not identify all risk situations, it is not sensible to perform a manual treatment without previously assessing, in a controlled manner, the patient's response to different stress situations similar to those suffered by the cervical arteries during the manipulation. As indicated by Refshauge et al.[256] and others, although the tests do not identify those patients that may suffer an adverse event, it would be negligent to discard them, since in some cases they

actually help identify patients with insufficient arterial perfusion.[29,76,257,258]

> Before a manual treatment, it is necessary to assess, in a controlled manner, the patient's response to different stress situations similar to those suffered by the cervical arteries during the manipulation.

Richter and Reinking,[259] after reviewing the studies regarding the effects of the functional tests of the perfusion of the vertebral artery, and the relevance of teaching them to physical therapy students, have shown that their sensitivity and specificity are low. Even so, they still recommend their practice as long as the decision to use a manipulative technique or not is based primarily on an analysis of the clinical history of the patient.

With the information available today, and given the controversial clinical value of the pre-manipulative tests, it is evident that the emphasis should be placed on the detection of the possible risk indicators in the clinical history of the patient.[29,257,258] For this reason, the clinical guidelines and reasoning guidance published in the last few years emphasize the importance of the medical history and the subjective examination as the first step of the pre-manipulative protocol.[257,258,260] Therefore, it is recommended to include functional tests of the vertebral artery in a wider clinical exploration, in which the clinical history of the patient and the subjective examination play a predominant role.

- The first step of the pre-manipulative protocol is the medical history and the subjective examination, with the aim of identifying potential risk indicators in the clinical history of the patient.
- The therapist should have enough knowledge to recognize signs or symptoms of a possible arterial dissection or VBI.

Subjective examination

The purpose of the subjective examination is to rule out, as far as possible, those clinical situations that contraindicate a manipulative treatment. The important issues of the medical history that may suggest a risk situation with a manipulation are:

- Personal clinical history of a pathology that may weaken the arterial walls, such as a collagen disorder, fibromuscular dysplasia, Marfan syndrome or Ehlers–Danlos syndrome, and even systemic hyperlaxity. In this regard, family history is very important, both of arterial dissection and arteriopathy, as many of these pathologies are congenital or have a familial prevalence.

- Symptoms that may be suggestive of an arterial dissection, such as sudden severe suboccipital or temporal neck pain or a severe and acute headache or an unusual headache that has never been experienced by the patient, especially if it was triggered by a sharp, rapid or high-amplitude movement of the neck, or by intense physical activity. It is important to bear in mind that an arterial dissection may be manifested exclusively with acute cervical pain or headaches, with no associated signs of ischaemia.
- Signs or symptoms of cerebrovascular ischaemia, such as facial and perioral paraesthesias, lip anaesthesia, dysarthria/dysphasia, dysphonia, diplopia, blurry vision, alteration of the visual field, paralysis of cranial nerve VI, loss of the corneal reflex, hypoacusis, tinnitus, instability, ataxia, sudden loss of balance, disorientation, Horner syndrome, nystagmus, dizziness, nausea or vomiting. If the patient suffers any of the symptoms described, the clinician must establish if they have appeared due to a trauma, and especially if they are aggravated by movements or positions of the cervical spine.
- Acquired stenosis of the cervical arteries, such as atherosclerosis, and hypertrophic articular degenerative changes that may induce an arterial stenosis.
- Traumatic injuries, even of low intensity. It is necessary to carefully analyse the signs and symptoms, since the symptoms of artery dissection often simulate those usually suffered after a trauma, such as a cervical whiplash.
- Respiratory infection, fever or malaise.
- Whether the patient has received previous treatments, especially of the cervical spine, both manipulative and non-manipulative, and their effect on the symptoms.[257]

When the information obtained from the subjective examination does not show any clear signs of arterial

dissection or neurovascular insufficiency, the functional tests of the artery are performed. Any sign that is potentially related to an arterial dissection, or a neurovascular insufficiency, absolutely contraindicates the pre-manipulative functional tests, since this would put the patient at risk unnecessarily. In this situation, the patient should be immediately referred to a specialized facility. When the signs and symptoms are uncertain, a neurological examination can be performed previously (Table 10-1).

- Any possible sign related to an arterial dissection or a neurovascular insufficiency absolutely contraindicates the pre-manipulative tests.
- If the patient shows vertigo or dizziness, and only if there are no other associated symptoms, a physical examination should be conducted to find out if the origin is VBI or any other aetiology.

If the patient shows vertigo or dizziness, and only if there are no other associated symptoms, a physical examination should be conducted to find out if the origin is a VBI or any other aetiology such as a vestibular disorder.

Physical examination

Functional examination of the cervical arteries

Currently, there are different protocols and clinical guidelines aimed at avoiding neurovascular accidents with the use of manipulation. These guidelines include the pre-manipulative protocol of the Australian Physiotherapy Association,[257] initially written in 1988 and revised in 2000, 2004 and 2006 by Rivett et al.,[257] and which is currently under review. The International Federation of Orthopaedic Manipulative Physical Therapists (IFOMPT) recently published a clinical reasoning framework to guide clinicians in assessment prior to treatment of the cervical region for potential neurovascular dysfunction.[258] This document supports the position of the Australian Physiotherapy Guidelines concerning functional testing, although it includes suggestions about other testing – for example, for carotid palpation and cervical ligament testing – which may not be so well supported by the literature. In addition there are other recent revisions to guidelines for other groups: Carey's protocol,[261] published by the

TABLE 10-1
Indications and contraindications for functional testing of the cervical arteries

Before performing the functional cervical artery tests (FCATs)

Information from the history, signs or symptoms that contraindicates the functional tests of the vertebral artery:

Absolute:

- Arterial dissection symptoms (headaches or high or suboccipital cervical pain of sudden appearance, acute nature and never experienced before by the patient)
- Signs or symptoms of cerebrovascular ischaemia
- Suspicion of congenital or acquired cervical or craniocervical instability

FCATs are contraindicated

Relative:

- Information from personal clinical history that may alert of a pathology that weakens the arterial walls, such as a collagen disorder
- Arteriosclerosis
- Acute degenerative changes of the cervical spine
- Cervical trauma
- Respiratory infection, fever or malaise
- Confusing symptoms ──▶ **Neurological exploration**

FCATs are performed carefully and progressively
Vertiginous or dizziness symptoms with no other associated symptom

Functional tests of the vestibular system
(Dix–Hallpike manoeuvre)

Journal of the Canadian Chiropractic Association and largely superseded by a clinical practice guideline[262] in 2005; the clinical guideline of the Ontario College of Physiotherapists, published previously in the *Manual Therapy* journal by Gross et al.[263]; and the guide adopted by the Manipulative Association of Chartered Physiotherapists and the Society of Orthopaedic Medicine[260] and revised by Kerry et al.[213] in 2008.

Functional examination of the cervical arteries should be conducted in every patient before any therapeutic procedure involving the cervical spine, and especially in all those cases where a high-velocity manipulation or a technique with high-amplitude movements is used.[257] This does not involve additional or excessive time, since the positions employed are part of the normal procedures used during a treatment session of the cervical spine. This examination is not recommended when the subjective assessment indicates the possibility of a pathology or neurovascular insufficiency, or when craniovertebral instability

is suspected. When there are confusing symptoms or a history of recent trauma, it is necessary to conduct a careful and gradual assessment to avoid any undesired effects during the evaluation. Importantly, it should be noted that the tests are not free of risks.[27,264] There have been cases in which, by simply placing the cervical spine in rotation, a cerebrovascular incident was triggered.[109,170]

- Functional examination of the cervical arteries should be performed in every patient before any therapeutic procedure.
- This exploration is not recommended when the medical history indicates the possibility of a pathology or neurovascular insufficiency, or when craniovertebral insufficiency is suspected.
- When the symptoms are confusing or there is a history of a recent trauma, it is necessary to conduct a careful and gradual assessment to avoid undesirable effects during the evaluation.

It is also important to note that the pre-manipulative functional test does not completely simulate the forces received by the cervical spine during the manipulative thrust. A negative functional provocative test in itself does not imply that a cervical artery is able to tolerate the forces and velocity applied during a manipulation.[75] In addition, this test does not predict the possibility of an injury: it evaluates the ability of collateral perfusion, and may serve as an indicator of the possible severity of the injury, should it occur.[70]

The functional examination of the cervical arteries should be preceded by an evaluation of the cervical mobility, initially in the seated position. The patient performs active and isolated physiological movements of the cervical spine in each sagittal, coronal and axial plane. The appearance of signs and symptoms potentially associated with the cervical arteries is carefully analysed, not only during the test but also after the test and the manipulative treatment.

- The functional tests of the vertebral artery are not free of risks, and they should be performed cautiously and gradually.
- The pre-manipulative test does not completely simulate the forces received by the cervical spine during the manipulation. A negative provocation test does not imply that cervical arteries are able to tolerate the forces and velocity applied during a manipulation.

- The pre-manipulative test does not predict the possibility of damage to the arteries.
- The appearance of signs and symptoms potentially associated with the cervical arteries is carefully analysed, not only during the test but also after the test and the manipulative treatment.

From the clinical recommendations of the Australian Physiotherapy Association, drafted by Rivett et al.,[257] and the studies of Arnold et al.[199] and Mitchell et al.,[189,198] the necessary functional tests include the following:

- Cervical rotation in its maximum range.
- Pre-manipulative position – simulation of placing the patient in the required therapeutic position (Fig. 10-16).
- In addition, the position in which the patient reports the appearance of the symptoms; for example, cervical extension.

It is recommended to achieve the maximum range of rotation gradually and not with a single movement.

All the positions are maintained for 10 seconds, unless the symptoms appear before. During this time, the appearance of nystagmus should be evaluated, and the patient should be asked to immediately report any symptoms such as dizziness or pre-syncope. After each test, there should be a 10-second wait since, on

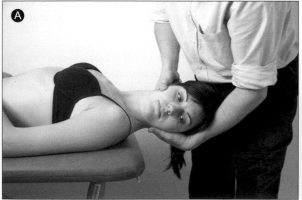
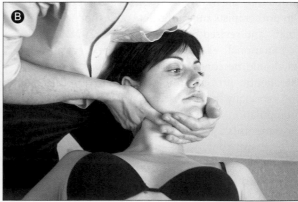

FIGURE 10-16 ■ The recommended functional tests are full-range cervical rotation (A) and simulation of the intended manipulative position (B).

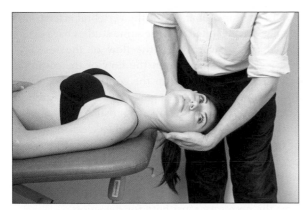

FIGURE 10-17 ■ If the functional tests of the vertebral artery are negative, a craniocervical extension can be performed in full-range rotation.

occasions, there is certain latency to symptom onset.[80,97,189,197] Latency is probably due to a gradual reduction in brain perfusion over time, in contrast to the immediate response of vestibular structures to head movement.

If the previous tests were negative, craniocervical extension can be added or the extension in its maximum range if necessary to identify the signs and symptoms related to VBI (Fig. 10-17). This position is obtained gradually and, similarly, will be maintained for 10 seconds.

If the cervical pain and stiffness restrict the examination of the complete mobility, it must be recorded that the examination was incomplete and, therefore, not all the necessary information is available to choose a modality of treatment.

If there is evidence of the signs and symptoms being related to an arterial injury or VBI, the patient must be referred immediately to a specialized *medical* facility.

If the signs and symptoms are confusing, both due to the clinical history and the functional examination, no manipulative technique or any technique that imparts large-range cervical mobilization should be applied. The response of the patient to manual treatment must be monitored and, when in doubt, the patient should be referred for medical evaluation.

During and after the treatment, the possible appearance of neurovascular signs and symptoms should be evaluated. The pre-manipulative test should be performed with each session of treatment.

Currently, all clinical guides recommend obtaining an informed consent from the patient. It is essential for the therapist to offer information regarding the procedures that are going to be used in the treatment, especially regarding the manipulative techniques.[257,258] However, as Cote et al.[195] point out, from an ethical point of view, it is not acceptable to alarm the patient unnecessarily. While recommendations for informed consent may vary between countries, it is generally considered that as a minimum the consent process should encompass advice to the patient on the risk and benefits of the treatment and include some discussion on treatment alternatives.[257,258]

Differentiation of vertiginous symptoms

When the subject in the subjective examination reports vertiginous symptoms, it is necessary to establish if they are actually of vertebrobasilar origin or have some other cause.[265] First, VBI is an uncommon entity, and the majority of vertiginous symptoms do not belong to this aetiology. Whereas vertigo or dizziness is often the main feature of VBI, it is possible that the vertigo in a VBI or arterial dissection may present itself isolated, with no other signs or symptoms of ischaemia in the areas irrigated by the basilar artery, such as the brainstem and the cerebellum, in addition to the central and peripheral vestibular system.

Grad and Baloh[225] found that, in VBI, vertigo may initially appear isolated, but its presence, with no other symptoms of ischaemia of the posterior circulation, for a period of more than 6 months, must imply another aetiology.

One of the types of vertigo that, due to its frequency, usually requires a differential diagnosis is BPPV.[241,266–268] This type of vertigo is rotational, acute but brief, and is triggered by quick movements of the head or trunk. The stimulus that triggers this vertigo is gravity and change of head position, and not the modification of the articular relationships, or its effects on the arterial perfusion. The specific tests, such as the Dix–Hallpike test,[269] are similar to those of the vertebral artery, especially if it is performed in the supine position. Therefore, it is quite possible that some patients, in whom a VBI has been suspected by the triggering of a vertiginous crisis during the tests of the vertebral artery, may suffer from vestibular vertigo instead. This would be considered more likely if the

TABLE 10-2

Protocol for functional testing of the cervical arteries

- If the clinical history indicates a possible VBI or vascular injury, functional cervical artery tests (FCATs) should not be performed
- The FCAT should be preceded by an examination of the full active mobility of the cervical spine
- If the history is not suggestive of vascular injury or VBI, the FCATs are carried out
- If the medical history is unclear, the FCATs are performed carefully and gradually:
  - If the FCATs are negative but the clinical history is unclear, manipulative treatment or one involving end-range mobilization should not be performed. The patient's response should be monitored and, when in doubt, the patient should be referred for a more thorough medical examination
  - If the FCATs are positive, the patient should be referred for a more complete medical examination
  - If the FCATs are negative, manipulative treatment may be initiated
- If symptoms only cause vertigo, vestibular function tests are performed:
  - If vestibular function tests are positive, this problem must be evaluated and resolved before commencing treatment with mobilization or manipulation
  - If vestibular function tests are negative, the patient should be referred for evaluation of possible VBI
- *Only* if the FCATs are negative and there is no clinical history suggestive of VBI or vascular injury may the manipulative treatment be initiated

Adapted with permission from Rivett D, Shirley D, Magarey M, Refshauge K. 2006. Clinical guidelines for assessing VBI in the management of cervical spine disorders. Appendix 2. Clinical flowchart. Australian Physiotherapy Association.

vertigo continued or got worse and did not settle quickly during the stages of the test. It is then recommended to perform the Dix–Hallpike test or other vestibular test to identify the cause of this vertigo (Table 10-2). The differential diagnosis of cervicogenic dizziness is discussed in Chapter 8.

If the functional examination of the vertebral artery causes vertigo exclusively, vestibular function tests must be performed.

Palpation and auscultation of the carotid pulses

Some authors have recommended the palpation or auscultation of the carotid pulses as an interesting pre-manipulative test.[258,270] This test detects a modification in the pulse between the neutral position and the posi-

tion of the functional test of the vertebral artery. This test has been justified because some studies have determined that a decrease in the flow of the vertebral artery causes an increase in the flow of the common carotid artery, especially in the contralateral artery[271] and carotid palpation is part of a normal carotid examination.[213] However, its diagnostic significance is unclear and it is unlikely to provide a clear indication of the risk of an adverse event.[258] Moreover, there are recorded cases of accidents after a manipulation in which the auscultation of the carotid pulses was negative[170,272] and, therefore, this test does not appear to have the necessary sensitivity for detection.

Hautant's test

Hautant's test is another test that can be included in the physical exploration, as it demonstrates an alteration in proprioception of cerebellar aetiology as the consequence of a reduction in blood flow in the vertebral arteries and subsequent perfusion of the posterior fossa.[243,273] It can potentially provide a more objective measure of vascular dysfunction than the vertebral artery test. However, the validity of this test is questioned as the sensitivity and specificity is low.

The patient sits on an examining table, with the forearms in supination, fingers extended and elbows in 90° of flexion. Then, the patient is asked to close her eyes for 15–30 seconds, and the therapist sees if the patient can maintain the position of both arms symmetrically. If this part of the evaluation is negative, the cervical spine is placed in rotation and extension, as in the functional test of the vertebral artery, while the therapist again observes the symmetry of the position of the arms. The loss of symmetry in one or both arms, loss of pronation or elbow flexion, may indicate a cerebellar condition related to the vertebral artery (Fig. 10-18).

NEUROVASCULAR ACCIDENTS AND CERVICAL MANIPULATION

The first question that the specialist must ask after this review is whether the use of manipulative techniques in the cervical spine is recommended. Some authors consider that, despite having small risks, the benefits of the manipulation do not exceed the risks, and therefore they recommend exclusively the use of the mobilization techniques.[22,97,108,256,274,275] Although such a

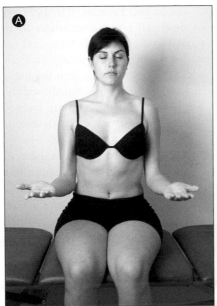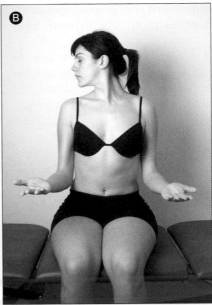

FIGURE 10-18 ■ Hautant's test: neutral position (A) and cervical rotation (B).

recommendation tends to be based on the fact that there is evidence that shows that the cervical manipulation has a greater number of adverse effects than the mobilization,[21] manipulative techniques have proven to be effective in the treatment of cervical pain and headaches[276–281] and, therefore, their use is justified, excluding those manipulations whose parameters have been shown to carry a higher risk of injury.

Obviously, when the data provided by the medical history are conflicting, it is preferable to use mobilization techniques. It is not advisable to use a high-velocity technique or one that imparts high-amplitude movements at the first visit or treatment of a patient. High-velocity techniques should be the final step in the progression of a manual treatment and they are never the first choice during the first visit.

High-velocity techniques are usually the final step in the progression of the manual treatment and are never the first choice during the first visit.

For some professionals, high-velocity techniques seem to be the only therapeutic tool. The relationship between the professional that practices the manipulation and the occurrence of accidents has been studied.[25,108,170] Rothwell[25] estimated that the risk of

a cerebrovascular accident in patients under 45 years old was 1.3 in 100,000 visits to a chiropractor. In these studies, it is clear that the occurrence of accidents after a manipulation is much higher among chiropractors, but this is probably because they use manipulation more frequently. While the incidence in physical therapists does not reach 2%, it as high as 70% among chiropractors.[108]

Jull[280] has compared the type of manipulative technique (high-velocity manipulation or mobilization) chosen by Australian physical therapists to treat patients with headaches. The conclusions of this study show that physical therapists in that country are aware of the possible risks of using a high-velocity manipulation, and they use it sparingly, less than mobilizations. Although in 42% of patients, during some sessions, a high-velocity manipulation was used, this technique was only used in approximately 20% of all treatments performed, and only in 10% of cases was it chosen in the first visit. In another study, conducted by Grant and Niere,[282] investigating the modalities of treatment used by physical therapists in the treatment of headaches, although manipulation was used in more than 40% of patients, it was more frequently at the C2–C3 level, and to a lesser extent was used in the upper segments C0–C1 and C1–C2. It has been recommended that chiropractors should use mobilization techniques more, due to their fewer adverse effects.[21]

Another aspect that seems to be related to cases of adverse incidents after a manipulation is the number of previous manipulations received by the patient. The literature of previous cases shows the high frequency, which in some reviews reaches 50%,[108] of manipulation sessions that the patients had received previously.[124] In Di Fabio's review,[108] only 10% of subjects that suffered an adverse event had received manipulation for the first time. There is enough data to show that a large number of visits were associated with a higher risk of arterial dissection.[25] In addition, many patients had received multiple manipulations in the same session,[97] although other authors argue that healthy arterial tissue should be capable of withstanding repeated strain.[86,179]

Some reviews also showed that there were patients with a clinical history that contraindicated the treatment, and that should have never received a manipulative treatment.[283,284] Terrett[170] described cases of subjects with signs of arterial dissection that were manipulated several times. A minimal adverse effect after a manipulation should be considered a complete contraindication for a new manipulation.[123,285]

A minimal adverse effect after a manipulation should be considered a complete contraindication for a new manipulation.

In order to obtain insight into the risk/benefit ratio of cervical manipulation, compared to other types of treatment commonly used in the same clinical situations, several interesting studies have been conducted. The risks of a manipulation have been compared to the risks associated with the intake of non-steroidal anti-inflammatory drugs (NSAIDs), since they can be considerably higher than the use of manipulation techniques.[286] In 2001, Graumlich[287] analysed the gastrointestinal complications caused by NSAIDs in the United States, and found that these drugs were responsible for more than 100,000 hospital admissions and approximately 16,500 deaths each year. However, such comparisons may be somewhat overstated, given the substantial differences in efficacy and clinical testing between the two modalities.[4]

Dabbs and Lauretti,[288] in 1995, compared the risk of death after a manipulation to the risk of death related to the use of NSAIDs, and found that the risk of death with cervical manipulation was 1 in 400,000, while the risk of death with the use of NSAIDs was 1 in 40,000. Carey[289] has established the risk of death at 3 in 10 million manipulations. Tramer et al.,[290] in 2000, showed that the risk of death due to gastroduodenal complications was 1 in 1200 when the subject takes NSAIDs daily for a period of 2 months.

Surgery of the cervical spine is not free of risks either, and it is estimated that 15.6 of 1000 interventions lead to neurological complications, and the mortality rate is 6.9 of 1000 interventions.[20]

Technical aspects of the manipulation and accident prevention

Current knowledge regarding adverse events following manipulation allows us to make some observations about the technical aspects.

The first observation to be highlighted is that articular mobilization techniques and muscular energy techniques are not entirely free of risks themselves, since it is known that, in subjects with structural weakness of the arteries, any manoeuvre has the potential to cause a dissection.[108] even the most gentle manipulation.[291]

The second observation is that, in order to avoid risks, not only the force and amplitude of the technique should be moderated but also, contrary to what was thought previously, the velocity. The arterial tunicas may be more prone to suffer a dissection with higher velocities and, therefore, it is suggested the velocity should be no greater than that which is needed to obtain the articular gapping.

Rotation is the other parameter that should be moderated, since there is sufficient evidence that a manipulation in rotation is potentially dangerous in vulnerable patients.[40,121] Not only should the amplitude of the impulse in rotation be reduced but also, when positioning the patient before the manipulation, it is advisable to limit this to less than 45°, although some authors suggest that a lateral thrust, since it generates a lower arterial stretching, could minimize the risks.[206,209,224] The cause of the arterial injury is not only the thrust but also the rotational position prior to the application of the manipulation. The other parameter, extension, has shown a potential risk of dissection of both the vertebral and carotid arteries, and probably should be avoided.[81] Paradoxically, many therapists use manipulation manoeuvres with the cervical spine in a significant degree of extension.

Some experts consider that the application of traction during the manipulation decreases the risks.[292] However, this suggestion cannot be confirmed, as the information provided by one study conducted in specimens showed that axial traction may induce the clogging of the vertebral artery,[63] yet ultrasound and MRI studies have shown no effect on cervical arterial blood flow.[184,193]

Every high-velocity manipulation technique or any technique that involves significant stress for the tissues should be preceded by a preparatory treatment for the soft tissues, as well as physiological mobilizations in which greater amplitude of movement is applied progressively, since it might improve the elastic capacity of the arterial walls, decreasing the risks of dissection. While care should be taken with all manipulative procedures, it is likely that most techniques are performed well within the limits of safety for a normal, healthy cervical artery.[179,293] However, the situation with an unhealthy artery or one which is otherwise damaged is not so certain and even safe application of manipulative or mobilization techniques may not offer any protection to clinicians.[20,80,193]

Different situations can contraindicate high-velocity techniques and not only the discovery a risk factor. These can be patient's discomfort, a headache or an acute neck pain, especially if there is a history of trauma[18] and vertiginous symptoms, even if the aetiology is not of vascular origin.

In conclusion, regarding the technical aspects:

1. Manipulation should never be performed during an acute episode of vertigo, headache or acute neck pain.
2. Any manoeuvre that causes vertigo or unpleasant symptoms for the patient should be avoided.
3. The functional test of the vertebral artery and the simulation of cervical manipulation position should be performed before every treatment and not only at the first session.
4. The pre-manipulative tests and their response should be documented in the patient history notes.

5. Manipulation should not be undertaken on older patients with degenerative changes.
6. Passive mobilization techniques should be used as initial treatment, and their effect should be observed during the first 24 hours, before considering any type of manipulation of the cervical spine.
7. When the manipulation is going to be applied, a single gentle manipulation should be used, as long as the functional tests are negative.
8. The force and velocity of the manipulation should be moderate.
9. The range of rotation should not exceed 45°.
10. There should be no traction components during the manipulation.
11. Extreme caution should be applied when manipulating the upper, craniocervical spine.
12. Informed consent should be obtained from the patient.

CONCLUSION

According to the current clinical knowledge and the importance of the clinical history and the subjective examination, in any clinical situation the therapist must decide if the high-velocity manipulation or techniques that involve high range of movement are suitable and appropriate therapeutic options. The most important risk factors for an arterial injury due to a manipulation are a previous trauma of the cervical spine that involves a subclinical injury of a cervical artery and disorders or alterations that involve weakening of the arterial walls. The development of an arterial dissection does not seem to depend on the forces applied during the manipulation, but on the arterial vulnerability in the patient, as the consequence of a trauma or previous pathology. With the available knowledge today, it is not possible to predict all subjects at risk for cerebrovascular accident caused by manipulation, and there are no guarantees that the negative results in the functional tests can avoid an adverse complication. Pre-manipulative functional tests and a thorough clinical examination do not absolutely guarantee that a manipulation will have no risks. With the purpose of minimizing the number of accidents, it is not enough to simply avoid potentially dangerous manoeuvres, but good technical skills are necessary, and most importantly a good clinical understanding of all the signs and symptoms that contraindicate such manoeuvres.

REFERENCES

1. Albuquerque FC, Hu YC, Dashti SR, et al. Craniocervical arterial dissections as sequelae of chiropractic manipulation: patterns of injury and management. J Neurosurg 2011;115(6):1197–205.

2. Biller J, Sacco R, Alberquerque F, et al. Cervical arterial dissections and association with cervical manipulative therapy. A statement for healthcare professionals from the American Heart Association/American Stroke Association. Stroke 2014;45:3155–74.

3. Cassidy D, Boyle E, Cote P, et al. Risk of vertebrobasilar stroke and chiropractic care. Results of a population-based case-control and case-crossover study. Spine 2008;33(4S):S176–83.

4. Ernst E. Adverse effects of spinal manipulation: a systematic review. J R Soc Med 2007;100(7):330–8.

5. Lord RS. Vertebrobasilar ischaemia and the extracranial arteries. Med J Aust 1973;2(1):32–7.

6. Moore K, Dalley A. Clinically oriented anatomy. 5th ed. Philadelphia: Lippincott Williams & Wilkins; 2006.

7. Fujita N, Ueda T, Yamanaka T, et al. Clinical application of ultrasonic blood rheography in vertebral artery for vertigo. Acta Otolaryngol Suppl 1995;519:178–83.

8. Stayman A, Noguiera RG, Gupta R. The diagnosis and management of vertebrobasilar insufficiency. Curr Treat Options Cardiovasc Med 2013;15:240–51.

9. Paciaroni M, Bogousslavsky J. Cerebrovascular complications of cervical manipulation. Eur Neurol 2009;61:112–18.

10. Debette S, Leys D. Cervical-artery dissections: predisposing factors, diagnosis and outcome. Lancet Neurol 2009;8(July):668–78.

11. Frumkin LR, Baloh RW. Wallenberg's syndrome following neck manipulation. Neurology 1990;40(4):611–15.

12. Haldeman S, Carey P, Townsend M, et al. Arterial dissections following cervical manipulation: the chiropractic experience. CMAJ 2001;165(7):905–6.

13. Okawara S, Nibbelink D. Vertebral artery occlusion following hyperextension and rotation of the head. Stroke 1974;5(5):640–2.

14. Debette S, Grond-Ginsbach C, Bodenant M, et al. Differential features of carotid and vertebral artery dissections: the CADISP study. Neurology 2011;77(12):1174–81.

15. Choi S, Boyle E, Cote P, et al. A population-based case-series of Ontario patients who develop a vertebrobasilar artery stroke after seeing a chiropractor. J Manipulative Physiol Ther 2011;34(1):15–22.

16. Lee KP, Carlini WG, McCormick GF, et al. Neurologic complications following chiropractic manipulation: a survey of California neurologists. Neurology 1995;45(6):1213–15.

17. Lee VH, Brown RD, Jayawant N, et al. Incidence and outcome of cervical artery dissection. A population-based study. Neurology 2006;67(Nov):1809–12.

18. Norris JW, Beletsky V, Nadareishvili Z. Sudden neck movement and cervical artery dissection. The Canadian Stroke Consortium. CMAJ 2000;163(1):38–40.

19. Rivett D, Milburn P. Complications arising from manipulative therapy in New Zealand. Physiotherapy 1997;83:626–32.

20. Hurwitz E, Aker P, Adams AH, et al. Manipulation and mobilization of the cervical spine. A systematic review of the literature. Spine 1996;21(15):1746–60.

21. Hurwitz EL, Morgenstern H, Vassilaki M, et al. Adverse reactions to chiropractic treatment and their effects on satisfaction and clinical outcomes among patients enrolled in the UCLA Neck Pain Study. J Manipulative Physiol Ther 2004;27(1):16–25.

22. Klougart N, Leboeuf-Yde C, Rasmussen RL. Safety in chiropractic practice. Part 1: The occurrence of cerebrovascular accidents after manipulation to the neck in Denmark from 1978-1988. J Manipulative Physiol Ther 1996;19:371–7.

23. Vickers A, Zollman C. ABC of complementary medicine. The manipulative therapies: osteopathy and chiropractic. BMJ 1999;319(7218):1176–9.

24. Kapral MK, Bondy SJ. Cervical manipulation and risk of stroke. CMAJ 2001;165(7):907–8.

25. Rothwell DM. Chiropractic manipulation and stroke: a population-based case-control study. Stroke 2001;32(5):1054–60.

26. Engelter S, Grond-Ginsbach C, Metso A, et al. Cervical artery dissection: trauma and other potential mechanical trigger events. Neurology 2013;80(21):1950–7.

27. Mann T, Refshauge KM. Causes of complications from cervical manipulation. Aust J Physiother 2001;47:255–66.

28. Rivett D, Milburn P, Chapple C. Negative pre-manipulative vertebral artery testing despite complete occlusion: a case of false negativity. Man Ther 1998;3(2):102–7.

29. Thomas LC. Cervical arterial dissection: an overview and implications for manipulative therapy practice. Man Ther 2016;21:2–9.

30. Caso V, Paciaroni M, Bogousslavsky J. Environmental factors and cervical artery dissection. In: Baumgartner RW, Bogousslavsky J, Caso V, et al., editors. Handbook on cerebral artery dissection. Basel: Karger; 2005. p. 44–53.

31. Argenson C, Franke JP, Sylla S, et al. The vertebral arteries (segments V1 and V2). Anat Clin 1980;2:29–41.

32. Warwick R, Williams PL, editors. Gray's anatomy. 35th ed. Edinburgh: Longman; 1975.

33. Chopard RP, de Miranda Neto MH, Lucas GA, et al. The vertebral artery: its relationship with adjoining tissues in its course intra and inter transverse processes in man. Rev Paul Med 1992;110(6):245–50.

34. Franke JP, Di Marino V, Pannier M, et al. The vertebral arteries (arteria vertebralis). The V3 atlanto-axoidal and V4 intracranial segments-collaterals. Anat Clin 1981;2:229–42.

35. George B, Laurian C. Vertebro-basilar ischaemia with thrombosis of the vertebral artery: report of two cases with embolism. J Neurol Neurosurg Psychiatry 1982;45(1):91–3.

36. Johnson C, Grant R, Dansie B, et al. Measurement of blood flow in the vertebral artery using colour duplex Doppler

ultrasound: establishment of the reliability of selected parameters. Man Ther 2000;5(1):21–9.

37. Thiel HW. Gross morphology and pathoanatomy of the vertebral arteries. J Manipulative Physiol Ther 1991;14(2):133–41.

38. Haynes M. Vertebral arteries and cervical movement: Doppler ultrasound velocimetry for screening before manipulation. J Manipulative Physiol Ther 2002;25(9):556–67.

39. Lamberty BGH, Zivanovic S. The retro-articular vertebral artery ring of the atlas and its significance. Acta Anat (Basel) 1973;85:113–22.

40. Haldeman S, Kohlbeck FJ, McGregor M. Risk factors and precipitating neck movements causing vertebrobasilar artery dissection after cervical trauma and spinal manipulation. Spine 1999;24(8):785–94.

41. Haneline M, Triano J. Cervical artery dissection. A comparison of highly dynamic mechanisms: manipulation versus motor vehicle collision. J Manipulative Physiol Ther 2005;28(1):57–63.

42. Nibu K, Cholewicki J, Panjabi MM, et al. Dynamic elongation of the vertebral artery during an in vitro whiplash simulation. Eur Spine J 1997;6(4):286–9.

43. Reddy M, Reddy B, Schoggl A, et al. The complexity of trauma to the cranio-cervical junction: correlation of clinical presentation with Doppler flow velocities in the V3-segment of the vertebral arteries. Acta Neurochir (Wien) 2002;144(6):575–80, discussion 580.

44. Giuffre R, Sherkat S. The vertebral artery: developmental pathology. J Neurosurg Sci 1999;43(3):175–89.

45. Macchi C, Giannelli F, Cecchi F, et al. The inner diameter of human intracranial vertebral artery by color Doppler method. Ital J Anat Embryol 1996;101(2):81–7.

46. Davis JM, Zimmerman RA. Injury of the carotid and vertebral arteries. Neuroradiology 1983;25(2):55–69.

47. Haneline M, Croft A, Frishberg B. Association of internal carotid artery dissection and chiropractic manipulation. Neurologist 2003;9(1):35–44.

48. Sturzenegger M. Spontaneous internal carotid artery dissection: early diagnosis and management in 44 patients. J Neurol 1995;242(4):231–8.

49. Taylor AJ, Kerry R. Neck pain and headache as a result of internal carotid artery dissection: implications for manual therapists. Man Ther 2005;10(1):73–7.

50. Dadsetan MR, Skerhut HE. Rotational vertebrobasilar insufficiency secondary to vertebral artery occlusion from fibrous band of the longus coli muscle. Neuroradiology 1990;32(6):514–15.

51. Healy AT, Lee BS, Walsh K, et al. Bow hunter's syndrome secondary to bilateral dynamic vertebral artery compression. J Clin Neurosci 2015;22(1):209–12.

52. Scheenan S, Bauer R, Meyer J. Vertebral artery compressions in cervical spondylosis. Neurology 1969;10:968.

53. Pollanen MS, Deck JH, Boutilier L, et al. Lesions of the tunica media in traumatic rupture of vertebral arteries: histologic and biochemical studies. Can J Neurol Sci 1992;19(1):53–6.

54. De Kleyn A, Nieuwenhuyse A. Schwindelanfalle und Nystagmus bei einer bestimmten Stellung des Kopfes. Acta Otolaryngol 1927;VII:155–7.

55. Sim E, Schwarz N, Biowski-Fasching I, et al. Color-coded Duplex sonography of vertebral arteries. 11 cases of blunt cervical spine injury. Acta Orthop Scand 1993;64(2):133–7.

56. Kuether TA, Nesbit GM, Clark WM, et al. Rotational vertebral artery occlusion: a mechanism of vertebrobasilar insufficiency. Neurosurgery 1997;41(2):427–32, discussion 432–3.

57. Bogduk N, Mercer S. Biomechanics of the cervical spine. I: Normal kinematics. Clin Biomech (Bristol, Avon) 2000;15:633–48.

58. Mimura M, Moriya H, Watanabe T, et al. Three-dimensional motion analysis of the cervical spine with special reference to the axial rotation. Spine 1989;14(11):1135–9.

59. Selecki BR. The effects of rotation of the atlas on the axis: experimental work. Med J Aust 1969;1(20):1012–15.

60. Hufnagel A, Hammers A, Schonle PW, et al. Stroke following chiropractic manipulation of the cervical spine. J Neurol 1999;246(8):683–8.

61. Andersson R, Carleson R, Nylen O. Vertebral artery insufficiency and rotational obstruction. Acta Med Scand 1970;188(6):475–7.

62. Barton JW, Margolis MT. Rotational obstructions of the vertebral artery at the atlantoaxial joint. Neuroradiology 1975;9(3):117–20.

63. Brown BSJ, Tatlow WF. Radiographic studies of the vertebral arteries in cadavers. Effects of position and traction on the head. Radiology 1963;81:80–8.

64. Grossmann RI, Davis KR. Positional occlusion of the vertebral artery: a rare cause of embolic stroke. Neuroradiology 1982;23(4):227–30.

65. Toole JF, Tucker SH. Influence of head position upon cerebral circulation. Studies on blood flow in cadavers. Arch Neurol 1960;2:616–23.

66. Yang PJ, Latack JT, Gabrielsen TO, et al. Rotational vertebral artery occlusion at C1-C2. AJNR Am J Neuroradiol 1985;6(1):96–100.

67. Di Duro JO. Stroke in a chiropractic patient population. Cerebrovasc Dis 2003;15(1–2):156. author reply 156.

68. Zaidi HA, Albuquerque FC, Chowdhry SA, et al. Diagnosis and management of bow hunter's syndrome: 15-year experience at Barrow Neurological Institute. World Neurosurg 2014;82(5):733–8.

69. Grego F, Lepidi S, Cognolato D, et al. Rationale of the surgical treatment of carotid kinking. J Cardiovasc Surg (Torino) 2003;44(1):79–85.

70. Rivett D, Sharples K, Milburn P. Effect of premanipulative tests on vertebral artery and internal carotid blood flow: a pilot study. J Manipulative Physiol Ther 1999;22:368–75.

71. Beatty RA. Dissecting hematoma of the internal carotid artery following chiropractic cervical manipulation. J Trauma 1977;17(3):248–9.

72. Parwar BL, Fawzi AA, Arnold AC, et al. Horner's syndrome and dissection of the internal carotid artery after chiropractic

manipulation of the neck. Am J Ophthalmol 2001;131(4): 523–4.

73. Peters M, Bohl J, Thomke F, et al. Dissection of the internal carotid artery after chiropractic manipulation of the neck. Neurology 1995;45(12):2284–6.

74. Herzog W, Tang C, Leonard T. Internal carotid artery strains during high-speed, low-amplitude spinal manipulations of the neck. J Manipulative Physiol Ther 2015;38(9):664–71.

75. Refshauge KM. Rotation: a valid premanipulative dizziness test? Does it predict safe manipulation? J Manipulative Physiol Ther 1994;17(1):15–19.

76. Thomas L, McLeod L, Osmotherly P, et al. The effect of end-range cervical rotation on vertebral and internal carotid arterial blood flow and cerebral inflow: A sub analysis of an MRI study. Man Ther 2015;20(3):475–80.

77. Etheredge SN, Effeney DJ, Ehrenfeld WK. Symptomatic extrinsic compression of the cervical carotid artery. Arch Neurol 1984;41(6):672–3.

78. Flis CM, Jäger HR, Sidhu PS. Carotid and vertebral dissections: clinical aspects, imaging features,and endovascular treatment. Eur Neurol 2007;17:820–34.

79. Ozdoba C, Sturzenegger M, Schroth G. Internal carotid artery dissection: MR imaging features and clinical-radiologic correlation. Radiology 1996;199(1):191–8.

80. Haneline MT, Rosner AL. The etiology of cervical artery dissection. J Chiropr Med 2007;6(3):110–20.

81. Stringer WL, Kelly DL Jr. Traumatic dissection of the extracranial internal carotid artery. Neurosurgery 1980;6(2): 123–30.

82. Lepojarvi M, Tarkka M, Leinonen A, et al. Spontaneous dissection of the internal carotid artery. Acta Chir Scand 1988;154(10):559–66.

83. Fabian TC, Patton JH Jr, Croce MA, et al. Blunt carotid injury. Importance of early diagnosis and anticoagulant therapy. Ann Surg 1996;223(5):513–22, discussion 522–5.

84. Dobrin PB. Mechanical properties of arterises. Physiol Rev 1978;58(2):397–460.

85. Piffer CR, Zorzetto NL. Microscopy anatomy of the vertebral artery in the suboccipital and intracranial segments. Anat Anz 1980;147(4):382–8.

86. Austin N, DiFrancesco L, Herzog W. Microstructural damage in arterial tissue exposed to repeated tensile strains. J Manipulative Physiol Ther 2010;33:14–19.

87. Kawchuk GN, Wynd S, Anderson T. Defining the effect of cervical manipulation on vertebral artery integrity: establishment of an animal model. J Manipulative Physiol Ther 2004;27(9):539–46.

88. Symons B, Leonard T, Herzog W. Internal forces sustained by the vertebral artery during spinal manipulative therapy. J Manipulative Physiol Ther 2002;25(8):504–10.

89. Wynd S, Anderson T, Kawchuk GN. Effect of cervical spine manipulation on a pre-existing vascular lesion within the canine vertebral artery. Cerebrovasc Dis 2008;26:304–9.

90. Debette S. Pathophysiology and risk factors of cervical artery dissection: what have we learnt from large hospital-based cohorts? Curr Opin Neurol 2014;27:20–8.

91. Dunne JW, Conacher GN, Khangure M, et al. Dissecting aneurysms of the vertebral arteries following cervical manipulation: a case report. J Neurol Neurosurg Psychiatry 1987;50(3): 349–53.

92. Nagasawa S, Handa H, Naruo Y, et al. Biomechanical study on aging changes and vasospasm of human cerebral arteries. Biorheology 1982;19(3):481–9.

93. Dorfler P, Puls I, Schliesser M, et al. Measurement of cerebral blood flow volume by extracranial sonography. J Cereb Blood Flow Metab 2000;20(2):269–71.

94. Berczi V, Toth P, Kovach AG, et al. Biomechanical properties of canine vertebral and internal carotid arteries. Acta Physiol Hung 1990;75(2):133–45.

95. Bevan JA. Sites of transition between functional systemic and cerebral arteries of rabbits occur at embryological junctional sites. Science 1979;204(4393):635–7.

96. Wilkinson IM. The vertebral artery. Extracranial and intracranial structure. Arch Neurol 1972;27(5):392–6.

97. Frisoni G, Anzola G. Vertebrobasilar ischaemia after neck motion. Stroke 1991;22:1452–60.

98. Caplan LR. Vertebrobasilar embolism. Clin Exp Neurol 1991; 28:1–22.

99. Anson J, Crowell RM. Cervicocranial arterial dissection. Neurosurgery 1991;29(1):89–96.

100. Ehrenfeld WK, Wylie EJ. Spontaneous dissection of the internal carotid artery. Arch Surg 1976;111(11):1294–301.

101. Hart RG, Easton JD. Dissections of cervical and cerebral arteries. Neurol Clin 1983;1(1):155–82.

102. Mokri B, Houser OW, Sandok BA, et al. Spontaneous dissections of the vertebral arteries. Neurology 1988;38(6):880–5.

103. Zetterling M, Carlstrom C, Konrad P. Internal carotid artery dissection. Acta Neurol Scand 2000;101(1):1–7.

104. Sherman DG, Hart RG, Easton JD. Abrupt change in head position and cerebral infarction. Stroke 1981;12(1):2–6.

105. Hoshino Y, Kurokawa T, Nakamura K, et al. A report on the safety of unilateral vertebral artery ligation during cervical spine surgery. Spine 1996;21(12):1454–7.

106. Stahmer SA, Raps EC, Mines DI. Carotid and vertebral artery dissections. Emerg Med Clin North Am 1997;15(3):677–98.

107. Bassetti C, Carruzzo A, Sturzenegger M, et al. Recurrence of cervical artery dissection. A prospective study of 81 patients. Stroke 1996;27(10):1804–7.

108. Di Fabio RP. Manipulation of the cervical spine: risks and benefits. Phys Ther 1999;79(1):50–65.

109. Daneshmend TK, Hewer RL, Bradshaw JR. Acute brain stem stroke during neck manipulation. Br Med J (Clin Res Ed) 1984;288(6412):189.

110. Easton JD, Sherman DG. Cervical manipulation and stroke. Stroke 1977;8(5):594–7.

111. Katirji MB, Reinmuth OM, Latchaw RE. Stroke due to vertebral artery injury. Arch Neurol 1985;42(3):242–8.

112. Parkin PJ, Wallis WE, Wilson JL. Vertebral artery occlusion following manipulation of the neck. N Z Med J 1978;88(625): 441–3.

113. Fast A, Zinicola DF, Marin EL. Vertebral artery damage complicating cervical manipulation. Spine 1987;12(9):840–2.

114. Horn SW 2nd. The "Locked-In" syndrome following chiropractic manipulation of the cervical spine. Ann Emerg Med 1983;12(10):648–50.

115. Kanshepolsky J, Danielson H, Flynn RE. Vertebral artery insufficiency and cerebellar infarct due to manipulation of the neck. Report of a case. Bull Los Angeles Neurol Soc 1972;37(2):62–5.

116. Vaccaro AR, Klein GR, Flanders AE, et al. Long-term evaluation of vertebral artery injuries following cervical spine trauma using magnetic resonance angiography. Spine 1998;23(7):789–94, discussion 795.

117. Marshall LF, Bruce DA, Bruno L, et al. Vertebrobasilar spasm: a significant cause of neurological deficit in head injury. J Neurosurg 1978;48(4):560–4.

118. Apsatarov EA, Balmagambetov BR, Liubinskii VL. [Angiographic diagnosis and rheologic properties of blood in vertebrobasilar insufficiency caused by scalenus anticus syndrome]. Kardiologiia 1988;28(9):74–7.

119. Seric V, Blazic-Cop N, Demarin V. Haemodynamic changes in patients with whiplash injury measured by transcranial Doppler sonography (TCD). Coll Antropol 2000;24(1):197–204.

120. Arning C, Schrattenholzer A, Lachenmayer L. Cervical carotid artery vasospasms causing cerebral ischemia: detection by immediate vascular ultrasonographic investigation. Stroke 1998;29(5):1063–6.

121. Assendelft WJJ, Bouter LM, Knipschild PG. Complications of spinal manipulation. A comprehensive review of the literature. J Fam Pract 1996;42(5 (May)):475–80.

122. Carnes D, Mars T, Mullinger B, et al. Adverse events and manual therapy. Man Ther 2010;15:355–63.

123. Ernst E. Manipulation of the cervical spine: a systematic review of adverse events, 1995-2001. Med J Aust 2002;176(8):376–80.

124. Haldeman S, Kohlbeck FJ, McGregor M. Stroke, cerebral artery dissection, and cervical spine manipulation therapy. J Neurol 2002;249(8):1098–104.

125. Rubinstein S, Peerdeman S, van Tulder M, et al. A systematic review of the risk factors for cervical artery dissection. Stroke 2005;36:1575–80.

126. Stevinson C, Ernst E. Risks associated with spinal manipulation. Am J Med 2002;112(7):566–71.

127. Jentzen JM, Amatuzio J, Peterson GF. Complications of cervical manipulation: a case report of fatal brainstem infarct with review of the mechanisms and predisposing factors. J Forensic Sci 1987;32(4):1089–94.

128. Hedera P. Influence of extreme head rotations on brainstem auditory evoked potentials (BAEP). Clin Neurol Neurosurg 1995;97(4):290–5.

129. Sedat J, Dib M, Mahagne MH, et al. Stroke after chiropractic manipulation as a result of extracranial postero-inferior cerebellar artery dissection. J Manipulative Physiol Ther 2002;25(9):588–90.

130. Jackson RS, Wheeler AH, Darden BV 2nd. Vertebral artery anomaly with atraumatic dissection causing thromboembolic ischemia: a case report. Spine 2000;25(15):1989–92.

131. Friedman D, Flanders A, Thomas C, et al. Vertebral artery injury after acute cervical spine trauma: rate of occurrence as detected by MR angiography and assessment of clinical consequences. AJR Am J Roentgenol 1995;164(2):443–7, discussion 448–9.

132. Schwarz N, Buchinger W, Gaudernak T, et al. Injuries to the cervical spine causing vertebral artery trauma: case reports. J Trauma 1991;31(1):127–33.

133. Veras LM, Pedraza-Gutierrez S, Castellanos J, et al. Vertebral artery occlusion after acute cervical spine trauma. Spine 2000;25(9):1171–7.

134. Beletsky V, Nadareishvili Z, Lynch J, et al. Cervical arterial dissection: time for a therapeutic trial? Stroke 2003;34(12):2856–60.

135. Beaudry M, Spence JD. Motor vehicle accidents: the most common cause of traumatic vertebrobasilar ischemia. Can J Neurol Sci 2003;30(4):320–5.

136. Dittrich R, Heidbreder A, Rohsbach D, et al. Connective tissue and vascular phenotype in patients with cervical artery dissection. Neurology 2007;68(24):2120–4.

137. Thomas L, Rivett D, Attia J, et al. Risk factors and clinical presentation of cervical arterial dissection: preliminary results of a prospctive case-control study. J Orthop Sports Phys Ther 2015;45(7):501–11.

138. Mokri B. Traumatic and spontaneous extracranial internal carotid artery dissections. J Neurol 1990;237(6):356–61.

139. Schellinger PD, Schwab S, Krieger D, et al. Masking of vertebral artery dissection by severe trauma to the cervical spine. Spine 2001;26(3):314–19.

140. Prabhakar S, Bhatia R, Khandelwal N, et al. Vertebral artery dissection due to indirect neck trauma: an underrecognised entity. Neurol India 2001;49(4):384–90.

141. Micheli S, Paciaroni M, Corea F, et al. Cervical artery dissection: emerging risk factors. Open Neurol J 2010;4:50–5.

142. Endo K, Ichimaru K, Shimura H, et al. Cervical vertigo after hair shampoo treatment at a hairdressing salon: a case report. Spine 2000;25(5):632–4.

143. Nwokolo N, Bateman DE. Stroke after a visit to the hairdresser. Lancet 1997;350(9081):866.

144. Shimura H, Yuzawa K, Nozue M. Stroke after visit to the hairdresser. Lancet 1997;350(9093):1778.

145. Weintraub MI. Beauty parlor stroke syndrome: report of five cases. JAMA 1993;269(16):2085–6.

146. Hanus SH, Homer TD, Harter DH. Vertebral artery occlusion complicating yoga exercises. Arch Neurol 1977;34(9):574–5.

147. Thomas L, Rivett D, Levi C. Risk factors and clinical features of craniocervical arterial dissection. Man Ther 2011;16:351–6.

148. Nagler W. Vertebral artery obstruction by hyperextension of the neck: report of three cases. Arch Phys Med Rehabil 1973;54(5):237–40.

149. D'Anglejan-Chatillon J, Ribeiro V, Mas JL, et al. Migraine – a risk factor for dissection of cervical arteries. Headache 1989;29(9):560–1.

150. Guillon B, Tzourio C, Biousse V, et al. Arterial wall properties in carotid artery dissection: an ultrasound study. Neurology 2000;55:663–6.

151. Brandt T, Hausser I, Orberk E, et al. Ultrastructural connective tissue abnormalities in patients with spontaneous cervicocerebral artery dissections. Ann Neurol 1998;44:281–5.

152. Sato T, Sasaki T, Suzuki K, et al. Histological study of the normal vertebral artery – etiology of dissecting aneurysms. Neurol Med Chir (Tokyo) 2004;44(12):629–35, discussion 636.

153. Majamaa K, Portimojarvi H, Sotaniemi KA, et al. Familial aggregation of cervical artery dissection and cerebral aneurysm. Stroke 1994;25(8):1704–5.

154. Mokri B, Mokri B, Piepgras DG, et al. Familial occurrence of spontaneous dissection of the internal carotid artery. Stroke 1987;18(1):246–51.

155. Perez-Higueras A, Alvarez-Ruiz F, Martinez-Bermejo A, et al. Cerebellar infarction from fibromuscular dysplasia and dissecting aneurysm of the vertebral artery. Report of a child. Stroke 1988;19(4):521–4.

156. Schievink WI, Wijdicks EF, Michels VV, et al. Heritable connective tissue disorders in cervical artery dissections: a prospective study. Neurology 1998;50(4):1166–9.

157. Vega Molina J, Chiras J, Poirier B, et al. Fibromuscular dysplasia of the vertebral artery (angiographic features). A review of 85 cases. J Neuroradiol 1985;12(2):123–34.

158. Mondon K, de Toffol B, Georgesco G, et al. [Ehlers Danlos type IV syndrome presenting with simultaneous dissection of both internal carotid and both vertebral arteries]. Rev Neurol (Paris) 2004;160(4 Pt 1):478–82.

159. North KN, Whiteman DA, Pepin MG, et al. Cerebrovascular complications in Ehlers-Danlos syndrome type IV. Ann Neurol 1995;38(6):960–4.

160. Vles JS, Hendriks JJ, Lodder J, et al. Multiple vertebro-basilar infarctions from fibromuscular dysplasia related dissecting aneurysm of the vertebral artery in a child. Neuropediatrics 1990;21(2):104–5.

161. Schievink WI, Michels VV, Piepgras DG. Neurovascular manifestations of heritable connective tissue disorders. A review. Stroke 1994;25(4):889–903.

162. Schievink WI, Parisi JE, Piepgras DG, et al. Intracranial aneurysms in Marfan's syndrome: an autopsy study. Neurosurgery 1997;41(4):866–70, discussion 871.

163. Youl BD, Coutellier A, Dubois B, et al. Three cases of spontaneous extracranial vertebral artery dissection. Stroke 1990;21(4):618–25.

164. Schievink WI. Spontaneous dissection of the carotid and vertebral arteries. N Engl J Med 2001;344(12):898–906.

165. Giossi A, Ritelli M, Costa P, et al. Connective tissue anomalies in patients with spontaneous cervical artery dissection. Neurology 2014;83(22):2032–7.

166. Pezzini A, Del Zotto E, Archetti S, et al. Plasma homocysteine concentration, C677T MTHFR genotype, and 844ins68bp CBS genotype in young adults with spontaneous cervical artery dissection and atherothrombotic stroke. Stroke 2002;33(3):664–9.

167. Arauz A, Hoyos L, Cantú C, et al. Mild hyperhomocysteinemia and low folate concentrations as risk factors for cervical arterial dissection. Cerebrovasc Dis 2007;24(2–3):210–14.

168. Kloss M, Metso A, Pezzini A, et al. Towards understanding seasonal variability in cervical artery dissection. J Neurol 2012;259:1662–7.

169. Fragoso YD, Adoni T, Amaral LL, et al. Cerebrum-cervical arterial dissection in adults during sports and recreation. Arq Neuropsiquiatr 2015:Oct 6.

170. Terrett AGJ. Vertebrobasilar stroke following spinal manipulation therapy. In: Murphy DR, editor. Conservative management of cervical spine syndromes. New York: McGraw-Hill; 2000. p. 533–78.

171. Pezzini A, Caso V, Zanferrari C, et al. Arterial hypertension as risk factor for spontaneous cervical artery dissection. A case-control study. J Neurol Neurosurg Psychiatry 2006;77(1):95–7.

172. Sasaki O, Ogawa H, Koike T, et al. A clinicopathological study of dissecting aneurysms of the intracranial vertebral artery. J Neurosurg 1991;75(6):874–82.

173. Ask-Upmark E, Bickerstaff ER. Vertebral artery occlusion and oral contraceptives. Br Med J 1976;1(6008):487–8.

174. Crawford JP, Hwang BY, Asselbergs PJ, et al. Vascular ischemia of the cervical spine: a review of relationship to therapeutic manipulation. J Manipulative Physiol Ther 1984;7(3):149–55.

175. Tzourio C, Benslamia L, Guillon B, et al. Migraine and the risk of cervical artery dissection: a case-control study. Neurology 2002;59(3):435–7.

176. Paciaroni M, Georgiardis D, Arnold M, et al. Seasonal variability in spontaneous cervical artery dissection. J Neurol Neurosurg Psychiatry 2006;77(5):667–79.

177. Schievinck W, Wijdicks EF, Kuiper J. Seasonal pattern of spontaneous cervical artery dissection. J Neurosurg 1998;89(1):101–3.

178. Grau AJ, Brandt T, Buggle F, et al. Association of cervical artery dissection with recent infection. Arch Neurol 1999;52(7):851–6.

179. Herzog W, Herzog W, Leonard TR, et al. Vertebral artery strains during high-speed, low amplitude cervical spinal manipulation. J Electromyogr Kinesiol 2012;22(5):740–6.

180. Goldstein SJ. Dissecting hematoma of the cervical vertebral artery. Case report. J Neurosurg 1982;56(3):451–4.

181. Schneider RC, Gosch HH, Taren JA, et al. Blood vessel trauma following head and neck injuries. Clin Neurosurg 1972;19:312–54.

182. Buzzatti L, Provyn S, Van Roy P, et al. Atlanto-axial facet displacement during rotational high-velocity low-amplitude thrust: an in vitro 3D kinematic analysis. Man Ther 2015;20(6):783–9.

183. Haynes M. Internal forces sustained by the vertebral artery during spinal manipulative therapy: letter to the. J Manipulative Physiol Ther 2004;27(1):67–8.

184. Smith RA, Estridge MN. Neurologic complications of head and neck manipulations. JAMA 1962;182:528–31.

185. Petersen B, Von Maravic M, Zeller JA, et al. Basilar artery blood flow during head rotation in vertebrobasilar ischemia. Acta Neurol Scand 1996;94(4):294–301.

186. Husni EA, Bell HS, Storer J. Mechanical occlusion of the vertebral artery. A new clinical concept. JAMA 1966;196(6):475–8.

187. Bowler N, Shamley D, Davies R. The effect of a simulated manipulation position on internal carotid and vertebral artery blood flow in healthy individuals. Man Ther 2011;16(1):87–93.

188. Haynes M, Hart R, McGeachie J. Vertebral arteries and neck rotation: Doppler velocimeter interexaminer reliability. Ultrasound Med Biol 2000;26(8):1363–7.

189. Mitchell J, Keene D, Dyson C, et al. Is cervical spine rotation, as used in the standard vertebrobasilar insufficiency test, associated with a measureable change in intracranial vertebral artery blood flow? Man Ther 2004;9(4):220–7.

190. Sakaguchi M, Kitagawa K, Hougaku H, et al. Mechanical compression of the extracranial vertebral artery during neck rotation. Neurology 2003;61(6):845–7.

191. DeMaria AA Jr. Positional compression of vertebral artery shown by magnetic resonance angiography. South Med J 1995;88(8):871–2.

192. Dumas JL, Salama J, Dreyfus P, et al. Magnetic resonance angiographic analysis of atlanto-axial rotation: anatomic bases of compression of the vertebral arteries. Surg Radiol Anat 1996;18(4):303–13.

193. Thomas L, Rivett D, Bateman GA, et al. Effect of selected manual therapy interventions for mechanical neck pain on vertebral and internal carotid arterial blood flow and cerebral inflow. Phys Ther 2013;93(11):1563–74.

194. Weintraub MI, Khoury A. Critical neck position as an independent risk factor for posterior circulation stroke. A magnetic resonance angiographic analysis. J Neuroimaging 1995;5(1):16–22.

195. Cote P, Kreitz BG, Cassidy D, et al. The validity of the extension-rotation test as a clinical screening procedure before neck manipulation: a secondary analysis. J Manipulative Physiol Ther 1996;19(3):159–64.

196. Thiel H, Wallace K, Donat J, et al. Effect of various head and neck positions on vertebral artery blood flow. Clin Biomech (Bristol, Avon) 1994;9(2):105–10.

197. Zaina C, Grant R, Johnson C, et al. The effect of cervical rotation on blood flow in the contralateral artery. Man Ther 2003;8(2):103–9.

198. Mitchell JA. Changes in vertebral artery blood flow following normal rotation of the cervical spine. J Manipulative Physiol Ther 2003;26(6):347–51.

199. Arnold C, Bourassa R, Langer T, et al. Doppler studies evaluating the effect of a physical therapy screening protocol on vertebral artery blood flow. Man Ther 2004;9(1):13–21.

200. Rivett D. Vertebral artery blood flow during pre-manipulative testing of the cervical spine [PhD thesis]. Dunedin: University of Otago; 2000.

201. Licht PB, Christensen HW, Hojgaard P, et al. Triplex ultrasound of vertebral artery flow during cervical rotation. J Manipulative Physiol Ther 1998;21:27–31.

202. Licht PB, Christensen HW, Hoilund-Carlsen PF. Is there a role for pre-manipulative testing before cervical manipulation? J Manipulative Physiol Ther 2000;23(3):175–9.

203. Erhardt JW, Windsor BA, Kerry R, et al. The immediate effect of atlanto-axial high velocity thrust techniques on blood flow in the vertebral artery: a randomized controlled trial. Man Ther 2015;20(4):614–22.

204. Quesnele J, Triano J, Noseworthy M, et al. Changes in vertebral artery blood flow following various head positions and cervical spine manipulation. J Manipulative Physiol Ther 2014;37(1):22–31.

205. Weintraub MI, Khoury A. Cerebral hemodynamic changes induced by simulated tracheal intubation: a possible role in perioperative stroke? Magnetic resonance angiography and flow analysis in 160 cases. Stroke 1998;29:1644–9.

206. Michaud TC. Uneventful upper cervical manipulation in the presence of a damaged vertebral artery. J Manipulative Physiol Ther 2002;25(7):472–83.

207. Haynes M, Milne N. Color duplex sonographic findings in human vertebral arteries during cervical rotation. J Clin Ultrasound 2001;29(1):14–24.

208. Schievinck WI. Spontaneous dissection of the carotid and vertebral arteries. N Engl J Med 2001;344(12):898–906.

209. Haynes MJ. Doppler studies comparing the effects of cervical rotation and lateral flexion on vertebral artery blood flow. J Manipulative Physiol Ther 1996;19(6):378–84.

210. Terret AGJ. Vertebrobasilar stroke following spinal manipulation therapy. In: Murphy D, editor. Conservative management of cervical spine syndromes. New York: McGraw Hill; 2000.

211. Licht PB, Christensen HW, Hoilund-Carlsen PF. Carotid artery blood flow during premanipulative testing. J Manipulative Physiol Ther 2002;25(9):568–72.

212. Brandt T, Orberk E, Weber R, et al. Pathogenesis of cervical artery dissections: association with connective tissue abnormalities. Neurology 2001;57(1):24–30.

213. Kerry R, Taylor A, Mitchell J, et al. Cervical arterial dysfunction and manual therapy: a critical literature review to inform professional practice. Man Ther 2008;13:278–88.

214. Arnold M, Bousser M. Carotid and vertebral artery dissection. Pract Neurol 2005;5:100–9.

215. Sturzenegger M. Headache and neck pain: the warning symptoms of vertebral artery dissection. Headache 1994;34(4):187–93.

216. Arnold M, Cumurciuc R, Stapf C, et al. Pain as the only symptom of cervical artery dissection. J Neurol Neurosurg Psychiatry 2006;77(9):1021–4.

217. Krespi Y, Gurol ME, Coban O, et al. Vertebral artery dissection presenting with isolated neck pain. J Neuroimaging 2002;12(2):179–82.

218. Nichols FT 3rd, Mawad M, Mohr JP, et al. Focal headache during balloon inflation in the vertebral and basilar arteries. Headache 1993;33(2):87–9.

219. Munari LM, Belloni G, Moschini L, et al. Carotid pain during percutaneous angioplasty (PTA). Pathophysiology and clinical features. Cephalalgia 1994;14(2):127–31.

220. Maruyama H, Nagoya H, Kato Y, et al. Spontaneous cervicocephalic arterial dissection with headache and neck pain as the only symptom. J Headache Pain 2012;13(3):247–53.

221. Silbert PL, Mokri B, Schievink WI. Headache and neck pain in spontaneous internal carotid and vertebral artery dissections. Neurology 1995;45(8):1517–22.

222. Asavasopon S, Jankosi J, Godges JJ. Clinical diagnosis of verte-brobasilar insufficiency: resident's case problem. J Orthop Sports Phys Ther 2005;35:645–50.

223. Smith WS, Johnston SC, Skalabrin EJ, et al. Spinal manipula-tive therapy is an independent risk factor for vertebral artery dissection. Neurology 2003;60(9):1424–8.

224. Dziewas R, Konrad C, Drager B, et al. Cervical artery dissection – clinical features, risk factors, therapy and outcome in 126 patients. J Neurol 2003;250(10):1179–84.

225. Grad A, Baloh RW. Vertigo of vascular origin. Clinical and electronystagmographic features in 84 cases. Arch Neurol 1989;46(3):281–4.

226. Hicks PA, Leavitt JA, Mokri B. Ophthalmic manifestations of vertebral artery dissection. Patients seen at the Mayo Clinic from 1976 to 1992. Ophthalmology 1994;101(11):1786–92.

227. Saeed AB, Shuaib A, Al-Sulaiti G, et al. Vertebral artery dissec-tion: warning symptoms, clinical features and prognosis in 26 patients. Can J Neurol Sci 2000;27(4):292–6.

228. Milandre L, Lucchini P, Khalil R. [Lateral bulbar infarctions. Distribution, etiology and prognosis in 40 cases diagnosed by MRI]. Rev Neurol (Paris) 1995;151(12):714–21.

229. Nagahata M, Hosoya T, Fuse T, et al. Arterial dissection of the vertebrobasilar systems: a possible cause of acute sensorineural hearing loss. Am J Otol 1997;18(1):32–8.

230. Koyuncu M, Celik O, Luleci C, et al. Doppler sonography of vertebral arteries in patients with tinnitus. Auris Nasus Larynx 1995;22(1):24–8.

231. Yokota M, Ito T, Hosoya T, et al. Sudden-onset tinnitus associ-ated with arterial dissection of the vertebrobasilar system. Acta Otolaryngol Suppl 2000;542:29–33.

232. Pelkonen O, Tikkakoski T, Luotonen J, et al. Pulsatile tinnitus as a symptom of cervicocephalic arterial dissection. J Laryngol Otol 2004;118(3):193–8.

233. Mas JL, Bousser MG, Hasboun D, et al. Extracranial vertebral artery dissections: a review of 13 cases. Stroke 1987;18(6):1037–47.

234. Mas JL, Goeau C, Bousser MG, et al. Spontaneous dissecting aneurysms of the internal carotid and vertebral arteries – two case reports. Stroke 1985;16(1):125–9.

235. Ausman JI, Diaz FG, de los Reyes RA, et al. Posterior cir-culation revascularization. Superficial temporal artery to supe-rior cerebellar artery anastomosis. J Neurosurg 1982;56(6):766–76.

236. Pessin MS, Gorelick PB, Kwan ES, et al. Basilar artery stenosis: middle and distal segments. Neurology 1987;37(11):1742–6.

237. Rigueiro-Veloso MT, Pego-Reigosa R, Branas-Fernandez F, et al. [Wallenberg syndrome: a review of 25 cases]. Rev Neurol 1997;25(146):1561–4.

238. Moubayed SP, Saliba I. Vertebrobasilar insufficiency presenting as isolated positional vertigo or dizziness: a double-blind retrospective cohort study. Laryngoscope 2009;119(10):2071–6.

239. Nunez RA, Cass SP, Furman JM. Short- and long-term out-comes of canalith repositioning for benign paroxysmal posi-tional vertigo. Otolaryngol Head Neck Surg 2000;122(5):647–53.

240. Parnes LS, Agrawal SK, Atlas J. Diagnosis and management of benign paroxysmal positional vertigo (BPPV). CMAJ 2003;169(7):681–93.

241. Kim JS, Zee DS. Clinical practice. Benign paroxysmal posi-tional vertigo. N Engl J Med 2014;370(12):1138–47.

242. Treleaven J. Sensorimotor disturbances in neck disorders affecting postural stability, head and eye movement control. Man Ther 2008;13(1):2–11.

243. Meadows J, Magee J. An overview of dizziness and vertigo for the orthopedic manual therapist. In: Boyling J, Palastanga N, editors. Grieve's modern manual therapy. Edinburgh: Church-ill Livingstone; 1994.

244. Conman W. Dizziness related to ENT conditions. In: Grieve G, editor. Modern manual therapy of the vertebral column. Edinburgh: Churchill Livingstone; 1986.

245. Bonkowsky V, Steinbach S, Arnold W. Vertigo and cranial nerve palsy caused by different forms of spontaneous dissections of internal and vertebral arteries. Eur Arch Otorhinolaryngol 2002;259(7):365–8.

246. Crum B, Mokri B, Fulgham J. Spinal manifestations of verte-bral artery dissection. Neurology 2000;55(2):304–6.

247. Hetzel A, Berger W, Schumacher M, et al. Dissection of the vertebral artery with cervical nerve root lesions. J Neurol 1996;243(2):121–5.

248. McGillion SF, Weston-Simons S, Harvey JR. Vertebral artery dissection presenting with multilevel combined sensorimotor radiculopathy: a case report and literature review. J Spinal Disord Tech 2009;22(6):456–8.

249. Barinagarrementeria F, Amaya LE, Cantu C. Causes and mech-anisms of cerebellar infarction in young patients. Stroke 1997;28(12):2400–4.

250. Barbic D, Levine Z, Tampieri D, et al. Locked-in syndrome: a critical and time-dependent diagnosis. CJEM 2012;14(5):317–20.

251. Izquierdo-Casas J, Soler-Singla L, Vivas-Díaz E, et al. Disección vertebral como causa del síndrome de enclaustramiento y opciones terapéuticas con fibrinólisis intraarterial durante la fase aguda. Rev Neurol 2004;38(12):1139–41.

252. Licht PB, Christensen HW, Hoilund-Carlsen PF. Vertebral artery volume flow in human beings. J Manipulative Physiol Ther 1999;22(6):363–7.

253. Westaway MD, Stratford P, Symons B. False-negative extension/rotation pre-manipulative screening test on a patient with an atretic and hypoplastic vertebral artery. Man Ther 2003;8(2):120–7.

254. Bolton PS, Stick PE, Lord RSA. Failure of clinical tests to predict cerebral ischemia before neck manipulation. J Manipu-lative Physiol Ther 1989;12(4):304–7.

255. Thiel H, Rix G. Is it time to stop functional pre-manipulative testing of the cervical spine? Man Ther 2005;10:154–8.

256. Refshauge KM, Parry S, Shirley D, et al. Professional responsi-bility in relation to cervical spine manipulation. Aust J Physi-other 2002;48:171–9.

257. APA. Clinical guidelines for assessing vertebrobasilar insuffi-cency in the management of cervical spine disorders. <www

.physiotherapy.asn.au>: Australian Physiotherapy Association; 2006.

258. Rushton A, Rivett D, Carlesso L, et al. International framework for examining of the cervical region for cervical arterial dysfunction prior to orthopaedic manual therapy intervention. Man Ther 2014;19(3):222–8.

259. Richter RR, Reinking MF. Evidence in practice. How does evidence on the diagnostic accuracy of the vertebral artery test influence teaching of the test in a professional physical therapist education program? Phys Ther 2005;85(6):589–99.

260. Barker S, Kesson J, Turner G, et al. Guidance for pre-manipulative testing of the cervical spine. Man Ther 2000;5(1):37–40.

261. Carey P. A suggested protocol for the examination and treatment of the cervical spine: managing the risk. J Can Chiropr Assoc 1995;39(1):35–40.

262. Canadian Chiropractic Association, Canadian Federation of Chiropractic Regulatory Boards, Clinical Practice Guidelines Development Initiative, et al. Chiropractic clinical practice guideline: evidence-based treatment of adult neck pain not due to whiplash. J Can Chiropr Assoc 2005;49(3):158–209.

263. Gross AR, Kay TM, Kennedy C, et al. Clinical practice guideline on the use of manipulation or mobilization in the treatment of adults with mechanical neck disorders. Man Ther 2002; 7(4):193–205.

264. Dunne J. Pre-manipulative testing: predicting risk or pretending to? Aust J Physiother 2001;47:165.

265. Yacovino DA, Hain TC. Clinical characteristics of cervicogenic-related dizziness and vertigo. Semin Neurol 2013;33(3):244–55.

266. Baloh RW. Differentiating between peripheral and central causes of vertigo. J Neurol Sci 2004;221(1):3.

267. Furman JM, Cass SP. Benign paroxysmal positional vertigo. N Engl J Med 1999;341(21):1590–6.

268. White J. Benign paroxysmal positional vertigo: how to diagnose and quickly treat it. Cleve Clin J Med 2004;71(9):722–8.

269. Dix MR, Hallpike CS. The pathology, symptomatology and diagnosis of certain common disorders of the vestibular system. Proc R Soc Med 1952;45(6):341–54.

270. Meadows J. Diagnóstico diferencial en fisioterapia. Madrid: McGraw-Hill Interamericana; 2000.

271. Hardesty WH, Whitacre WB, Toole JF, et al. Studies on vertebral artery blood flow in man. Surg Gynecol Obstet 1963;116:662–4.

272. Murthy JM, Naidu KV. Aneurysm of the cervical internal carotid artery following chiropractic manipulation. J Neurol Neurosurg Psychiatry 1988;51(9):1237–8.

273. Miller KJ, Sittler MD, Corricelli DM, et al. Combination testing in orthopedic and neurologic physical examination: a proposed model. J Chiropr Med 2007;6(4):163–71.

274. Raskind R, North CM. Vertebral artery injuries following chiropractic cervical spine manipulation – case reports. Angiology 1990;41(6):445–52.

275. Wand B, Heine P, O'Connell N. Should we abandon neck manipulation for mechanical neck pain? Yes. BMJ 2012; 345(7869):e3679.

276. Boline PD, Kassak K, Bronfort G, et al. Spinal manipulation vs. amitriptyline for the treatment of chronic tension-type headaches: a randomized clinical trial. J Manipulative Physiol Ther 1995;18(3):148–54.

277. Bronfort G, Evans R, Nelson B, et al. A randomized clinical trial of exercise and spinal manipulation for patients with chronic neck pain. Spine 2001;26(7):788–97.

278. Gross A, Miller J, D'Sylva J, et al. Manipulation or mobilisation for neck pain: a Cochrane Review. Man Ther 2010;15(4): 315–33.

279. Hurwitz EL, Morgenstern H, Harber P, et al. A randomized trial of chiropractic manipulation and mobilization for patients with neck pain: clinical outcomes from the UCLA neck-pain study. Am J Public Health 2002;92(10): 1634–41.

280. Jull G. Use of high and low velocity cervical manipulative therapy procedures by Australian manipulative physiotherapists. Aust J Physiother 2002;48(3):189–93.

281. Nilsson N. A randomized controlled trial of the effect of spinal manipulation in the treatment of cervicogenic headache. J Manipulative Physiol Ther 1995;18(7):435–40.

282. Grant T, Niere K. Techniques used by manipulative physiotherapists in the management of headaches. Aust J Physiother 2000;46(3):215–22.

283. Puentedura E, March J, Anders J, et al. Safety of cervical spine manipulation: are adverse events preventable and are manipulations being performed appropriately? A review of 134 case reports. J Manipulative Physiol Ther 2012;20(2):66–74.

284. Stevinson C, Honan W, Cooke B, et al. Neurological complications of cervical spine manipulation. J R Soc Med 2001; 94(3):107–10.

285. Vautravers P, Maigne JY. Cervical spine manipulation and the precautionary principle. Joint Bone Spine 2000;67(4): 272–6.

286. Ellrodt A. Assessing the risks of cervical manipulation for neck pain. CMAJ 2002;166(9):1134–5.

287. Graumlich JF. Preventing gastrointestinal complications of NSAIDs. Risk factors, recent advances, and latest strategies. Postgrad Med 2001;109(5):117–20, 123–8.

288. Dabbs V, Lauretti WJ. A risk assessment of cervical manipulation vs. NSAIDs for the treatment of neck pain. J Manipulative Physiol Ther 1995;18(8):530–6.

289. Carey P. A Report on the occurrence of cerebral vascular accidents in chiropractic practice. J Can Chiropr Assoc 1993;57(2): 104–6.

290. Tramer MR, Moore RA, Reynolds DJ, et al. Quantitative estimation of rare adverse events which follow a biological progression: a new model applied to chronic NSAID use. Pain 2000;85(1–2):169–82.

291. Schneider G. Vertebral artery complications following gentle cervical treatments. (Comment on Mann T and Refshauge KM, Aust J Physiother 47:255-66.) Aust J Physiother 2002; 48(2):151.

292. Cyriax J, Cyriax P. Cyriax's illustrated manual of orthopaedic medicine. 2nd ed. London: Butterworth Heinemann; 2000.

293. Symons B, Bruce S, Walter H. Cervical artery dissection: a biomechanical perspective. J Can Chiropr Assoc 2013;57(4): 276.

THE COMPLEX PAIN PATIENT

11

RAFAEL TORRES CUECO

THE PROBLEM OF PAIN

This chapter is intended solely as a brief introduction to a topic, the understanding of which covers multiple aspects as well as the treatment of chronic pain. Addressing this issue is critical for several reasons: it is one of the most common problems faced by health professionals in their daily clinical practice, it has considerable impact at both the individual and socioeconomic levels and, finally, because usual therapeutic approaches offer disappointing results. Despite remarkable development in recent years of new therapeutic tools in the treatment of musculoskeletal disease, chronic pain is becoming a serious health problem in Western countries.

The prevalence of chronic pain is extremely high in industrialized countries. An epidemiological study conducted in 2006 in Europe showed that the prevalence of moderate to severe chronic pain amounted to 19% of the population, seriously affecting the quality of their social and working lives.[1] Among the various types of chronic pain, musculoskeletal pain is the most common and disabling[2] The most prevalent chronic pain conditions are back and neck pain,[2,3] headache[4] and fibromyalgia.[5]

- The prevalence of moderate to severe chronic pain in Europe is 19%.[1]
- Chronic pain has a significant impact on activities of daily living, personal relationships, and mental health.[2]
- Musculoskeletal pain is the most common and the most disabling.[4]
- The most prevalent sites are back and neck,[4,5] headache[6] and fibromyalgia.[7]

- Treatment is very limited, resulting in client dissatisfaction, which can be up to 60%.[13]

Chronic pain is also a social problem due to the high economic and social costs involved, as a result of the increased use of health care services, expenditure on drug treatments and invasive procedures, hours of work lost, and costs associated with compensations. In Europe, data published in 2009 on the impact of pain on employment reveal that musculoskeletal pain is responsible for 49% of absenteeism, 60% of permanent disability, and the costs amount to 240 billion euros.[6] Despite the exponential increase in health expenditure, the prevalence of back and neck pain, for example, in Western societies has continued to increase.[7,8]

A recent study has shown that US health costs arising from the treatment of chronic pain reach US$635 billion, exceeding the total amount of expenses for cancer, diabetes and heart disease.[24] This study also shows the current trend involving an increased use of invasive procedures while physiotherapy and other conservative approaches would be more beneficial for the patient.[9] An important aspect revealed in this study is the discrepancy between current knowledge on pain and its therapy. This study also goes on to note that it will only be possible to reduce the impact of chronic pain through a cultural transformation, which is only achievable through education of health professionals and of society.[9]

Musculoskeletal pain is not only the most prevalent pain but also that which has the highest impact throughout an individual's life. The Global Burden of Disease Study[2] published in 2012 shows that the leading causes of years lived with disability worldwide are low back pain, ranking first, and neck pain fourth.

It would not be an overstatement to say that Western countries are experiencing a real epidemic, despite our better understanding of the neurophysiological mechanisms of pain and better therapeutic tools for its treatment.[10] As David Morris pointed out, 'Today we face the paradox that although biomedical research has greatly expanded our knowledge of the anatomy, physiology and pharmacology of pain, never before, especially with regard to chronic pain, had pain reached its current epidemic proportion.'[11]

The problem, as John Bonica noted, is that the medical system has addressed the diagnosis and treatment of chronic pain in the same manner as acute pain, which has had little effect and in many cases iatrogenic complications.[12] Many chronic pain patients show a pattern of central hyperexcitability plus psychosocial components, which usually explains why the strategies used in acute pain fail in these patients.

CHRONIC PAIN AND THE BIOMEDICAL PARADIGM

Pain has historically been viewed as a clear symptom of disease.[13] At present, however, it is clear that pain can be experienced without any tissue damage.

Failure in the treatment of chronic pain is therefore the result of understanding pain as a sensation necessarily associated with tissue damage. As pointed out by Jacobson and Mariano,[14] the difficulty of treating chronic pain stems mainly from the philosophical and structural principles of biomedicine. From the seventeenth century to the mid-twentieth century, the concept of pain has been derived directly from the Cartesian conception of man. According to Descartes, humans had two components – soul and body – acting as separate entities. In his view the activity of the mind was the result of the activity of the soul. Descartes thought that the perception of pain occurs in a special place where the mind observes the body and interprets its signals. Pain, as a signal coming from the body, is perceived by the mind (Fig. 11-1).

This dualistic concept, which has been dominant in Western countries, has supported the biomedical paradigm of pain. This paradigm has considered pain as a sensory perception generated in the central nervous

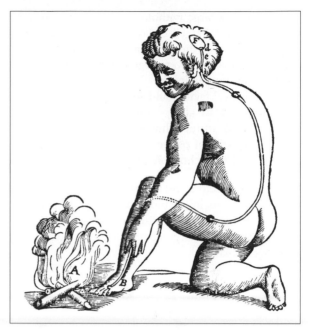

FIGURE 11-1 ■ René Descartes (1596–1650) De L'homme.

system (CNS) as the result of an injury of the peripheral tissues. Therefore, the traditional model of care that has governed for decades is 'organ-based medicine'. The diagnosis requires specific tests that target the affected organ or system, and treatment addresses that particular organ or system. We continue to consider that pain is the direct result of a tissue injury. This means that we continue to address pain mechanistically. In fact, today, both undergraduate and postgraduate training for doctors and physical therapists dedicated to pain is excessively oriented to learning techniques and procedures. Moreover, a patient's treatment depends more on the preferences and affinities of the therapist for a particular technique or 'school' than on the patient's real needs.

According to the biomedical paradigm, which Haldeman[15] called the *classical pathological model*, there is a direct linear correlation between pain and tissue damage. Therefore, greater tissue injury would proportionally imply more severe pain. An appropriate therapeutic intervention on the injured tissue would be sufficient to ease the pain. However, this is only so in cases of severe pain lasting a short time. Paradoxically, we note that there are many patients reporting severe pain with minor injuries, and conversely, patients with a large pathological deterioration with few symptoms[16] (Fig. 11-2). For decades there has been ample evidence of the fact that completely asymptomatic subjects show severe degenerative changes in the cervical and lumbar spine.[17,18]

Psychological factors and social issues, in this biomedical model, are always considered secondary phenomena.[19] This attitude thus leads to the establishment of two categories of patients: those with organic pain and those with psychogenic pain.

Psychological factors and social issues are always secondary factors in the biomedical paradigm. This attitude thus leads to establishing two categories of patients: those with organic pain and those with psychogenic pain.

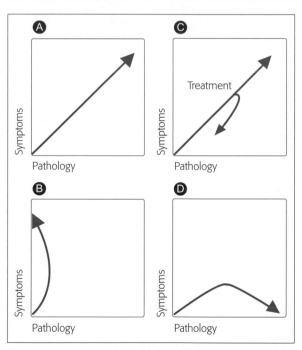

FIGURE 11-2 ■ Paradox of pain. In the biomedical model it is assumed that there is a direct correlation between pain and tissue injury. Therefore, greater tissue damage would be related to a proportionately more severe pain (A). An appropriate therapeutic intervention on injured tissues would be sufficient to eliminate the pain (B). However, paradoxically, what is observed is that there are many patients reporting severe pain with minor injuries (C), and on the other hand, patients with a large pathological deterioration that show few symptoms (D). *Redrawn with permission from Butler D. The sensitive nervous system. Adelaide: Noigroup Publications; 2000.*

The biomedical model represents an important contribution to health, mainly in the treatment of acute illnesses. However, its sole interest in biological factors, although necessary, is insufficient for the treatment of chronic pain. Many patients suffering this type of pain will achieve no improvement even with the most advanced biomedical contributions, and will develop a severe disability. There are, therefore, other variables involved in the experience of pain, especially in patients with chronic pain. These variables are related to CNS neuroplasticity and psychosocial aspects, and are of major importance in constructing painful experiences.[20]

PAIN REVOLUTION

In the last 20 years there has been a genuine revolution in the understanding of pain, leading to a paradigm shift. Significant factors in this change have included progress in the neurobiology of pain and the inclusion of the biopsychosocial paradigm in clinical practice. There has been a shift from a model in which nociception and pain were considered almost as synonymous terms, to a more complex, but more attractive view, wherein pain is interpreted as a response of the brain, and where nociception can play a varying role. As we have often stressed, the problem of pain does not lie primarily in its treatment, but rather, in a poor or inadequate understanding of what pain essentially is. And this means continuing to consider pain as a perception always associated with injury.[21] Today we know that there is no correlation between injury and pain. Many patients develop severe pain with minor injuries, and, on the contrary, other patients with a large pathological deterioration manifest few symptoms[16] (Fig. 11-3).

For decades, there have been attempts to explain the development of a chronic pain from a pathoanatomical perspective, and although this should not be completely ruled out, it is clearly insufficient.[22]

The problem of pain does not lie primarily in its treatment, but rather, in a poor or inadequate understanding of what pain essentially is.

The proposal of the gate control theory by Melzack and Wall[23] was crucial to begin to contemplate pain

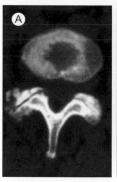
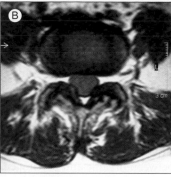

FIGURE 11-3 ■ There are different entities that occur chronically, such as lumbar facet joint degenerative changes. However, most subjects do not develop chronic pain. CT images (A) and MRI (B) of a patient with severe degenerative hypertrophy of lumbar facet joints.

from a multidimensional perspective. Pain could be modulated by substantially varying afferent and efferent mechanisms able to determine the subjective experience of pain in each individual.

A crucial change in the understanding of pain relates to the recognition of the importance of CNS neuroplasticity as a fundamental mechanism in the transition from acute pain to chronic pain[24-27] The development of chronic pain can be associated with profound structural and functional changes in the CNS. It should be noted that there is no necessary correlation between central neuroplastic changes and the pain and disability the patient may develop. Still, in many subjects, the central sensitization is an important aspect which explains the clinical manifestations associated with chronic pain. Central sensitization has been defined by Woolf[25] 'as an amplification of neural signalling within the central nervous system that elicits pain hypersensitivity'.

Central sensitization (CS) involves plastic changes to the neurons of the central nervous system, resulting in reorganization, decreased threshold activation and decommissioning of inhibitory interneurons. CS has been studied widely in different chronic pain conditions such as chronic low back pain,[28-31] widespread musculoskeletal pain,[32] whiplash -associated disorder,[27,33-37] complex regional pain syndrome,[38] chronic pelvic pain,[39-43] fibromyalgia,[28,44-48] chronic fatigue syndrome,[49] epicondylalgia,[50] osteoarthritis[51] and postsurgical pain.[52]

It should be noted that, despite the fact that CS explains many mechanisms in the transition from acute to chronic pain, the role in chronic pain is not yet clear. For instance, a systematic review and meta-analysis published in 2013 about the relationship between quantitative sensory testing (QST) and pain or disability has reported that this association is inconsistent. This review concludes that pain threshold assessment, for example, is a not a good marker of CS and that sensitization does not play a major role in patients' reporting of pain and disability.[53]

The developing of a maladaptive central sensitization involves not only changes associated with the processing of nociceptive information but also motor changes, dysregulation of the neuroendocrine and immune systems and cognitive behavioural factors in response to a perceived threat.[54] The aversive emotional component of pain aims to trigger a stress response that facilitates the fight or flight behaviours. This emotional component implies a state of physiological arousal mediated by the autonomic and neuroendocrine nervous system.[55,56] The magnitude of the emotional component of pain is proportional to its perception as a threat.[57,58] This stress response can also be triggered by a psychological threat.

As mentioned before, the immune system plays an important role in stress response.[59-62] Immune changes, secondary to injury, not only increase the perception of pain[63] but also cause changes in behaviour, mood, motivation and cognition.[63-65] The CNS responds not only in terms of stimulus intensity but also based on the context in which the physiological response occurs.[66] The development of a complex and chronic pain condition, such as chronic whiplash, fibromyalgia, etc., is often associated with a dysfunctional processing in the CNS.[35,67-70] So many chronic pain syndromes can be explained as consecutive to anomalies in the central modulation of pain.[69] Neuroplastic deep changes force us to consider chronic pain differently from acute pain.

One of the advances in the understanding of the central changes associated with chronic pain has been the development of functional neuroimaging techniques.[71-77] Brain imaging technologies can be used to test hypotheses about the CNS mechanisms underlying pain perception and chronification (Fig. 11-4).

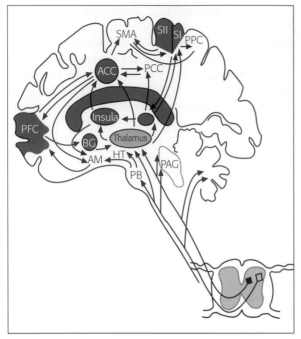

FIGURE 11-4 ■ Subcortical and cortical structures involved in pain processing. ACC, anterior cingulate cortex; AM, amygdala; BG, basal ganglia; HT, hypothalamus; PAG, periaqueductal grey; PB, parabrachial core of the projection; PCC, posterior cingulate cortex; PFC, prefrontal cortex; PPC, posterior parietal complex; SI, primary somatosensory area; SII, secondary somatosensory area; SMA, supplementary motor area. *Modified with permission from Price DD. Psychological and neural mechanisms of the affective dimension of pain. Science 2000;288(5472):1769-72.*

The factors that best explain the transition from acute to chronic pain are two:

- The set of neuroplastic changes that lead to abnormalities in central pain modulation, known as central sensitization.
- The influence of psychosocial factors in establishing such dysfunctional CNS changes.

Our understanding of chronic pain has also undergone a significant change through the development of explanatory models of pain based on psychological and social perspectives.[78] It is evident how different kinds of psychosocial factors play a crucial role in the development of chronic pain.[79]

The biopsychosocial paradigm seeks to integrate all biological, psychological, social and cultural factors, considering that they are all essential in the development, maintenance and exacerbation of pain. The biopsychosocial approach has signified a fundamental change in the consideration of chronic pain. Unlike the reductionism of the classical model, chronic pain and its various manifestations are explained as the interaction between the pathophysiological changes, psychological characteristics and social and cultural factors that affect the patient's perception and response to a situation of distress. From this perspective, the division between organic and psychogenic pain is eliminated.

The biopsychosocial model involves understanding that the patient's clinical presentation, evolution, prognosis and response to treatment does not depend solely on a specific disease or physical dysfunction, but also on their beliefs, behaviours and social context. Pain is a perceptual experience influenced by the individual's unique past history, and the meaning assigned to the experience of pain, including the potential consequences for the future.[80] As stated by Waddell,[81] a patient's demand for medical care depends largely on the patient's interpretation of the symptoms, and learned cultural behaviour patterns associated with pain experience.

Pain is a perceptual experience influenced by the individual's unique past history, and the meaning assigned to the experience of pain, including the potential consequences for the future

---

The biopsychosocial model involves considering the patient's problem within his or her context and perception of the disease, and therefore helps in understanding pain as a multidimensional phenomenon, which, to varying degrees in each patient, biomedical, psychological, cultural and social factors are involved. The adoption of a biopsychosocial approach has caused a change among clinicians and researchers.

The publication by the WHO of the International Classification of Functioning, Disability and Health (WHO 2001) reflects this need for a change in the conceptual framework of health. The therapeutic goal cannot solely consist in eliminating pain, but must also address the patient's resumption of professional, social and recreational activities. The personal and social factors involved, therefore, are particularly relevant in patient assessment as well as the patient's beliefs and behaviours. Pain management should be based both on recent advances in the field of pathophysiology of pain, as well as on the role of the various cognitive, emotional, behavioural and social aspects.[21,82]

PAIN AS A MULTIDIMENSIONAL EXPERIENCE

Pain is defined by the International Association for the Study of Pain (IASP) as 'An unpleasant sensory and emotional experience associated with actual or potential tissue damage, or described in terms of such damage'.[83] This definition specified that although pain may be associated with tissue damage, there may be pain without injury. Also, the emotional component was included as an indivisible part of the pain experience. This definition means understanding pain as an existentially complex subjective experience, covering three dimensions:

1. **Discriminative-Sensory.** Its function is to transmit the painful stimulation and describe its intensity and spatiotemporal characteristics.
2. **Motivational-Affective.** Involves the experience of pain as unpleasant and aversive, qualities that can cause anxiety and impaired emotional responses of the subject as well as escape behaviours.
3. **Evaluative-Cognitive.** The role that thoughts, beliefs, attributions, meaning and value have in the experience of pain. Also the role of attention, anticipation, expectation, catastrophism, memory, etc.

Pain, however, has many other dimensions:

■ **Motor.** Pain is associated with changes in motor activity, such as dysfunctional motor patterns, decreased muscle mass and motor pseudo negligence phenomena.
■ **Multisystemic.** Pain generates multisystem responses involving the sympathetic nervous system, the sympathetic-adrenal system, neuroendocrine and immune system. Thus, many patients with chronic pain can express dysregulation of these systems.
■ **Behavioural.** Pain also has a behavioural function. Examples include the development of the sick role and fear-avoidance behaviours.

■ **Social and Cultural.** Finally, pain is not understood without regard to its social and cultural aspects such as the role of the family, the work environment, different social structures, the concept of welfare society, the role of the medical system and its influence on the media, religious beliefs, etc. (Fig. 11-5).

Pain encompasses the whole individual. Melzack and Wall[80] wrote,

> The psychological evidence strongly supports the view of pain as a perceptual experience whose quality and intensity is influenced by the unique past history of the individual, by the meaning he gives to the pain-producing situation and by his 'state of mind' at the moment. In this way pain becomes a function of the whole individual, including his present thoughts and fears as well as his hopes for the future.

Pain is a result of a combination of biological, psychological and social afferents with the existing neural architecture in the individual.[84] Therefore,

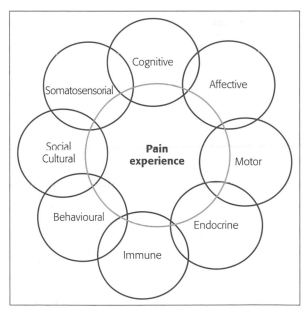

FIGURE 11-5 ■ Pain as a complex subjective experience, covering multiple dimensions.

understanding pain involves addressing its many facets: biomedical, psychological, social and cultural. And it follows that those who devote their efforts to the management of patients with complex pain need to possess transdisciplinary expertise.

One of the problems in the management of chronic pain is derived from the various professional biases. Therefore, in recent decades the need for interprofessional education for all those who care for patients with chronic pain has been stressed in order to improve collaboration and quality of care.[85] The IASP recognized this necessity, and in 2010 created the Special Interest Group in Pain Education (http://www.iasp-pain.org/SIG/Education) and developed the IASP Interprofessional Pain Curriculum Outline (http://www.iasp-pain.org/Education/CurriculumDetail.aspx?ItemNumber=2057) with the aim of enabling shared opportunities for the different professions involved in pain management in order to learn together. Also, recently, the World Confederation for physical Therapy has established a Physical Therapy Pain Network (http://www.wcpt.org/ptp) to facilitate communication and encourage exchange of information and ideas not only between physical therapists but also among all professionals interested in pain. Many interest groups and societies interested in pain in the physiotherapy profession, such as the Spanish Society on Physiotherapy and Pain (SEFID), the Physiotherapy Pain Association UK, Pain Science Division of the Canadian Physiotherapy Association, etc., have been established in a number of countries.

GENERAL CONSIDERATIONS ABOUT PAIN

Pain and its biological function

Pain is more than just an unpleasant sensory experience associated with actual or potential tissue damage, and this is why the IASP definition is insufficient to qualify the biological purpose of pain and its complex dimensions.[86] Pain should no longer be regarded as a symptom, considered as a reflex consequence of a tissue injury or dysfunction. Pain is always a brain response with a clear biological function, critical to prevent injury. Pain has to be unpleasant; this aversive emotional component of pain is

what allows the generation of behavioural protection responses so that the individual avoids stimuli that can potentially trigger the pain. Pain, therefore has an important evolutionary function as it is essential for survival.[87]

Both acute and chronic pains are not a direct reflection of tissue condition. Pain serves to prevent damage, to provide information that damage has been caused, and ultimately to promote the healing process. From a didactic perspective, though not strictly scientific, we could distinguish three types of pain in their biological function:

- An initial pain, Aδ pain, which is characterized by severe disproportionate pain to tissue injury. Its mission is clearly to generate a response of immediate withdrawal to prevent damage.
- A second pain, C pain, which warns that an injury has occurred. Often, once warned, the pain tends to disappear. Both pains are primary pains (Fig. 11-6).
- Finally, a third pain, the secondary pain, which aims to promote healing processes and tissue repair generating behaviours that limit movement or load.

The mission of primary pain would be to avoid injury and give a warning, while secondary pain has a behavioural function, thus promoting tissue healing.

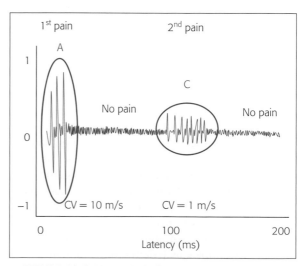

FIGURE 11-6 ■ Drawing of a neurographic recording.

The '3 pains' and their biological function:

- 1st pain – prevent damage
- 2nd pain – a warning signal that an injury has occurred
- 3rd pain – promote healing processes and tissue repair generating behaviours that limit movement or load.

The immune system is very similar to the pain system: it is also a protection system. The immune system and the nervous system must jointly and continually assess and decide whether to activate the protection mechanisms. Therefore, both systems need to learn throughout life about potential new threats requiring a protective response. But, in addition, all senses such as sight, hearing, smell and taste are involved in detecting potential threats to our biological integrity.

Pain can also be classified as adaptive and maladaptive pain. Adaptive pain contributes to survival, preventing injury and promoting healing. Maladaptive pain is the expression of an abnormal processing in the nervous system. Examples of adaptive pain are nociceptive and inflammatory pain, whereas maladaptive examples include neuropathic are complex pain.

Pain depends on the degree of excitability of the central nervous system at the time the stimulus occurs

The activity of the nociceptive system and pain perception depend not only on the stimulus but also on the sensitivity of the nervous system at each given time. Many phenomena are associated with increased or decreased central excitability. Examples include changes in the perception of olfactory, gustatory or auditory stimuli that some women experience during the hormonal cycle. Sensory perception is strongly influenced by the activity of the sympathetic-neural, neuroendocrine and immune systems.

From a therapeutic point of view, it is crucial to consider the excitability of the patient's nervous system at the moment in which the pain or the stimulus that triggers the pain is produced. If the patient has a high central hyperexcitability, all excessively vigorous therapeutic techniques or those which cause pain are usually contraindicated. As noted by Nijs and Van Houdenhove[88] 'herapists unaware of, or ignoring the processes involved in the development and maintenance of chronic pain (....), may cause more harm than benefit to the patient by triggering or sustaining central sensitization'.

In addition, central excitability is dependent on the emotional situation and cognitive elaborations of the individual at the time. The patient's interpretation and attribution about pain determines their degree of perception. Also, the individual's expectations about the treatment applied are crucial to its outcome, activating the descending pain-controlling pathways.

Pain does not require nociception

Pain is always an output of the brain: therefore, pain and nociception are not synonymous terms. Nociception may be the mechanism involved in many patients with pain, but many others can suffer a severe and disabling pain with no evident nociceptive mechanism.

Nociception refers to biological phenomena triggered by noxious stimuli that act in the body and their transmission from the periphery to the CNS before the individual becomes consciously aware (Fig. 11-7). Nociception can cause brain responses that are painless, while not reaching consciousness.[89] The CNS is not a pain receptor, but it builds the painful experience.[58] Indeed, nociception does not necessarily lead to perception of pain and it can be present without any nociceptive input. Osborn and Derbyshire[90] have shown in a functional magnetic resonance imaging (fMRI) study that simply observing someone else in pain produces an actual noxious somatic experience as well as an emotional one. These experiences were correlated with an activation of the emotional and sensory brain regions associated with pain. A hypnotic induction may cause the activation of the brain regions belonging to a pain network equivalent to that experimentally produced with nociceptive stimulation.[91,92]

The correlation between pain and injury can vary considerably from one individual to another or there may even be no correlation at all. Although this view is widely recognized by experts in pain research and treatment, it is not often shared by professionals treating the patient. They still consider pain as a direct reflex of tissue injury and, consequently, there remains a significant gap between our current understanding of chronic pain and therapeutic approaches that often patients undergo.[93]

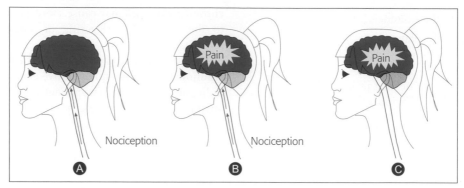

FIGURE 11-7 ■ Nociception does not necessarily result in the perception of pain (A). Pain is usually the result of the activation of nociceptors (B), but there may be pain without nociception (C).

- Nociception is the result of biological phenomena triggered by the action of noxious stimuli on the organism and its transmission from the periphery to the CNS before that information becomes conscious.
- Pain is the perception of the individual involving not only sensory aspects but also cognitive and affective aspect.
- There may be nociception without pain and pain without nociception.

Pain as a product of consciousness

Pain experience, as any other human experiences, is not a sensation, but is a phenomenon of consciousness, an interpretation of the nociceptive by the individual.

Consciousness is an emergent property of the brain as the result of communication between multiple brain networks operating dynamically. The brain thus builds an internal representation of reality (individual experience of pain) from the sensory information, contextual cues that interact at the time, cognitive processing and the stored memory.

In many cases of chronic pain, the brain's pain generation is often not related to any nociceptive input.

Pain can be considered as a projection of the brain to consciousness, like a film projected on a screen and observed by the subject. Understanding pain as a perception means that its experience is common to any other perception. Perception does not occur automatically with a stimulus, whether auditory, olfactory and nociceptive. In fact, our brain is constantly

cancelling perceptions when these are not new or relevant or when performing activities that involve the activation of the *brain default mode network*, such as evoking memories, planning activities or future situations, mind wandering, internal mentation, etc. The real possibility of modulating perception is an aspect of considerable interest in the management of chronic pain.

Pain as complex reasoning

Pain is always the result of a complex and unconscious reasoning. It is the result of the analysis of both external and interoceptive sensory stimuli, as well as CNS processes that are processed simultaneously.

The result of this complex reasoning, which is pain, is determined by the previous experiences of the individual, the anticipation of future consequences, family and social learning, and the context in which the stimulus occurs.[94] All these aspects refer to a meaning that is based on the perception of a threat to the biological integrity of the individual. As Ramachandran said: Pain is an opinion on the organism's state of health rather than a mere reflective response to an injury.[95] In the same way that an opinion is a result of information gained from childhood in the family, in our social and cultural context and contrasted with our own experience, so also is pain.

Pain always refers to meaning

Pain is an interpretation not only of nociceptive input but also of contextual clues and especially their significance.[96,97] The patient's attribution about the meaning of symptoms, particularly their perception as a sign of a serious problem, their beliefs about the potential impact on their lives and worries about the future, are all critical in pain perception.[98,99]

Patients' beliefs about pain determine their emotional and behavioural responses, disability and response to treatment.[100,101] An increased perception of the threatening meaning of pain is expressed in increased catastrophism, hypervigilance and anxiety, which in turn increases the pain intensity.[96,102,103]

Patients' attributions about the meaning of symptoms, their beliefs about the potential impact on their lives and worries about the future, are all critical in pain perception.

The meaning is determined by cognitions, emotions, previous experiences, memory and learning of the individual, by the social environment, and by cultural constructions. Religious conceptions and the role of experts such as health care professionals are also involved in developing the meaning of the painful experience. Health care professionals can become the

'real culprits' in the development of chronic pain when providing threatening interpretations to the patient's clinical condition. Understanding how all these complex issues are able to change the experience of pain is absolutely essential in the treatment of patients with chronic pain.

The crucial importance of meaning in the patient's perception of pain and disability justifies the use of strategies that modify its threatening meaning (Fig. 11-8). This is the central component of education in the biology of pain proposed by Moseley and Butler,[104] a change in the conceptualization of pain as an indicator of tissue damage to its consideration as a need for protection of body tissues.[105]

Pain: attention, salience and relevance

Pain as a sign of a real or potential threat demands attention. Attention to a nociceptive stimulus is one of the most studied aspects, based on its ability to increase pain severity.[106] Attention operates by biasing the processing and by selecting the most appropriate information. Distracting a subject's attention from a nociceptive stimulus not only decreases the subjective

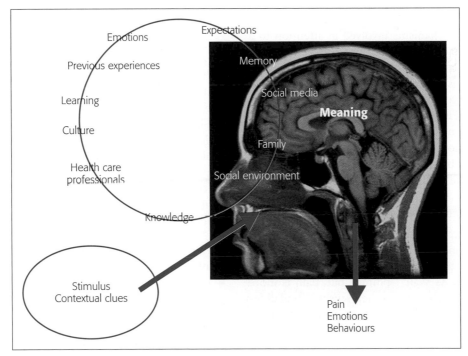

FIGURE 11-8 ■ Pain always refers to meaning.

perception of pain but also entails a decrease in the magnitude of evoked brain responses.[107–109]

Pain requires bottom-up, top-down mechanisms, or both at the same time, to direct attention. Bottom-up mechanisms are directly related to the salience of the stimulus, while top-down mechanisms relate to its relevance. Salience is not dependent on voluntary control, and is determined by the intensity of the stimulus and its novelty. Salience implies that the ability of a nociceptive stimulus to attract attention not only depends on its intensity but also on competition with other stimuli that occur at that time.[86,110] The salience of a stimulus derives therefore from its ability to draw attention to it. It is also dependent on previous experience and its contrast with the subject's expectations. Salience plays a critical role by prioritizing the processing of those stimuli against which there is a need to develop an appropriate behaviour, which in the case of pain corresponds to a motor or behavioural action to a threat against physical integrity.

- Pain as a sign of a real or potential threat demands attention.
- Pain directs attention by bottom-up (salience) and top-down (relevance) mechanisms.

Top-down mechanisms involved in attention to a stimulus are determined by their relevance. The relevance of the stimulus is specific to each individual – their previous experiences – and is dependent on emotional and cognitive elaborations of their own personal history (Fig. 11-9). The relevance of pain therefore depends on very different aspects. For example, the interpretation that pain is a sign of a serious or potentially disabling disease, competing explanations a patient receives from health care professionals, etc.

Pain as an action-targeted response

Pain is a coherent response directed to action. Pain only appears once the decision that this response is appropriate to the biological needs of the individual has been taken. As Wall[111] pointed out, pain is more like thirst or hunger than other sensory modalities such as hearing or sight. Therefore, pain is produced by the brain when it deems necessary to prevent damage or avoid further damage, whether real or potential. It is the meaning of the nociceptive input or

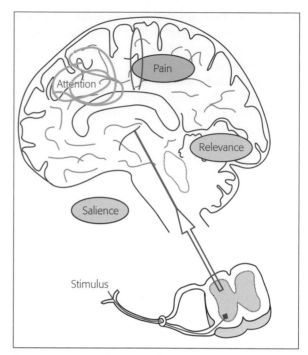

FIGURE 11-9 ■ Pain requires bottom-up (salience) and top-down mechanisms (relevance) to direct attention.

of the context which is capable of generating a pain response or not, at a given time.

In addition, every experience of pain is associated with behavioural responses that are specific to each individual based on what is considered appropriate at that particular time.[112] All dimensions of pain, cognitive, emotional, motor, behavioural, etc., are to promote the individual's survival.[113] In some cases, an amplification of pain will be necessary to prevent damage or avoid further damage. In other cases, intense activation of descending noradrenergic modulatory systems is required to allow the fight or flight response, or in contexts where damage is unavoidable, serotonergic modulator mechanisms will be activated.

- Pain as a sign of a real or potential threat demands attention.
- Pain directs attention by bottom-up (salience) and top-down (relevance) mechanisms.

Pain as a response to threat

Pain as a response to a threat has already been noted by Sanders[114] and by Price.[115] For Sanders,[114] pain is a sensory and emotional experience of discomfort, typically associated with a threat of injury. Price[115] defines pain as a somatic perception consisting of a body sensation similar to those reported for tissue injury, the experience of a threat, and discomfort or a negative emotion based on the perception of threat. As noted by Moseley, pain is characterized by the 'simplicity of its modus operandi: the body is in danger and an action is required'.[116] Pain is a biologically consistent conclusion to the perception of a real or potential threat that requires an adapted behavioural response. Pain therefore is produced by the brain when it perceives a danger to the individual and an action is required to prevent it.[116] All dimensions of pain are directed towards this goal. Pain is also expressed in behaviour, determined by many contextual, social and cultural aspects.

Pain is a biologically consistent conclusion to the perception of a real or potential threat that requires an adapted behavioural response.

Pain requires a somatic and spatial framework

Pain is felt in the body and in a specific physical space, since its aim is to identify and respond to potentially threatening stimuli. Hence pain requires a somatic representation and that of the peripersonal space around the body.[117] These aspects and the possible brain areas involved in somatic and peripersonal space representation have been reviewed by various authors. (For a review, see Legrain et al.[118] and Moseley et al.[119]) It is the concept of a representation framework including not only the 'virtual body' but also the body's near reference space.[117] Without these brain representations the individual is unable to bodily and spatially recognize where the aggression occurs or may occur. Without this representation the subject is also unable to select the most appropriate motor response against an aggression. Pain therefore requires the activation of those brain areas that have a somatotopic organization, such as the ventral posterior nucleus of the thalamus, S1, S2, portions of the insula and the posterior parietal cortex. These somatotopic and peripersonal space representations do not occur in isolation, but are linked to motor, homeostatic and emotional representations.[119]

Pain may be a maladaptive response

Pain has not only a protective function. Many patients suffer from complex pain not secondary to tissue or nervous system injury that results in the individual's serious deterioration. Pain, as emphasized, can be an entirely dysfunctional maladaptive brain response, which instead of helping to maintain the integrity of the individual determines his or her deterioration. Right now it is essential to properly identify when pain is not associated with a significant nociceptive source. Subsequently, those aspects that can help identify complex pain will be addressed. Much of the iatrogenicity stems from the inability of health care professionals to identify this complex and maladaptive pain.

Pain is associated with emotions

Emotions are central to human experience and are decisively involved in consciousness. As noted by Chapman,[55] emotion is often confused with feelings. Emotions are primarily physiological reactions and are only secondarily subjective. Emotions have an objective component, such as the activation of the autonomic nervous system and hormonal system. The subjective aspects of emotions are feelings and are a phenomena of consciousness.[56] The role of emotions is to generate relevant information (emotional valence) for selecting among several behaviours. Emotion represents within awareness the biological significance or meaning that a stimulus acquires at a given time.

Pain-related emotions represent within awareness the biological significance or meaning that a stimulus acquires at a given time.

Pain, to be biologically useful, needs to be aversive, unpleasant and determine an avoidance response. However, these psychological and behavioural responses that are adaptive in acute pain may become maladaptive when the injury is in a clear recovery phase or when there is no material injury. As clinicians, it is critical to recognize when these responses become maladaptive and can lead to a complex pain.

Chronic pain is associated with anxiety, depression and low self-efficacy. Also, patients with anxiety and depression experience more pain and are more likely to develop chronic pain.[120] Patients with chronic pain exhibit negative and pessimistic thoughts, often obsessively, both about pain and their life. Emotions and negative thoughts, therefore, play a crucial role in both the perception of pain and the development of avoidance behaviours, and finally on patient's disability. From a therapeutic point of view it is essential to assess these psychological aspects as they may determine the therapeutic response.

Pain and body perception

Chronic pain may cause significant cortical neuroplastic changes.[121] Cortical reorganization in patients with chronic pain can distort body perceptions. In fact, the amount of cortical reorganization appears to correlate with pain severity and chronicity.[122] The role of distorted body perception in persistent pain has been a new and interesting area of research in the last few years.[121,123,124] This research has led to emerging treatment approaches to improve this distorted body perception and to restore normal cortical reorganization. To achieve this goal different strategies are being developed such as manipulating the flow of sensory inputs, activation of the areas of sensory and motor cortical representation from gradual exposure programmes, training of sensory skills, mirror therapy, laterality recognition, two points discrimination, graded motor imagery, etc.[125] The aim is to act on the cortical representation of the body area where the subject perceives pain. In different clinical conditions the recovery of function and improvement in pain requires the normalization of sensory and motor cortical representations.

Pain is not just pain

Pain does not only include sensory aspects, but is always associated with emotional, motor, behavioural and multisystem responses such as endocrine and immune responses. In fact, pain in itself is an output of the CNS. All these multisystem responses, including the behavioural response, are highly variable and depend on what the subject considers appropriate or not to a particular situation.

- Pain does not only include sensory aspects, but is always associated to emotional, motor, behavioural and multisystem responses such as endocrine and immune responses.

- Chronic pain is associated with significant comorbidity.

Considering pain as a multisystem response is important because chronic pain is associated with significant comorbidity. Many patients with musculoskeletal pain also suffer from other chronic conditions such as headache, irritable bowel syndrome, painful bladder syndrome and chronic pelvic pain, in addition to such psychological problems as depression, low mood and anxiety.

Pain and cognitive functions

Chronic pain can determine deleterious effects on cognitive processes.[120,126] These processes include attention, learning and memory, psychomotor ability and executive function. In turn, cognitive processes can modulate pain perception. This alteration in cognitive functions aggravates the patient's clinical condition and can be a significant barrier to interventions involving cognitive re-elaboration of the pain experience. An interesting area of study is the analysis of the correlations between chronic pain, cognitive dysfunctions and altered brain activity and brain neural networks connectivity.[127,128]

Pain as memory

The aversive nature of pain promotes learning. It is critical for survival to learn what stimuli can be hazardous to biological integrity. Individuals from infancy accumulate nociceptive experiences which in the future will allow them to develop more consistent and appropriate responses to potentially dangerous stimuli. It is essential that the pain system, like other protection systems such as the immune system, continue learning throughout life, as they must constantly evaluate and decide whether to activate the protection mechanisms.

The memory of pain, like other memories, depends directly on the emotional significance of the stimulus. Man, from childhood and throughout life, only stores relevant and meaningful experiences, which have been accompanied by an aversive or hedonistic emotional impact. External or internal aversive stimuli, especially if associated with a negative meaning, can facilitate the acquisition of a painful memory. The activation of various systems such as the immune system and the hypothalamic–pituitary axis, associated with a fear or stress response, promotes memory consolidation. Also, activation of the amygdala, a key component of the limbic system, is able to determine neurogenesis in the hippocampus.[129]

The relationship between memory and learning has been a central point in the research of chronic pain from the early work of Fordyce.[130,131] Currently, many researchers, based on the plastic changes observed in brain circuits, argue that the persistence of pain in the absence of evidential pathology stems from a memory of pain in the CNS.[132–135]

Chronic pain has been defined by Apkarian,[135] 'Chronic pain is a persistence of the memory of pain and/or the inability to extinguish the memory of pain evoked by an initial inciting injury.' Chronic pain would thus be the inability to extinguish aversive pain-related memories.[133] Chronic pain and associated maladaptive changes in body perception, then, would

be associated to learning-related and memory-related plastic changes of the central nervous system.[136]

Chronic pain is a persistence of the memory of pain and/or the inability to extinguish the memory of pain

Generating long-term pain memories can occur by different mechanisms, such as explicit and implicit memory. As noted by Flor,[136] explicit memory corresponds to those processes based on the conscious reproduction of events stored in the memory. Implicit memory would be one that is acquired in a non-conscious manner and includes non-associative learning such as habituation and sensitization phenomena and associative learning, Hebbian learning, classical conditioning, operant conditioning and social learning or modelling (Fig. 11-10). These mechanisms lead to a reorganization of limbic areas, and medial pre-frontal areas of the amygdala and hippocampus. These

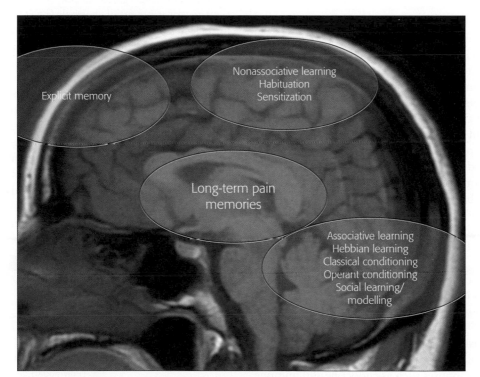

FIGURE 11-10 ■ Generating long-term pain memories can occur by different mechanisms, such as explicit and implicit memory. The explicit memory are processes based on the conscious reproduction of events stored in the memory. Implicit memory includes non-associative learning (habituation and sensitization phenomena) and associative learning (Hebbian learning, classical conditioning, operant conditioning and social learning/modelling).

neuroplastic changes would alter the processing in somatosensory and cognitive areas, which, in turn, would alter the modulation capabilities of both afferent and interoceptive stimuli.[137]

Fear is the main mediator of pain memory.

Fear is the main mediator of pain memory. An experience of pain can be intense enough to generate a memory of pain for life, as well as fear of experiencing pain. Predicting the damage is a crucial aspect of the pain system. Therefore, all those stimuli that are present during the experience of pain can be stored in the memory as predictors of pain. The relationship between fear of pain and learning is a fundamental aspect of Vlaeyen's fear-avoidance model.[138,139]

To consider chronic pain as a memory codified in the CNS has considerable therapeutic implications; it implies that this 'pain memory' can be reversed, so that it is possible to extinguish the chronic pain.

Pain is social

Pain is not only an individual but also a social experience. All pain is expressed in behaviour. Pain is accompanied by external verbal, gestural, behavioural and physical manifestations of pain-related emotion, which are a useful form of communication to obtain social support in situations that pose a risk to survival. Pain and pain behaviours are social responses learned from childhood. Besides, the pain experience is shaped by culture and social environment, which explains why the perception of pain and its expression is clearly determined by culture. It is unacceptable that at present many professionals who treat patients with pain fail to understand the complex familial and sociocultural pain framework.

Pain and pain behaviours are social responses learned from childhood and shaped by culture and social environment.

In conclusion, pain necessarily implies cognitive and affective factors, motor and behavioural responses, multisystem responses such as endocrine and immune responses, and it is significantly influenced by learning, previous experiences and culture. Pain, therefore, is a complex subjective experience influenced by the

characteristics of the nociceptive stimulus, the higher or lower CNS sensitivity, physical and psychological condition of the individual at that time and the context in which it occurs.[140] Pain is an inherently subjective phenomenon that is introduced into the individual's life, entailing associated emotional, behavioural, etc., responses. It is subjected to cognitive assessment, and is dependent on social and cultural coordinates.

CHRONIC PAIN AND CENTRAL SENSITIZATION

Pathogenesis of chronic pain

Nociceptors and pain

Nociceptors are high-threshold sensory receptors of the peripheral somatosensory system capable of transducing and encoding noxious stimuli. Nociception is thus evoked by high-intensity stimulus. Nociceptors transduce intense mechanical, thermal or chemical stimuli via voltage-gated Na channels (NaV) and transient receptor potential channels (i.e. TRPV1; TRPA1) into electrical activity. These primary nociceptors are thinly myelinated Aδ fibres (group III) and unmyelinated C fibres (group IV). Somatic pain is primarily mediated by C fibres, most of them polymodal nociceptors, as these are capable of responding to different thermal, mechanical and chemical stimuli (Table 11-1). The transmission of information from peripheral nociceptors to higher centres undergoes considerable modulation, which depends on many factors: activity of the primary nociceptor itself, descending modulatory pathways, the activity of glial cells and the central nociceptive processing state, all in turn dependent on the activity in multiple brain areas.[141,142] For a

TABLE 11-1	
Afferents groups III and IV	
Aδ (III)	Aδ (N) acute pain (shooting pain) Aδ (T) innocuous cold
C (IV) C Non-nociceptive	C (T) heat C (T) cold
C (IV) C Nociceptive	C (N Cutaneous) burning pain C (Polymodal) deep pain C (MN) C (MT) C (MT) silent

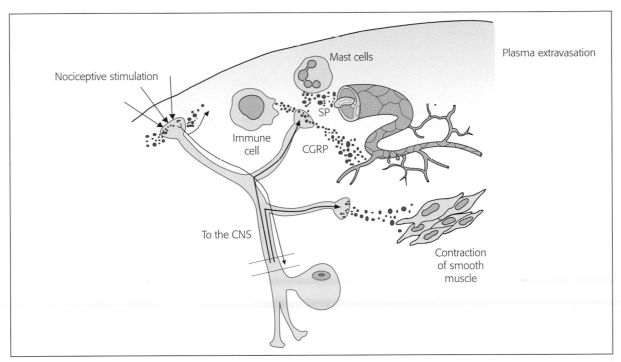

FIGURE 11-11 ■ Stimulation of C fibres triggers an action potential that propagates in an orthodromic manner to the central nervous system and in an antidromic manner to its terminal branches. These antidromic action potentials trigger the release of neuropeptides such as SP, CGRP and neurokinin A. These neuropeptides stimulate, among other cells, mast cells to release histamine, which, in turn, triggers vasodilation and increased capillary permeability, to immune cells. These reactions triggered by the activity of C fibres plus allogenic substances released into the medium due to tissue injury, such as bradykinin and prostaglandins, determine neurogenic inflammation.

review of the mechanisms of peripheral sensitization, see Chapter 5 in Volume 1 (Fig. 11-11).

Second-order neurons and central sensitization

The first synapse of the nociceptive pathway is in the dorsal horn of the spinal cord or in sensory nuclei of the corresponding cranial nerves. The dorsal horn contains six histological layers, referred to as lamina by Rexed, from lamina I (the most superficial) to VI (the deepest).

Second-order nociceptive neurons (SONN) are mainly located in lamina I and II (Fig. 11-12). These neurons are classified into two types: nociceptive-specific (NS) neurons responsive only to noxious stimuli, and wide dynamic range (WDR) neurons, which can respond to low-threshold as well as nociceptive stimuli, in a wide range of intensities.

Lamina I (marginal zone) and lamina II (substantia gelatinosa) receive the afferent axons of the peripheral nociceptors, especially peptidergic C fibres and Aδ fibres. Lamina II contain regulatory interneurons, which modulate the intensity of both noxious and non-noxious stimuli, and act as filters that pass signals from the periphery to the brain (Fig. 11-13). Lamina III and IV contain neurons that respond to non-noxious stimuli from Aß fibres. Therefore, these neurons receive non-noxious stimuli from the periphery, and have small receptive fields, topographically organized. Lamina V neurons are basically wide dynamic range (WDR) neurons receiving information from Aß, Aδ and C non-peptidergic fibres. Finally, lamina VI neurons receive non-noxious mechanical impulses from muscles and joints.

Lamina I spinothalamic tract (STT) neurons largely project to the ventral posterior (VP) nucleus, the posterior part of the ventral medial nucleus (VMpo), the ventral posterior inferior VPI) nucleus and the ventral

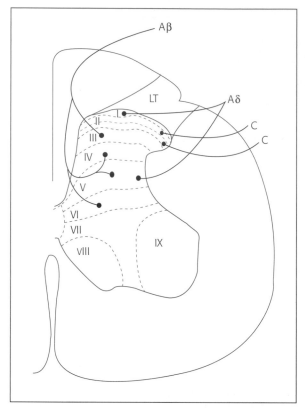

FIGURE 11-12 ■ Rexed laminae. Diagram of the projection of afferent fibres in the dorsal horn. Nociceptive Aδ and C fibres synapse with second-order nociceptive neurons primarily in laminae I and II. Laminae III and IV contain neurons that respond to non-noxious stimuli from Aß fibres. Lamina V neurons are basically WDR neurons that receive information from Aß, Aδ and C fibres. Finally, neurons in lamina VI receive non-noxious mechanical impulses from muscles and joints.

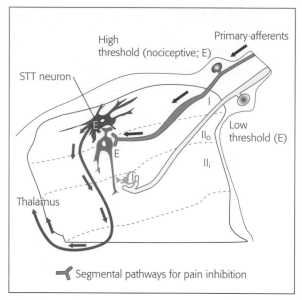

FIGURE 11-13 ■ Lamina II (substantia gelatinosa) contain regulatory interneurons, which modulate the intensity of both noxious and non-noxious stimuli, and act as filters that pass signals from the periphery to the brain. E, excitatory; In, inhibitory; STT, spinothalamic tract.

caudal division of the medial dorsal nucleus (MDvc). Lamina V STT axons terminate in VP, VPI, ventral lateral nucleus and intralaminar nuclei.

Most of the lamina I SONN are nociceptive-specific. These neurons also receive small-amplitude synaptic inputs from low-threshold afferents and nociceptive inputs from outside their receptive fields; however, under normal conditions these inputs do not determine depolarization of nociceptive-specific neurons. However, the sensitization of these neurons can determine the recruitment of these subthreshold inputs with profound changes in receptive field threshold and spatial and temporal properties.[24]

WDR neurons respond gradually, first to low-intensity non-noxious stimuli, which become noxious when the intensity increases. WDR neurons project to the brainstem and parts of the thalamus and upper centres. They receive type C, Aδ and Aß fibres, often originating from deep visceral and somatic structures (Table 11-2).

SONN in the dorsal horn are activated by the neurotransmitter release by first-order afferents. The main neurotransmitters in this level are glutamate, which binds to AMPA and NMDA receptors, and substance P (SP) that binds to the neurokinin-1 (NK 1) G-protein-coupled receptor and brain-derived neurotrophic factor (BDNF) to the tyrosine kinase receptor.

Glutamate is the main neurotransmitter of primary afferents in the dorsal horn, both for nociceptors and non-nociceptors; it acts upon receptors for AMPA glutamate (Na^+), and produces fast synaptic potentials in dorsal horn neurons. Unmyelinated peptidergic nociceptors also release SP and calcitonin gene-related peptide (CGRP). Glutamate and other neurotransmitters, such as SP, have different effects on postsynaptic neurons. Glutamate acts only in the synapse, and its

		TABLE 11-2	
	Rexed lamina, first- and second-order neurons and functions		
Lamina	**Input**	**Second-order neuron**	**Function**
I	C Aδ	NS	Pain
II	C Aδ Non-nociceptive afferents	Excitatory interneurons Inhibitory interneurons	Modulation of afferent signalling
III + IV	Aβ	Small receptive field receptors	Tactile stimulus transmission
V	C Aδ Aβ	WDR	Pain, temperature, tactile stimulus

recapture in the synapse by the glial cells is rapid and highly effective.

Neuropeptides have a different role, determining the amplification and prolongation of the effect of glutamate. Neuropeptides have no recapture mechanisms and have a great dissemination ability, which can exert a powerful influence on many postsynaptic dorsal horn neurons, exerting their effect remotely. The increased excitability of the dorsal horn and diffuse pain location in many clinical situations is partly due to non-recapture of neurotransmitters and an increase in the release of neuropeptides. SP causes a long-lasting membrane depolarization and contributes to the temporal summation of C-fibre–evoked synaptic potentials, and contributes to central sensitization.[24] CGRP contributes to central sensitization through postsynaptic CGRP1 receptors, which activate protein kinase C (PKC) and protein kinase A (PKA), also enhancing the release of BDNF, involved in the development of central sensitization.[24] Raised levels of these peptides contributes to increased excitability of dorsal horn neurons as well as the widespread nature of many chronic pain entities.[143]

Central sensitization and chronic pain

Considerable progress in recent decades has led to the recognition of the importance of neuroplastic changes occurring in the CNS, involved in pain amplification and in the transition from acute to chronic pain.[47,67,69,144,145] Central sensitization has shifted the pain paradigm from tissues to the central nervous system plasticity. Pain is not merely a consequence of peripheral nociceptor activity, but it is also a dynamic reflection of the state of excitability and plasticity of the CNS. The basic assumption is that nociceptive information in the spinal cord induces changes, in the long term, at the dorsal horn synapses, similar to a learning process. Second-order neurons thus increase their excitability and express amplified responses, both to painful and to normal stimuli.[145] Central sensitization maintains the activity of nociceptive neurons even after the healing of the peripheral lesion without therefore a nociceptive stimulus. Thus, a subject, without significant tissue damage and, hence, with few findings on physical examination, can suffer severe and chronic pain. Central sensitization is not only involved in the transition from acute to chronic pain but also it[25,36,67,69,145–148] can determine treatment outcomes.[33,149] Accordingly, it is crucial to identify the contribution of central sensitization in a patient's clinical condition.

Pain is not merely a consequence of peripheral nociceptor activity, but it is also a dynamic reflection of the state of excitability and plasticity of the central nervous system.

Central sensitization at spinal level

SONN) can modify their activity as a result of neuroplastic changes, which initially being transient functional changes, may become stable morphological changes. Central sensitization has attracted much interest in recent years, as it explains the transition from acute to chronic pain.

Some of these changes at the spinal level include long-term potentiation and 'wind-up'. These phenomena mean that SONN, after intense or persistent stimulation of C fibres, suffer lasting functional changes, amplifying their activity, which is maintained without the need of stimuli from peripheral tissues.[150,151] The 'wind-up' phenomenon occurs as a result of the action of glutamate on the N-methyl-D-aspartate (NMDA) ion channels (Fig. 11-14). These NMDA ion channels do not normally participate in the transmission of pain; however, a sustained release of glutamate causes

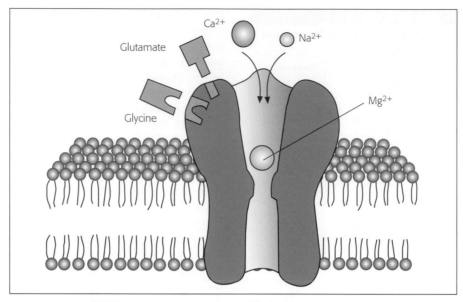

FIGURE 11-14 ■ NMDA receptor, blocked by a magnesium ion.

an alteration in the inner operation of the WDR second-order neuron and leads to the opening of these receptors.[144,152–154]

The process develops in the following manner: when glutamate is released by primary afferents in the synapse, it binds to SONN. This triggers the depolarization by sodium influx into the cell. The NMDA receptor is normally blocked with a magnesium ion, so the glutamate is unable to open the ion channel. However, continuous depolarization, leads to the elimination of the magnesium in the NMDA receptors, allowing calcium into the cytoplasm. Ca^{2+} ions are second messengers that trigger a multitude of intracellular enzymes. The increase in intracellular Ca^{2+} is one of the main triggers initiating activity-dependent central sensitization.

One of its many effects is the phosphorylation of ion channels present in the postsynaptic membrane. Phosphorylation determines that the receptor remains open for longer, preventing the magnesium from reclosing the channel. Long-term gene expression in the nucleus of the neuron is modified, leading to a synthesis of new ion channels (Fig. 11-15). The increase in intracellular Ca^{2+} concentration increases the production of nitric oxide (NO). NO, besides stimulating adjacent neurons, is capable of activating glial cells of

the immune system, increasing the synthesis of cytokines which, in turn, favours central sensitization. The neuron thus sensitized becomes hyperexcitable both to painful and non-painful stimuli. Central sensitization has many other effects: besides the secondary hyperalgesia and allodynia, it can cause an increase in spontaneous activity and an expansion of the receptive fields, which causes pain spreading beyond the edges of the corresponding spinal segment.[67,152,155]

Nociceptor afferents innervating muscles or joints produce a longer-lasting central sensitization than those that innervate skin.[156] The transition from acute to chronic pain at the spinal level includes morphological changes in the circuits of the dorsal horn, such as the generation of new synapsis.[157] Such changes that occur in lamina I and V neurons have been demonstrated in other parts of the CNS such as the amygdala[158] and anterior cingulate cortex (ACC).[159]

A phenomenon considered to favour the formation of a situation of chronic pain is the excitotoxicity neuronal hyperexcitation or neurodegeneration in the dorsal horn.[160] This implies that abnormal primary afferent activity increases glutamate levels simultaneously releasing large amounts of SP and other neuropeptides. Thus, excessive activity of NMDA receptors increases the Ca^{2+} levels in the dorsal horn neurons,

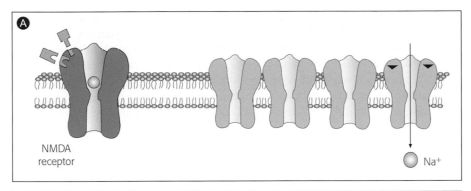

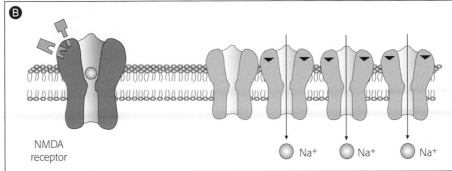

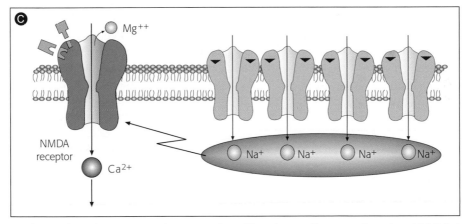

FIGURE 11-15 ■ The wind-up phenomenon. Glutamate released by primary afferents and continued NNSO depolarization (A and B), leads to the elimination of the magnesium-blocking NMDA receptors, allowing Ca^{2+} into the cytoplasm (C). Ca^{2+} ions trigger phosphorylation of ion channels, which determines that, on the one hand, the receptor remains open for longer and, secondly, that new ion channels are synthesized.

going beyond the capacity of the mitochondria, which determines apoptosis of GABA interneurons. As a result of this process the dorsal horn is devoid of inhibitory interneurons, which triggers chronic hyperactivity and disinhibition of nociceptive neurons

Central sensitization can also determine the conversion of nociceptive-specific neurons to wide-dynamic neurons that now respond to both innocuous and noxious stimuli and the expansion of the dorsal horn receptive fields.[24,161]

In the last decade, research has led to the increased recognition of the importance of glial cells (such as microglia and astrocytes) in central sensitization phenomena, playing a key role in the maintenance of persistent pain.[162–164] Glial cells are actively involved in the integration of neural information, they modulate synaptic activity and communicate in different ways with neurons.

A peripheral injury and the subsequent release of neuropeptides from the presynaptic terminals of neurons, such as CGRP, SP and glutamate, can determine 'glial activation'. Activated glial cells produce proinflammatory cytokines (TNF-α, IL-1, IL-6) and brain-derived neurotrophic factor that further increase the neuronal excitability[165] (Fig. 11-16). It has also been shown that TNF-α and IL-1β can directly modulate spinal cord synaptic transmission to induce central sensitization and enhance pain conditions.[166] Such glial activation is believed to play an essential role in the pathogenesis of chronic pain.[167–171] Glial cell activation might also be involved in the phenomenon of pain sensation on the contralateral side (i.e. mirror image pain).[172] Likewise, an increase in brain glial activation in chronic pain patients has been evidenced recently.[173]

Different neuroplastic spinal level changes lead to central sensitization:

- permanent change of the sensitivity of the second-order neurons WDR and NS

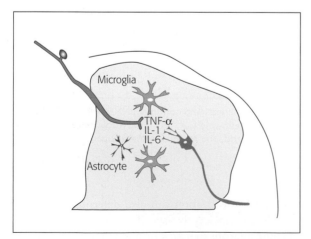

FIGURE 11-16 ■ Glial activation. Activated glial cells produce proinflammatory cytokines (TNF-α, IL-1, IL-6) and brain-derived neurotrophic factor that further increase the neuronal excitability.

- altered levels of neurotransmitters
- creation of new synapses
- expansion of the receptive fields of neurons in the dorsal horn: referred pain
- apoptosis of inhibitory neurons
- glial activation at spinal level
- alteration of descending modulation
- increase in brain glial activation.

In conclusion, sensitization of the nociceptive system, reducing the activation thresholds of the nociceptive system, amplifies the protection of the individual responses. Peripheral sensitization implies reduced activation thresholds of peripheral nociceptors after exposure to inflammatory mediators. It contributes to an increase in the excitability of the nociceptive system but, unlike central sensitization, it is only expressed at the site of the tissue injury (primary hyperalgesia). Central sensitization is therefore of an adaptive response which allows increased sensitivity (secondary hyperalgesia) to stimuli which are potentially indicative of injury and provided the state of hypersensitivity returns to its baseline status once the tissue has healed. However, sensitization may be maladaptive when it is perpetuated after the nociceptive input has disappeared. As stated by Woolf[25] 'Pain could in these circumstances become the equivalent of an illusory perception, a sensation that has the exact quality of that evoked by a real noxious stimulus but which occurs in the absence of such an injurious stimulus'.

- Central sensitization as an adaptive response: increased sensitivity (secondary hyperalgesia) to stimuli which are potentially indicative of injury and provided the state of hypersensitivity returns to its baseline status once the tissue has healed.
- Central sensitization as a maladaptive response: when it is perpetuated after the nociceptive input has disappeared.

Clinical chronic pain is not simply the consequence of the sustained activation of the 'pain system' by a particular peripheral input due to a specific injury, but it also reflects a state of altered excitability of the central nervous system.[25] Any pain expressed having a longer duration, greater severity or a greater distribution than those justified by a nociceptive input or occurring after stimulation of low threshold Aβ fibres suggests a central amplification phenomenon due to increased excitation or reduced inhibition.[25]

Nociceptive pathways

Nociceptive information ascends to the thalamus in the contralateral spinothalamic tract (STT) and to the medulla and brainstem via spinoreticular and spinomesencephalic tracts. Other tracts, such as the spinolimbic tracts, do not project to the thalamus but to the amygdala and the hypothalamus.[55,174–176]

There are five fundamental pathways in nociceptive transmission (Fig. 11-17):

- The spinothalamic tract is the most important nociceptive pathway, but it is also implicated in the transmission of temperature and tactile stimuli. The axons of this pathway end in different thalamic nuclei, such as the ventral posterior lateral (VPL) nucleus, the ventral posterior inferior (VPI) nucleus, the ventral posteromedial (VPM) nucleus, the central lateral (CL) nucleus, and other intralaminar and medial thalamic

nuclei.[177] The afferent terminals in the VPL nucleus are organized somatotopically. The axons that reach the lateral thalamic nuclei are mainly projected to the primary (S1) and secondary (S2) somatosensory cortex and the middle and posterior section of the insula, and are involved in discriminative-sensory pain components, such as pain intensity and spatial localization. This route maintains the specificity and discrimination of the nociceptive message.

- The spinoreticular tract provides connections to the brainstem reticular formation and medial thalamic nuclei and project to the hypothalamus and the limbic system. This transmission pathway is polysynaptic, its somatotopic organization is rough, and it has a high degree of convergence, losing the specificity of nociceptive modality. Due to its projections to the frontal lobe and limbic neocortex, this pathway is involved in emotional and affective components of the painful experience (Fig. 11-18).

- The spinomesencephalic tract ends in the reticular formation and the periaqueductal grey (PAG) matter of the midbrain (Fig. 11-19). This tract provides connections to the amygdala, one of the main constituents of the limbic system, contributing therefore to the affective component of pain. Its role is critical in pain modulation mechanisms.

- The cervicothalamic tract originates from the neurons of the external cervical nucleus, located in the white matter of the two upper cervical segments and reaches the midbrain and thalamus.

- There are two spinolimbic tracts: the spino-amygdalar tract, which is projected directly to the amygdala and assists in the development of emotional responses, and spinohypothalamic tract, which is projected directly to the control centres of the autonomic nervous system (ANS), activating complex neuroendocrine and cardiovascular responses.

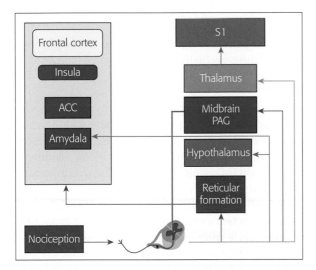

FIGURE 11-17 ■ In nociceptive transmission several pathways are involved (spinothalamic, spinoreticular, spinomesencephalic, cervicothalamic, spino-amygdalar and spinohypothalamic) that project to different central nervous system structures such reticular formation, hypothalamus, PAG, thalamus, S1, S2, insula, ACC, amygdala and prefrontral cortex. ACC, anterior cingulated cortex; PAG, periaqueductal grey.

Supraspinal centres and pain

Thalamus

The *thalamus* receives information from all sensory systems with the exception of the olfactory system and projects this information into the specific cortical

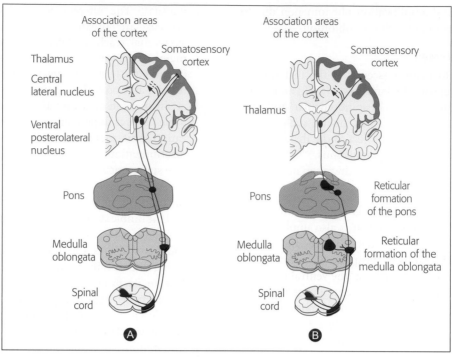

FIGURE 11-18 ■ Main pathways in nociceptive transmission: spinothalamic tract (A) and spinoreticular tract (B).

representation areas. This is why the thalamus is often considered the 'gate to consciousness'. The thalamus is a citoarchitecturally complex structure and it is subdivided in different nuclei. Regarding its role in nociceptive information, some thalamic nuclei have usually been considered as belonging to the *lateral pain system* involved in the sensory-discriminative aspects of pain and some other nuclei belonging to the *medial pain system* related to the affective-motivational pain components.

The nuclei of the lateral system, receiving axons from the spinothalamic pathway, are the VPL and VPM nuclei and the VPI nucleus and project to the contralateral S1 and bilateral S2 and mid and posterior sections of the insula. Intralaminar and medial thalamic nuclei receive information from the spinoreticular, spinomesencephalic, and spino-parabrachial pathways. These medial thalamic nuclei project densely into crucial structures of the limbic system, such as the ACC, the amygdala, the hippocampus, the anterior insula and prefrontal cortex.[142] They represent the

perceived pain threat and are related to the affective and cognitive-evaluative determinants of pain.

Brainstem

The spinal projections to the brainstem play an important role integrating nociceptive activity with homeostatic arousal and autonomic circuits. The brainstem processes all the information jointly before sending it to the forebrain regions.[112] The brainstem is important in mediating changes in pain perception.

The *reticular formation (RF)* in the brainstem comprises important ascending and descending projecting systems and a multitude of local interneuronal connections within the brainstem. It is anatomically and functionally divided into three vertical zones and contains the *ascending reticular activating system*, the *raphe nuclei of serotonergic neurons* and many afferents from the amygdala and hypothalamus. The RF is connected with many cortical and subcortical structures such as locus coeruleus, ventral tegmentum and raphe pathways. It has an important role in mediating motor,

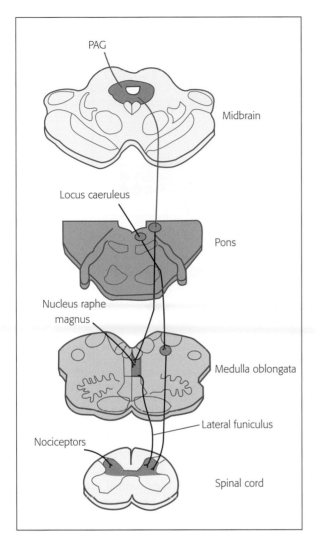

FIGURE 11-19 ■ The spinomesencephalic tract projects to the raphe magnus and through the lateral funiculus, reaching the dorsal horn of the spinal cord. Another pathway goes from the locus caeruleus, projecting into the same region of the posterior horn.

respiratory and cardiovascular functions and pain modulation. The activity of the RF is implicated in the circadian rhythm; it is an important mediator of consciousness and facilitates escape behaviour following acute painful stimuli.

Descending pain modulatory system

Chronic pain, as noted, can also be the result of central changes in the processing of nociceptive information.

SONN activity receiving deep nociceptive information is subject to a powerful modulating influence of supraspinal centres.[178,179] Specific pathways suppress (descending inhibition) or potentiate (descending facilitation) nociceptive transmission from the spinal cord to the brain.[180] In addition, the descending modulatory mechanisms are important, as they are involved in the neural circuits, allowing the emotional and cognitive aspects of painful experience to affect their transmission. Descending pathways modulate nociception via an interaction with several neuronal elements in the dorsal horn: the terminals of primary afferent fibres, the projection neurons to supraspinal centres, the intrinsic excitatory and inhibitory interneurons and terminals of other descending pathways[180] (Fig. 11-20).

The anatomical structures of the descending system can be implicated in the development and maintenance of central sensitization conditions.[181,182] The descending pain modulatory systems are implicated in chronic pain, either due to a dysfunctional descending inhibitory system or an enhanced descending facilitatory system.[182,183] The descending pain controlling pathways can, thus, be activated 'top-down' from brain to brainstem or 'bottom-up' from peripheral and spinal cord nociceptive activity to the brainstem.[184]

Chronic pain can be associated with dysfunctional a descending inhibitory system or an enhanced descending facilitatory system.

The bottom-up control system explains analgesia by counter-irritation and was named by Le Bars et al.[185] as *diffuse noxious inhibitory control* (DNIC), which implies the mechanism whereby dorsal horn neurons responsive to nociceptive stimulation from one location of the body may be inhibited by noxious stimuli applied to another remote location in the body. This mechanism allows the sensory system to focus on the most salient and most recent stimulus.[186] A group of neurons has been identified: namely, the subnucleus reticularis dorsalis (SRD), also known as the dorsal reticular nucleus, which is the key structure for the DNIC.[185,187] SRD receives nociceptive input from both somatic and visceral tissue and projects directly to superficial and deep lamina of the dorsal horn.[186] SRD has been suggested as a major supraspinal site

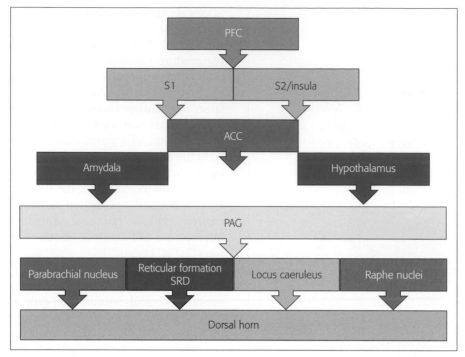

FIGURE 11-20 ■ Pain modulatory systems involve many cortical and subcortical structures: prefrontal cortex (PFC), primary (S1) and secondary (S2) somatosensory cortex, insula, anterior cingulate cortex (ACC), amygdala, hypothalamus, periaquaductal grey matter (PAG), parabrachial nucleus, subnucleus reticularis dorsalis (SRD), locus caeruleus, raphe nuclei and dorsal horn.

mediating in the 'pain-inhibits-pain,' or counter-irritation phenomenon.

Conversely, a group of neurons in the subnucleus reticularis dorsalis can elicit hyperalgesia. The SRD, like the rostroventromedial medulla (RVM), exerts both facilitatory and inhibitory actions. Therefore modulation of dorsal horn nociceptive information can be obtained through descending inhibitory control, but also enhancing facilitatory descending activity.[183]

DNIC is responsible for a tonic level of widespread inhibition throughout the body under normal conditions. It has been proposed that a loss of inhibition could be responsible of the unusual widespread distribution of spontaneous pain and tenderness in patients with fibromyalgia (FM).[76] The term 'conditioned pain modulation' (CPM) is presently preferred to refer to the protocols for evaluating the DNIC-like phenomena.[188]

These CPM changes may occur soon after the noxious stimulus.[189] As noted by Yarnitsky,[184] these

findings raise the question of whether an inefficient CPM is secondary to pain or if less efficient pain inhibition is a risk factor for the development of chronic pain. Some longitudinal studies suggest that dysfunctional CPM is primary to acquisition of pain.[190,191] The association between pro-nociceptive states and idiopathic pain syndromes can be interpreted as a 'cause-and-effect' relationship.[192] Therefore, subjects with 'pro-nociceptive' pain modulation can become more prone to developing a chronic pain syndrome.

Another important aspect is the relationship between CPM and other pain modulator phenomena, such as expectation or placebo. It has been shown that a suggestion of change in the intensity of the conditioning stimulus can alter CPM efficiency.[193] Thus, CPM efficiency can be enhanced by suggestion to its efficiency.[194] Goodin et al.[195,196] have shown how having an optimistic attitude improves CPM efficiency. Therefore, the CPM is, in turn, modulated top-down by the activity in different brain regions.

The top-down descending modulating system is also formed by various noradrenergic and serotonergic components of the brainstem, such as RVM, the raphe magnus nucleus, tractus solitarius nucleus, the locus caeruleus and the PAG. These brainstem pain control centres send projections to the spinal cord, which can be either inhibitory or facilitatory of the incoming nociception from the periphery. There is no absolute anatomical separation between structures involved in the activation of descending inhibition as compared to descending facilitation. For example, common anatomical structures in both the RVM and nucleus tractus solitarius (NTS) give rise to descending pathways producing inhibition or facilitation.[180]

PAG is the key structure in the modulation of pain. It is organized in a number of longitudinal columns that run parallel to the aqueduct. It receives input from the spinomesencephalic tract and is reciprocally interconnected with the hypothalamus, RVM, the parabrachial nucleus (PBN), the NTS, the nucleus raphe magnus, locus caeruleus as well as with the A5 and A7 noradrenergic nucleus of the medulla.[197] It is connected with diverse cortical and limbic structures such as the prefrontal cortex, ACC, amygdala and hypothalamus, consistent with their key roles in emotions such as anxiety and fear. Forebrain input to the PAG mediates contextual information from the prefrontal cortex, the amygdala, the ACC, and the hypothalamus in connection with behavioural goals, past experience and bodily needs of the moment. The PAG can be divided into two distinct regions: the dorsolateral PAG (PAGd) and ventrolateral PAG (PAGv). The PAGd runs from the dorsolateral pons and the ventrolateral medulla, which is involved in controlling the autonomic nervous system. The ventrolateral PAG connects to the raphe magnus nucleus and adjacent reticular formation. The connections between the PAG and the RVM are critical in modulating pain since the modulatory action of the PAG is transmitted largely through the RVM. Stimulation of PAGd induces antinociception, sympathoexcitation, activation of alpha motor neurons, increased heart rate and blood pressure, lower limb vasodilation, increased respiratory rate and increased motor activity (i.e. fight-or-flight responses). The neurotransmitter is noradrenaline and its analgesic effect is mediated by opioid analgesia of mechanical nociceptive stimuli. PAGd activation produces analgesia in situations that pose a threat to the individual and in which a fight-or-flight response is needed.

The PAGv runs to the raphe magnus nucleus. Stimulation thereof causes inhibition of the sympathetic nervous system and inhibition of the alpha motor neuron. Its activity determines passivity, quiescence, decreased vigilance, decreased reactivity, hypotension and bradycardia. Its neurotransmitter is serotonin and its analgesic effect is opioid analgesia to nociceptive stimuli. PAGv activation produces analgesia in recovery situations following injury. Nociception modulation also occurs in higher levels by complex interactions in the thalamus, hypothalamus, brainstem reticular formation, limbic system and other cortical regions. Different routes inform the brain of the nature and meaning of pain and activate regions of the forebrain, which activate a different response mechanism in the PAG. These response mechanisms are different ways of behavioural adjustment depending on whether the pain is escapable or inescapable.[198] Escapable pain is associated with the activation of PAGd and noradrenergic systems and trigger patterns of autonomic, motor and sensory changes that enable an animal to escape or confront a transient threat. Inescapable nociceptive inputs activate neurons in the ventrolateral PAG and serotoninergic systems that coordinate patterns of quiescence and sympathoinhibition.

Rostroventromedial medulla is a heterogeneous region incorporating distinct populations of neurons, each of which provides descending pathways to dorsal horn lamina I, II and V. RVM has dense connections with relevant forebrain structures, both directly as well as via the PAG. These structures include the ACC and insular (IC) cortices and certain subcortical amygdala and hypothalamic nuclei. Brainstem input from the ACC is particularly significant since the ACC has been invested with a pivotal role in integrating sensory and affective aspects with attentional, cognitive and emotional aspects of pain.[115] RVM exerts inhibitory and facilitatory actions through respective 'OFF' and 'ON' cells. The OFF cells are (indirectly) excited by opioids and inhibited by nociceptive input: they display a transient interruption in their discharge immediately prior to a nociceptive reflex and participate in the induction of descending inhibition. The ON cells are inhibited by opioids and excited by nociceptive input, triggering descending facilitation.

The *parabrachial nucleus* (PBN) in the brainstem integrates autonomic and somatosensory information and is interlinked with higher structures involved in the emotional and cognitive dimension of pain. Various subdivisions of the parabrachial nucleus project to the *nucleus tractus solitarius* (NTS), RVM and dorsal horn. Stimulation of the PBN suppresses the response of dorsal horn neurons to both nociceptive and non-nociceptive input.

The NTS processes visceral information, receiving a major input from the vagal nerve, as well as afferents from superficial and deep dorsal horn neurons. Like the PBN, with which it is interconnected, the NTS behaves as an interface between autonomic and sensory systems. It is reciprocally linked with the hypothalamus and limbic and cortical regions and provides a major input to the PAG and monoaminergic nuclei of the brainstem, and directly projects to the spinal cord.

The *dorsolateral pontine tegmentum (DLPT)* projecting noradrenergic neurons to the dorsal horn contributes significantly to pain modulation. The major sources of noradrenergic projections are the locus caeruleus and A5 and A7 (subcaeruleus) regions. These noradrenergic neurons are a parallel pathway for PAG and RVM pain modulation on the spinal cord nociceptive activity.

The *locus caeruleus* (LC) is the principal site for brain synthesis of norepinephrine and is responsible for many of the sympathetic effects during a stress response. The LC receives inputs from the medial prefrontal cortex (MPC) and hypothalamus and sends projections to many areas such as the spinal cord, amygdala, hippocampus, cerebellum and to the frontal cortex. The LC is implicated in responses to sensory stimuli that potentially threaten the biological integrity of the individual.[55] The LC activation and the consequent release of norepinephrine activates the hypothalamic–pituitary–adrenal axis, stimulating the release of a corticotrophin-releasing factor (CRF) from the hypothalamus, which in turn induces the release of adrenocorticotrophic hormone (ACTH) from the anterior pituitary gland that provokes the release of cortisol by the adrenal glands. LC activation influences the prefrontal cortex, modifying cognitive functions and increasing motivation through its action in the nucleus accumbens.

Primary somatosensory cortex

The primary somatosensory cortex (S1) is located in the parietal lobe and includes the Brodmann areas 1, 2, 3a, and 3b. S1 and S2 cortices receive input from lateral thalamic nuclei, and are responsible for sensory-discriminative processing.[199] S1 is organized somatotopically and is important for the perception of location and duration of the nociceptive stimulus. The pattern of activity in S1 is elicited identically either from nociceptive and non-nociceptive somatosensory stimuli. This does not imply that both stimuli activate the same group of neurons in S1, but different subgroups of neurons which at the moment are spatially difficult to distinguish with the available technology.[200]

Secondary somatosensory cortex

The secondary somatosensory cortex (S2) is situated lateral and posterior to S1 and occupies the posterior parietal operculum. Due to its anatomical location and its strong connectivity, S2 is in a unique position to link nociceptive information to limbic cortical regions, such as the ACC and medial prefrontal cortex.[55,201] Therefore, S2 is involved in generating somatosensory representation of the body and linking this representation with affective appraisal.[55]

Insular cortex

The insular cortex is an anatomically complex structure located adjacent to S2, and plays a key role in the somatosensory and interoceptive representation of the body and integrates this multimodal sensory information with affective pain components.[202,203] In neuroimaging studies of pain, the insula is the most frequently activated structure.[142]

The insula can be divided into three subregions: the posterior, middle and anterior insula.

The insula, according to Craig,[204] is like a serial processing system that from the posterior portion of the insula to its anterior portion, and adding various information, allows the integration of somatosensory, homeostatic and emotional information (Fig. 11-21).

The posterior insula integrates interoceptive (homeostatic) and exteroceptive signals from the thalamus.[205] The mid insula receives posterior insular input and integrates this information with inputs from the amygdala and the nucleus accumbens. This

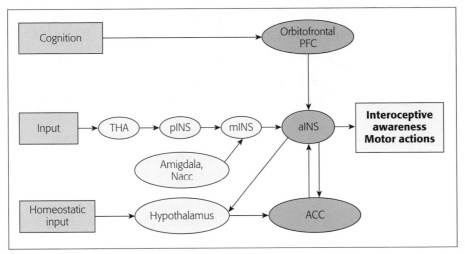

FIGURE 11-21 ■ The insula is like a serial processing system that from the posterior portion of the insula to its anterior portion, and adding various information, allows the integration of somatosensory, homeostatic and emotional information. ACC, anterior cingulate cortex; aINS, anterior insula; mINS, mid insula; Nacc, nucleus accumbens; PFC, prefrontal cortex; pINS, posterior insula; THA, thalamus.

connection to the amygdala increases pain awareness and vigilance and helps to generate the emotional valence, either aversive or hedonic, of both interoceptive and exteroceptive information. The connection to the nucleus accumbens adds motivational and reward components to the body perceptions. All this information reaches the highest integrative level in the anterior insula, which in turn receives information from ACC and from the orbitofrontal and ventrolateral prefrontal cortex. This important top-down control system would facilitate the process of selective attention to potential threat situations and its memory storage.

The insular cortex is crucial for integrating all subjective feelings related to the body, and especially to its homeostatic conditions, into emotional experiences and conscious awareness of the environment and the self.[204]

Cingulate cortex

The cingulate cortex is considered a key structure of the limbic system and is divided into distinct areas: anterior cingulate cortex (ACC), midcingulate cortex (MCC), posterior cingulate cortex (PCC) and the retrosplenial cortex (RSC)[206] (Fig. 11-22).

A major input to ACC comes from medial and intralaminar thalamic nuclei, which places the ACC into the centre of the previously considered medial pain system, subserving affective-motivational pain components.[115,207,208] Together with S2 and the insula, ACC is the most consistent region activated by pain. ACC is considered to have a central role in integrating sensory and affective aspects with attentional, cognitive and emotional aspects of pain.[115]

Hypothalamus

The *hypothalamus* receives nociceptive inputs from the spinohypothalamic tract, and is extensively interlinked with brainstem and corticolimbic structures. The hypothalamus represents the connection between the nociceptive and the neuroendocrine system, and is involved in the generation of multisystem responses to actual or potential threat.

Amygdala

The important contribution of the amygdala to the perception of pain, especially in its affective dimension, is becoming increasingly more evident.[93,209,210] The amygdala is implicated in negative emotions such as stress, anxiety and fear. The amygdala is activated in threatening situations to facilitate a defensive behaviour. The amygdala plays a key role in memory consolidation, so it is critical for fear conditioning, but

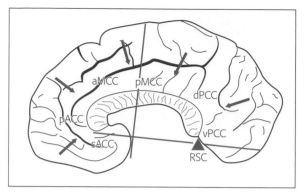

FIGURE 11-22 ■ The cingulate cortex is considered a key structure of the limbic system and is divided into distinct areas: anterior cingulate cortex (ACC), midcingulate cortex (MCC), posterior cingulate cortex (PCC) and the retrosplenial cortex (RSC).[3] Each of these areas is subdivided into subregions: ACC in subgenual (sACC) and pregenual (pACC), the MCC in anterior (aMCC) and posterior (pMCC), and PCC in dorsal (dPCC) and ventral (vPCC).

also in other forms of associative learning, including reward and appetitive learning.[211,212]

The amygdala sends projections to the PAG that might initiate antinociceptive action during emotional stress, being implicated in stress and expectation-induced analgesia.[209,213]

Hippocampus

The hippocampus is considered the primary brain structure for storage and retrieval of long-term explicit memories.[214] Regarding its adaptive value, the hippocampus is important in learning pain and pain-related behaviour and can play an important role in chronic pain and chronic pain-related avoidance behaviour.

Prefrontal cortex

The anterior part of the frontal lobe, the prefrontal cortex (PFC), contains 30% of brain mass. It can be subdivided into the mid-dorsal, dorsolateral (dlPFC), ventrolateral, orbitofrontal and medial frontal parts.[215] The PFC is involved in higher-level cortical functions that characterize human beings, such as abstract thinking, the traits of individual personality, decision-making and planning behaviours and actions (see Fig. 11-24).

Prefrontal pain-evoked activity may be related to cognitive, attentional and emotional aspects of pain perception, rather than directly to pain sensation.[216] dorsolateral prefrontal cortex (DLPC) has been considered the key structure of the 'top-down' endogenous pain control system and is therefore implicated in placebo analgesia.[217,218] The vlPFC activation is also involved in analgesia, as it appears related to cognitive modulation of the pain experience.[99]

The brain and chronic pain

Neuroimaging studies have shown marked differences between the brain processing of acute and chronic pain. These differences relate to functional and structural changes in different brain areas in patients with chronic pain. As already mentioned, neuroimaging has helped shape the concept of chronic pain covering not only a response of the somatosensory system but also a condition in which emotional, cognitive and modulatory areas of the brain are implicated.[120]

Chronic pain and augmented central pain processing

One of the brain changes observed in chronic pain is an increase in central pain processing. Early neuroimaging studies in patients with fibromyalgia (FM), for example, showed increased brain activity in pain-related areas (S1, S2, ACC, IC and cerebellum).[72]

Chronic pain patients subject to the same stimulus intensity referred more pain and showed greater cortical activity in these areas. This increased activity was interpreted as a reflection of increased sensitivity in these patients[72] (Fig. 11-23). If the stimulus intensity was increased in healthy control subjects, to achieve the same painful intensity as that perceived by patients with FM, the brain activation patterns were equated.

Chronic pain and inhibitory systems dysfunction

Patients with chronic pain often refer to widespread pain in different body areas. This widespread pain may be due to a lower tonic level of inhibition that can be evaluated with 'conditioned pain modulation' (CPM) protocols.[188] The loss of inhibition may also occur in the brain. Jensen et al.[74] observed that fibromyalgia patients, unlike controls, showed no activation in the rostral anterior cingulate cortex, which is a region involved in pain inhibition.

Although perceived pain intensity was the same in both patients and control subjects, rostral ACC (rACC) activation was lower in patients.[74] As previously

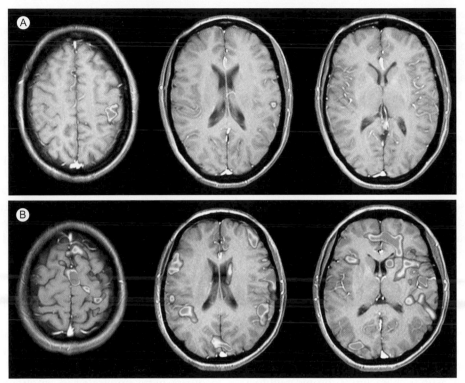

FIGURE 11-23 ■ Brain activation pattern obtained with fMRI. Activation pattern by applying 4-kg thumb pressure in a control subject. Activation of the contralateral sensorimotor area 1 (A) is observed. Activation pattern by applying the same pressure to a subject with fibromyalgia. A broad pattern of activation is observed, showing significant activity in different parietal and frontal regions, the insula and the anterior cingulate cortex (B). *Courtesy of Deus et al.*[231] *and the Institute for Advanced Technology (IAT) of the Barcelona Biomedical Research Park (PRBB) of CRC Mar (Health Corporation).*

discussed, the activation of the rACC is related to the DLPC-attentional and placebo antinociceptive network. The loss of inhibition in FM patients might be related to changes in these cerebral–midbrain–spinal pain modulation mechanisms.[219]

Pain matrix and the salience network

Currently the concept of 'pain matrix' is being contested as many previously believed pain-related areas respond to multimodal relevant stimuli. Recent studies conducted by Iannetti et al.,[220] Mouraux et al.[200,221] and Legrain et al.[118] have called into question the specificity of brain responses to pain. Some brain regions such as the ACC, insula and S2 have been shown to respond to multimodal stimuli with no evidence of a nociceptive specific response.[200] The anterior insula as well the cingulate cortex are considered[222] a multimodal

sensory stimulus salience detection network, whereby salient stimuli are encoded and processed to appropriately orient attention.[118,200,222–226] Therefore, activity in these areas is not specific to pain and may actually represent a general salience response.[118,224] This has led to the recognition of a specific brain network known as the *salience network* (SN), which includes the anterior insula (aINS), ACC, MCC, temporoparietal junction (TPJ) and dlPFC. The activity in the SN is dependent on the degree to which an external stimuli is able to capture attention.[200,224,227] It should be noted that attention to a stimulus is not only determined by its salience but also by its relevance; the relevance of the stimulus is specific to each individual, their previous experiences, and is dependent on emotional and cognitive elaborations of their own personal history. The relevance of pain therefore depends on very different aspects: for example, the interpretation that pain is a sign of a serious or potentially disabling disease, competing explanations from health care professionals, etc. Thus, the increased activity of these brain areas in some experimental pain conditions on chronic pain patients may be related to a greater pain salience and relevance for them.

Chronic pain and changes in brain activity patterns

Although the aforementioned studies are indeed interesting, chronic pain cannot be simply and exclusively understood as an increase in the responses of the 'pain matrix' as observed in acute pain.[228] The brain activity pattern that characterizes chronic pain is not equivalent to the brain responses observed in these patients when a stimulus is induced experimentally. Acute painful stimuli generally activate somatosensory and cingulate cortical regions, while spontaneous pain and allodynia activate prefrontal cortex and limbic regions such as ACC, anterior insula and basal ganglia.[229–235] The activation of these brain regions is associated with the attentional component, hypervigilance, and the emotional component of pain. These studies highlight that 'emotional' aspects characterize chronic pain to a greater extent than somatosensory aspects.[236] Schweinhardt et al.[237] observed that the activation of the anterior insula in patients with chronic neuropathic pain occurred in a more rostral area, more involved in the integration of emotional aspects, compared to healthy subjects in which experimental pain were induced. Also observed in FM patients is an increased activation in areas that encode emotional aspects such as the anterior insula and cingulate cortex.[232,233]

Acute and chronic pain are different regarding the many different brain activity patterns

---

Parks et al.[235] analysed the differences in cortical responses between evoked and spontaneous pain in subjects with osteoarthritis of the knee. The most significant difference was that spontaneous pain engaged the prefrontal limbic structures, more associated with an emotional state, whereas evoked experimental pain did not. According to the authors, this means that mechanical and thermal pain thresholds do not measure the same construct as that of the pain experienced by patients. This would also explain why there is frequently a poor correlation between pain thresholds and the pain reported and pain-related disability in patients with chronic pain.

Baliki et al.[229] analysed the brain activity patterns in patients with chronic low back pain and found that pain intensity was not constant but varied from time to time. They separately analysed brain responses at times when a rapid increase in the pain occurred and at times when the intensity remained high. These authors showed that the brain activity pattern when pain rapidly increases is similar to that observed in healthy patients undergoing experimental acute pain. This pattern is characterized by the activation in the anterior insula, mACC, supplementary motor area (SMA), primary somatosensory (S1), and motor (M1) regions, secondary somatosensory cortex (S2) and cerebellum. However, at times when the pain intensity remained even, the pattern was different, with an especially marked activation of the medial prefrontal cortex (mPFC). The activation of the amygdala, rACC, posterior thalamus and ventral striatum was also observed. Therefore, pain perception involves a shift in the areas of brain activation from regions involved in acute pain to others more implicated in emotional processing. This different pattern of brain activity, characterized by a marked activation of mPFC, implicated in emotional processing relative to the self, would explain how chronic pain is qualitatively different from acute pain. Chronic pain is therefore more aversive and unpleasant and corresponds to an experience of suffering.

Chronic pain involves a shift in the areas of brain activation from regions involved in acute pain to others more implicated in emotional processing.

On the other hand, mPFC activation is antithetical to the activation of dlPFC, the latter involved in attentional capacity and working memory. This could also explain dlPFC atrophy, observed by some authors in patients with chronic pain and the frequent cognitive dysfunction in these patients. The mPFC activation has also been observed in patients with rheumatoid arthritis when experiencing their pain, while this did not occur when they were subjected to experimental pain.[238] This study also found that the magnitude of mPFC activation correlated with depressive symptoms. It has been suggested that depressive disorders and persistent pain share the same central neuroplastic changes,[239] which makes it difficult to determine at this time whether they correspond to pain or emotional disorders associated with it.

Chronic pain and cortical reorganization

One of the areas of study in chronic pain relates to the different neuroplastic changes observed in S1.[132,240–244] The cortical representation of any part of the body is directly proportional to the sensitivity of that area. Areas of the body with greater sensitivity and hence a higher density of receptive fields have greater representation in S1. Changes in the somatosensory area can be described as an abnormal reorganization in the cortical representation of the area of the virtual body corresponding to the body region where the patient perceives pain.[245–247]

Somatosensory cortical reorganization has been observed in clinical conditions such as phantom limb pain,[248–253] chronic low back pain[254] and complex regional pain syndrome (CRPS).[245–247,255–258] The amount of cortical reorganization seems to correlate with pain severity and pain chronicity.[122] Neuroimaging studies have shown that the cortical area where the patient experiences referred pain overlaps with neighbouring cortical areas.[245,246,258] For example, in patients with chronic low back pain, the representation of the lower back shifts toward the representation of the legs in S1.[254] The study carried out by Juottonen et al.[245] observed a reduction in the distance between S1 thumb representation and little finger one of the affected side. In upper limb amputees and in subjects with CRPS, lip stimulation triggers the activation of the S1 area corresponding to the hand.[246,248,259]

Changes in the somatosensory area can be described as an abnormal reorganization in the cortical representation of the area of the virtual body corresponding to the body region where the patient perceives pain.

These alterations in the representation could explain why patients with chronic pain frequently perceive the stimulation in territories that do not correspond to the area of the affected limb stimulated or report that the size of the affected limb is larger than the contralateral.[260–262] For example, Soler et al.[263] observed

in 48 patients with complete spinal cord injury that it was possible to reproduce painful and non-painful referred sensations in very remote areas below the injury level, being body parts with total anaesthesia, by touching various body points above the injury level.

The degree of somatotopical reorganization seems to correlate directly with the severity of pain and hyperalgesia[246] and the severity of alteration in sensory discrimination.[122] Interestingly, cortical reorganization correlates with impaired sensory discrimination evaluated with two-point discrimination.[122]

Cortical reorganization is also observed in the primary motor area (M1) and the supplementary motor area, showing an asymmetry between the two hemispheres in CRPS.[264–266] Decreased inhibitory mechanisms and increased excitability in contralateral M1 has also been shown.[264] Maihofner et al.[266] analysed cortical activity during the performance of motor tasks and observed a significant reorganization of central motor circuits with increased activation of M1 and supplementary motor cortex. Therefore, in patients with CRPS there are extensive changes in the function of cortical motor areas. This alteration of the representation may explain the difficulty of movement dissociation and the dystonia in patients with CRPS. Gieteling et al.[267] have analysed the cortical changes in patients with CRPS that specifically showed dystonia. The cortical activation between subjects with CRPS and control subjects was compared during implementation and during the imagination of hand movements of the affected and non-affected hands. It was noted that there were no differences between subjects with CRPS and controls in the execution of hand movements and imagination of hand movements of the not-affected hand. However, in patients with CRPS compared with control subjects, the imagination of hand movements of the affected hand provoked a lesser activation in the prefrontal cortex and ipsilateral premotor cortex.

A lesser activation in postcentral gyrus and in inferior parietal cortex was also observed. This study shows that subjects with CRPS1 with dystonia have a decreased activation of areas involved in planning movements, somatosensory integration and autonomic responses. This interesting study supports the use of motor imagery in the treatment of patients with CRPS. Therefore, the reorganization of cortical representations of the body disrupts body perception and can be strongly implicated in persistent painful conditions.[121,124,268] These changes may lead to inconsistency between the virtual body and the real body and may be the basis of impaired motion perception and motor performance observed in subjects with chronic pain.[269-271]

Cortical reorganization can be at the basis of negligence phenomena frequently observed in patients with chronic pain. Neglect phenomena can be classified into sensory neglect and distortion in body perception, motor and cognitive neglect. One most studied form of neglect is the hemineglect often seen in subjects after an acquired brain lesion.[266,272] Hemineglect has been defined as 'a deficit in processing corresponding to sensory stimuli in the contralateral hemispace, a part of the own body, the part of an imagined scene, or may include the failure to act with the contralesional limbs despite intact motor functions'.[273]

Cortical reorganization can be at the basis of sensory, motor and cognitive neglect phenomena frequently observed in patients with chronic pain.

Chronic pain patients show significant changes in higher-order cognitive representations. Patients with CRPS, for example, develop a neglect syndrome, so that the affected limb is perceived as strange (cognitive negligence) and requires attentional and visual focus to move the limb (motor neglect).[123,274] A study by Galer and Jensen[274] in 242 patients with CRPS, revealed some symptoms of neglect in 84% and both cognitive and motor neglect in 47%. Lewis et al.[123] conducted a qualitative research observing that patients with CRPS show cognitive neglect: they experience a distortion of the mental image of their limb, perceiving it as strange, as if not belonging to their body and they have difficulty recognizing their spatial position. Patients express feelings of hostility towards their limb and in some cases would prefer amputation. Moseley[275] has also shown how patients with CRPS have difficulty recognizing image laterality when it corresponds to the side where they perceive pain. These somatosensory and cognitive neglect phenomena have also been documented in patients with chronic low back pain.[276] Symptoms of neglect can aggravate disability experienced by patients with chronic pain.

Neglect has classically been considered as a protective response of the painful limb aimed at avoiding the pain associated with movement or touch. However, it seems that this neglect is rather the result of changes in the cortical representation of the limb.

Various studies have strived to confirm that the changes in the representation are not only the result but also the cause of perceptual disturbances. In subjects with CRPS, pain and oedema of the limb increase if they see a magnified image of the limb.[277]

Alterations in the cortical representation can be normalized after effective treatment.[278] As demonstrated by Maihofner et al.,[278] there is a correlation between improvement of symptoms and normalization of cortical reorganization. Also, Pleger et al.[279] demonstrated that a programme of sensory and motor rehabilitation adapted to CRPS patients can normalize cortical reorganization in S1 and S2, showing a correlation between this normalization of cortical maps and improved discrimination between two points. Therefore, sensory disorders do not involve exclusively peripheral changes but also profound changes in cortical maps. Hence, retraining sensorimotor discrimination may be an important aspect in the treatment of some chronic pain conditions, not only in enhancing perceptual abilities but also in improving pain.[280-282]

Changes in brain representation may induce pain, sensory disturbances, impaired proprioception, vasomotor changes, dystonia, abnormal movement patterns and phenomena of neglect of the body area where the patient reports pain.

Research conducted in the past decade based on clinical studies and functional neuroimaging studies has led to a thorough review of the relationship between peripheral and central changes in chronic pain entities. Certainly, nociceptive information can lead to central neuroplastic changes, with the consequent alteration of the perception of the affected body area. But alterations in cortical representation are not only the result but also the cause of the signs and symptoms experienced by the individual with chronic pain. Alterations in representation are alone capable of inducing pain, sensory disturbances, impaired proprioception, vasomotor changes, dystonia, abnormal movement patterns and phenomena of neglect of the body area where the patient reports pain. These findings have significant implications for treatment, paving the way to new strategies capable of reversing these neglect phenomena and thus improving cortical reorganization.[280,281]

Chronic pain as a memory

Central neuroplastic changes associated with chronic pain share molecular, neurophysiological and structural similarities with plasticity in other regions of the brain such as the hippocampus and cerebral cortex that are involved in associative learning and memory.[283–285] Many researchers, based on these plastic changes in brain circuitry, maintain that the persistence of pain in the absence of evidential pathology stems from a memory of pain in the CNS.[132–135,286]

Chronic pain in the absence of evidential pathology may stem from a 'pain memory' in the brain.

Generating long-term pain memories can occur by different mechanisms, such as explicit and implicit memory. As noted by Flor,[136] explicit memory corresponds to those processes based on the conscious reproduction of events stored in the memory. Implicit memory would be one that is acquired in a non-conscious manner and includes non-associative learning such as habituation and sensitization phenomena as well as associative learning, Hebbian learning, classical conditioning, operant conditioning and social learning or modelling.

Pain memory can be activated not only after nociceptive stimulation but also with very different stimuli. In subjects with chronic pain, merely the sight of touching a painful limb can evoke the pain and swelling even when it is not actually being touched,[287] as well as imagining movements of a painful limb without any movement at all.[288]

Considering chronic pain as a memory codified in the CNS has considerable therapeutic implications; it implies that this 'pain memory' can be 'extinguished' or at least reduce its 'activation', so it may be possible to reduce the chronic pain.

Chronic pain, resting state networks and connectivity

One of the most relevant functional characteristic of the nervous system is clearly communication. Connectivity is imperative in neuronal function. It is the principle 'connect or die': neurons that fail to receive and send signals undergo a process of apoptosis.[289] Pain is a multidimensional experience and, as already suggested by Melzack[290] in his theory of the neuromatrix, the conscious experience of pain, like any other perception, requires activation of many brain areas. Therefore, a considerable progress in understanding the relationship between brain activity and pain has been the ability to analyse the connectivity between different brain networks involved. The 'network analysis' can identify brain regions with similar co-varying activity during a specific condition, like perceiving pain.

Until recently the majority of functional neuroscience studies have aimed to record and analyse brain responses to a task or stimulus. However, the brain remains active even in the absence of any explicit input or output.[291] In fact, the majority of the activity of the brain is related to intrinsic neuronal signalling and it has been established that any specific task accounts for less than 5% of brain energy.[292] As noted by Zhang and Raichle,[293] that in the same way that 75% of the total mass-energy in the cosmos is dark energy, the spontaneous neuronal activity can be considered the *brain's dark energy*. This 'brain resting state' activity entailed a critical change in the consideration of the patterns of brain activity.[294]

The first resting state network to be recognized was the *default mode network (DMN)*,[295–297] so-called because it is deactivated during tasks that require external attention. The main areas that are part of the DMN are the mPFC, posterior cingulate cortex (PCC), inferior parietal lobe (IPL), medial temporal lobe and the hippocampal formation (HF).[295,297,298]

The first study showing the impact of chronic pain in brain networks was carried out by Baliki et al.[299] in patients with chronic low back pain. These authors found that patients with chronic back pain, during the execution of a simple visual task, showed reduced deactivation in several key DMN regions. In these patients with spontaneous pain an enhanced activation of the mPFC, a brain region that modulates emotional evaluation relative to the self, was observed.[229] The reduced deactivation during task performance, mainly in the mPFC,[299,300] is interpretable as suggesting patients with chronic pain are 'stuck' in a state of self-referential thought or focus on their pain.[77]

The main finding is that chronic pain is different from acute pain in terms of the brain activity pattern evoked. The activity in brain areas important for affective and self-relevant processing such as the mPFC may also play an important role in mediating the relationship between depressive symptoms and pain severity.[238] Therefore, chronic pain is more 'emotional'. Moreover, as the mPFC is anatomically connected with the PAG, it may be the most important node within the DMN that mediates communication with the antinociceptive system.[301]

Since DMN is crucial for internal self-monitoring, the aberrant activity can be interpreted as a failure to disengage attention from pain. These findings show that chronic pain has a significant impact on many brain functions and suggest that alterations in the DMN may be responsible for the emotional distress and cognitive and behavioural dysfunctions observed in these patients.

Aberrant activity in the DMN can be interpreted as a failure to disengage attention from pain.

Pain and the brain dynamic pain connectome. Resting state studies have shown that brain activity analysis needs to focus on what best expresses its nature: namely, connectivity. The comprehensive map of neural connections in the brain has been termed *connectome*.[302–304]

The dynamic behaviour of the brain is determined by the dynamic fluctuations related to attention to pain, dependent, as mentioned above, on its salience and relevance.

There is a well-known interaction between pain and attention: pain interferes with attention and cognitive processing, while engagement in a cognitive task reduces pain.[305] Therefore, the experience of pain is determined by the activity and dynamic connectivity between different networks: the salience network (SN), the antinociceptive network, the DMN and cognitive networks involved in the relevance.

> Pain can be modulated by other stimuli that compete with the nociceptive stimulus (salience) and by different mental processes that require directed attention, thoughts and context that are able to modify its relevance.

The SN plays a crucial role as it identifies the most biologically relevant internal and external stimuli in

order to generate an adaptive behavior.[306] It plays a major role as it mediates the activity between the central executive network and the DMN.

Activation of the SN is dependent on the degree to which an external stimulus is able to capture the attention.[200] DMN activation is inversely proportional to the activation of the salience network. Kucyi et al.[301] have shown that when a subject draws attention to pain, the SN is activated more strongly than when the subject is distracted. The activation of the DMN is produced when the subject's mind wanders and is deactivated when the subject focuses attention on pain. These two patterns are related to a different functional connectivity with the antinociceptive system. When the subject is mind-wandering away from pain, the antinociceptive system shows an increased functional connectivity between the mPFC and PAG. This study suggests that the dynamic communication between the DMN and antinociceptive system may underlie the spontaneous fluctuations in attention to pain. It also shows that there is variability between subjects in terms of the ability to 'disconnect from pain'. While some subjects tend to mind-wander easily and thus to divert attention from pain, others, by contrast, tend to focus attention on pain. This suggest, therefore, that subjects who have difficulty to disengage from pain have less functional connectivity between the DMN and the antinociceptive system.

Therefore, a possibility of chronic pain management may lie in training in the ability to 'disengage' attention from pain. For example, the effects of mindfulness on pain may be due to a learning process to mind-wander away from pain. But attention is strongly driven by the meaning and interpretation of pain. A direct intervention directed to change the patient's beliefs about pain such as the *Explain Pain* approach may also disengage the patient from pain.

Cognitive pain modulation. As already mentioned, different areas of the prefrontal cortex, and based on different mechanisms, play a role in pain modulation. The activation of the dlPFC and the ventrolateral prefrontal cortex (vlPFC) are associated with analgesic modulation. Conversely, the activation of the mPFC and orbitofrontal cortex (OFC) is associated with increased pain perception.

The activation of the dlPFC or of the vlPFC involve different mechanisms. The mechanisms dependent on dlPFC-induced analgesia are related to attentional pain control[216] and are implicated in placebo analgesia.[217,218,307] As shown by Wiech et al.,[99] the mechanisms that underlie vlPFC analgesia are much more 'cognitive'. The vlPFC is involved in reappraisal of the emotional significance of a stimulus leading to a decreased perception of the pain severity[99] (Fig. 11-24).

Chronic pain and structural brain changes

Patients with chronic pain not only process pain differently but also may exhibit structural brain changes in both the grey and white matter. Grey matter changes in brain structure that can be quantified in MRI are

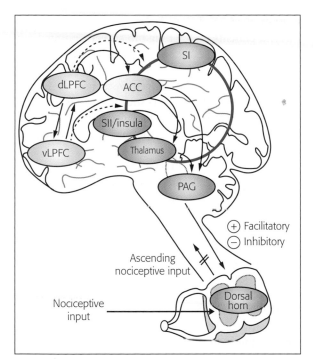

FIGURE 11-24 ■ Different areas of the prefrontal cortex, and based on different mechanisms, play a role in pain modulation. The mechanisms dependent on dlPFC-induced analgesia are related to attentional pain control. The vlPFC is involved in reappraisal of the emotional significance of a stimulus leading to a decreased perception of the pain severity. ACC, anterior cingulate cortex; dlPFC, dorsolateral prefrontal cortex; PAG, periaqueductal grey matter; vlPFC, ventrolateral prefrontal cortex. *Reproduced with permission from Wiech et al.*[99]

grey matter density and volume using voxel-based morphometry (VBM) and voxel-based cortical thickness (VBCT).[308] Although both VBM and the cortical thickness analysis are used to quantify grey matter, they are not based on the same processing techniques and results are not interchangeable.[309]

The first clinicians to show differences in brain morphometry associated with chronic pain were Apkarian et al.[310] They found that patients with chronic back pain showed 5–11% less neocortical grey matter volume (GMV) than control subjects. This decrease in GMV occurred mainly within the bilateral dorsolateral prefrontal cortex (dlPFC) and right anterior thalamus. The decrease in GMV seemed related to pain duration. The decrease in the dlPFC, an area involved in the top-down inhibitor system and in higher cognitive functions, seems to correlate with cognitive impairment present in patients with chronic pain.[311,312]

These structural changes have been observed in other studies with different clinical conditions: chronic low back pain patients,[313] fibromyalgia,[314–319] complex regional pain syndrome (CRPS),[320] irritable bowel syndrome (IBS),[321,322] chronic pelvic pain,[323] migraine,[324–329] chronic tension type headache,[330] chronic facial pain[331] and temporomandibular disorders.[332,333] These alterations in morphometry have also been observed in patients with chronic fatigue syndrome[334] and with post-traumatic stress disorder (PTSD).[335]

The decrease in grey matter was mainly observed in central processing or pain modulation areas such as the frontal cortex, ACC, IC and thalamus. Other regions in which such changes have also observed are the parahippocampus, basal ganglia, S1, S2, the temporal lobe, posterior cingulate cortex and brainstem. It has been speculated whether these structural changes are the cause or the consequence of pain.[336]

It is not clear whether brain structural changes are the cause or the consequence of pain.

Initially, these findings suggest, according to some authors, that the cause of the development of chronic pain would be a neurodegeneration process as seen in the ageing brain. Kuchinad et al.[314] showed that individuals with FM exhibit an age-associated decrease in grey matter volume 3.3 times greater than healthy controls. Therefore, each year of FM was equivalent to 9.5 times the normal loss of grey matter with age. Some authors began to suggest that entities such as fibromyalgia were the result of a brain disorder characterized by accelerated ageing.[337]

Some studies seem to confirm that the decrease in grey matter is associated with a longer duration of pain over time.[310,314,320,324–326,329,330,338–340] Other studies, however, indicate that these changes in the grey matter are not correlated with the duration of pain but with its intensity and affective components of pain, such as anxiety and emotional distress.[313]

Longitudinal studies seem to suggest that they are the consequence of pain and not its cause. Rodriguez-Raecke et al.[341] performed an MRI before and after hip replacement for osteoarthritis, observing a return to baseline grey matter levels, although not entirely, when the pain disappeared. However, as we will discuss later, long-term follow-up of these patients resulted in very different conclusions. Gwilym et al.[342] did a similar study in patients with unilateral hip osteoarthritis before surgery and 9 months after hip arthroplasty, also being compared with control subjects. The changes observed in brain volume before surgery normalized 9 months later. Therefore, these changes could not be interpreted as an accelerated ageing process, but were related to pain.

The functional implications of these structural changes are unclear. Some authors suggest that they are the expression of altered endogenous pain inhibition systems[343] because volume reduction is observed in regions considered crucial in these mechanisms such as the rACC or dlPFC.[339,340]

Structural changes when affecting areas such as the prefrontal cortex and hippocampus may be correlated, according to some authors, with cognitive deficits often observed in subjects with chronic pain.[316,319,337,343] This would justify, for example, memory deficits and 'fibrofog' reported by FM patients.[337]

However, despite the influence of these studies, their interpretation is complex and problematic for several reasons. First, not all structural MRI studies that examined the same brain areas found the same changes. Areas with structural changes reported in the studies vary greatly, which could be explained by the fact that studies have been conducted in different pain conditions. However, there should be a greater coincidence in terms of brain areas where these changes have been detected, since the common feature of all these clinical conditions is chronic pain. Some studies have even found no significant differences in grey matter volume in patients with chronic pain and pain-free controls.[344,345]

The second problem is the unknown pathophysiology of changes in the grey matter. These changes may not only be a consequence of neuronal loss but also due to the decreased density in dendritic spines, changes in glial cells, neuroinflammation, or to changes in extracellular fluids or blood volume.[77,346]

Another problem is that the results are based on correlation analyses derived almost exclusively from cross-sectional studies. Without evidence of causation, it is not possible to know whether these morphological changes are actually the cause of chronic pain, if they are the result of prolonged pain over time or multiple confounders.

Rodriguez-Raecke et al.,[341] in their longitudinal study in patients undergoing hip surgery, pointed out that normalization in brain volume obtained after surgery, besides being possibly related to the elimination of the peripheral nociceptive source, could be related to many other aspects such as the effects of the investment in treatment and resulting positive expectations, as well as changes in the level of patient activity and in their lifestyle after surgery.

Possible factors also related to the decrease in the volume of grey matter are affective disorders such as a high level of stress, depression, anxiety and catastrophism.[77,345] It is known that stress associated with chronic pain can cause neurohormonal changes that can determine the changes observed in the PFC, hippocampus, amygdala, etc., in subjects with chronic pain.[347,348] Gianaros et al.[349] have shown that a chronic stress situation can be predictive of a decrease in the volume of grey matter in the hippocampus.

Jensen et al.,[340] in a study of functional and structural changes in fibromyalgia (FM) patients, have shown that decreases in cortical thickness are correlated with higher scores of depression. Therefore, an improvement in mood as a result of a decrease in pain could explain the partial remission of grey matter abnormalities.[77] Other studies have shown that changes in the grey matter relate to personality traits like neuroticism or catastrophism.[350–352] Hsu et al.[345] conducted a study in patients with FM, whereby the reduction in grey matter volume in the left anterior insula was present only in those patients with an affective disorder. The structural differences observed in FM patients compared to healthy control subjects disappeared after controlling the affective disorder.

Another aspect to consider is the effect of consuming some analgesics, such as anti-inflammatory drugs and opiates, which may cause structural brain changes[353,354] that disappear when the patient improves clinically and stops taking them.

Rodriguez-Raecke et al.[355] published a second study in 2013, including more patients undergoing hip surgery, and assessed the structural brain changes in four time slots with a follow-up 12 months after surgery. In this study the increase in the grey matter over time was quite subtle and effect sizes were small. These authors suggested that the observed changes in patients with chronic pain are not due to neuronal atrophy, but may be related to a decrease in nociceptive input, a change in lifestyle, improvement in motor function, better state of mind and greater welfare of subjects after surgery.

In this regard, a recent study by Dolman et al.[356] found no association between chronic low back pain and cortical decline. These authors suggest that the decrease in cortical volume can be attributed to comorbid affective disorders rather than to the pain itself. Their results indicate that if other variables such as affective aspects, age and drug consumption are controlled, differences in grey matter between patients with pain and control subjects are removed. As the authors note, there remain significant doubts regarding a relationship between chronic pain and changes in grey matter.

Pain and cognitive functions

In recent years, the effects of chronic pain in a series of cognitive processes have been researched.[120,126,128] These processes include attention, learning and memory, processing speed, psychomotor ability and executive function. These cognitive functions can be assessed by neuropsychological tests. Patients with chronic pain show attention deficits,[357,358] especially in performing complex tasks.[359] Patients with fibromyalgia evidenced alterations in working memory and attentional control.[312,360,361] A recent review has shown how subjects with chronic pain have a poorer performance in working memory tests than healthy control participants. However, it is not clear if there are physiological differences between patients and

controls during working memory tests.[127] Executive function and decision-making are also altered in different chronic pain conditions.[311,312,362]

These cognitive deficits can be exacerbated if the subject is treated with opioids over a long term.[363] This alteration in cognitive functions aggravates the patient's clinical condition and can be an obstacle to interventions involving the cognitive re-elaboration of pain. For an updated review of the effect of chronic pain on the cognitive and executive functions, the meta-analytical review by Berryman et al.[128] is recommended.

Clinical implications of brain changes

Progression of both spinal and supraspinal neuroplastic changes may be the neurophysiologic mechanism which explains the chronic pain experience with no active nociceptive source. Neuroimaging techniques have opened a door that can help us to understand the brain mechanisms involved in chronic pain.

Chronic pain is associated with increased central processing in different brain areas, including the salience network, and may be accompanied by an extensive cortical reorganization. In addition, brain activity for chronic pain shifts away from the pattern shown for acute pain to more prefrontal and limbic circuitry.[136,364,365] It can also be associated with changes in brain connectivity between brain regions (Fig. 11-25). Patients with chronic pain have shown an increase in changes in activation (increased pain sensitivity) (greater emotional responses) as well as in the structure and connectivity between brain regions, particularly in regions implicated in antinociception. Neuroimaging studies support the notion that pain is not only pain, but is often accompanied by changes in body perception and emotional problems and cognitive deficits.[336,366]

Chronic pain may be associated with:

■ increased central processing in different brain areas, including the salience network
■ extensive cortical reorganization
■ changes in connectivity between different brain regions
■ a shift in brain activity to more prefrontal and limbic circuitry.

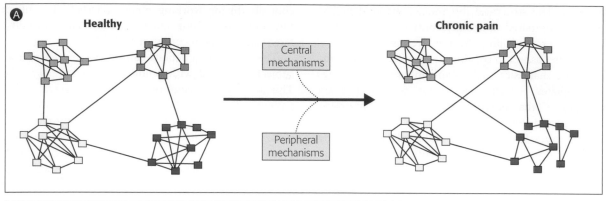

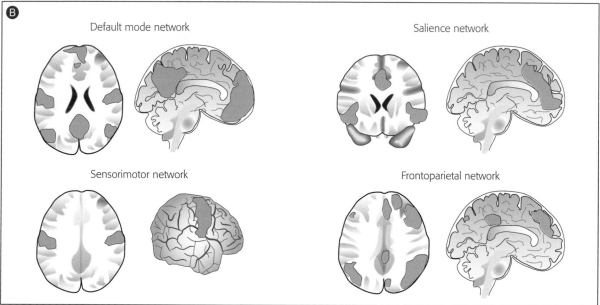

FIGURE 11-25 ■ (A, B) The brain can be represented as different interrelated networks where the nodes correspond to constitutive elements, or nodes. The presence of chronic pain may alter the properties of these modules through changes in inter- or intramodular interactions, through peripheral and central mechanisms. *Reproduced with permission from Farmer et al.*[365]

Chronic pain is associated with increased central processing in different brain areas, including the salience network, and may be accompanied by an extensive cortical reorganization. In addition, brain activity for chronic pain shifts away from the pattern shown for acute pain to more prefrontal and limbic circuitry.

The explanation of complex pain in the absence of significant pathology could be found in these brain changes. Therefore, if the problem is not in the tissues yet in the brain, therapeutic strategies must ultimately be focused on reversing these changes.

Despite the impressive development of neuroimaging techniques in recent years, the knowledge we have today is partial and limited and does not provide clinical biomarkers that can be used in the diagnosis of chronic pain patients. Moreover, pain is a complex experience that cannot be reduced to biomarkers from a mechanistic perspective.

In conclusion, as stated by Baliki et al.,[367] the brain of a chronic pain patient is not merely a healthy brain processing pain information, but rather a brain altered by the persistent pain in a manner reminiscent of other neurological conditions associated with cognitive impairments.

PAIN AND NEUROBIOLOGICAL MODELS

The gate control theory of pain proposed by Melzack and Wall[23] in 1965 can be considered to be the beginning of the development of modern current neurobiological models of pain.

The gate control theory of pain

Melzack and Wall[23] developed the gate control theory to explain that there is no linear and direct relationship between nociceptive input and pain (Fig. 11-26). This theory represented a crucial change in the understanding of pain, not only in giving an explanation to the central modulation of nociceptive signals but also because it regarded pain as the result of an interaction between physical and psychological aspects. This theory, although modified over the years, maintains its basic concepts.[67,368]

Melzack and Wall's theory proposed that at different CNS levels, and mainly in the dorsal horn of the spinal cord, there are mechanisms modulating the transmission of nociceptive input. It suggested that a large number of both nociceptive and Aß primary afferent fibres, excitatory and inhibitory interneurons and descending fibres coming from the higher CNS centres, converge in the gelatinous substance. The theory is based on the following:

1. The transmission of nociceptive stimuli of afferent fibres to the second-order nociceptive neurons (SONN) can be removed or amplified by a gate mechanism in the dorsal horns.
2. The control mechanism is dependent on the stimuli reaching the dorsal horn. An increase in the activity of nociceptive fibres tends to facilitate transmission (opens the gate), while activity in large-diameter non-nociceptive fibres, such as Aß touch fibres, tends to inhibit transmission (closes the gate).
3. The control gate mechanism is influenced, in turn, by supraspinal stimuli. Stimulation of large-diameter fibres determines activity of the central control system on the spinal gate system, modulating transmission.

This theory represented a revolution in the conception of pain as, from then on, pain was not merely seen as a physical reflex sensation, the result of nociceptive stimulation. Peripheral nociceptive information is being continuously modulated both by other peripheral non-nociceptive information and by the influence of the CNS.[369]

The theory forced clinicians and researchers to understand the CNS, not as a mere receiver of information, but as an active system that filters, selects and modulates inputs. The dorsal horns were not merely passive transmission stations but sites at which dynamic activities such as inhibition, excitation and modulation occurred.[370]

The gate control theory of pain was the first model that attempted to explain how different sensory and psychological factors could activate the modular and descending inhibitory systems and therefore the perception of pain. This theory attempts to design an integrative theoretical model able to explain the lack of direct correlation between injury, nociception and pain as well as different individual responses, including psychological responses, to injury and pain.

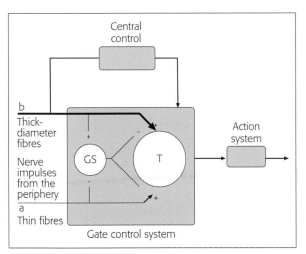

FIGURE 11-26 ■ Gate control theory. Nociceptive neurons (a) and non-nociceptive neurons (b) projecting in lamina II (gelatinous substance – GS) and in the central transmission fibres (T). The increase in activity of thick-diameter non-nociceptive fibres (b) exerts an inhibitory effect on GS which reduces the activation of T fibres. These fibres also trigger increased CNS modulating activity.

Melzack[370,371] postulated for the first time that different brain areas that determine the experience of pain after nociceptive activation could evoke that same pain perception even in the absence of an active nociceptive source.

The parallel processing theory

In 1968, Melzack and Casey[372] developed an extension of the gate control theory: namely, the parallel processing theory. This theory suggested that there were different systems involved in the various sensory, emotional and cognitive aspects that characterize the pain experience. In this theory the stimuli that reach the dorsal horn are simultaneously transmitted through different channels: some give sensory-discriminative information and others affective-motivational information of pain. The higher centres of central modulation and cognitive control influence both systems (sensory-discriminative and affective-motivational) once they have evaluated all the information, checking it against past experiences and determining an adapted response (Fig. 11-27). The experience of pain could be modulated by sensory, cognitive and emotional mechanisms.

This theory of parallel processing has been supported by later research showing how the different components of the pain experience use different pathways and end in different brain structures. Sensory-discriminative components depend primarily on the spinothalamic tract or trigeminothalmic tract, in the case of the cephalic extremity, establishing a synapse with the posterior ventral nucleus of the thalamus and from there reaching the primary and secondary somatosensory cortex. Affective-motivational components use other pathways that project to the reticular formation, particularly the parabrachial nucleus, and intralaminar nuclei of the thalamus and also to the cingulate cortex, insula, frontal lobe, amygdala and hypothalamus (Figs 11-28 and 11-29). Finally, Melzack[373] in 1990 developed the model that has had more influence as a paradigm of pain with the *neuromatrix theory*.

Body-self neuromatrix concept

Melzack developed the concept of body-self neuromatrix as a new theoretical model of perception which, among other things, was able to reveal the complexity of pain and could serve as a model explaining many situations of pain such as phantom limb pain or pain experienced in the lower limbs by subjects who have suffered a complete spinal cord section.[290,370,371,374]

Melzack proposed that the brain possesses a widespread network of neurons in many areas, the body-self

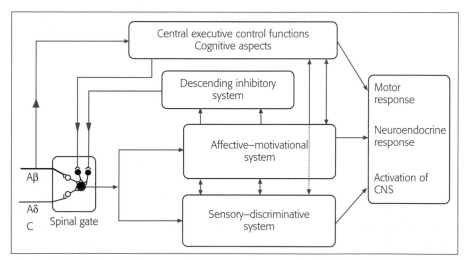

FIGURE 11-27 ■ The parallel processing theory emphasizes that the painful information ascends by different pathways: some give sensory-discriminative information and others give affective-motivational information of pain. Higher centres influence both systems (sensory-discriminative and affective-motivational) once they have evaluated all the information against past experiences and determined an appropriate response.

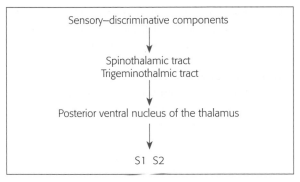

FIGURE 11-28 ■ Sensory-discriminative components depend primarily on the spinothalamic tract or trigeminothalmic tract, establishing a synapse with the posterior ventral nucleus of the thalamus and from there reaching the primary and secondary somatosensory cortex.

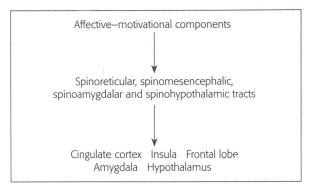

FIGURE 11-29 ■ Affective-motivational components use other pathways that project to the reticular formation, particularly the parabrachial nucleus, and intralaminar nuclei of the thalamus and also to the cingulate cortex, insula, frontal lobe, amygdala and hypothalamus.

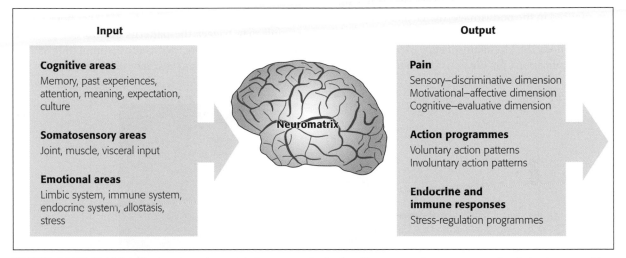

FIGURE 11-30 ■ Melzack's neuromatrix model. Inputs to the body-self neuromatrix are sensory discriminative, cognitive-evaluative and emotional. Outputs of the body-self neuromatrix are pain, action programmes and endocrine and immune responses.

neuromatrix, from which all bodily perceptions derive and finally produces the pattern that is felt as a whole body possessing a sense of self.[375] The neuromatrix not only creates the perception but also is responsible for the different motor, emotional, behavioural and sensory responses associated with each body experience. Synaptic architecture of the neuromatrix is determined by genetic inheritance, but it suffers profound modifications by individual somatosensory and emotional experiences, learning and the cognitive functions of the brain.[370] The neuromatrix consists of different parallel somatosensory, limbic and thalamocortical components responsible for sensory-discriminative, affective-motivational and evaluative-cognitive dimensions of the experience of pain (Fig. 11-30). The areas of the brain involved in pain experience and behaviour are widespread as, in addition to the somatosensory system, they must include the homeostatic, visual and vestibular system, the limbic system as well as cognitive areas of the brain.[375]

Synaptic architecture of the neuromatrix is determined by genetic inheritance, but it suffers profound modifications by individual somatosensory and emotional experiences, learning and cognitions.

The various components constituting the neuromatrix diverge to permit parallel processing and converge to permit the interactions between the output products of processing. These responses are triggered by the activation of a specific neurosignature, which determines the particular qualities of experience and of pain behaviour. Different neurosignatures can be triggered by nociceptive stimuli, but also independently of them.

The neuromatrix theory assumes that this pain is experienced in the body image, the virtual body, which has the brain. As Melzack said, 'You do not need a body to feel a body'.[376] The neuromatrix concept has profound implications for the consideration of pain and opens the door to the development of new clinical and therapeutic approaches. Pain is not a reflex response to a nociceptive stimulus but a multidimensional experience produced by specific neurosignatures generated by an extensive cerebral neural network. This theory moves away from the pathoanatomical model of pain. Pain is not the consequence of a stimulus but a response generated by the CNS.

Pain is not a reflex response to a nociceptive stimulus but a multidimensional experience produced by specific neurosignatures generated by an extensive cerebral neural network

Nociceptive stimuli, according to this model, are not able to generate the experience of pain and its associated response but can only activate a specific neurosignature that triggers a pattern of response, of which pain is a part (Fig. 11-31). The nociceptive stimuli may trigger the patterns but do not produce them.[375] Furthermore, nociceptive stimulation is one of the many different stimuli that can act on the

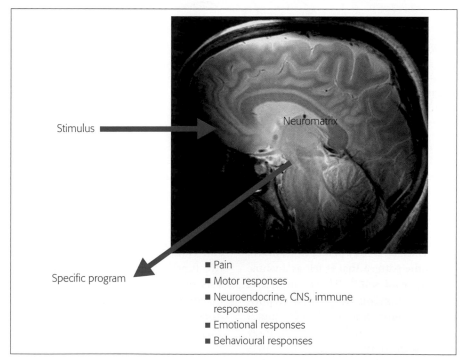

FIGURE 11-31 ■ Nociceptive stimuli, according to this model, are not able to generate the experience of pain and its associated response, but can only activate a specific neurosignature that triggers a pattern of response, of which pain is a part.

neuromatrix and trigger a specific neurosignature. The brain is, therefore, an active system which filters, modulates and selects those responses that it then considers most appropriate. Hence, the neural networks in the brain can produce all of the body's perceptive experiences, including pain, without a nociceptive stimulus. Research data have demonstrated how a painful experience can occur without an active nociceptive input.[91,92,377–379]

The result can be summarized in the statement that 'nociception does not hurt'. Pain, as each of the perceptual experiences, is already stored in the brain as a programme (neurosignature); only the presence of a consistent stimulus for the activation of this programme is required. That explains how the response to various types of pain such as cutaneous, somatic and visceral pain is similar among individuals, especially in early childhood. Individuals also express very different responses that are determined by the individual's previous experiences, learning, social environment and culture. The social and family environment, as well as culture, are critical in giving a full 'meaning' to the individual experience of pain. Another fundamental aspect is that the neurosignature not only involves the perception of pain but also a series of complex responses: neuroendocrine, behavioural and motor responses due to activation so-called 'action-neuromatrix' according to Melzack.[376] Also, the psychological responses are no longer reactions secondary to pain and are viewed as an integral part of the experience. Thus, an explanation is given to the biological effects of those forms of intervention in pain capable of modulating these psychological responses.[370]

Inputs to the body-self neuromatrix are sensory-discriminative, cognitive-evaluative such as own cognitions, past experiences, cultural learning, etc., and motivational-affective, including emotions, hypothalamic–pituitary–adrenal system, noradrenaline-sympathetic system, immune system and all brain limbic structures.

The various stimuli that can trigger a pain neurosignature include:

1. Nociceptive sensory stimuli.
2. Non-nociceptive sensory stimuli that the subject has associated with pain.
3. Visual stimuli or other sensory stimuli that influence the interpretation of the situation.
4. Cognitive stimuli such as the relationship established by the patient between a stimulus and the perception of pain, fear of pain or of injury.
5. Affective stimuli associated with the painful experience.
6. The activity of the stress-regulation systems of the body.

The cognitive and emotional aspects of this model are as valuable as nociceptive and somatosensory stimuli in the activation of a neurosignature and in triggering the pain response.

Neuromatrix responses can be divided, according to Melzack,[374,375] into pain perception, action programmes and stress-regulation programmes (Fig. 11-32).

The pain perception programmes include the whole pain experience in all its cognitive-evaluative, sensory-discriminative and affective-motivational dimensions. The action programmes comprise the voluntary and involuntary motor patterns and behavioural responses, coping strategies and social communication of the experience. The stress-regulation programmes include all the homeostatic responses, including the endocrine, autonomic, immune and opioid systems. Therefore, the output patterns from the neuromatrix produce the multiple dimensions of pain experience as well as concurrent and behavioural dimensions.

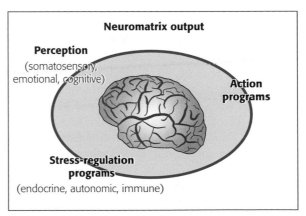

FIGURE 11-32 ■ Neuromatrix outputs can be divided into pain perception, action programmes and stress-regulation programmes.

All potentially threatening stimuli trigger the simultaneous activation of different neural networks, including basic responses such as motor protection and immune neuroendocrine responses, activation of somatosensory areas, limbic networks and cognitive areas. The 'switch' concept is useful for the patient to understand that the physical stimuli, which reproduce their pain, are not the 'cause' but the trigger. Actions or movements that cause pain are simply individual learned 'switches'. The fact that a movement causes pain in no way implies that there is 'injury' in the body, but that movement in that particular individual is assessed as a consistent stimulus to trigger activation of the pain programme.

The neuromatrix theory proposes that brain mechanisms may underlie chronic pain and points to new forms of treatment.[375] This theory establishes that the neuromatrix output determines whether pain will be experienced or suppressed. Pain suppression can be determined not only by the release of endorphins and other opioids but also by sensory, discriminative and evaluative processes.

Melzack stressed that pain can no longer be regarded as a purely sensory phenomenon, as it also disrupts the homeostatic regulation systems of the brain, thereby producing stress and initiating complex programmes to restore homeostasis. Acknowledging the role of the stress system in pain processes offered new understandings in terms of homeostasis for the development of chronic pain and disability. Different stressors can activate programmes of neural, hormonal and behavioural activity aimed at restoring homeostasis. If stress responses continue, they lead to immune system suppression and activation of the limbic system (which has a role in the emotional, motivational and cognitive processes). Therefore stress and pain perception possess overlapping mechanisms. Prolonged activation of the stress-regulation systems can lead to the development of chronic pain conditions as well as depression. Pain in itself can be a strong stressor if it implies danger and threat to the self, physically or psychologically.

The neuromatrix theory has been considered one of the most important contributions to pain research because it challenged profoundly seated assumptions about the nature of pain and somatosensory perception.[380] Nociceptive input may initiate pain but, it is not the only, or even the dominant, causal mechanism. Pain is not the consequence of a passive brain registering tissue trauma, but rather the product of an active brain forming subjective experience in response to sensory signalling or any other contextual clue.[380]

Pain is not the consequence of a passive brain registering tissue trauma, but rather the product of an active brain forming subjective experience in response to sensory signalling or any other contextual clue.

The neuromatrix concept has been very influential among researchers and clinicians dedicated to pain. The literature of pain has popularized different terms that seemed to mean the same as 'pain matrix',[381,382] 'pain neuromatrix'[383] or 'pain signature'.[112] However, Melzack did not restrict the neuromatrix to the perception of pain, but made it extensive to any perception and, above all, to the concept of generating self-awareness.[374]

Melzack,[374] in his neuromatrix theory, introduced the role of awareness in self-perception. One of the important aspects of this theory was the unifying concept of perception of the body as a unit, the 'self', different from other individuals and the environment. Melzack[374] defined the body-self neuromatrix as a distributed cerebral system but functionally integrated which works as a whole and allows us to feel the body as a unit with different qualities at different times. The neuromatrix would be the anatomical substrate of the body-self. The experience of the self is thus generated by central neural processes, as it cannot be produced by the peripheral nervous system or the spinal cord.

The body-self neuromatrix generates a continuous outflow, the neurosignature, which is projected to areas in the brain, 'the sentient neural hub', wherein the stream of nerve impulses becomes a continuous flow of awareness. The neurosignature patterns bifurcate, some to the sentient neural hub (where the pattern is converted into the experience) and others to activate the action programmes (motor, endocrine or immune responses). According to Melzack,[375] the four components of this new conceptual nervous system are (1) the body-self neuromatrix; (2) cyclical processing and synthesis in which the neurosignature is produced; (3) the sentient neural hub, which transforms the flow of neurosignatures into awareness; and (4) activation of an action neuromatrix to provide the motor, neuroendocrine and behavioural responses.

As stated by Melzack[384] the future of pain implies the shift from a bottom-up to a 'top-down strategy that begins with brain function, and conscious experience will expand the field of pain research by incorporating the rapidly growing knowledge of cognitive neuroscience and the evolution of the brain'. As Chapman and Nakamura[385] emphasized, the study of consciousness should enhance the study of pain. Although the neural mechanisms implicated in nociception and consciousness are clearly different, pain as a phenomenal experience is a 'constructed subset of consciousness'.

The mature organism model

This model was developed by Gifford[386] as a tool to help give both clinicians and patients a broader under-

standing of pain, in its biological context, integrating the knowledge outlined above. This model integrates the three levels involved in the pain experience: input level (uptake of nociceptive information); processing level (the central pain processing); and output level (elaboration of responses). The body detects the information from both tissues and environmental changes, it processes the information obtained, and prepares responses tailored to address the perceived aggression.

Instead of a 'linear' model (tissue injury – central pain perception) this 'circular' model emphasizes how the experience of pain can start at any level determining impact on the rest.[84] (Fig. 11-33).

One aspect emphasized by the model is the close relationship between pain and stress response. The stress response biology analyses the physiological mechanisms and behavioural strategies that equip organisms for survival and the maintenance of

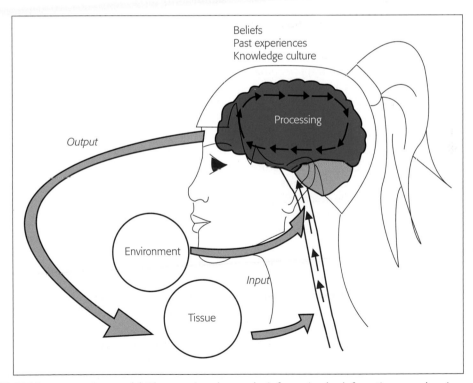

FIGURE 11-33 ■ Mature organism model. The organism detects the information both from tissues and environmental changes (input), it processes the information obtained (central processing) and prepares responses adapted to address the perceived aggression (output). The information is processed both consciously and unconsciously, comparing it with past experiences and responses that include changes in motor activity and in the autonomic, neuroendocrine and neuroimmune nervous systems. *Adapted from Gifford.[386] Reproduced with permission.*

homeostasis. Pain is one of the sensory components of the stress response whose first adaptive purpose is to encourage the body to modify its behaviour in order to facilitate recovery and survival. The nociceptive system, instead of being described as a system directed to pain, becomes, together with the endocrine and immune system, part, firstly, of a system for analysing the state of tissues and innervated structures and, secondly, of a system able to develop adapted motor or behavioural responses.

The information is processed both consciously and unconsciously, it is compared to past experiences, and responses are developed that include changes in motor activity and in the autonomic, neuroendocrine and neuroimmune and motor systems.[387]

So, in the case of an injury to the tissues, the CNS of the mature organism can access information stored in the conscious and unconscious memory, past experiences and successful behaviours that may be relevant to the situation and can help develop a response directed to restore homeostasis.[388] When there has been tissue injury or the subject perceives that this is possible, this produces pain, an emotional, motor and behavioural response and physiological responses that facilitate recovery. These responses have, in turn, a consequence on the peripheral tissues and determine neuroplastic changes in the CNS.

Any pain experience is divided into three levels: uptake of nociceptive information; pain; and preparation of responses. Based on the model of the mature organism, three pathobiological mechanisms and three distinct categories of pain can be described: pain related to input information; pain related to central processing; and pain related to response systems.

These categories facilitate the analysis of the patient's type of pain. Instead of only thinking of the anatomical structure which is the source of pain, attention is directed to pathobiological processes or mechanisms which are dominant in the clinical picture.[84]

- **Pain related to input information** – the pain associated with a nociceptive input. This model also shows that the input capacity to evoke a pain response is context-dependent.
- **Pain related to central processing** – the pain is the consequence of central processing so that there is no nociceptive input or it is irrelevant.

The central processing is dependent on cognitive aspects (interpretation, previous experiences, consequences evaluation) and affective (emotional distress, mood).

- **Pain related to response systems** – the pain is secondary to response mechanisms and involves an impaired response of the motor system, autonomic nervous system, neuroendocrine or neuroimmume systems. Examples of this type of pain include the complex regional pain syndrome and pain associated with inflammatory and immune arthropathy.

Although all these mechanisms interact and occur in every experience of pain, in some subjects one will be dominant. In acute pain, the dominant mechanism is related to the input information. In chronic pain, the dominant mechanism may be related to central processing, in which cognitive and affective aspects are significantly involved, and response mechanisms.[389] For patient evaluation and treatment, it is essential to determine which mechanism is dominant.

Pain, emotions and stress response

Chapman,[56,58,390] from a psychophysiological perspective, developed the relationship between emotional components of pain and stress response. As noted by this author, many health professionals consider emotions as epiphenomena of mental activity, of a subjective nature and scarcely important for physical health.[390] However, emotions are the result of complex physiological responses, and conscious recognition is a secondary aspect.

Emotions are primarily physiological reactions, only being secondarily subjective. They consist of two aspects: an objective aspect (the activation of the autonomic nervous and neuroendocrine systems) and a subjective aspect (feelings).

Emotion is not the consequence of the sensation of pain, which arises after a noxious sensory message reaches the somatosensory cortex, but rather is a fundamental part of the experience of pain. It is therefore important to consider pain as an emotion. Thus considered, pain is interpreted as a threat to the individual's biological integrity. The magnitude of the emotional component of pain is proportional to its perception as a threat.[56–58] As stated by Moseley,[116] pain is produced by the brain when it perceives a threat to the individual and therefore requires an action to avoid it. All dimensions of pain are aimed at this goal.

Emotions intervene decisively in consciousness and their function is to generate information that is important when making a selection from among several behaviours. They provide subjective information that is useful to develop a necessary behaviour, such as fight or flight, for the preservation of the individual and the species.[56,58] In addition, the emotions aroused by pain have a social function. The external verbal, gestural, behavioural and physical manifestations of emotion are a useful form of communication to obtain social support in situations that pose a threat to survival.[56]

The magnitude of the emotional component of pain is proportional to its perception as a threat signal. Emotions intervene decisively in consciousness to generate information important in selecting homeostatic behaviours.

The intense negative emotion that pain implies is expressed in a sympatho-neural and sympatho-adrenal response and with the activation of the hypothalamic–pituitary–adrenal (HPA) axis. The secretion of adrenaline and other catecholamines in the adrenal medulla is stimulated by acetylcholine of the preganglionic sympathetic fibres. Activity in the spinothalamic pathways, as well as in the ponto-hypothalamic pathways also activates the HPA axis.[177] The stimulation of the paraventricular nucleus of the hypothalamus triggers the release of the corticotrophin-releasing factor (CRF), initiating a complex adaptive neuroendocrine stress response in the HPA axis that triggers the release of cortisol[391–394] (Fig. 11-34).

The CRF is a neurotransmitter that activates the descending locus caeruleus–noradrenergic modulator system which also causes the release of noradrenaline.[54,394–396] Cortisol maintains high glucose levels necessary for a stress response. This response prepares the body for an emergency response and promotes survival in threatening circumstances for a limited time. These factors involved in stress response intervene in memory consolidation of emotionally adverse experiences.[397–402]

The stress response becomes maladaptive when the stressor persists, partly because the actions of glucocorticoids are fundamentally catabolic. An increased and maintained sympathomimetic response such as increased heart rate is a predictor of later development of PTSD.[403–406]

The development of a chronic pain syndrome is the result of the interaction between a dysregulation of the stress response system and cognitive-behavioural factors.

Maladaptive stress is a self-sustaining cascade of neural, endocrine and immune responses that degrade health and physical and mental well-being of the individual. Chronic pain, therefore, is not an isolated symptom, but is often accompanied by other problems such as chronic fatigue, sleep disturbance, decreased physical activity, altered endocrine and immune function and altered mood.[65] Maladaptive stress may favour a situation of generalized sensory hypersensitivity, which can be expressed as photophobia, phonophobia, osmophobia, intolerance to cold or heat, stress intolerance, etc.

The immune system plays an important role in stress response and pain perception.[59–62] Immune changes, secondary to injury, not only increase the perception of pain[63] but also cause changes in behaviour, mood, motivation and cognition.[63–65] Thus, the activity of the immune system is responsible for the generalized sickness response, including secondary changes in mood, but cognitive and emotional aspects can also have a powerful effect on the immune system.

THE CONCEPT OF REPRESENTATION AND THE CORTICAL BODY MATRIX

Moseley et al.,[119] in a review of different body illusions, have recently developed the concept of the 'cortical body matrix'. The brain has neural representations responsible for mapping our body. These representations are distributed in different areas of the brain, including every area with a somatotopic organization. These somatotopic representations allow us to perceive the localization of any stimulus our body receives. Classical somatotopic areas include S1, S2 and ventral posterior nucleus of the thalamus. However, the

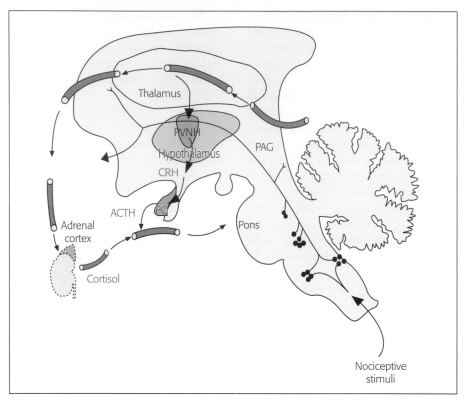

FIGURE 11-34 ■ The neuroendocrine stress response. Nociceptive information reaches different nuclei of the medulla oblongata and of the projection reaching the paraventricular nucleus of the hypothalamus (PVNH). Excitation triggers the production of corticotrophin-releasing hormone (CRH), which stimulates the release of adrenocorticotrophic hormone (ACTH) from the apophysis into the general circulation. This hormone stimulates the adrenal cortex to release corticosteroids to that general circulation. *Modified from Chapman.*[390] *Reproduced with permission.*

activation of these areas is not sufficient for conscious stimulus perception. As shown by Schubert et al.,[407] conscious perception depends on additional access of the input into higher-order cortical areas such as parietal and frontal cortices. As these areas have been related to spatial selective attention, it is clear therefore that attention is needed in conscious perception. Our body representation continuously receives information from different brain areas that encode visual, exteroceptive, proprioceptive and input information. So this representation is multisensorial, and is being continuously modulated by all this information. It also includes objects with which we 'live with'.

The brain, besides somatosensory information, has also neural representations responsible for mapping the space around the body.[119] The representation of this 'peripersonal space' provides information about the position of objects in the surrounding environment with respect to the body. This representation permits the planning and execution of movements to protect the body from any physical threat in the immediate environment. This representation is also included in the cortical body matrix. A characteristic of this peripersonal space representation is that the body matrix is aligned with a body-centred rather than a hand-centred frame of reference. It means that when a stimuli arises from the right side of external space it is mapped in the body matrix as 'right', even though it is applied to the left part of the body. Therefore, changes in normal representation may be more dependent on the space than on somatotopy.

The cortical body matrix is not only somatosensorial but also motor, emotional and homeostatic. It is flexible and context-dependent, so what and how we feel in a moment can be radically different at another moment. What we feel in a certain moment is our synchronical representation, but this can shift in a second to a diachronical one, how we felt at another moment, and it can even recreate a representation we had many years ago.

A crucial aspect is that cortical body matrix would be responsible for the cognitive aspects of self-perception: our body awareness and our sense of ownership. So it could be considered as the anatomical substrate of our body-self. Many brain areas would be involved in these mechanisms of multisensory integration of self-perception and action such as posterior parietal cortex (sensorimotor integration and spatial perception), and insular cortex (interoceptive awareness, emotional experience, homeostasis, body temperature).[119,408,409] Representational changes would explain the phenomena of cognitive, sensory and motor pseudo-neglect frequently seen in chronic pain patients.

DEVELOPMENT OF CHRONIC PAIN: PREDISPOSING AND TRIGGER FACTORS

Pain is an inherent human experience. Everyone experiences acute pain; however, just a small proportion of people develop chronic pain, and a lower percentage of these will evolve towards disability. In the development of chronic pain and pain-related disability, various physical and psychosocial aspects can act as predisposing and trigger factors.

The existence of predisposing physiological and psychological factors, as well as the need for early identification to prevent chronic pain,[94,410–414] has been the subject of many studies.

Physiological predisposing factors

The existence of a physiological predisposition may be due to genetic variables. There seems to be a genetic influence on inter-individual differences in sensitivity to pain and the response to analgesics.[415] Genetics is an emerging discipline and, as often happens in these cases, perhaps too many answers in the field of chronic pain are expected. Research that in principle can provide information on the role of genes relates to studies in twins and in animals, mostly conducted with transgenic knockout mice.

Multiple genes may be involved with genetic interactions, but also with gene–environment interactions and epigenetic variants. More than 200 candidate genes have been proposed in the modulation of pain, but of all of them, only a few have been associated with phenotypes of pain in humans. Those proposed include polymorphisms in the genes involved in the catecholaminergic systems (COMT), serotoninergic and dopaminergic systems, and genes involved in the expression of ion channels. A few years ago, the group of Jeffrey S. Mogil[416] launched a database of genes involved in pain (http://www.jbldesign.com/jmogil/enter.html). Currently it is difficult to make a reliable estimate of the genetic component of chronic pain syndromes, because of the complex interactions between gene–environment, psychological comorbidity and aspects of family learning.[417,418]

Prior physical and psychological trauma

Adverse experiences in childhood, either physical or psychological, as well as child abuse, sexual abuse and neglect, are factors that increase the vulnerability of individuals and may predispose them to the development of chronic pain in adulthood.[419–424] Among the types of abuse, sexual abuse in both men and women most influences the development of chronic pain.[423] In this case, pain in the pelvic area is the most prevalent complaint.[425,426] However, this issue has also been controversial. A prospective study based on documented cases of child abuse and neglect found no evidence of a relationship between victimization and pain complaints in adulthood.[427] These same authors, 10 years later, in a long-term follow-up of these subjects, showed that childhood experience of a PTSD as a result of early childhood abuse or neglect was a significant predictor in the development of chronic pain.[428] It is therefore important to understand that the crucial factor and predictor of increased chronic pain is not trauma, but the PTSD related to it.

Stressors in childhood are not only a risk factor for developing chronic pain in adulthood but also in the development of various chronic diseases such as inflammatory arthropathies, heart disease, diabetes and autoimmune diseases.[429–431] Neurobiological mechanisms involved are derived from a high-stress situation in childhood capable of producing long-term changes in hypothalamic–pituitary–adrenocortical activity, sensitization of central pain processing mechanisms and somatic hypervigilance.[430,432–435]

It is essential, therefore, in the evaluation of patients with pain, to explore not only the current history but also aspects such as premorbid conditions or prior physical and psychosocial traumatic events that may contribute to understanding the patient's experience of pain.[431]

As discussed later, the patient's near environment, and foremost, the family, is directly related to the development of a chronic pain syndrome. The social and family learning and memory are key variables in perception and tolerance and in establishing behaviours of pain and disability.[414]

Trigger factors

The most important physical and psychosocial triggering factors include high severity of pain at the onset of the symptoms.[436] Sometimes the pain is not severe, but has a high emotional impact for the subject. At other times the development of chronic pain is due to a concomitant and emotional situation not directly related to pain. Today we have ample evidence of the fact that difficult emotional experiences, traumas and interpersonal conflicts contribute to the perpetuation of pain.[93,437]

Problematic emotional experiences, traumas and interpersonal conflicts contribute to the perpetuation of pain.

This is even more evident in patients with complex pain or pain secondary to maladaptive central sensitization. A recent systematic review has shown a significant association between a traumatic psychological experience and the development of a functional somatic syndrome.[438]

Pain and personal conflicts

A key aspect, without which it would be difficult to understand why a patient has developed chronic pain, lies in the patient's personal biography. Many cases of pain show underlying personal or interpersonal conflicts that, unless they emerge, make it hardly possible

to obtain stable results with a pain programme. As Van Houdenhove[419] points out, it is very important to create feelings of trust with patients, asking questions non-intrusively and respectfully, so that they can 'open up' and tell their 'whole story'. Asking about issues of a personal nature is justified only if they are relevant to the patient's pain management. Unfortunately, at present, many patients are offered only analgesic drugs and interventional techniques without attempting to understand the role played by different social, psychological or family aspects in their experience. In other cases, patients are handled with a 'standard cognitive-behavioural approach', despite the evidence implying that traumatic experiences and personal conflicts can be the source of pain. An approach that fails to address the personal problems of these patients will probably offer a scarce reduction of pain and disability.[439]

Post-traumatic stress and pain

Pain may be associated with a post-traumatic stress disorder (PTSD) as a result, for example, of experiencing a road traffic accident, having witnessed a war scenario, surviving torture, having been abused, etc.[438,440,441] For example, 80% of veterans who have PTSD suffer from chronic pain.[442] The symptoms that characterize PTSD are the intrusive re-experiencing of symptoms associated with the traumatic event, cognitive avoidance of memories or situations that evoke it, cognitive and emotional disturbances that begin or get worse after the traumatic event and physiological hyper-reactivity.[443]

The high comorbidity between PTSD and chronic pain can be explained by the fact that both conditions share similar mechanisms, such as selective attention to certain stimuli, avoidance behaviours, etc., which promote its self-perpetuation.[444] Importantly, PTSD is often diagnosed in patients who show a high level of distress after a traumatic event, such as a road traffic accident, without the diagnostic criteria actually being met.

Physical abuse, intimate partner aggression and sexual abuse are associated with significant psychological distress and, as previously mentioned, are involved in the development of chronic pain and other physical and psychological health problems.[445–452] (Fig. 11-35).

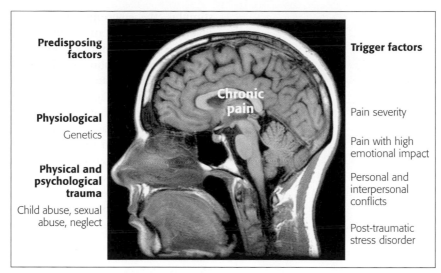

Predisposing factors

Physiological
Genetics

Physical and psychological trauma
Child abuse, sexual abuse, neglect

Chronic pain

Trigger factors

Pain severity

Pain with high emotional impact

Personal and interpersonal conflicts

Post-traumatic stress disorder

FIGURE 11-35 ■ Development of chronic pain: predisposing physiological (genetics), physical and psychological factors, trigger factors (acute injury or disease, personal conflicts, post-traumatic stress).

PAIN AND PSYCHOLOGICAL ASPECTS

It is important to focus on the role of different psychological aspects and chronic pain for four reasons: persistent pain can induce a cascade of neurological processes capable of modifying physiological responses; pain perception is highly modifiable by psychological aspects[453,454]; different psychological aspects involved in the experience of pain can act as mediators in the transition from acute to chronic pain[413]; and, finally, a preliminary psychological condition can increase the risk of pain becoming chronic due to a 'cross-sensitization' mechanism.[282] For example, having suffered a stress situation in the past, such as having suffered abuse in childhood, can lead to greater sensitivity, causing pain to become chronic.[430] Therefore, it is of considerable interest to know which factors are involved in the development of chronic pain such as attention, beliefs, emotions and past experiences.

PSYCHOLOGICAL FACTORS AND CHRONIC PAIN

- Persistent pain can induce a cascade of neurological processes capable of modifying physiological responses.
- The perception of pain is extremely changeable, based on psychological aspects.

- Different psychological aspects involved in the experience of pain can act as mediators in the transition from acute to chronic pain,
- A previous psychological condition can increase the risk of pain becoming chronic by a 'cross-sensitization' mechanism.

Linton and Shaw[94] describe a possible sequence of the processes involved in the development of chronic pain. After the initial awareness of a noxious stimulus, the subject develops a cognitive processing, both conscious and unconscious, in which the interpretation of pain determines certain pain behaviours. These pain behaviours will be determined by the individual's interpretation of the meaning of pain based on previous experiences and social and cultural learning (Fig. 11-36). The processing is often not dependent on the intensity of the nociceptive stimulus, but on its relevance for the patient at a given time and in a given context.

Attention

Pain, as a biologically relevant stimulus, demands attention.[113] Attention is a critical protection mechanism because it leads to adaptive responses to potential injury. Ignoring the pain, especially when having characteristics that generate a major alarm such as severe

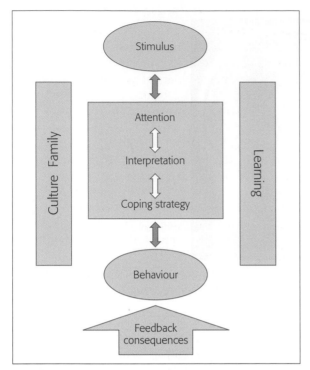

FIGURE 11-36 ■ Possible sequence of the processes involved in the development of chronic pain. *Reproduced with permission from Linton and Shaw.*[94]

pain or different from any other pain previously experienced, is not a biologically adaptive behavior.[94] The function of attention is therefore to motivate appropriate behaviour against a real or potential threat.

Attention can significantly modulate both sensory and affective aspects of the pain experience.[108,455,456] It has been demonstrated that attention not only modulates the intensity of the stimulus but also that it can modulate its temporal perception. Zampini et al.[457] presented a painful stimulus and a visual stimulus randomly at different stimulus onset asynchronies. It was shown that when attention was directed toward the painful stimulus, it was perceived as occurring earlier than when it was directed toward the visual stimulus. This phenomenon is known as the 'prior-entry effect.'[458]

Attention, as already mentioned, is primarily dependent on two different aspects: stimulus salience and relevance.[86] Salience involves a bottom-up capture of attention and depends on the novelty of the stimulus, the environmental context, etc. Relevance involves top-down attentional control and depends on subjective cognitions, motivations, etc. Patients with chronic pain show a selective attention to pain and high hypervigilance, the degree of attention being dependent on the painful stimulus when perceived as potentially threatening.[113,459] The greater the perceived threat, the greater the attention, fear and anxiety and, therefore, the greater the awareness of pain. Attention to pain, in this case, is a top-down phenomenon that relates to the degree of relevance for biological integrity that the subject gives the stimulus. Attention is then dependent on real or imagined previous experiences, the reappraisal of the experience and the meaning of pain.[99]

Distraction is a classic therapeutic strategy in pain. However, intentional efforts to 'be distracted' from pain can be counterproductive.[460] A more useful strategy in patients with chronic pain is to 'involve' them in carrying out tasks and achieving personal goals. Strategies requiring attention can help to reduce pain in chronic pain patients,[461] especially if they involve an 'immersion' in the task. Examples include the paradigm of *virtual reality distraction*. But what provides a more 'distracting' effect to a task or activity is its affective-motivational valence: it must be pleasant, meaningful or emotionally important to the subject.[106] Therefore, an important aspect in a pain management programme is to encourage the patient to seek and try to achieve significant goals in everyday life and to participate in valued activities. This strategy significantly reduces the attention focused on pain and its perception as something threatening, and therefore improves daily performance.[462]

An important aspect in a pain management programme is to encourage the patient to seek and try to achieve significant goals in everyday life and to participate in valued activities.

The effect of attention on perception has been the subject of numerous neuroimaging studies. Attention can exert a powerful modulation of pain not only in its sensory aspects but also in its emotional aspects in multiple brain areas that encode sensory, cognitive and affective aspects of pain.[108,109,113,455,456,463–465] During distraction, activation is observed in areas involved in

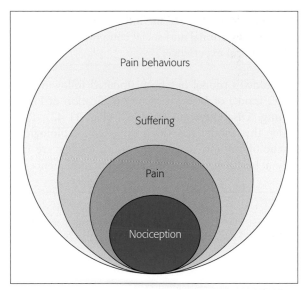

FIGURE 11-40 ■ Loeser's model establishes four hierarchical levels: nociception, pain, suffering and pain behaviours.

are already coming into play, and this is what explains why two individuals exhibit different responses to the same painful stimulation. Also, a single individual may not feel pain or otherwise experience unbearable pain, depending on his or her emotional state and the circumstances at the time. As Bausbaum and Jessell[663] point out, pain more than any other sensory modality is influenced by the emotional state and environmental contingencies.

Suffering is a negative affective response generated at the higher levels of the CNS by pain or other unpleasant emotional situations, which trigger a more or less intense stress response. There may, therefore, be pain without suffering and suffering without pain. Pain from a teleological perspective is perceived as a threat to the biological integrity.[56–58] Suffering involves a sense of loss of control, helplessness, intolerability and meaninglessness.[540]

Pain behaviours are all those behaviours or external manifestations observed in the subject and associated with the experience of pain. These behaviours include the verbal or non-verbal communication of the painful experience by the subject, such as facial expression denoting pain; analgesic consumption; seeking medical attention; requesting time off work; and changes in family relationships.

Fordyce's model

Fordyce[130,131] developed a model based on a behavioural perspective, focused almost exclusively on operant learning and pain behaviour. The application of operant learning theory on chronic pain by Fordyce has had a huge impact on chronic pain research and management.[664] Fordyce emphasized that despite the pain experience being private and individual, it is expressed in publicly observable behaviours that are modulated by the context and reinforcement. According to Fordyce, there are two types of painful experiences: respondent pain and operant pain. The first type would be all those behaviours that arise as a result of tissue damage and which are perfectly explained from the classical pain model. By contrast, in the case of operant pain, tissue injury would be insufficient as a factor explaining the continuance of pain.

In this case, the pain behaviours would be maintained based on their consequences in the subject's life, on environmental factors and on learning processes. Respondent pain characteristics would be those of acute pain, while operant pain would relate to chronic pain. According to Fordyce,[130,131] in an intact organism the nociceptive stimulus almost always triggers a form of pain behaviour. Pain interrelates with other stimuli that are active at that time, with the mood and perceived or expected consequences of any action taken. It is the processing of nociceptive stimuli together with other cognitive and sensory phenomena which enables learning.

Learning involves the reinforcement or inhibition of a response over time. Reinforcement is the basis of *classical conditioning* described by Pavlov. In classical conditioning, behaviour appears as a consequence of a previous stimulus. In *operant conditioning*, so named because the behaviour operates in the environment, learning occurs based on what happens afterwards or what is expected to happen. For example, complaints or facial expressions that indicate pain can trigger responses of support or attention from the environment. In operant conditioning, pain behaviours are maintained or reduced by the persistence of favourable or unfavourable consequences.

Two profiles of operant conditioning that have significance in pain can be distinguished: (1) behaviour as a result of positive reinforcement and (2) escape or avoidance behaviour as a result of negative reinforcement. An example of the former would be behaviours that get more attention from medical staff and a caring attitude from the family. The latter would be those behaviours that prevent activities as they may aggravate the pain. The patient approach is aimed, therefore, to modify their pain behaviours, using the principles of stimulus reinforcement and control, including those from the individual's social and family environment.

Pain, disability and Waddell's model

Waddell's model[81] emphasizes the relationship between chronic pain and disability. This model, in addition to including the elements described by Loeser, adds cognitive aspects and the social environment. According to this model, pain and disability are therefore dependent on five elements: pain, cognitive components, affective components, pain behaviours and social interactions (Fig. 11-41).

There is not a proportional relationship between pain and disability

Chronic pain can be extremely severe, thus determining a greater or lesser disability. Disability may initially be the result of a tissue injury, but its progression to chronic disability is subject to powerful psychosocial influences.[561] There is no direct correlation between the severity of pain and disability, so the degree of disability is unique to each individual.

Disability is the result of the interaction of all cognitive, emotional and social components involved in the painful experience.

Waddell's model has been updated following the WHO model of International Classification of Functioning, Disability and Health[665] (Fig. 11-42). Pain under this model has three dimensions: biological, psychological and social. Pain and disability are not only a health problem but also the consequence of

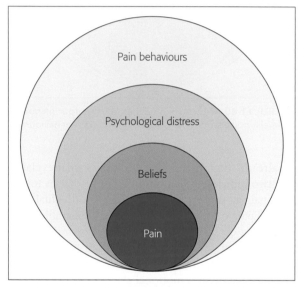

FIGURE 11-41 ■ Waddell's model emphasizes the relationship between pain and disability.

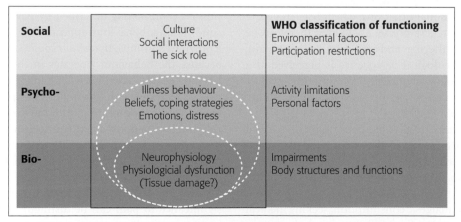

Social	Culture Social interactions The sick role	**WHO classification of functioning** Environmental factors Participation restrictions
Psycho-	Illness behaviour Beliefs, coping strategies Emotions, distress	Activity limitations Personal factors
Bio-	Neurophysiology Physiologicial dysfunction (Tissue damage?)	Impairments Body structures and functions

FIGURE 11-42 ■ Waddell's model has been updated following the WHO model of International Classification of Functioning, Disability and Health. *Reproduced with permission from Waddell and Burton.*[561]

psychological and social aspects. The biological dimension is related to physiological dysfunctions or neurophysiological changes and is expressed as impairments and changes in body function. The psychological dimension is related to beliefs, emotional distress, coping strategies and pain behaviours and is expressed as how the subject lives the experience and as limitations in their activity. The social dimension has to do with family relationships, culture and social interactions and is expressed as changes in work and in recreational and social activities.

Fear-avoidance behaviour and vlaeyen's model

The 'cognitive-behavioural fear-avoidance model' and 'in vivo exposure treatment' proposed by Vlaeyen and colleagues have gained much interest among researchers and clinicians.[138,518,666] The weight of this model is based on its ability to explain how psychological aspects generate behaviours which jointly mediate in the transition from acute to chronic pain.

Vlaeyen et al.[138,518] have shown how fear-avoidance behaviours are primarily responsible for the establishment of disability, disuse and depression in patients with chronic pain (Fig. 11-43). This model describes how these three aspects (disuse, disability and negative emotions) are the result of learned protective behaviours. These behaviours can involve excessive attention and hypervigilance towards pain-related stimuli, obvious escape-avoidance behaviour or less obvious safety behaviours.

The model proposes two possible contrasting behaviours, avoidance and confrontation, and establishes the vicious circle responsible for the patient's deterioration.[667] This 'road to perdition' begins with negative appraisals, such as catastrophic thinking about the pain and its consequences, negative emotions, fear of pain, and hypervigilance, which lead to

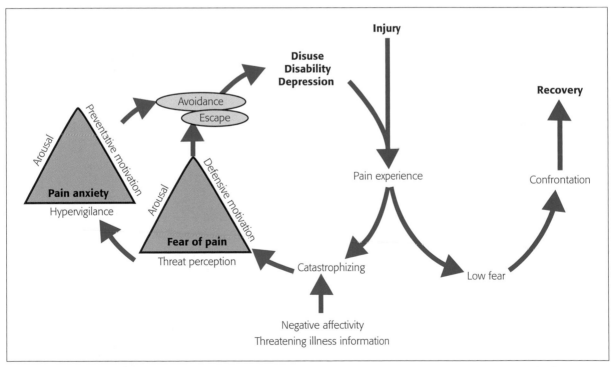

FIGURE 11-43 ■ Fear-avoidance model. Based on the fear-avoidance model of Vlaeyen and Linton (2000) and the fear-anxiety-avoidance model of Asmundson et al. (2004). *Reproduced with permission from Vlaeyen and Linton*[138] *and Asmundson G, Norton P, Vlaeyen J. Fear-avoidance models of chronic pain: an overview. In: Asmundson G, Vlaeyen J, Crombez G, eds. Understanding and treating fear of pain. Oxford: Oxford University Press; 2004. p. 3-24.*

fear-avoidance behaviours that determine the establishment of a disuse syndrome, depression and disability. Fear of pain, hypervigilance and low mood determine decreased activity tolerance and pain amplification. Fear of pain and hypervigilance intersects with the patient's cognitive abilities so that the patient becomes ever less able to divert attention from pain, which interferes in work, recreational and family activity, leading the patient to a situation of work disability, family problems and social self-exclusion.

Disability and main and spanswick's model

Main and Spanswick[661] developed a model covering the different aspects which in subjects with chronic pain lead to disability. These various aspects are divided into seven levels: (1) disuse and deconditioning; (2) fear-avoidance; (3) depression; (4) anger and frustration; (5) iatrogenics; (6) family; and (7) socio-occupational factors. These levels aim to reflect the various aspects that are often involved in the development of disability in patients with pain. Each of these levels can occur cumulatively in the history of the patient (Fig. 11-44).

Patients can easily recognize themselves in this model, which allows them to understand how their disability is not a direct consequence of pain, but the interaction of multiple physical and psychosocial factors. This model also emphasizes the importance from a therapeutic point of view of addressing each of the factors involved. The first level shows how pain generates guarded movements that may favour a disuse syndrome and deconditioning. At the second level, the patient's incorrect interpretation of the relationship between pain and injury determines the fear of movement and therefore an avoidance behaviour. The third level signals the importance of depression in the perception of pain and how it can mediate between pain and disability. The fourth level reveals how disability is aggravated by the frustration associated with suffering chronic pain and anger associated with the lack of pain relief even after receiving explanations and treatments. Iatrogenics, which is common in chronic pain, at the fifth level, significantly contributes to the development of disability. The family, at the sixth level, especially if it is overprotective and solicitous, can strongly hinder the patient in any attempt to return to an active life. And, finally, socio-occupational aspects, the seventh level, can be a major barrier preventing patients from returning to their working lives. Psychosocial factors are better predictors of the ability to return to work than the pathology or physical demands.[599]

CHRONIC PAIN? WHAT IS IT ABOUT? THE RELEVANCE OF A TAXONOMY OF CHRONIC PAIN

The problem of defining chronic pain

As mentioned earlier, in the last 20 years there has been a paradigm shift in the consideration of pain. Relevant factors in this new paradigm have been the advance in

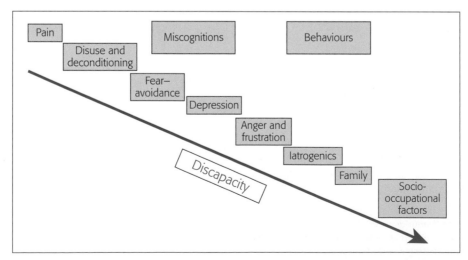

FIGURE 11-44 ■ Main and Spanswick model of pain and disability. *Reproduced with permission from Main and Spanswick.*[606]

the neurobiology of pain and the inclusion of the biopsychosocial paradigm in clinical practice.

As we have often stressed, the problem of chronic pain management does not lie primarily in its treatment, but rather, in a poor or inadequate understanding of what chronic pain essentially is.

One of the main topics of interest among researchers and pain clinicians is chronic pain.

Although clinicians and researches use the term 'chronic pain', two issues are fundamental: What does this term actually mean? Is all chronic pain essentially the same? As discussed herein, the answers to these two questions can be quite different, and the understandings of what pain essentially is, are entirely dissimilar. It must be emphasized that these questions are absolutely decisive because the responses may determine very different therapeutic decisions. While some authors still believe that the persistence of pain always requires a persistent nociceptive source, others focus on the central neuroplastic changes and believe nociception to be irrelevant. In the development of chronic pain, some authors emphasize the role of changes in the endocrine and immune systems, others stress the importance of genetic polymorphisms and yet others, finally, focus on psychological factors. In addition, all chronic pain by the mere fact of being such, is often seen as a single entity.

However, the recognition of pain as a response of the central nervous system, not necessarily dependent on an active nociceptive source, and the integration into practice of the biopsychosocial model, has led to some misunderstandings in the clinical practice. For example, some have mistakenly assumed that pathoanatomical aspects are of little importance in clinical decision making in patients with chronic pain.[668] There has even been an unwarranted and unjustified belief that diagnosis and treatment based on the patient's pathology offer limited clinical utility and that instead of improving results, these become worse.[7,669] Chronic pain patients should, thus, be contemplated under the anthropological and sociological construct of illness as opposed to disease. Psychosocial factors are clearly essential for the classification and treatment of patients with chronic pain. However, arguments justifying the exclusion of pathoanatomical factors both in the clinical practice and in research are not compatible with the current literature.[670–672] Controversies in the treatment of chronic pain and their

objectives are relevant and are basically derived from the interpretation of what chronic pain is in itself. Can one of the treatment's goal, besides improving the quality of life of patients, be to eliminate the pain? Or, conversely, when pain is chronic, could eradicating it be a feasible target? The lack of consensus on the definition of chronic pain is a major barrier both for the progress of knowledge and for the treatment of chronic pain. This lack of consensus as to what chronic pain is in itself makes it difficult for both researchers and health professionals to compare their results and clinical observations. What follows is a review of the current concepts of chronic pain.

Chronic pain based on timeline

A definition of chronic pain can be based pragmatically on the timeframe after the onset of pain. The IASP chose the period of 3 months as the dividing line between acute and chronic pain, although for research purposes a 6-month period is preferable.[673]

Chronic pain has also been defined as a pain that persists beyond the normal time of tissue healing.[673] In this definition it is assumed, therefore, that in chronic pain there is no active pathology, or that it is insufficient to justify the patient's pain.[674] Based on this definition, clinical conditions lasting several weeks may be considered chronic pain conditions, when pain persists despite the tissues having completely healed. This definition is also insufficient, as in many chronic painful conditions such as rheumatoid arthritis or osteoarthritis an active pathology exists. In some entities considered as chronic pain, such as complex regional pain syndrome (CRPS), there are severe tissue changes as well as peripheral and central sensitization phenomena. There are other chronic conditions, such as in chronic migraine, which are not related to any tissue injury, and the symptoms may persist for years with acute episodic exacerbations.

Chronic pain has also been defined as a pain that persists beyond the normal time of tissue healing, but in many chronic painful conditions an active and persistent pathology exists.

Chronic pain as maladaptive

Chronic pain has also been defined as pain that has lost its biological function. According to this view, while acute pain is adaptive because it contributes to survival, preventing injury and promoting healing, chronic pain is maladaptive, the expression of a pathological process in the nervous system without any biological function. According to Chapman and Nakamura,[56] chronic pain should be considered as pain that is severe, that persists over time, ceases to serve a protective function and degrades health and functional capabilities, becoming a source of suffering and disability. However, many patients experience pain for long periods of their life and show no disability. Besides, all chronic pain is not necessarily maladaptive, since in some cases it may reflect a persistent inflammatory or nociceptive source and need not be severe.

All chronic pain is not necessarily maladaptive, since in some cases it may reflect a persistent inflammatory or nociceptive source.

In order to differentiate between adaptive and maladaptive pain, the American Academy of Pain Medicine introduced the terms eudynia and maldynia.[675] Eudynia is defined as pain related to nociceptive activity, and thus a symptom of an underlying pathological disorder. Maldynia is considered a maladaptive pain secondary to changes in the central nervous system.[676–678] Maladaptive pain is either the result of a dysfunction of the nervous system, or secondary to an inadequately relieved nociceptive source. The problem, once again, with the definition of maldynia, is that it does not contemplate the possibility of persistent pain without nociceptive activity. Therefore, a category that includes those pain conditions not associated with nociception or where it is unable to fully explain the patient's symptoms, is needed.

Chronic pain as a syndrome

Most patients attending a pain clinic are not simply subjects with persistent pain, but many of them have high emotional distress and severe disability and are often refractory to any therapeutic modality. As early as 1984, Crook and Tunks[679] had already proposed the term *chronic pain syndrome* as a conceptual model that could define these chronic pain patients.

The concept of chronic pain syndromes has been supported by several authors, and different names have been used to define clinical complex pain conditions in which nociception fails to fully explain patient symptoms such as functional pain syndrome, idiopathic pain syndrome, chronic pain syndrome, unexplained pain syndromes, central sensitivity syndromes and somatoform disorder.[438,680–682]

The American Medical Association[683] described the characteristics of chronic pain syndromes on '8D's' list:

Duration: pain is considered chronic when it persists beyond the normal healing time.

Dramatization: patients exhibit unusual behavior, use terms to describe their pain with a strong emotional character and manifest expressions like groans, grimacing and awkward postures.

Diagnostic dilemma: extensive history of clinical examinations with multiple diagnoses. The patient has undergone multiple diagnostic studies. The diagnostics are vague, inconsistent and inadequate.

Drugs: dependence and substance abuse, including alcohol and prescribed and non-prescribed medications.

Dependence: dependence on health care professionals and excessive demand for medical care. Patients hope to get improvement with passive treatment modalities. Dependence on the spouse and relatives and abandonment of their domestic and social responsibilities.

Depression: common symptoms of depression or low mood. Decreased ability to cope and low self-esteem leads to a decrease in self-confidence and increased dependence on others.

Disuse: low physical activity level responsible for the appearance of secondary musculoskeletal symptoms. Inadequate advice of health care providers, including recommending rest, leading to a progressive physical deconditioning that perpetuates the cycle of pain and pain behaviours.

Dysfunction: low activity levels. Inadequate advice of health practitioners, including recommending rest, leading to progressive physical deconditioning and perpetuating the cycle of pain and pain behaviours.

Progressive loss of active coping strategies results in a gradual social self-exclusion, including work, recreational activities, friends and family. Increased isolation reduces the activity to the minimum essential for life. Deprived of social contacts, rejected by the medical system and private financial resources, the patient becomes disabled in the broad sense of the word: physical, emotional, social and economic. In this guide, it was considered that the presence of at least four of the eight characteristics could establish the diagnosis of chronic pain syndrome.

THE 8 DS CHARACTERISTICS OF A CHRONIC PAIN SYNDROME

- Duration
- Dramatization
- Diagnostic dilemma
- Drugs
- Dependence
- Depression
- Disuse
- Dysfunction

Chronic pain and central sensitivity syndromes

The concept of *central sensitivity syndromes* (CSS) has been advocated in the last decades as a new nosological category, among others, by authors that previously defended the term 'fibromyalgia'.[682] This category includes chronic and not fully understood clinical pain conditions such as fibromyalgia, chronic fatigue syndrome (CFS), irritable bowel syndrome (IBS) and tension-type headaches (TTH), among others. According to the authors that support the concept of central sensitivity syndromes, these syndromes show objective markers of disease, including central sensitization phenomena, brain activity changes observed in neuroimaging techniques, changes on levels of neurotransmitters or neuromodulators, sympathetic overactivity and changes in neuroendocrine immune systems. Most of the symptoms of the CSS would be secondary to biological changes, mainly in the neuroendocrine immune system, which in a subgroup of patients would be enhanced by psychological factors.

A similar construct is the *idiopathic pain disorder*, in which the same chronic pain conditions would be the consequence of a state of pain amplification and psychological distress.[680] Pain amplification and psychological distress would be mediated by an individual's genetic polymorphic variations and by exposure to environmental factors such as physical or emotional stress. It has been proposed, for example, in patients with back pain that, besides subgrouping according to psychological and behavioural factors, it can also be grouped based on genetic factors.[684] One problem with this model, although it does consider the predisposing psychosocial factors, is that it gives too much importance to genetic factors, while the current level of knowledge about them is still scarce. It can also generate the convictions that, first, the patient will always be 'vulnerable' to developing chronic pain and that, secondly, it will hardly be possible to eradicate the pain.

The concepts of pain syndromes such as central sensitivity syndromes and idiopathic pain disorder have some disadvantages: we may assume that the patient will always be 'vulnerable' to developing chronic pain and that it will hardly be possible to prevent or eradicate the pain.

Chronic pain as a disease

Siddall and Cousins[13] propose that chronic pain should be considered a disease entity, as it meets disease criteria: its own pathology, symptoms, and signs. They differentiate between three types of pathologies: primary, which generates nociception; secondary, the neuroplastic changes in the central nervous system; and tertiary, the environmental factors (psychological and social) that may contribute to pain pathology. Depending on the 'type' of pathology, treatment should address the tissues or modulate central responses or to psychosocial aspects. However, although this construct is comprehensive because it includes aspects related to neuroplastic changes and the effect of environmental factors, it seems to support the notion that in a patient with chronic pain, although it may improve, pain will always be present.

As already mentioned, one of the advances in the understanding of pain has been the development of functional neuroimaging techniques.[71-76] Hence some authors propose that pain is a 'disease' based on brain functional and structural changes observed in chronic pain patients using neuroimaging techniques.[685] Chronic pain has thus been considered a disease of the brain.[314,686] However, it cannot be said that such brain changes are the cause of chronic pain, as they could be a secondary normal response to pain prolonged over time.[687,688]

As pointed out by Sullivan et al.[689] to consider chronic pain as a brain disease can have negative consequences for pain research, but above all for the treatment of patients. The main consequence would be to understand pain as an exclusively medical problem, caused by pathological changes on the patient's brain, forgetting the important role of psychological, personal and social factors.[690] Once again, it is the problem of the medicalization of the human experience, under which political rather than scientific aspects underlie. The interpretation of pain as a problem affecting the brain also leads to the so-called mereological fallacy, whereby only what can be attributed to the person as a whole is attributed to the brain.[689] In short, although functional neuroimaging is a tool that can help us to better understand the pathophysiologic brain changes, it cannot reduce the complex experience of pain to these changes.[691]

Chronic pain and the DSM-5

Many patients with chronic pain have considerable emotional distress and report disproportionate pain and disability. Some of chronic pain conditions suffered have been considered as 'medically unexplained symptoms', 'somatization disorder', or 'functional somatic syndromes'. Hence they can be included in different categories of the Diagnostic and Statistical Manual of Mental Disorders (DSM-5) of the American Psychiatric Association (APA). This new classification has established the term somatic symptom disorder to replace somatoform disorders terms such as somatization disorder, hypochondriasis and pain disorder that were listed in the DSM-IV and often overlapped.[692] Somatic symptom disorder (SSD) is defined as a disorder characterized by persistent somatic symptoms (≥6 months) that are either very distressing or result in significant disruption of functioning, as well as excessive and disproportionate thoughts, feelings and behaviors regarding those symptoms (Table 11-11).

While a key feature for many of these disorders in DSM-IV is medically unexplained symptoms, a SSD can be associated with another medical condition in the new classification. The emphasis of DSM-5 criteria in this category is that patient's thoughts, feelings and

TABLE 11-11
Somatic symptom disorder diagnostic criteria (DSM-5)

A. One or more somatic symptoms that are distressing or result in significant disruption of daily life

B. Excessive thoughts, feelings, or behaviours related to the somatic symptoms or associated health concerns as manifested by at least one of the following:
1. Disproportionate and persistent thoughts about the seriousness of one's symptoms.
2. Persistent high level of anxiety about health or symptoms.
3. Excessive time and energy devoted to these symptoms or health concerns

C. Although any one somatic symptom may not be continuously present, the state of being symptomatic is persistent (typically more than 6 months)

Specify if:

With predominant pain (previously pain disorder): this specifier is for individuals whose somatic symptoms predominantly involve pain

Specify if:

Persistent: a persistent course is characterized by severe symptoms, marked impairment, and long duration (more than 6 months)

Specify current severity:

Mild: only one of the symptoms specified in Criterion B is fulfilled

Moderate: two or more of the symptoms specified in Criterion B are fulfilled

Severe: two or more of the symptoms specified in Criterion B are fulfilled, plus there are multiple somatic complaints (or one very severe somatic symptom)

Reproduced with permission from the American Psychiatric Association.[712]

behaviors about their somatic symptoms are disproportionate or excessive.

The problem with this category, although it gives further clarification, is that it belongs to a classification of psychiatric disorders, which may be mistakenly understood as synonymous of 'psychogenic pain' without any physical or neurophysiological substrate. Any perceptual experience has a clear biological substrate.

The psychological / psychiatric taxonomies are of interest and emphasize the role of psychological and behavioral responses, the role of learning, and social context. However, they are insufficient as they do not consider the neurobiological aspects inherent to the experience of pain. The risk, as pointed out by

Merskey[693] in referring to the term somatization, is that 'it automatically implies actively producing physical symptoms, whether indirectly or from some 'unconscious' motive". As has been noted by Main et al.[516] 'somatization' should be considered a normal phenomenon, a biological response depending on the patient's pain interpretation. The term somatic symptom disorder, in the same way as it occurs with terms such as somatization, may involve from a mere concern in somatic symptoms to a severe psychiatric disorder. Continuing to maintain the mind-body dichotomy poses a risk. As stated by Sullivan[690] 'pain thus originates, not in mind or body, but between mind and bodies'. Once again, from a practical perspective, a taxonomy that could differentiate pain associated with nociception, from pain in which no relevant nociceptive source is present, is important.

Chronic pain IASP classification

The IASP Task Force has developed a pragmatic classification of chronic pain for the upcoming 11th revision of the International Classification of Diseases (ICD) of the World Health Organization (WHO).[694] This new ICD category for 'Chronic Pain' defines it as persistent or recurrent pain lasting longer than 3 months. Chronic pain disorders are divided into seven groups: (1) chronic primary pain; (2) chronic cancer pain; (3) chronic post-traumatic and postsurgical pain; (4) chronic neuropathic pain; (5) chronic headache and orofacial pain; (6) chronic visceral pain; and (7) chronic musculoskeletal pain.

Classification of chronic pain (IASP Task Force)

- Chronic primary pain
- Chronic cancer pain
- Chronic post-traumatic and postsurgical pain
- Chronic neuropathic pain
- Chronic headache and orofacial pain
- Chronic visceral pain
- Chronic musculoskeletal pain

Chronic primary pain is defined as pain in one or more anatomic regions that persists or recurs for longer than 3 months, and is associated with significant emotional distress or significant functional disability, and that cannot be better explained by another chronic pain condition. In this group, for example,

back pain that cannot be identified as musculoskeletal or neuropathic pain, chronic widespread pain, fibromyalgia and IBS are included. Therefore, the category of *chronic musculoskeletal pain* is limited to nociceptive or inflammatory pain that arises as part of a disease process directly affecting musculoskeletal tissues. This group includes metabolic, infectious and autoimmune disorders such as rheumatoid arthritis and disorders secondary to a structural or degenerative aetiology such as symptomatic osteoarthrosis. When pain is apparently musculoskeletal but its causes are not completely understood, such as chronic widespread pain and non-specific back pain, it should be included in the chronic primary pain group. This differentiation is interesting in the clinical setting as it differentiates two types of chronic pain: chronic pain associated with tissue injuries (post-traumatic, postsurgical, visceral, malignant pain, etc.), and chronic primary pain that has three characteristics – no relevant nociceptive source, significant emotional distress and significant functional disability.

A mechanism-based view of chronic pain

Chronic pain can also be characterized based on the mechanisms underlying pain. A pain mechanism approach to chronic pain could also explain the persistence of pain for long periods of time. The management of chronic musculoskeletal disorders which formerly focused on pathoanatomical diagnoses has evolved in recent years to a broader approach based on the understanding of pathophysiological pain mechanisms.[47,695] Therefore, one of the key issues in patient management is to identify the dominant neurophysiological mechanisms implicated: nociceptive, inflammatory, or neuropathic.

In many patients, the lack of evidence of injury or diseases in the tissues has led many clinicians and researchers to thinking that chronic pain may be of a neuropathic origin. This meant that in clinical practice any painful presentation difficult to categorize, such as fibromyalgia or chronic low back pain, should be considered as *central neuropathic pain*.[696–698] However, the definition of neuropathic pain adopted by IASP in 2008 required it to be a direct consequence of an injury or disease affecting the somatosensory system.[699] This definition which is more restrictive than the former 1994 one[700] has two advantages: it prevents any confusion regarding terms such as 'dysfunction', and pain is not labelled as neuropathic when symptoms are an expression of neuroplastic changes of the nociceptive system secondary to an acute injury or inflammatory process.

Central sensitization pain construct

Several authors have proposed that in addition to the classic pain mechanisms such as the nociceptive, inflammatory or neuropathic pain mechanisms, a new category should be established, and it has been termed '*central sensitization pain*'.[49,701–705]

A clinical algorithm has recently been developed to identify patients with central sensitization pain.[706] This algorithm accounts for aspects such as the severity of pain and its relationship with disease or tissue injury, the distribution of pain and hyperalgesia, sensory hypersensitivity and some other clinical features.

This classification requires 2 major steps: the exclusion of neuropathic pain and the differential classification of nociceptive versus central sensitization pain. The first step requires the utilization of the IASP diagnostic criteria of neuropathic pain.[699] In the second, clinicians screen their patients for 3 major classification criteria. The first is a mandatory criterion that entails disproportionate pain, implying that the severity of pain and perceived disability are disproportionate to the nature and extent of injury or pathology. The 2 remaining criteria are 1) the presence of diffuse pain distribution, allodynia, and hyperalgesia; and 2) hypersensitivity of senses unrelated to the musculoskeletal system.

Criterion 1: Pain experience disproportionate to the nature and extent of injury or pathology. This first criterion implies that the severity of pain and disability are disproportionate to the alleged pathology or injury.

Criterion 2: Diffuse pain distribution, allodynia and hyperalgesia. This criterion considers as a common feature observed in these patients that they refer pain, allodynia and hyperalgesia in diffuse and widespread body areas. As some examples: widespread pain, pain in the whole lower or upper extremity, allodynia/hyperalgesia outside the segmental area of (presumed) primary nociception, etc.

If criteria 1 and 2 are both met, then the classification of central sensitization pain can be established. In the event only the first criterion (disproportionate pain) is met and not the second criterion, further screening of the remaining criteria is required.

Criterion 3: Hypersensitivity of senses unrelated to the musculoskeletal system. The patient with a central sensitization pain frequently shows a general sensory hypersensitivity to different stimuli such as mechanical stimuli,[35,707,708] odors, temperature,,[709] electric stimuli.[70,707] Due to the frequent central hyperexcitability in these patients, many different environmental stimuli are capable of triggering pain. It is also frequent that they show a reduced tolerance to stress[54,710] to emotional or mental load.[54,710] The isolated presence of these symptoms is common in anxious subjects, and although their premorbid presence does not exclude the possibility of developing central sensitization pain, it makes them unreliable for diagnosing it. This algorithm is not intended to be all-inclusive of all those characteristic features of a patient with a chronic pain, but only those that can facilitate central sensitization pain identification.

The algorithm already presented can be an initially interesting clinical tool, but for a broader understanding of the clinical picture of a patient's experience we need a more comprehensive clinical reasoning. . Since central sensitization would be the pathophysiological mechanism that could explain many chronic pain syndromes such as fibromyalgiaMoreover, it seems to us that the term 'central sensitization pain' can be confusing. Since central sensitization can be the neurophysiological mechanism implicated in the transition from acute to chronic pain, central sensitization has been erroneously equated with chronic pain[691,692,711,712]. It is also assumed that subjects with increased sensitivity report higher levels of pain and disability.[713,714] Moreover, many patients with chronic pain refer pain away from the primary area of pain.[73,715] Certainly the mechanisms of central sensitization such as facilitation and disinhibition are common features in chronic pain.[27,49,716,717]

It is also assumed that subjects with increased sensitivity report higher levels of pain and disability.[693,694] Certainly the mechanisms of central sensitization such as facilitation and disinhibition are common features in chronic pain.[27,49,695,696]

Many patients with chronic pain refer pain away from the primary area of pain.[73,697] Thus, according to this model, central sensitization is the key neurophysiological mechanism of chronic pain, and the evaluation of pain sensitivity could be a valid marker to identify patients with chronic pain. Hence, in recent years, various methods have been used in order to determine changes in the central sensitivity in chronic pain conditions, such as pressure pain thresholds (PPTs) in remote areas away from the site of the primary injury or lesion, quantitative sensory testing (QST) and conditioned pain modulation (CPM).[34,718–721] However, recently, some doubts have arisen as to whether an increase in the central sensitivity is relevant as an explanation of chronic pain. It has even been posited that differences in pain thresholds may be more related to psychological distress and fear-avoidance of the patients evaluated.[713,722]

In a recent systematic review, Hubscher et al.[53] have shown that in patients with spinal pain there is no consistent evidence linking the severity of pain and disability with the measurements obtained with QST. These authors suggest that many other factors, such as psychological factors related to pain, can better explain patients' pain severity and disability. Different studies have shown that the most important predictors of pain and disability are related to catastrophizing, depression, anxiety, pain self-efficacy, illness perceptions, etc.[502,723] Moreover, while central sensitization can play an important role in the development of chronic pain, it is not yet clear whether in some cases these changes in central pain processing are primary or are secondary to prolonged pain, or secondary to the emotional distress to pain or its interpretation.[39]

In addition, although many patients with chronic pain have widespread hyperalgesia and allodynia, these features can also be observed in entities characterized by nociceptive or inflammatory pain such as osteoarthritis or rheumatoid arthritis.[724–729]

- Central sensitization is NOT present in all patients with chronic pain.
- Acute and subacute musculoskeletal pain DOES NOT exclude the possibility of a central sensitization.
- Central sensitization is not the differential characteristic of chronic pain conditions and does not seem to play a major role in patients' reporting of pain and disability.

Patients with such clinical conditions can refer symptoms usually attributed to neuropathic pain presenting the same high scores on scales assessing neuropathic pain, such as painDETECT score,[726,730] whereas in some pain conditions such as chronic idiopathic neck pain, central sensitization does not seem to be a characteristic feature in all patients.[731] Therefore, central sensitization is not the differential characteristic of chronic pain conditions and does not seem to play a major role in patients' reporting of pain and disability.[53]

- Chronic pain is not always maladaptive.
- Chronic pain may be associated with a persistent nociceptive mechanism.
- Chronic pain is not necessarily the result of an inadequately relieved nociceptive source nor necessarily involves dysfunction of the nervous system.
- Chronic pain is not necessarily associated with disability.
- Chronic pain cannot be defined as central neuropathic pain.
- Chronic pain cannot be interpreted as the expression of a 'syndrome' secondary to biological, neuroendocrine, or genetic changes, etc.
- The term *central sensitization pain* is not an appropriate category.
- Chronic pain does not necessarily imply central sensitization.
- Chronic pain does not necessarily mean brain reorganization.
- Chronic pain is not a 'disease of the brain'.
- Chronic pain is not a 'disease entity'.

Complex pain category

DysfunctionalComplex pain category

As it has been noted, understanding of neurophysiological mechanisms is useful to identify the dominant pain mechanisms implicated. The recognition of pain as a response of the central nervous system, not necessarily dependent on an active nociceptive source, and the integration into practice of the biopsychosocial model, has led to some misunderstandings in the clinical practice. For example, some have mistakenly assumed that pathoanatomical aspects are of little importance in clinical decision making in patients with chronic pain.[721] There has even been an unwarranted and unjustified belief that diagnosis and treatment based on the patient's pathology offer limited clinical utility and that instead of improving results, these become worse[7,722] But as central sensitization is not the differential characteristic of chronic complex pain patients, it is needed another more adequate term. Furthermore, understanding. Chronic pain patients should, thus, be contemplated under the anthropological and sociological construct of illness as opposed to disease. Psychosocial factors are clearly essential for the classification and treatment of patients with chronic pain. However, arguments justifying the exclusion of pathoanatomical factors both in the clinical practice and in research are not compatible with the current literature.[723–725]

In many chronic pain conditions an active and persistent nociceptive source exists, while in conditions such as rheumatoid arthritis, osteoarthritis, etc. it does exist. Therefore, chronic pain does not necessarily imply that it always lasts beyond the normal time of healing or that it is always maladaptive. the problem of patient's pain requires then to differentiate whether this is the result of active disease or an abnormal response not associated with nociception. Therefore, it is necessary to include a new category for those with chronic pain (but also with acute pain) in which there is no relevant nociceptive input.

Wolf proposed the term *complex pain* as a new category for this type of pain. Complex pain is defined as pain that is not the consequence of a tissue injury, any detectable inflammation or damage to the nervous system.[732,733] As stated by Woolf,[25] pain 'in these circumstances becomes the equivalent of an illusory perception, a sensation that has the exact quality of that evoked by a real noxious stimulus but which occurs in the absence of such an injurious stimulus'.

However, terms such as functional or dysfunctional have classically been misinterpreted as a 'psychogenic pain', and on the other hand in Wolf's definition many other aspects observed in chronic complex pain patients such as behavioral and psychosocial responses are not included in this definition. In this sense, we propose the term 'complex pain'.

Complex pain is characterized by a pain severity and duration inconsistent with the alleged injury or pathology, has a natural history that does not match any known clinical pattern, widespread pain distribution, allodynia and hyperalgesia not related to a nerve injury or disease, generalized hypersensitivity to many stimuli such as thermal, chemical, weather, stress stimuli, etc., frequently shows an abnormal therapeutic response to the habitual treatment and is associated with psychological distress, significant functional disability and illness behaviors. Complex pain can be initiated by an afferent input or without any input, and is associated to some degree of central hyperexcitability, and it persists despite there no longer being a nociceptive peripheral input.

COMPLEX PAIN CHARACTERISTICS

- No known structural nervous system lesion or disease or active peripheral inflammation.
- Pain severity and duration incoherent with an injury or pathology.
- Natural history does not match any known clinical pattern.
- Often widespread pain distribution, allodynia and hyperalgesia.
- Often neuropathic-like symptoms.
- Generalized hypersensitivity to many stimuli (thermal, chemical, weather, stress, etc.).
- Abnormal therapeutic response.
- Psychological distress
- Functional Disability
- Illness behaviors

Symptoms of central sensitization, such as spontaneous electric shock pain, mechanical hyperalgesia and thermal and mechanical allodynia, enhanced temporal summation and sensory abnormalities are common in patients with an ongoing inflammatory process and neuropathic pain, but also in complex pain conditions. A relevant proportion of patients with complex pain show high scores in some neuropathic pain screening tools.[730] These common features with neuropathic pain are associated with central sensitization phenomena that may also be present in a complex pain. These neuropathic-like symptoms have confounded clinicians into believing in a neuropathic component in complex pain conditions. But it must be emphasized that the degree of central sensitization in patients with complex chronic pain can be very variable in the same way as it is with inflammatory and neuropathic pain.

- In addition, complex pain may also present as an acute pain
- It is not uncommon that patients with complex pain can present breakthrough pain with minimal stimulus or spontaneously

Salomons et al.[734] report two cases of patients experiencing pain flashbacks that persisted for years after the patients suffered a traumatic episode of awareness under anaesthesia. Pain can be a 'memory' that may be activated by a learned conditioned stimulus. In clinical practice it is common for many patients to report the onset of chronic pain after an innocuous stimulus but associated with a pain experience. The brain keeps diachronic representations of pain that can be activated with a stimulus associated with them.

A new proposal for chronic pain classification

The adjective 'chronic' only defines a temporal quality of pain. Therefore a classification is needed that could better explain the various aspects involved in a chronic pain experience.

IASP has published a multiaxial classification of chronic pain which attempts to standardize the descriptions of the most relevant painful syndromes.[673]

This taxonomy groups patients with chronic pain according to 5 axes. This system establishes a five-digit code that corresponds to each chronic pain diagnosis. For a review of definitions and taxonomies of pain it is recommended.[674]

IASP MULTIDIMENSIONAL CLASSIFICATION OF PAIN

- Axis I: Region of the body
- Axis II: System whose abnormal functioning could produce the pain
- Axis III: Temporal characteristics of pain and pattern of occurrence
- Axis IV: Patient's statement of intensity and time since onset of pain
- Axis V: Presumed etiology

However, this classification fails to incorporate some important aspects in the development of chronic pain, such as pain mechanisms involved and the degree of central sensitization. Accordingly, a pain classification that incorporates the mechanisms involved (nociceptive, inflammatory, neuropathic and complex mechanisms) is proposed (Fig. 11-45 and 11-57). All these types of pain can be acute, subacute, recurrent or chronic. Complex pain is often experienced by patients with chronic disabling pain. But, as previously mentioned, complex acute pain may appear

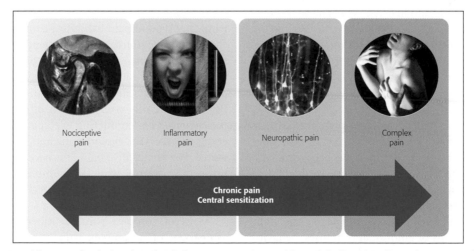

FIGURE 11-45 ■ All types of pain (nociceptive, inflammatory, neuropathic and dysfunctional) can be acute, subacute, recurrent or chronic and the degree of central sensitization can be very variable in all types.

spontaneously or following somatic, cognitive or emotional stimuli capable of triggering the activation of a 'painful memory'. It is also wrong to equate acute pain with peripheral mechanisms, and therefore with scarce central sensitization, and chronic pain with central processing mechanisms. Central sensitization can play an important role in the perception of acute pain. Examples include the phenomena of hyperesthesia, associated hyperalgesia and allodynia which are common after posttraumatic injuries and inflammatory processes. Therefore, central sensitization may be expressed to a greater or lesser extent in all types of pain.

- It is wrong to equate acute pain with peripheral mechanisms and chronic pain with central processing mechanisms.
- Central sensitization can play an important role in the perception of acute pain
- All types of pain (nociceptive, inflammatory, neuropathic and complex) can be acute, subacute, recurrent or chronic.
- Complex pain is often experienced by patients with complex chronic pain.

According to the time axis, whenever the subject experiences pain beyond a certain period of time (about 3 months) we could consider pain as chronic or persistent. However, other taxonomic axes must be considered in order to define a patient's pain experience in a more comprehensive way and to provide treatment goals. For example, and considering the etiology, if chronic pain is the result of an active nociceptive source, it is imperative to treat the tissues. But if there is no nociception, the treatment should be directed to modulate the centrally generated pain responses.

Therefore, to better explain different aspects involved in a chronic pain experience, a new broader taxonomic classification, that includes behavioral and psychosocial aspects, is suggested that considers pain according to 9 axes: persistence over time, etiology, pain mechanisms, pain severity, physical impairments, degree of central sensitization, impact on the individual's life in terms of emotional responses, behavioral responses such as the presence of dysfunctional illness behaviors and associated disability, and finally all the psychosocial aspects involved (personal, family, work, etc.).

AXES OF A TAXONOMIC CLASSIFICATION

- Persistence
- Etiology
- Pain mechanisms
- Pain severity
- Physical impairments
- Central sensitization
- Emotional responses
- Behavioral responses and disability
- Psychosocial aspects

Pain identifiers

Clinical identifiers of pain conditions (acute and chronic) not related to relevant nociceptive input are much needed. In patients with complex pain, different aspects dominate the clinical picture and mediate treatment responses, such as central hyperexcitability, illness behaviours, psychological distress and disability.

The central sensitization pain algorithm, described above, provided criteria related to signs and symptoms of central sensitization. But, as already mentioned, central sensitization is not the only or the most important aspect for identifying subjects with complex pain. In addition, psychosocial aspects are often better indicators of complex pain than an increased central sensitization.

Recognition of this type of pain is critical because, while any type of pain exhibits a consistency between the nociceptive source and the patient's clinical expression, complex pain does not. The pattern of pain is either disproportionate to the severity of the injury or does not match any recognizable clinical pattern. Failure to identify complex pain often results in the patient receiving conflicting explanations and undergoing unnecessary explorations and ineffective treatments. For nociceptive pain, it is necessary to treat the nociceptive source, while for complex pain we must focus on the central modulation mechanisms and psychosocial aspects.

A list of complex pain identifiers for a broader assessment of a complex pain condition is offered. The aim of these is to promote the recognition of complex chronic pain situations not associated with a nociceptive input or, where this is not relevant, including both aspects of pain characteristics and the different associated behavioural and psychosocial aspects. These identifiers can be classified into the following: main identifiers (pain timeline, pain, clinical pattern, pain-related dysfunction and intolerance to daily activity); secondary identifiers which express a condition of central hyperexcitability, such as sensory hypersensitivity not related to the musculoskeletal system and comorbidity; confirmatory identifiers (diagnosis, physical assessment and therapeutic response); and associated identifiers such as cognitive and emotional aspects and psychosocial issues (Table 11-12).

The main feature of a complex pain is the presence of **inconsistency** between signs and symptoms and any known pattern of injury or disease. This initially forces the clinician to rule out any known pathologies, especially if signs and symptoms are secondary to a severe condition (e.g. myelopathy, cauda equine, polyneuropathy, multiple sclerosis, etc.). The clinical presentation of complex pain is not only chronic but also may be acute or subacute (Fig. 11-46).

TABLE 11-12
Identifiers of complex pain

Main identifiers

Identifier 1: Pain timeline
Identifier 2: Pain and other symptoms, localization and clinical pain pattern
Identifier 3: Severity of related dysfunction and intolerance to everyday activity

Secondary identifiers

Identifier 4: Hypersensitivity of senses unrelated to the musculoskeletal system (hypersensitivity to odours, bright light, sound, taste, height fluctuations, etc.)
Identifier 5: Comorbidity

Confirmatory identifiers (diagnosis, assessment and treatment)

Identifier 6: Diagnosis
Identifier 7: Physical assessment
Identifier 8: Abnormal therapeutic response to previous or ongoing treatments

Associated identifiers (personal and psychosocial)

Identifier 9: Cognitive and emotional aspects
Identifier 10: Psychosocial issues

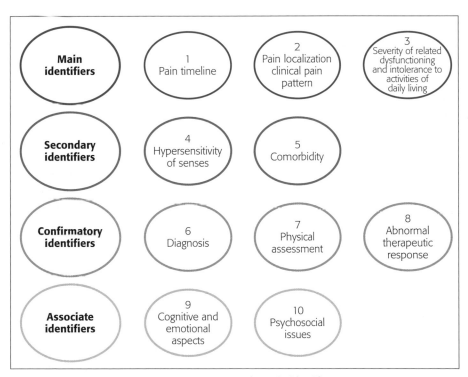

FIGURE 11-46 ■ Complex pain identifiers.

Identifier 1: pain timeline

The pain timeline does not match the natural history of a recognized clinical condition. Examples include: pain persisting beyond expected tissue healing, persistent pain for more than 3 months without any remission; complaints of continuous pain for years; cyclical pain related to seasonal or weather changes, or stressful or adverse life events; the cyclic or acute onset cannot be explained by a recognized clinical condition.

Identifier 2: clinical pain presentation

The clinical pain presentation does not match a recognized clinical condition. The patient's symptoms are inconsistent in the sense that either there is no active disease or its severity does not justify the pain intensity or the degree of disability. In the first scenario, despite the absence of a discernible tissue injury, patients report severe pain. This criterion is met, therefore, in conditions such as fibromyalgia and irritable bowel syndrome. In the second scenario, the injury or pathology is not enough to explain the pain and disability experienced by this patient.

It is obviously critical that the clinician is able to rule out an active disease and to know what is considered proportionate or disproportionate to a clinical condition.

This criterion addresses: pain pattern, pain behaviour, subjective sensory symptoms, subjective motor symptoms and neglect of signs or symptoms. In addition, or instead of pain, some patients may have symptoms such as muscle weakness or paralysis, numbness, paraesthesia, dysaesthesia and even anaesthesia with no plausible neuroanatomical distribution and not justified by a pathology. These patients with dysfunctional chronic pain may also meet the criteria for a conversion disorderin which the patient refers neurological symptoms (sensitive or motor) that are incompatible with neurological pathophysiology.

Pain pattern

- Large pain area with non-anatomical or segmental distribution.
- Widespread pain.
- Atypical pain pattern.
- 'Paraplegic pain'.

- Pain on half of the body, hemilateral pain ('hemiplegic pain').
- Bilateral pain/mirror pain (Fig. 11-47).
- Pain in the whole lower or upper extremity.
- Pain varying in (anatomical) location ('travelling pain').
- Any new painful condition never disappears.
- Association of different painful syndromes throughout the body.
- Clinical pattern that combines pain of a different nature: musculoskeletal, neuropathic and visceral.

Pain behaviour

- Pain disproportionate to the nature and extent of injury or pathology.
- Pain disproportionate to the intensity of the mechanical stimulus.
- Pain of high severity and irritability.
- Spontaneous pain, stimulus independent pain, paroxysmal or breakthrough pain.
- Latent pain: there is a distortion between stimulus/response.
- Pain can be present spontaneously but not after a strong stimulation.
- Pain occurs without any known cause and can disappear for months or years, to then reappear later on.

Subjective sensory symptoms

- Allodynia outside the segmental area of primary nociception.
- Subjective hypoaesthesia.
- Hemiplegic or paraplegic allodynia or hyperaesthesia.
- Numbness or paraesthesia without neurological injury or disease.
- Subjective feeling of oedema in the whole limb.
- Glove or sock numbness or paraesthesia without a painful polyneuropathy.

Subjective motor symptoms

- 'Paralysing pain'.
- Pain associated with functional impotence of the whole member (faults throughout the leg or in the arm).
- Claudicating pain (after eliminating neurogenic or vascular claudication).

Neglect signs or symptoms

- Any sign or symptom of cognitive, sensory or motor neglect.

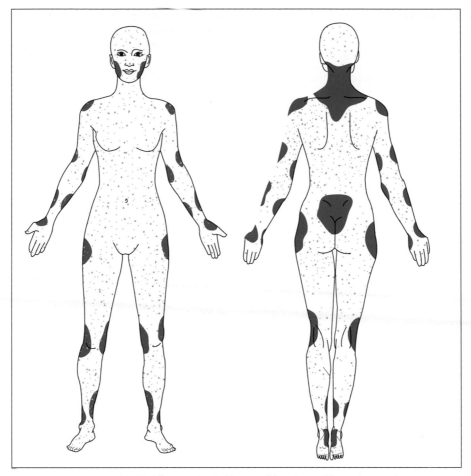

FIGURE 11-47 ■ (A, B) Mirror pain. A 40-year old patient with a mirror pain pattern.

Identifier 3: severity of related dysfunction and intolerance to daily living activity

Severity of related dysfunctioning and intolerance to daily living activity are disproportionate to the amount and/or severity of tissue damage. Many chronic pain patients show adverse responses to low-intensity physical activities. Fear-avoidance behaviours are also common features in chronic complex pain patients and contribute directly to disability.[529,530,534,535] A decreased frequency of sexual intercourse is also common.

The daily living activity intolerance could be assessed with simple questions such as:

■ bending and lifting weight (heavy suitcase or child 3–4 years old)
■ sitting (< 30 minutes)
■ standing (<30 minutes)
■ walking (<30 minutes)
■ travelling (by car or bus in <30 minutes)
■ difficulty performing daily tasks of low intensity
■ need help dressing.

Identifier 4: hypersensitivity of senses unrelated to the musculoskeletal system

The complex pain patient frequently shows a general sensorial hypersensitivity to different stimuli such as mechanical stimuli,[35,707,708] odours, temperature[709] and electric stimuli.[70,707] Some patients also refer intolerance to a certain type of fabric used in garments, to chemicals, to multiple drugs and taste hypersensitivity.

For instance, Small and Apkarian[735] showed that patients with chronic back pain have an increased sense of taste.

Hypersensitivity of senses unrelated to the musculoskeletal system:

- photophobia
- phonophobia
- osmophobia
- cold or heat intolerance
- intolerance to a certain type of clothes
- intolerance to chemicals
- intolerance to multiple drugs
- gustatory hypersensitivity.

Identifier 5: comorbidity

Another important additional criterion is comorbidity. Many patients with complex pain also suffer from other chronic conditions such as headache, dizziness, irritable bowel syndrome, painful bladder syndrome and chronic pelvic pain. Patients should be then questioned about any other clinical condition. Some patients report a past history of other clinical conditions that also correspond to a complex pain; therefore, they should be asked about any premorbid pain.

Comorbid clinical condition:

- IBS
- painful bladder syndrome
- vulvodynia
- dysuria
- headaches
- nausea
- instability
- abdominal chronic discomfort or pain
- allergic symptoms.

Premorbid pain: some patients report a past history of other clinical conditions that also correspond to a complex pain.

Identifier 6: diagnosis

The diagnosis either fails to match a known clinical pattern or fails to render a clear conclusion. History of diagnostic dilemma: the patient has undergone multiple diagnostic studies. The diagnoses are vague, inconsistent and inadequate. Diagnosis of clinical conditions

with no obvious pathogenic aetiological evidence such as FM, chronic fatigue syndrome, IBS, late whiplash, vulvodynia, etc., are included in this criterion.

- Diagnostic dilemma.
- Diagnoses are vague or inconsistent.
- Diagnosis of clinical conditions with no obvious pathogenic aetiological evidence.

Identifier 7: physical assessment

Physical assessment shows abnormal responses that are incompatible with a recognized clinical pattern.

- Anodyne or weird.
- Physical assessment intolerance.
- Diffuse/non-anatomic areas of pain/tenderness on palpation.
- Jump sign.
- Severe hyperaesthesia
- Mechanical allodynia.
- Thermal allodynia.
- Hypersensitivity not anatomical.
- Pain in the amplitude without inflammatory condition.
- Reduction on the range of movement without objective stiffness.
- Aberrant mobility pattern.
- Guarded movements.
- Weakness that does not follow neuroanatomical pattern.
- During the assessment patients show incongruent clinical responses: they do not tolerate a minimal manual examination (i.e. the foot) while able to jump on one leg without any pain.
- Hyperactive behaviours during the assessment: rubbing the affected area, holding it, a grimace, sweating, sighs.

Identifier 8: abnormal therapeutic response

Many patients with complex pain show abnormal therapeutic responses to previous or ongoing treatments. These typical abnormal therapeutic responses are: non-responders to any treatment; inconsistent or unpredictable response to treatment; and intolerance to various treatment approaches, including symptom exacerbation beyond what is regularly seen in patients with nociceptive pain.[703,736]

- Non-responders.
- Inconsistent/unpredictable response to treatment. What appear a successful treatment technique one day cannot obtain any response the other day.
- Intolerance to various treatment approaches.
- Adverse responses: significant worsening of the symptoms, fatigue, nausea after treatment
- Adverse responses to treatment in previous pain conditions.
- History of prior surgeries with negative outcomes (failed surgery).
- High effectiveness of 'miraculous' and 'alternative' treatment modalities.
- Visits to the emergency services.
- Acute increase in hypersensitivity to various stimuli in response to (new) treatment, including symptom exacerbation beyond what is regularly seen in patients with local musculoskeletal pain disorders.

Identifier 9: cognitive, emotional and behavioural aspects

Cognitive, emotional and behavioural factors are commonly involved in complex pain conditions. Patients with chronic pain exhibit negative and pessimistic thoughts, often obsessively, both about pain and their life. The patient's interpretation of the cause of pain determines the intensity with which it is experienced.[96] If the pain is interpreted as an indicator of something serious and threatening, the perception of pain is amplified.[103,474] Common emotions to the pain experience are depression, anxiety, fear, anger and frustration. Emotions and negative thoughts, therefore, play a crucial role in both the perception of pain and the development of avoidance behaviours and, finally, in the patient's disability. Common cognitive and emotional factors are erroneous cognitions about pain, catastrophizing, hypervigilance, low self-efficacy, illness perception, fear related to pain, depression and anxiety. These cognitive-affective factors can be the mediating mechanisms responsible for the differences in levels of self-reported emotional well-being and physical function. Chronic complex pain patients commonly show behavioural responses such as disproportionate disability, fear-avoidance and illness behaviours, reduced sexual intercourse and social self-exclusion.

- Misconceptions about pain
- Hypervigilance
- Catastrophism
- Emotional distress
- Anxiety
- Low mood/depression
- Low self-efficacy

Identifier 10: psychosocial issues

Different psychosocial aspects may be implicated in the development and maintenance of chronic pain such as adverse early-life experiences, immediate family members with chronic pain, sexual abuse, low socioeconomic and educational level and work-related issues. It is essential, therefore, in the evaluation of patients with complex pain, to explore not only the current history but also aspects such as premorbid conditions and psychosocial traumatic events that may contribute to understanding the patient's experience of pain.[431] Moreover, difficult emotional experiences, traumas, post-traumatic stress and interpersonal conflicts contribute to the perpetuation of pain.[93,437] Lower levels of education, low socioeconomic status and compensation issues are associated with higher rates of chronic pain and disability.[412,616]

- Adverse early-life events
- Immediate family members with chronic pain
- Post-traumatic stress disorders
- History of previous sick leave
- History of claims due to other injuries
- Low socioeconomic status
- Low educational background
- Compensation issues

In these patients the target of treatment no longer relates to the tissues, yet rather to the 'pain memory' and dysfunctional behaviours. Treatment strategies must be capable of reducing 'memory' activation and should also address maladaptive cognitions, behaviours, disability and all the biopsychosocial aspects implicated in the patient pain experience.

Conclusion and clinical implications

The biopsychosocial model and knowledge in central neuroplasticity mechanisms provide a more complete picture of complex chronic pain. The term 'chronic pain' can have very different interpretations, including definitions which only consider a pain duration of over 3 or 6 months, or as being one that persists beyond the normal healing time and therefore a maladaptive pain. Clinical complex pain conditions in which nociception fails to fully explain patient symptoms have been considered as chronic pain syndromes, known under various names, such as central sensitivity syndromes, hypersensitivity pain disorders, idiopathic pain syndrome, etc. In these cases, when pain aetiology is not completely understood, such as chronic widespread pain and non-specific back pain, the IASP proposes the term 'chronic primary pain'.

It has also been proposed that, in addition to the classic pain mechanisms such as nociceptive, inflammatory or neuropathic pain, a new category should be established, and it has been called '*central sensitization pain*'. Despite the fact that sensitization phenomena can be one of the mechanisms involved in chronic pain, these phenomena are present in acute pain associated with a nociceptive input. Furthermore, this algorithm does not include behavioural and psychosocial aspects that are absolutely relevant to understand the complex experience of chronic pain. Therefore, a thorough and comprehensive taxonomy that incorporates both somatosensory and psychosocial identifiers is needed in clinical practice. It should also be able to clearly differentiate pain associated with a nociceptive source from that in which it is irrelevant or does not justify the patient's symptoms.

'Complex pain' may be a better term for pain that is not the consequence of a tissue injury, any detectable inflammation or damage to the nervous system. It is crucial to identify the nature of chronic pain: nociceptive or inflammatory, neuropathic or dysfunctional. It is also important to determine the role of central sensitization in each case, bearing in mind that it may be adaptive. Thus, a suitable pain taxonomy has the potential to improve clinical decision-making and has important consequences both for the diagnosis and treatment and prognosis of patients with pain.[737] If the patient's symptoms are secondary to a nociceptive input, tissue treatment is justified. However, if the clinical picture relates to complex pain, strategies are needed which are capable of modulating the altered central processing and aimed at changing cognitions and reducing fear-avoidance behaviour and disability.

TREATMENT APPROACH TO PATIENTS WITH CHRONIC COMPLEX PAIN

The therapeutic approach presented is mainly aimed at the management of patients with chronic complex pain. It is the result of many influences and takes into account the important contributions of different therapeutic models such as educational therapeutic models, treatment based on movement, systematic desensitization techniques, strategies for cortical representations, as well as cognitive and behavioural approach models such as operant conditioning, gradual exposure and in vivo exposure, cognitive behavioural therapy, acceptance and commitment therapy, etc.

Treatment programme for patients with chronic complex pain

Before proposing a chronic pain treatment programme to the patient, it is essential to conduct a high-quality assessment by a clinician experienced in the patient's clinical condition.

The issues that the clinician should initially consider are:

1. Identify the dominant neurophysiological mechanism implicated in the patient's pain: nociceptive, inflammatory, neuropathic or dysfunctional. This is one of the most important aspects which will determine the therapeutic strategies to use.
2. What are the patient's major specific physical impairments?
3. How severe is central sensitization and what is the degree of CNS hyperexcitability?
4. Do the patient's beliefs about their pain conform to reality?
5. Are the patient's behaviours adaptive or of fear-avoidance?
6. What psychosocial aspects are involved?

It is necessary to identify whether there is an active pathology and its correlation with the patient's pain. Once again, it is necessary to insist on the essential differentiation from the therapeutic point of view between dysfunctional chronic pain and nociceptive, neuropathic or inflammatory persistent pain.

Treatment of patients with chronic complex pain should be approached from a multidimensional perspective and must be based on cognitive-behavioural principles. Individuals continually process the internal and environmental information so that the response of each individual does not depend reflexively on stimuli but is based on the processing. This processing involves the subject's cognitions, previous experiences, consideration of future consequences, context and family and cultural learning. The processing of information will determine motor and multisystem responses, including behaviours and emotions that will also influence the perception of pain. Pain is always a biologically consistent response, although clearly maladaptive in patients with complex pain. This maladaptive response is also mediated by cognition and determines behaviours that aggravate the individual's impairment. Therefore, these two aspects, cognitions and behaviours, are crucial in the treatment of patients with chronic complex pain.

To address, therapeutically, cognitions and behaviours is crucial in patients with chronic complex pain.

The first step in the management of these patients should be aimed at modifying inadequate cognitions of patients about their pain. In this sense, one of the strategies that is showing promising results is pain biology education, also called pain neurophysiology/neuroscience education. The second essential strategy is aimed at changing fear-avoidance behaviours and disability based on a programme of gradual exposure/exposure in vivo and physical reactivation. Another interesting strategy, especially in patients with severe hyperalgesia and allodynia, is desensitization using peripheral stimulation. In recent years strategies have been developed with the intention of acting on 'the virtual body' and thus acting on the cortical reorganization, reducing pain and sensory distortion phenomena. Finally, in many patients, those psychosocial aspects that favour and perpetuate the pain behaviours and disability need to be addressed.

STRATEGIES IN THE MANAGEMENT OF PATIENTS WITH CHRONIC COMPLEX PAIN

- Education in pain neurobiology.
- Treatment of specific physical intolerance and disability: gradual exposure/exposure in vivo and general physical reactivation.

- Peripheral desensitization techniques.
- Strategies aimed at the 'virtual body'.
- Management of psychosocial aspects involved.

The two cornerstones of treatment in most patients are education in pain biology and design of a physical reactivation programme aimed at obtaining desensitization and reducing specific disability. Although some treatment principles can be outlined, it should be noted that treatment must be designed according to each individual.

FUNDAMENTALS OF TREATMENT OF PATIENTS WITH CHRONIC PAIN

- Pain education
- Physical rehabilitation:
  - desensitization
  - specific intolerance treatment.

Before addressing treatment, we must bring to mind two common conceptual errors. The first is to consider that the only goal of treatment is to relieve pain and the second is that symptomatic improvement will allow the patient to return to normal life.

Although reducing pain is one of the treatment goals, it should not be the sole or primary objective. Many patients clinically improve with treatment but do not return to work and continue to maintain a situation of disability. Therefore, the current clinical models focus on improving the functionality and quality of life. It is important for patients to understand that it is essential to guide their behaviours towards significant activities grounded on their values. Another aspect to note is the negative effect which passive treatment modalities may have in patients with a complex pain. Passive treatments, in this case, are not only irrelevant but also can be counterproductive, because they strengthen the patient's conviction that the source of pain lies in a pathology or physical dysfunction. Aspects that *do* make a difference in the outcome are patient education, addressing specific physical intolerance and fear-avoidance behaviour and increasing the level of activity.

- Eliminating pain is not the only goal of treatment.
- Passive treatment modalities can be counterproductive.

- The aim is that the patient may resume their work, family and recreational activities.
- It is necessary to address all biological, psychological and social aspects.
- It is essential to reduce the emotional impact of pain and modify the patient's behaviour.

A key aspect of this model is that the patients takes an active role throughout the process. Therefore, their classic role of passive recipients of treatment should be amended and they should become the main active promoters of their recovery process. The therapist should be involved in the demedicalization of the problem, assuming a completely different role from the usual biomedical role. The therapist, rather than applying techniques, acts as an educator, whose aim is to encourage cognitive and behavioural changes, transmitting information and designing a programme of physical rehabilitation and specific desensitization for the patient. In this therapist–patient relationship it is important to listen to patients, acknowledge their pain, offer support and get their confidence by demonstrating updated knowledge about their problem.

TREATMENT PRINCIPLES

- Collaborative patient-centred treatment.
- The therapist should be involved in the demedicalization of the patient's problem.
- Individualized conceptualization of the problem.
- Specific objectives for each patient.
- The patient should understand that pain is not the primary goal of treatment, but the most important thing is to resume a normal life.

The therapist–patient interaction is very important for positive outcomes. In controlled experimental studies, it has been shown that enhanced therapeutic alliance modulates pain intensity in patients with chronic pain.[738] To obtain therapeutic alliance, an essential aspect is to find a professional who knows the complex dimensions of chronic pain and understands the patient's situation, as many patients have been treated as 'psychosomatic patients' and even as simulators. It is necessary to create a warm and friendly therapeutic environment in which the patient feels supported at all times by the therapist.[739] Acknowledging the patient's pain and suffering is essential, however,

and from the beginning the sick role and maladaptive illness behaviours should be discouraged.[740]

A critical aspect is that patients should reconceptualize their problems. The point to focus on, and this is one of the fundamental aspects, is not the elimination of pain, but to resume work, family and social activities. The patient must understand that the problem is not only the pain but also many other aspects of their life, such as disability, deterioration in their family and social relationships, etc. It is therefore essential that the patient's and the therapist's conceptualization of the problem should coincide. It is critical that the therapist is capable of 'mapping' the patient's pain problem in all its physical, behavioural, personal and social dimensions. The therapist must be able to offer patients a broader and more comprehensive view of their problems. Therefore, a personalized approach covering the particular aspects of the patient's life is required.

This is a patient-centred and collaborative treatment model, where therapist and patient share decisions. Highly important aspects include patients' values, previous experience, perception of self, vision of the world and not just their pain, their own skills and expectations. Treatment should empower patients to take an active and responsible role in their recovery. The aspect that will ultimately determine the success of the programme is whether such a programme is capable of 'empowering' patients to manage their pain: it must get patients to develop their own coping strategies, which depend on their motivations, values and efforts.[561] A necessary objective is also to 'immunize' the patient against treatments not evidence-based, especially if they are interventional or surgical. For patients with complex pain, having high emotional distress and disability for many years, it is recommended that the therapist should be trained in cognitive-behavioural strategies.

IMPORTANT ASPECTS IN THE THERAPIST–PATIENT RELATIONSHIP

- It is critical to obtain a good therapeutic alliance with the patient.
- It is important to listen to the patient.
- Acknowledge the patient's pain and suffering.
- Identify the patient's meanings and attributions about their pain.

- Provide patient support.
- Do not judge the patient.
- Demonstrate current knowledge about their problem.
- Match patient–therapist conceptualization of the problem.
- Empower the patient to take an active and responsible role in recovery.

Planning the treatment programme

Assessment of mediators, moderator and prognostic factors

Treatment of patients with chronic pain is complex: it is essential to adjust the treatment to those most relevant aspects involved in the patient's pain. Before starting treatment, it is essential to evaluate the mediating and moderating variables of therapeutic response and prognostic factors. A mediator is defined as a variable responsible for all or part of the effects of treatment. For a variable to be a mediator there must be a causal relationship between treatment and outcomes. A moderator is a baseline characteristic that interacts with and affects treatment outcomes.[741] While mediators identify what and why a treatment is effective, moderators identify who and under what circumstances the treatments have different effects. Identifying response-moderating and -mediating variables allows us to design the most appropriate treatment strategies for the individual patient.

Expectations and motivations, obstacles and barriers in the treatment should be evaluated, assessing the various factors involved in the patient's pain and determining what is more decisive in the patient's pain experience. Identifying all those prognostic factors, especially when they are modifiable, allows their use as treatment goals, designing the treatment based on the patient's characteristics.[742]

Patients' expectations are important determinants of treatment outcomes.[508,742–744] Expectations and motivations that may determine a poor therapeutic prognosis are seeking a magical, quick and effortless solution, patients pushed by third parties (children, spouse) but who are not personally motivated or patients who are interested in understanding what is the matter but not in changing.

EVALUATING PROGNOSTIC ASPECTS

- Expectations and motivations.
- Obstacles and barriers in the treatment.
- Factors involved in the patient's pain.
- The most relevant factors in the patient's pain experience.

All sorts of obstacles and barriers hinder treatment such as deeply rooted erroneous cognitions regarding pain, extremely severe pain, high anxiety, obsessive thoughts about pain, emotional and affective situations, low cultural and socioeconomic status, dysfunctional behaviour over many years, dependence on and tolerance to drug treatment, especially prolonged use of opiates, family aspects, repeated sick leave and a high degree of disability.

Physical factors involved in the patient's pain must be assessed, determining specific physical intolerances and fear-avoidance behaviour, based on which the gradual exposure programme will be planned. The patient's level of physical activity, quality of sleep and general health should be taken into consideration.

A key issue is to assess the cognitive aspects: What are the patient's beliefs about the pain? What is the information received from health professionals? Does it conform to reality or not – patients' alarmist thoughts, fears about their pain and their future expectations? Knowing patients' erroneous beliefs about their pain is essential before any cognitive intervention. The negative interpretation of the cause of pain is able to focus attention on bodily symptoms, aggravating the patient's pain and disability: for example, the common belief that the spine is a vulnerable structure, that back injuries are serious and have a bad solution. It is therefore critical from the start to modify the patient's inappropriate beliefs in order to improve therapeutic results.[479]

OBSTACLES AND BARRIERS IN TREATMENT

- Erroneous cognitions about pain.
- Obsessive thoughts about pain.
- Extremely severe pain.
- Emotional and affective aspects: high anxiety and depression, low self-efficacy, passive coping style, high hypervigilance.
- Dysfunctional behaviour over many years.

- Occupational aspects: repeated sick leave.
- High degree of disability.
- Dependence on and tolerance to drug treatment.
- Low cultural and socioeconomic status.
- Family aspects: such as an overprotective spouse

As for the relevant emotional aspects, it is necessary to assess the mood, the degree of anxiety and depression, if the patient is angry, if they believe that something or someone is to blame for their situation, the patient's greater or lesser self-efficacy, passive or active coping ability, their degree of hypervigilance and their personality traits. Family relationships can play a significant role in the patient's pain and disability, especially regarding the spouse. It is necessary to establish if the spouse is punitive or solicitous, reinforcing the patient's pain behaviours. It is very important to know the patient's working status, whether they have been off work, the relationship with their employer and coworkers, as well as to identify disputes or issues relating to financial compensation and if the subject shows social self-exclusion behaviours. Managing psychological factors that are primarily related to a patient's pain and functional incapacity has to be part of all the health care providers' responsibility to the patient.[477]

Treatment expectations are critical to treatment outcomes. For example, those patients who expect to return to work show a global recovery nearly 50% earlier than those who did not have a positive expectation.[743] Also, an important aspect is to recognize that the therapist's beliefs, expectations and attitudes influence the patient.[745,746]

Initial assessment

Before approaching the patient with the programme, it is essential that the initial assessment should include a complete clinical examination, even if we are convinced that the patient's pain is dysfunctional and that there is no relevant active pathology. This strategy allows us to adjust to the patient's initial expectations and gives us arguments to help the patient understand that the pain is dysfunctional and does not need further investigation in search of a somatic disease. Patients must understand that their physical dysfunctions are not causing their pain but are the consequence of a pain memory, guarded movements, fear-avoidance behaviour, disuse and deconditioning, etc. Patients must also understand the need to evaluate

the various psychological and social aspects of their pain experience. They hardly accept, at least initially, the important role of these aspects in relation to their pain. One of the problems of the Cartesian mind–body dualism is that patients may consider that when we discuss the role of the CNS in pain, their pain is being interpreted as purely psychological. The need to assess psychosocial aspects can be justified simply by explaining to patients that there is no chronic pain without emotional suffering and without family and personal consequences. In this way, patients will accept being questioned specifically about their beliefs about pain and its causes, emotional responses, pain behaviours and coping styles and family, socio-economic and occupational aspects. Ideally, therefore, the perspective we initially offer the patient should be highly 'neurobiological' to then introduce those psychological and social aspects that are involved in pain.

The subjective assessment model we propose can be found in Chapter 8 of Volume 1. We always recommend splitting the subjective assessment into two parts. In the first part, the clinician obtains information in order to use clinical reasoning based on pattern recognition. Our main interest in this part is to get a first impression of the patient's condition to identify the clinical pattern and to explore what the painful experience has meant for the patient from a narrative perspective. It gives us information about the patient's beliefs, expectations, emotions, context and the significance of the problem for the patient.

The diagnostic procedure model comprises three stages: pattern recognition, hypothetical-deductive reasoning and interpretative reasoning. One of the main features of chronic complex pain is that it does not fulfil the principle of adequacy. This principle establishes that for the occurrence of a particular clinical situation (What?), the necessary conditions (Why?) must be met and this clinical situation must be expressed with its characteristic signs and symptoms (How?). The interpretative reasoning is aimed at understanding the significance of the problem for the patient in all its dimensions. Managing patients' pain problems requires an understanding of each patient's unique illness experience.[747]

In the subjective examination and physical assessment, the most relevant factors should be established at different domains: clinical condition and severity and type of associated dysfunction, if there are any physical impairments, pain mechanisms (nociceptive, inflammatory, neuropathic or dysfunctional), central sensitization phenomena, patients' beliefs (adaptive or maladaptive), patients' behaviours (fear-avoidance and illness behaviours) and psychosocial aspects involved. It is crucial to assess social participation and interactions, such as limitations in work or daily activities (e.g. inability to drive) and in activities that require social interaction (e.g. missing work due to sick leave or avoiding leisure activities).

ASSESSMENT OF RELEVANT FACTORS

■ Clinical condition.
■ Physical impairments.
■ Pain mechanisms (nociceptive, inflammatory, neuropathic or dysfunctional).
■ Central sensitization phenomena.
■ Patients' beliefs (adaptive or maladaptive).
■ Patients' behaviours (fear-avoidance and illness behaviours).

■ Psychosocial factors.
■ Social participation and interaction.

Personal aspects, both physical and psychological, as well as social and environmental aspects, such as family, occupational status, etc., are also important. These personal and contextual factors are often able to explain the patient's specific clinical picture, being key to patient management and treatment outcomes. Our objective as clinicians is not to 'fix' tissue impairment or to improve the patient's physical dysfunction but to help patients to resume work and social participation and interaction. Therefore, we must know all personal and contextual factors and it is imperative to assess the patient's cognitions and behaviours.

> Managing patients' pain problems requires an understanding of each patient's unique illness experience. Personal and contextual factors are often able to explain the patient's specific clinical picture, being key to the patient's management and treatment outcomes.

TABLE 11-13	
Patient ratings scales and questionnaires	
Dominion	**Scales and questionnaires**
Pain severity	NRS VAS
Pain unpleasantness	NRS VAS
Pain descriptors	
Pain location	Pain body map
Physical functioning and disability	**General** Brief Pain Inventory[748] Brief Pain Inventory[749] Brief Pain Inventory Short Form,[749,750] Graded Chronic Pain Scale[730] Multidimensional Pain Inventory[751] Multidimensional Pain Inventory Interference Scale (MPI-I).[752] Patient-Specific Functional Scale (PSFS)[753] SF-36,[754] SF-12.[755] Graded Chronic Pain Scale[751] Multidimensional Pain Inventory[752] Multidimensional Pain Inventory Interference Scale (MPI-I).[753] Patient-Specific Functional Scale (PSFS)[754] SF-36,[755] SF-12.[756] **Specific conditions** Oswestry Disability Index (ODI) 2.0[757] Roland-Morris Disability Questionnaire[758] Neck Disability Index (NDI)[759] Northwick Park Neck Pain Questionnaire[760]

Questionnaires for assessment

Different questionnaires may be useful in the initial evaluation. In addition, they are needed to measure treatment outcomes. They should cover different dominions such as pain severity and unpleasantness, pain location, patient's cognitions, emotional functioning, physical functioning and disability, fear-avoidance behaviours, coping styles and self-efficacy (Table 11-13).

Pain severity, unpleasantness and pain descriptors. *Pain severity* can be assessed by a 0–10 numerical rating scale (NRS) or 10-cm visual analogue scale

(VAS). It should be assessed as the average, the maximum and the minimum pain during the past week. It is considered that a decrease in individuals' pain intensity of approximately 1 cm (or 1.0 point) or 15–20% represent 'minimal change', whereas decreases of 2.0–2.7 points or 30–41% have more meaning to patients.[748]

Assessment of *pain unpleasantness* is important since the affective component of pain can be distinguished from pain intensity and its response to treatment can be very different. Pain unpleasantness can also be assessed with VAS and the NRS, grading from 'not unpleasant' to the 'most unpleasant feeling possible'.

TABLE 11-13
Patient ratings scales and questionnaires—Cont'd

Dominion	Scales and questionnaires
Emotional functioning	Beck Depression Inventory –II (BDI-II)[760] Hospital Anxiety and Depression Scale[761] Profile of Mood States (POMS)[762]Beck Depression Inventory –II (BDI-II)[761] Hospital Anxiety and Depression Scale[762] Profile of Mood States (POMS)[763]
Fear in relation to pain	Fear of Pain Questionnaire (FPQ)[763] Pain Anxiety Symptoms Scale (PASS)[764] Fear of Pain Questionnaire (FPQ)[764] Pain Anxiety Symptoms Scale (PASS)[765] Fear-Avoidance Beliefs Questionnaire (FABQ)[519] Fear Avoidance of Pain Scale (FAPS)[765] Tampa Scale for Kinesiophobia (TSK),[766] TSK- short version (TSK-11) Fear Avoidance of Pain Scale (FAPS)[766] Tampa Scale for Kinesiophobia (TSK),[767] TSK- short version (TSK-11)[767,768]. Photographs Series of Daily Activities (PHODA)[768] Pain Beliefs Screening Instrument (PBS),[769] Orebro Musculoskeletal Pain Questionnaire[770] Pain and Impairment Relationship Scale (PAIRS).[771] Photographs Series of Daily Activities (PHODA)[769] Pain Beliefs Screening Instrument (PBS),[770] Orebro Musculoskeletal Pain Questionnaire[771] Pain and Impairment Relationship Scale (PAIRS).[772] STarT Back[772,773].
Catastrophizing	Pain Catastrophizing Scale[773] Pain self-perception scale PSPS[774]Pain Catastrophizing Scale[774] Pain self-perception scale PSPS[775]
Coping styles	Vanderbilt Pain Management Inventory[775]Vanderbilt Pain Management Inventory[776]
Self-efficacy	Pain Self-Efficacy Questionnaire.[776]Pain Self-Efficacy Questionnaire.[777]
Pain acceptance	Chronic Pain Acceptance Questionnaire (CPAQ).[777]Chronic Pain Acceptance Questionnaire (CPAQ).[778]
Patient ratings of global improvement and satisfaction with treatment	Patient Global Impression of Improvement Scale (PGI-I)[778] Global Rating of Change Scale.[779]Patient Global Impression of Improvement Scale (PGI-I)[779] Global Rating of Change Scale.[780]

Pain descriptors are one of the key factors to determine the pain mechanisms involved. Whether pain is somatic, inflammatory, neuropathic or dysfunctional and not associated with an active nociceptive source. Patients should be asked to use descriptors to explain their pain. The quality of pain defined as dull, burning, stabbing, paroxysmal, pressing, etc., provides relevant information on the type of pain and the pathophysiological mechanisms involved. Importantly, many patients use descriptors of neuropathic pain when there is no injury or disease in the somatosensory system. Clinicians should be aware that these neuropathic-like symptoms have nothing to do with a neuropathy and are very frequent among patients with complex pain.

Pain location. In order to accurately record the area where the patient refers the pain symptoms, its location is drawn on a silhouette of the entire body. The *pain map* can be drawn by the therapist, as the patient is often unable to express the symptoms on the drawing. However, it is also interesting to ask patients to draw their own map of symptoms. Normally, a widespread pain, with non-anatomical distribution or a complex pattern, may suggest a complex pain. The manner in which the patient describes the symptoms and records them on the pain map allows therapists to understand how the patients perceive their own clinical situation and, often, provides information regarding the emotional impact that the problem has on the individual.

Phases in the development of the programme

The pain programme can be divided into: pain education, treatment of specific physical intolerance and disability, peripheral desensitization techniques, strategies aimed at the 'virtual body'' and management of psychosocial aspects involved.

Pain education

The most important aspect of treatment is patient education. The information held by patients is in many cases wrong, as they continue associating pain to tissue injury. The problem is this considerable misinformation is often transmitted by health professionals and social media. An example of education with counterproductive results is one commonly used in *back schools* in the management of patients with chronic low back pain, where anatomical and biomechanical factors responsible for low back pain are usually explained to the patients. This type of education has a negative effect, because it conceptualizes back pain in terms of a structural problem, so that the patient understands that this structure is vulnerable to injury. It also increases attention to the pain and the use of health resources.[781–784]

Other educational models have developed in the form of booklets for patients that are targeted at specific pain conditions: e.g. *The Back Book*,[785] *The Neck Book*,[786] *The Whiplash Book*[787] and *The Whiplash Injury Recovery.*[788] These publications clearly challenge the traditional advice based on a biomedical model and are clearly intended to encourage the patient to adopt an active attitude in their recovery, medicalizing the clinical condition and based on an active self-management approach.

The essential messages may be summarized as follows: pain does not mean a serious damage; pain improvement is usually rapid; basic analgesics can be used; avoiding activity slows recovery; it is recommended to do simple exercises; and early return to daily activities and work is not only safe but also can be very helpful for a full recovery.[789]

Education in the neurobiology of pain.

Education in the neurobiology of pain is a powerful strategy in the management of patients with chronic pain. This model developed by Butler[84] and Moseley[116] and popularized in *Explain Pain*[104] by Butler and Moseley has shown significant results in the management of chronic pain patients. Explaining pain (EP) has been defined as a range of educational interventions that aim to change patient understanding of the biology of pain in order to reduce it. EP is a therapeutic intervention that uses the explanation of pain neurophysiology, making use of the new contributions of pain science and neuroscience, to change maladaptive pain cognitions, illness perceptions or coping strategies, to further introduce normal movement and activity and reduce pain and functional disability. The core objective of the EP approach is to shift patient conceptualization of pain from that of 'a marker of tissue damage or disease to that of a marker of the perceived need to protect body tissue'.[105] As pain is fundamentally dependent on meaning, a new conceptualization of pain as a response to perceived threat and a need of protection can not only change maladaptive pain cognitions but also improve patients' perception of their ability to control and manage pain.[790] This change in the conceptualization of pain helps the patient to develop more adaptive emotional, motor and behavioural management strategies. However, for these changes to be transformed into attitudes and behaviours, in-depth patient learning involving a conceptual change is essential.[105,116]

The aspects that make pain education so powerful are, on the one hand, its ability to 'biologize' the pain experience for the patient: pain is not psychological but has a neurobiological explanation. On the other hand, it is the assumption of the paradigm of central sensitization and neuroplasticity, which means that the brain can 'relearn', become desensitized, change and stop generating pain. Unlike other strategies that are aimed at dealing with the consequences of pain in terms of disability, emotional responses, etc., the goal is much more ambitious: to reduce the pain memory activation.

Although patients when starting the programme only want the pain to go away, it must be explained to them, as previously mentioned, that pain is not the only the problem but a life of disability, emotional distress, social self-exclusion, etc. It is necessary to change the focus of attention to prevent them from just 'taking their temperature'. It is also advisable to focus the treatment on the elimination of any pain behaviours and on enabling the patient to return to normal life.

Combining education in the physiology of pain with therapeutic approaches to improve the physical abilities of the patient produces a significant change in beliefs, reduces pain and improves quality of life.

Pain education may be offered in different formats, including intensive one-to-one sessions, or in small or large groups. The format currently used by the author in patients with complex pain usually involves between 4 and 6 sessions of an hour and a half, distributed once a week. Follow-up of the patient is performed with revisions at 3 and 6 months and finally after 1 year. After the first visit the therapist has already identified if the patient suffers dysfunctional chronic pain and if that particular patient is capable of performing a pain programme. Before starting the programme, the therapist must explain to the patient how it will develop,

the therapist–patient roles, how they will assess progress and how follow-up is conducted.

Educational components of the programme are divided into different areas that include education in neurophysiology of pain, pain as a bodily perception, pain and physical performance, the relationship between thoughts, emotions and maladaptive behaviours and pain perception and, finally, pain-related psychosocial aspects.

The aim of this educational programme is not to provide information to patients on pain and the role of the CNS but to generate a consistent change in their beliefs, behaviour and perception of pain. To do so, messages must be coherent and credible, adjusting to the patient's experience of pain. They should also be presented eloquently and in a rhetorically convincing manner. Patients should be encouraged to reproduce, by themselves, the content presented in each session.

The first session is very important: the initial objective is that patients understand the reasons whereby they have been prompted to start a pain management programme. In this first session we must acknowledge their pain and convince them that more tests are not needed to identify a potential source of pain. It must be explained that unsuccessful therapeutic pilgrimages that many undergo has to do with the fact that, frequently, certain health professionals do not have updated knowledge about pain.

The main messages during this first session are that the pain is real, but that it is not the result of tissue injury or of a psychological origin. The concepts of dysfunctional maladaptive pain and central sensitization are introduced. The patient must understand that there is no linear relationship between injury and pain, but pain is always a brain response that is generated by the joint interaction of many factors, such as interpretation, context, emotional distress, previous experiences, learning and assessment of future consequences.

Many examples can be used to explain to the patient the scarce relationship between pain and injury, such as any of the following: serious injuries in which the patient experiences no pain at all; the phenomena of allodynia; secondary hyperalgesia and referred pain; and phantom limb pain.

The patient must understand that pain is not a sign of injury (pain does not mean damage), but the consequence of maladaptive central sensitization. Patients must realize that the neuroplastic changes of their SNC are capable of causing severe and persistent pain without any significant tissue damage. Changes in CNS processing can induce an increase in pain facilitatory mechanisms as well a reduction of central inhibitory mechanisms at supraspinal levels, activation of the pain neurosignature and changes in sensory and motor cortical representation.

This phenomenon should be seen as an individual response to a real threat or one perceived as such. Pain is aimed at action, so that all the sensory and emotional dimensions serve to develop behaviours that prevent injury.[116] Dysfunctional chronic pain is a 'memory' stored in the brain. The stimuli associated with the patient's pain do not 'cause' the pain: they are just learned triggers. Knowledge in the biology of pain, as an expression of a stress response to threat, provides a physiological basis that allows the patient to understand the role of psychological factors involved in chronic pain. The patient must also be aware that maladaptive central sensitization causes a decreased tissue tolerance to mechanical stress due to disuse and the establishment of dysfunctional motor patterns. The patient is also introduced to the paradigm of neuroplasticity and how changes in central processing that perpetuate pain may be reversible.

An important aspect in this session is that the patient understands the central role of beliefs about the perception of pain. A similar model to the Ellis's ABC model[791] can be used, wherein A is pain, B beliefs and C consequences. The patient is worried about the pain (A) and the consequences (C) of pain in his life, both in terms of emotional suffering and disability (work, family, friends, etc.). Ruminating thoughts continually oscillate between A and C, but never analyse B. However, the fundamental problem lies in the patient's beliefs about pain (B). B is the crucial link in a chain (ABC) of pain, suffering and disability.

UNDERSTANDING ABC

- ABC is a chain of pain, suffering and disability
- A = pain; B = belief; C = suffering and disability
- Your thoughts go from A to B, but do not analyse B
- Your real enemy is B

Positive expectations should be created, helping the patient to identify beliefs, emotions and dysfunctional behaviours. The patient must understand the impact of catastrophic thoughts and fear-avoidance behaviour

in the development of disability.[507,792] Knowing the nature of chronic pain reduces the feeling of threat and emotions associated with the pain experience, and also decreases the activation of alarm and defence responses, such as endocrine, neuroimmune, sympathetic and motor systems. It is essential to reduce the impact of pain on the patient's life. Other relevant cognitive factors in the therapeutic outcomes are reductions in fear of movement and catastrophizing, and increase in functional self-efficacy. It is therefore essential to target these cognitive factors when treating chronic pain patients.[793] The ultimate idea is that a new understanding of their pain will be able to generate new coping behaviours and changes in their complex pain processing.

- It is imperative that the patient understands that the nature of chronic pain is multidimensional and how changes in central pain processing, physical dysfunction and psychosocial aspects interact.

The second session deals with aspects of neurophysiology of pain such as neurons and transduction and transmission mechanisms, the role of ascending and descending pathways, central modulation mechanisms and how chronic pain is associated with changes in central pain processing. It is important to introduce the concept of pain as a maladaptive brain response in response to a perceived threat. 'Narratives' can be built based on pain neuroimaging studies that support our theory.

In the third session, the patient needs to understand pain as a projection of the brain to consciousness that generates a perceptual distortion. Understanding pain as a perception helps explain how it can be modulated by different aspects such as attention, cognitions regarding pain. Explicit examples of how the brain can override perceptions depending on the context should be presented. The aim of the third session is that the patient understands chronic pain as a dysfunctional memory capable of generating an alteration in somatic perceptions.

This 'dysfunctional memory' can be activated by different stimuli and contexts. An important message of this session is that those movements or postures that are associated with pain are not the cause directly but act as learned 'switches' capable of triggering a 'pain memory'. The concept of neuromatrix and virtual body is introduced and the various strategies aimed at the desensitization and retraining of the virtual body.

The fourth session focuses on the patient's comprehension of the relationship between fear-avoidance behaviours and loss of physical abilities. It exposes how the reduction in physical activity decreases tissue tolerance due to disuse; it can generate dysfunctional motor patterns, guarded movements and, eventually, lead to a deconditioning syndrome. This session justifies the gradual exposure programme.

The fifth session addresses the relationship between thoughts, emotions and pain perception and maladaptive response models. The patient must realize that the nature of chronic pain is multidimensional, and understand how changes in central pain processing, physical dysfunction and psychosocial aspects interact. The patient must understand that pain is contextual. Work, family and social situation can have a decisive influence on the persistence of pain.

A fundamental aspect in these sessions is to give patients the opportunity to reassess the meaning of their problem and the accuracy and adequacy of their thoughts, fears and behaviours. Patients need to understand how their own meaning and interpretation of pain are able to modify the attention, amplifying or decreasing it, and thus increasing or decreasing pain perception. Also, how the interpretation of pain is able to determine their adaptive or maladaptive emotional and behavioural responses, and therefore being critical in the emotional impact of pain and degree of disability. The patient must understand the impact of erroneous beliefs, anxiety, attention, expectation, fear, stress, catastrophic thoughts, mood, self-efficacy, self-esteem and self-perception in the perpetuation of pain.

Finally, in the last session, patients should be led to reflect on the meaning given to their painful situation from a broader perspective, including changes that pain produced in their lives, their work and in their personal and family relationships. Also, how these different psychosocial aspects, including family learning, previous experiences and the occupational and social context, may have influenced the development and chronicity of pain (Fig. 11-48). In this last session, the management of reactivations is also addressed (Table 11-14).

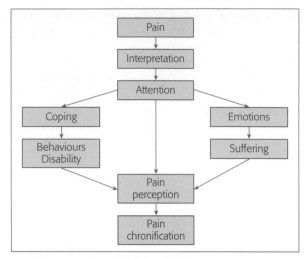

FIGURE 11-48 ■ The patient must understand the impact of erroneous beliefs, anxiety, attention, expectation, fear, stress, catastrophic thoughts, mood, self-efficacy, self-esteem and self-perception in the perpetuation from pain. They must understand how these different psychosocial aspects, including family learning, previous experiences and the occupational and social context, may have influenced the development and chronicity of pain.

A frequent source of failure is that during the pain programme, the patient continues to visit different health professionals with a pathomechanical vision opposed to the programme information. We must 'immunize' the patient against all 'peripheral' interventions, especially invasive techniques. To do this, we must offer the patient relevant and updated information on chronic pain. It should be an essential requirement to begin a pain treatment programme that the patient should desist from a 'medical pilgrimage' and not see other professionals who might dilute the strength of the treatment.

Intervention in maladaptive thoughts, emotions and behaviours

Many patients are unaware of the mental processes involved in the experience of pain. Cognitive-behavioural approaches are based on the assumption that the subjects are active processors of information whereby the responses, including pain, are never stereotyped or automatic. Importantly, the patient should realize that thoughts, knowledge, attributions and expectations can trigger or modulate pain and

TABLE 11-14	
Education sessions	
1. Picture of the problem	Reasons for implementing the programme
	Explanation of programme development
	Therapeutic targets
	Introduction to the concept of maladaptive central sensitization and central neuroplasticity
2. Neurophysiology of pain	Pain and nociception
	Neurons, synapses, ion channels
	Ascending and descending pathways
	Central sensitization: spinal and supraspinal changes
	Pain as a brain response to threat
	Central modulation mechanisms
	Chronic pain and changes in the central processing
3. Pain and body perception	Pain as a perceptual distortion
	Pain as a perceptual memory
	The concept of neuromatrix
	The concept of virtual body
	The role of desensitization strategies
	Retraining the virtual body
4. Pain and physical performance	Pain and physical performance
	Pain and deconditioning
	Fear-avoidance behaviour
	The vicious circle: pain, threatening information, fear of pain, avoidance, disuse, disability and depression
5. Pain, thoughts, emotions and behaviours of pain	Relationship between thoughts, emotions and pain perception
	Pain, erroneous cognitions and catastrophic thoughts
	The thought–emotion–perception–behaviour cycle
	Maladaptive patterns of thinking, feeling and responding
	Pain and emotions: stress, anxiety, low mood, self-perception, self-efficacy and self-esteem
6. Pain and psychosocial aspects	Pain and learning
	Pain and family aspects
	Pain and occupational issues
	Social self-exclusion

associated physiological responses, as well as their emotions and behaviours. All these responses are determined by learning, previous experiences, context and family and social environment.

Patients with chronic pain have learned maladaptive patterns of thinking, feeling and responding. Therefore, the aim of treatment should not only be to reduce pain but also to modify maladaptive pain behaviours, which necessarily requires addressing all cognitions, thoughts and emotions involved in the development of those responses. The patient should understand the relationship between their elaborations and cognitive interpretations, emotions that can be evoked and the perceptual experience of pain.

A useful strategy may be to 'uncover the hidden connections' that may be perpetuating pain. To do this,

using a form, during the first week, patients must identify, several times they experience pain during the day, what automatic thoughts are triggered, emotions that appear and how they respond behaviourally (Fig. 11-49). It is also interesting for the patient to note the visual image associated with the experience of pain. The patient should ask whether all these mental processes and behavioural responses conform to reality, whether or not they further exacerbate their pain and disability and if there are no other more adaptive ways to respond. It is generally helpful for the patient to fill out several times a day, a template listing these mental processes and behavioural responses.

The following week, patients repeat the same exercise, but they must develop an adaptive response to every thought, visual image, emotion and behavioural

Identification of thoughts, emotions and maladaptive behaviour **First week**				
Pain situation	Negative irruptive thoughts	Visual image	Negative emotions	Maladaptive behaviour

FIGURE 11-49 ■ Form for identifying thoughts, emotions and behaviour: first week.

Intervention in thoughts, emotions and maladaptive behaviour **Second week**								
Pain situation	Negative irruptive thoughts	Alternative adaptive thoughts	Visual image	Alternative visual image	Negative emotions	Alternative adaptive emotions	Maladaptive behaviour	Alternative adaptive behaviour

FIGURE 11-50 ■ Form for identifying thoughts, emotions and behaviour: second week.

response (Fig. 11-50). This exercise enables the patient to learn to observe the mental processes that underlie their responses, also helping them learn to distance themselves from their thought processes. In this way, they can begin to realize that the responses previously considered as normal and automatic are not so.

It may also be interesting for some patients to use training strategies that modify the relationship between thoughts and automatic responses such as those proposed by the ACT model, such as *cognitive defusion* and the *self-as-a-context*. *Cognitive defusion* training means that the patient understands that thoughts are just thoughts and not necessarily to be believed as 'real', and should not lead the patient away from personally important and meaningful activities. *Self-as-a-context* implies that patients are aware of their own thoughts and are able to 'contemplate them from the outside', as an observer.

Difficulties and obstacles in the pain programme

As already mentioned, pain education is one of the most powerful tools in the treatment of chronic pain; however, this approach sometimes fails to work. On some occasions, the patient shows a significant resistance to accepting that there can be pain without injury; others understand, but nothing changes, and they still have pain and disability; and in other cases, a significant initial improvement is obtained but after some months everything returns to the baseline situation. Why is there no change in some patients or, in others, after an initial 'huge success', pain returns months later?

Some issues are related to the quality of information we provide, others to the programme format, others to the therapist's training and skills and, lastly, others relate to the patient because it is he or she who must operate the change.

As already noted, it is necessary to initially assess *expectations and motivations* that may hinder the results from the inception of the programme. Some examples of common problems include the following:

1. Patients refuse to understand the message; they are still set on the idea that 'there must be something'.
2. Patients seem to understand the message but it fails to translate into any change. Learning is

superficial; patients are unable to 'apply' that message to their situation. When their coping style is clearly passive, they are still looking for magical, quick and effortless solutions.

3. Patients start the programme, pushed by others, but are not really interested; when they start the programme 'to try' something different but still visit other professionals who give conflicting messages.

4. When there is a clear often unconscious resistance to change the sick role when patients have suffered pain all their lives. Often, there is an irrational 'fear of emptiness' if they stop being sick. In some patients, being sick entails secondary gains.

We must also consider the *obstacles and barriers* we will find: the patient has cognitive difficulties and high levels of catastrophizing; subjects suffer a high emotional distress – they are anxious and desperate about pain, 'needing it to please go away', or their mood is in tatters, so much that they feel unable to do something for themselves. Patients are sometimes angry, perceiving that something or someone is responsible for their situation. The patient may have had very dysfunctional behaviours for many years. They often start the programme being dependent on pain drugs, having developed tolerance to opiates and needing help to give them up gradually. If, as already mentioned, these variables are not evaluated before starting treatment we cannot really know whether any results will be obtained.

One must also point out *difficulties related to the therapist*: insecurity when presenting information due to lack of knowledge or doubting their own abilities. We must insist that implementing a programme with complex pain patients needs a sufficiently trained therapist. Sometimes, in addition to *explaining pain*, cognitive-behavioural strategies are also required. Moreover, the therapist must have good communication skills and be able to achieve an excellent therapeutic alliance. And, as in any therapy, there is a necessary learning curve.

It is essential that the therapist has skills to 'map' the pain patient's problem in all its biological, behavioural, personal and social dimensions. Therapists must be able to offer patients a more comprehensive view of their problem. It should therefore be presented in a personalized way, picking out particular aspects of the patient's life.

Difficulties concerning the format: the educational programme can be implemented individually or in groups. When the latter option is chosen, a small group is recommended with members that have similar characteristics. In many patients, pain education has an almost 'immediate' effect. However, many other patients need more time and, above all, need long-lasting support. Very often, after an initial improvement, pain reappears forcefully. A therapist who can suitably handle these reactivations is required, offering different strategies, depending on the problems that arise and supporting the patient throughout the process. In our experience, complex patients need at least a 1-year follow-up.

DIFFICULTIES AND OBSTACLES IN THE PAIN PROGRAMME

- Related to the patient:
- Patient expectations and motivations
- Patient obstacles and barriers
- Related to the therapist
- Related to the format

Physical re-education

Pain education is useless if it fails to change the pain behaviour. It is therefore critical to treat fear-avoidance behaviour and activity intolerance. Physical re-education can be divided into two sections: (1) a specific section, aimed at treating specific patient intolerance and (2) another non-specific section, which aims to progressively increase the level of general physical activity. Chronic pain can determine physical dysfunctions such as joint stiffness, abnormal mobility patterns, etc., that sometimes need to be addressed initially.

Treatment of physical dysfunction

The treatment of physical dysfunction, when present, aims to further facilitate more functional rehabilitation programmes. Physical dysfunctions are often derived from fear-avoidance behaviours and are specific to each individual patient: in some cases, the most significant dysfunction is the loss of joint mobility; in other cases, deficit in balance control; and in others, the

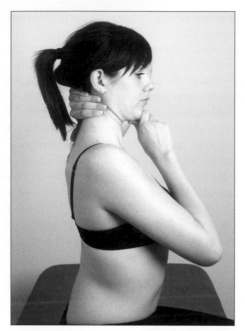

FIGURE 11-51 ■ Re-education of dysfunctional motor patterns.

development of dysfunctional motor patterns, etc. (Fig. 11-51). Treatment should be tailored to each patient, based on the patiemt's specific physical dysfunctions.

In patients with chronic or complex pain, although passive treatment modalities may be justified to reduce the symptoms, active techniques become more important. Therefore, from the start of treatment the patient should be taught self-treatment modalities for the physical dysfunctions found, such as active and functional exercises, primarily based on everyday activities, etc., to be carried out at home. The aim is that patients should learn to exert control over their pain. During the first stage it is highly important to achieve a reduction of symptoms in order to boost the patient's confidence, thus ensuring collaboration throughout the process. In that sense, it is initially important to adapt to the patient's expectations as to the type of treatment and establish strategies that favour the neuromodulation of pain.

Specific physical re-education and treatment of intolerance

The major problem in chronic pain is related to a syndrome of intolerance to a given movement, functional activity or posture. This intolerance is secondary to maladaptive central sensitization and fear-avoidance behaviors.[794] The goal is to eliminate intolerance so that the patient is able to resume work, social and family activities with as little disability as possible. In this regard, exposure strategies aimed at addressing those specific intolerances are proposed.

The exposure-based methods such as systematic desensitization, gradual exposure and in vivo exposure have been included for many decades in cognitive-behavioural approaches. Exposure treatments generally seek to increase the patient's contact with previously avoided experiences, such as bodily sensations, emotional experiences or specific social situations.

Treatment of intolerance may be approached using two types of exposure strategies: gradual exposure or in vivo exposure. The fundamental difference between the two strategies relates to the focus. While progression in gradual exposure is set according to the functional capabilities and pain, the focus of in vivo exposure is determined by the fear that various activities of daily life can evoke. As already mentioned, there is a strong positive association between pain-related fear and disability.[536] The patient must understand how fear-avoidance behaviour is a crucial pain-perpetuating factor that leads to a deconditioning syndrome, which, in turn, aggravates the pain, generates depression and leads to increased disability.

In vivo exposure involves systematic exposure to daily activities that the patient avoids due to fear of pain or re-injury. These activities are identified, establishing a hierarchy on a scale of 0 to 100 based on the patient's fear of them. For this purpose, the PHODA scale consisting of photos of functional activities is used.[769] Patients should perform *behavioural experiments*, progressing from the activity that causes less fear to the one they perceive as most dangerous or threatening. The patient is repeatedly exposed to specific activities of daily living until the fear disappears. For patients exhibiting a more significant fear of physical activity, it is more convincing to live the experience first hand, proving that the fears are unjustified, than a rational argument.[667]

One of the interesting aspects of this approach is that instead of using therapeutic exercises, functional activities of daily living are specifically chosen. Establishing functional goals has the advantage that patients stop focusing attention on the pain and begin to direct efforts towards resuming their activities of daily life and returning to their normal lives.

When planning the exposure programme, it is very useful if the patient completes the scheme by Vlaeyen et al.[518] (Fig. 11-52) to understand how the catastrophic thoughts, inadequate information received,

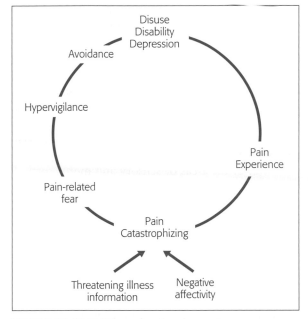

FIGURE 11-52 ▪ When planning the exposure programme, it is very useful if patients completes their personal pain problems following the Vlaeyen et al. scheme. *Reproduced with permission from Vlaeyen et al.[667]*

the fear of pain and avoidance behaviours are responsible for starting a 'vicious circle' responsible for the aggravation of pain, low mood and disability. To review the exposure model in the treatment of chronic pain, the book by Vlaeyen et al.[667] is recommended.

The essential and most complex aspect of this exposure programme is its planning. For a gradual exposure programme, the baseline level of activity should be well below the level which may trigger pain.[104,116] Activity may be increased slowly or more rapidly, but always in a progressive manner. It is essential to break the activity-dependent pain cycle that perpetuates the patient's perception of being defenseless against the pain and unable to control the symptoms. The pain should stop being the parameter that determines the performance of the exercises or any activity proposed. For the preparation of the exposure programme, an excellent metaphor is the 'Twin Peaks' explanation of the book *Explain Pain* by Butler and Moseley.[104]

Intolerance postures or movements should be specifically addressed with a gradual exposure or in vivo exposure

If, for example, the patient does not tolerate the sitting position, a daily programme will be designed gradually increasing the time in this position (Fig. 11-53). When the patient is working on postures or movements involving severe intolerance, neuromodulation techniques can be used. Peripheral neuromodulation implies the manipulation of sensory inputs in

Starting level	Rate	Week	Monday		Tuesday		Wednesday		Thursday		Friday		Saturday		Sunday	
			G	D	G	D	G	D	G	D	G	D	G	D	G	D
4	1 minute every day	1	4		5		6		7		8		9		R	
		2	10		11		12		13		14		15		R	
		3	15		16		17		18		19		20		R	
		4	20		21		22		23		24		25		R	
		5	25		26		27		28		29		30		R	

FIGURE 11-53 ▪ Treatment programme for intolerance to sitting. G, goal; D, done, R, rest.

order to obtain desensitization. Examples of such techniques include the use of thermal patches while performing physical activity. The patient can be trained in the use of desensitization strategies (Fig. 11-54). We must avoid dependence on the therapist and limit contact with health personnel. Self-massage, baths with hot water, active stretching and active joint mobilization are examples of tools that can be effective as long as the patient perceives them as beneficial and pleasant.

Those environmental aspects that may have a neuromodulator effect should also be addressed. In the above example, the patient can work on the sitting position in a bathtub with hot water (increased cutaneous afferents) while listening to music (modification of an environmental factor and distraction effect). The use of environmental sensory stimuli that promote a pleasant emotional state or distraction may favor the modulation of pain.[795] Sometimes intolerance is so severe that before starting gradual exposure, strategies aimed at the cortical representation are required.

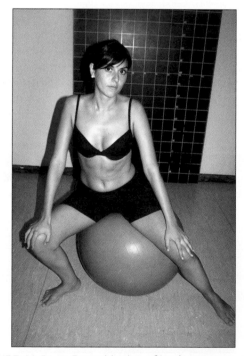

FIGURE 11-54 ■ Desensitization of intolerance to a sitting position with exercises using a ball.

Strategies for cortical representation

As has been pointed out, there is a complex interaction between pain, impairment of bodily perceptions and changes in cortical maps. Cortical reorganization in patients with chronic pain can be indicative of a distortion between the real body and the virtual body.[121] This situation would appear to indicate that the bodily proprioceptive information is not representing the real situation; therefore, motor activation patterns are not consistent with the functional needs of the individual.[246,248] Current research suggests that this inconsistency between virtual body and motor responses alone is capable of perpetuating chronic pain.[796] These findings support the use of treatments aimed at reversing cortical reorganization in order to reduce pain and perceptual and motor disturbances.[123]

Different strategies are being used to achieve this goal, such as manipulating the flow of sensory inputs, activation of the areas of sensory and motor cortical representation based on gradual exposure programmes, the imagination of movements, motor imagery and training of sensory skills.

All these strategies are aimed at stimulating the virtual body. The aim is to act on the cortical representation of the body area where the subject perceives pain. In principle, any technique that increases non-nociceptive afferent input over the area where the patient reports pain can have a neuromodulator effect, as neuroplastic changes occur in the cortical representation of the body part where the subject perceives pain. This suggests that the subject perceives pain in the body image he has built of himself.

A more intense neuromodulator effect can be obtained thanks to the activation of those elements that are part of the 'pain memory', provided that pain is not triggered. This constitutes the basis underlying the gradual exposure programmes described previously. However, in subjects with severe pain and a marked sensory hypersensitivity, gradual exposure can improperly reactivate the 'pain programme'. In some subjects even the imagination of a movement can cause pain and trophic changes in the tissue.[288] In order to initially address these clinical situations, different strategies based on sensory retraining have been proposed, such as imagined movements, re-education using mirror imagery, recognition of laterality and two-point discrimination training.[104,797–802]

The mechanisms underlying these techniques are not entirely known. It has been proposed that the improvement in pain and other symptoms may be due to the reconciliation between motor responses and sensory information, the activation of mirror neurons and the gradual activation of cortical motor circuits.

It is known that imagined movements activate the same cortical networks as real movements. It has been proposed that these are related to the system of 'mirror neurons' described by Gallese et al.[803] These researchers, while analysing the cortical activity in monkeys, found that a group of neurons in the premotor cortex was activated not only when they performed an action but also when they watched another monkey performing the same action. The neurons reflected as if in a mirror the activity they were observing. Therefore, these types of neurons are activated both during the development of an action and during the observation of the same action performed by another individual. So when we observe an action in another individual, a 'potential motor action', which is identical to that which would be activated spontaneously during our performance of that action, is evoked in our brain. These neurons allow us to interpret the intentionality of motor actions of other individuals, thanks to our' knowledge'. This knowledge enables us to immediately attribute an intentional meaning to the movement we observe. Therefore, in the absence of this meta-representation, we would be unable to understand the purpose of the actions of others.[804] These neural circuits are also the basis of empathic behavior.[805] Mirror neurons form a complex network comprising areas of the occipital and temporal visual cortices and two cortical areas located in the inferior parietal lobe and inferior frontal cortex, close to Broca's area, whose function is fundamentally motor.

Imagined movements

The aim is to imagine the movement of the limb or body part where the patient perceives pain. As already mentioned, imagined movements can activate similar cortical networks as actual movements and thus allow access to the sensorimotor virtual body without triggering pain. In cases of high irritability it is advisable to start imagining movement components before doing this with the whole movement.

Re-education using mirror imagery/virtual re-education

Re-education using mirror imagery (mirror box therapy) involves the mobilization of the limb contralateral to the one affected while the patient watches in a mirror how this movement is reflected, which visually simulates a mobilization of the affected limb (Fig. 11-55).

It has been proposed that visual mirror image feedback improves the symptoms of patients because they are able to reconcile the motor responses with the sensorial information and activate the premotor cortex, which has a close relation with visual processing areas.[244,797,806–809] It is also likely that mirror image therapy reduces the protection responses as a result of the exposition to the movement and that it promotes cortical reorganization as a result of the activity of the afflicted member.[275]

Mirror box therapy has proven effective in the treatment of type I complex regional pain syndrome (SDRCI),[805,806,809-812], CRPS II[812] V STE, pain after brachial plexus avulsion, in rehabilitation after tendon transfer and repair of the peripheral nerve, phantom limb pain,[813] and in motor recovery following hemiplegia , CRPS II[813] V STE, pain after brachial plexus avulsion, in rehabilitation after tendon transfer and

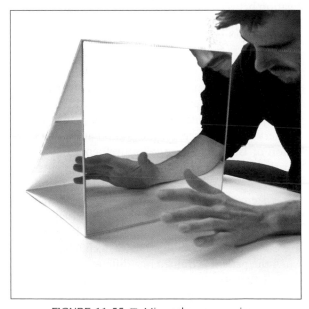

FIGURE 11-55 ■ Mirror therapy exercises.

repair of the peripheral nerve, phantom limb pain,[814] and in motor recovery following hemiplegia

Currently, virtual reality and augmented reality systems based on the same principles as the visual feedback methods are beginning to be used, and are showing promising results.[801,802] An example of this is the *virtual reality mirror visual feedback* (VRMVF), which replicates in a mirror the activity of the non-afflicted member using virtual reality technology. In this virtual environment a series of progressively difficult tasks can be added using augmented reality. The high efficiency of re-education using mirror therapy and virtual reality can be explained because the visual information dominates over somatosensory information in the development of cortical proprioceptive representation.[815–818]

Recognition of laterality

This therapeutic strategy seems to rely on the same mechanisms as those involved in re-education using mirror imagery. It entails recognizing whether the images of a body part seen in a photograph or on a computer screen correspond to the left or right (Fig. 11-56). Various studies show that subjects who suffer pain in a limb require more time and make more mistakes when they see an image that corresponds to the one in which they perceive pain.[275] Also, there is a correlation between the difficulty in recognizing laterality and the duration and intensity of pain.[275]

Moseley[818] has developed a treatment protocol called graded motor imagery (GMI) based on the combination of recognition of laterality, imagined movements and mirror box therapy. GMI has proven effective in patients with SDRCI Moseley[819] has developed a treatment protocol called graded motor imagery (GMI) based on the combination of recognition of laterality, imagined movements and mirror box therapy. GMI has proven effective in patients with SDRCI[797–799,818–820] and and phantom limb pain,[819] as the systematic revision on the efficacy of physiotherapy in the treatment of CRPS1 carried out by Daly and Bialocerkowski[821] has shown. Interestingly, the effect of this combination of techniques is lost when the patient is trained in a different order,[799] suggesting that its effects are dependent on the proper sequential activation of sensory or motor cortical networks.

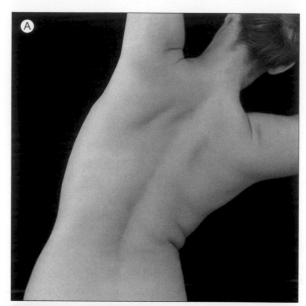

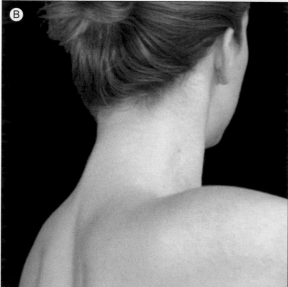

FIGURE 11-56 ■ Graded motor imagery. Lumbar spine (A) and Cervical spine (B).

Sensory discrimination training

Subjects with chronic pain are less able to distinguish the location and characteristics of a stimulus applied to the skin of the body region with pain.[822] There is also a relationship between a decrease of these sensory skills and pain intensity. Obviously, this alteration is derived from cortical reorganization of S1 associated with chronic pain.[248] The intensity of cortical reorganization is related to both pain intensity and decreased sensory discrimination.[278]

One of the first works that therapeutically used sensory discrimination was by Flor et al.[823] This study was conducted in the upper limb of amputees with phantom limb pain. Eight electrodes were placed on the trunnion, and short-lasting electrical stimuli were applied for 90 minutes daily for 2 weeks. Patients should distinguish the stimulus location and frequency. The results showed that sensory discrimination training improved phantom limb pain, and that this improvement was associated with a normalization of the reorganization of S1.

Moseley et al.,[125] in a study in patients with CRPS, compared the effects of sensory discrimination retraining against tactile stimulation. This study also demonstrates that sensory discrimination retraining is able to reduce chronic pain. This result is not being obtained solely with cutaneous stimulation (Fig. 11-57). In conclusion, strategies for re-education of the 'virtual body' have an enormous potential as a non-invasive analgesic alternative in the treatment of some chronic pain entities.

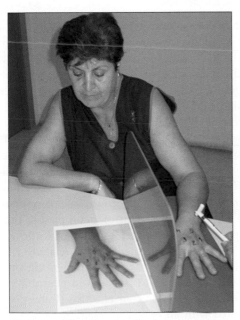

FIGURE 11-57 ■ Sensory discrimination training.

Physical reactivation

In addition to the specific treatment of intolerance, a gradual increase in the level of activity in general is proposed to the patient, choosing a sport or other physical activity. Which physical activities to be implemented according to the requirements of the patient's life should be analysed. All activities must therefore be aimed at achieving specific functional goals that are meaningful to the patient. In order to facilitate progressive adaptation to mechanical stress, the physical activity should be associated with a recreational component or carried out in a pleasant environment for the patient (Fig. 11-58). Those exercises or activities that the patient considers boring or unpleasant must be avoided.

The benefits of physical activity not only arise from an improvement in fitness but also from its effects on beliefs. It is very difficult to obtain a change in beliefs based solely on advice and information. It is the experience of success in physical performance, associated with education, which operates a change in pain-related beliefs and behaviours.[824,825] An improvement in the perception of self-efficacy can have a very powerful effect on pain behaviours. The most important message to be transmitted is that the progressive increase in the level of activity leads to a progressive reduction of pain[826] (Fig. 11-59).

■ The benefits of physical activity not only arise from improved fitness but also from its effect on beliefs.

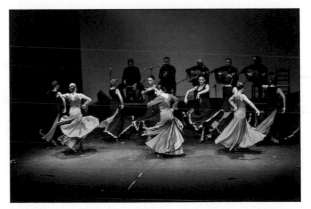

FIGURE 11-58 ■ For physical recovery, activities that combine a recreational component must be chosen. *Julia Grecos Spanish dance company. Courtesy of Marta Rubio.*

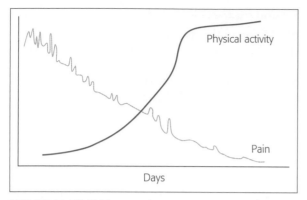

FIGURE 11-59 ■ The most important message to be transmitted is that the progressive increase in the level of activity leads to a progressive reduction of pain.

- The perception of self-efficacy can have a very powerful effect on pain behaviours and pain perception

Finally, patients should understand that they need to eliminate all pain behaviours. Playing down and ignoring all complaints of pain can be used as negative reinforcement of these behaviours. Positive reinforcement is to recognize and emphasize the progress made. It is important that patients understand that the results will be obtained if they undertake a commitment towards their recovery which ultimately depends on their motivation, values and effort. The ideal situation is when we observe that the patient is ahead of the therapist, comprehending that the message is consistent and identifies with their situation, while undertaking behavioural changes and initiating activities before being told to do so.

In addition to specific activities, patients should be encouraged to resume their social interaction and recreational activities. Social self-exclusion favours a low mood and depressive symptoms. Family should be involved in this process, as their collaboration can be a critical factor in the recovery of the subject. They can help the patients to be aware of their functional improvements and encourage them to do the exercises and proposed activities. If family members are not aware of the problem, they can sabotage the treatment.

At the end of the programme, therapist and patient should summarize the work done, evaluating the goals achieved. The patient's programme of activities during that year should be discussed, bearing in mind the final results to be achieved. Dates for reassessment must be scheduled. Sometimes it may be positive for the patient to write a short essay that reflects the therapeutic process from beginning to end.

> It is important to understand that we are not dealing with a dysfunctional nervous system but a person with a life history, a childhood, family relationships and specific personality traits.

The aspect that will ultimately determine programme success is whether it manages to empower patients in managing their pain. The therapist should help the patient to acquire not only practical and functional skills but also cognitive and emotional skills to reverse their situation of disability. It is necessary to reduce anxiety and depression symptoms, improve self-confidence and self-efficacy, help patients regain significant functional activities, promote the return to work and regain their social relations and finally, demedicalize the patient. A key aspect is that patients understands that the important thing is to guide their objectives towards achieving significant goals in their lives based on their values.

CONCLUSION

Complex chronic pain is not the result of a joint, muscular or neural dysfunction, but is derived from a maladaptive central sensitization. Chronic pain, as already noted, causes significant cortical neuroplastic changes. In recent decades new ways to act on central maladaptive neuroplasticity are being explored. The recovery of the functionality of the nervous system and improvement in pain require the normalization of sensory and motor cortical representation, decreased activation of areas related to the aversive emotional response using cognitive restructuring, suggestion, etc. The treatment of patients with chronic pain should be based on the compression of neuroplastic, physical and psychosocial changes associated with chronic pain. The goals of treatment should relate to all neurobiological and psychosocial components involved in the patient's disability. Education in neurobiology of pain is being shown as an effective strategy, which, associated with an exposure programme, can obtain excellent therapeutic results.

The close relationship between chronic pain, altered body perception and altered cortical representation justifies treatments aimed to 'remap the brain' to reduce pain and normalize the perception and regain motor function. Currently, new strategies are being explored with promising results for the control of complex pain situations which are difficult to treat.

Patients need expert clinicians in the treatment of chronic pain, able to recognize and modify erroneous beliefs and fear-avoidance behaviours, as well as to establish a programme to reverse the phenomena of sensory distortion that favours physical reconditioning, and an independent management of pain by the patient. New knowledge in the pathophysiology of chronic pain and a biopsychosocial approach allows us to better understand chronic pain and accompanying disability and enables us to evaluate and treat patients who suffer this and not just the dysfunctions reported. A treatment associating pain neurobiology education with an exposure programme and overall physical recovery can produce good therapeutic outcomes; it is able to radically change many miserable and painful lives. However, we need to conduct further research on how to increase the effectiveness of our treatment approaches in the largest possible number of patients.

REFERENCES

1. Breivik H, et al. Survey of chronic pain in Europe: prevalence, impact on daily life, and treatment. Eur J Pain 2006;10(4):287–333.
2. Vos T, et al. Years lived with disability (YLDs) for 1160 sequelae of 289 diseases and injuries 1990-2010: a systematic analysis for the Global Burden of Disease Study 2010. Lancet 2012;380(9859):2163–96.
3. Macfarlane G, Jones G, McBeth J. Epidemiology of pain. In: McMahon S, Koltzenburg M, editors. Wall and Melzack's Textbook of Pain. Philadelphia.: Elsevier Churchill Livingstone; 2006. p. 1199–214.
4. Bendtsen L. Central sensitization in tension-type headache–possible pathophysiological mechanisms. Cephalalgia 2000; 20(5):486–508.
5. Wolfe F, et al. The prevalence and characteristics of fibromyalgia in the general population. Arthritis Rheum 1995;38(1): 19–28.
6. Bevan S, et al. Fit For Work? Musculoskeletal Disorders in the European Workforce. London: The Work Foundation; 2009.
7. Deyo RA, et al. Overtreating chronic back pain: time to back off? J Am Board Fam Med 2009;22(1):62–8.
8. Martin BI, et al. Trends in health care expenditures, utilization, and health status among US adults with spine problems, 1997-2006. Spine 2009;34(19):2077–84.
9. Pizzo PA, Clark NM. Alleviating suffering 101–pain relief in the United States. N Engl J Med 2012;366(3):197–9.
10. Loeser JD. What is chronic pain? Theor Med 1991;12(3):213–25.
11. Morris DB. The Culture of Pain. University California Press; 1991.
12. Bonica J. General considerations of chronic pain. In: Bonica J, editor. The Management of Pain. Lea & Febiger; 1990.
13. Siddall PJ, Cousins MJ. Persistent pain as a disease entity: implications for clinical management. Anesth Analg 2004;99(2):510–20, table of contents.
14. Jacobson L, Mariano AJ. Consideraciones generales sobre el dolor crónico. In: Loeser JD, editor. Bonica Terapéutica del Dolor. Mexico DC: McGraw-Hill Interamericana; 2003.
15. Haldeman S. North American Spine Society: failure of the pathology model to predict back pain. Spine 1990;15(7):718–24.
16. Reid S, et al. Medically unexplained symptoms in frequent attenders of secondary health care: retrospective cohort study. BMJ 2001;322(7289):767.
17. Gore DR, Sepic SB, Gardner GM. Roentgenographic findings of the cervical spine in asymptomatic people. Spine 1986;11(6):521–4.
18. Gore DR, et al. Neck pain: a long-term follow-up of 205 patients. Spine 1987;12(1):1–5.
19. Weisberg MB, Clavel AL Jr. Why is chronic pain so difficult to treat? Psychological considerations from simple to complex care. Postgrad Med 1999;106(6):141–2, 145-8, 157-60; passim.
20. Torres-Cueco R. El problema del dolor crónico: abordaje biopsicosocial. In: Perez J, Fernandez J, editors. Fisioterapia y Dolor XV Jornadas de. Escuela Universitaria de Fisioterapia ONCE Madrid; 2005. p. 102–24.
21. Torres-Cueco R. La fisioterapia y el dolor: un cambio de modelo necesario y urgente [Editorial]. Cuestiones de fisioterapia 2011;40(2):85–6.
22. Torres-Cueco R. Dolor Miofascial Crónico: Patofisiología y aproximación terapéutica. Fisioterapia 2005;27(2):87–95.
23. Melzack R, Wall PD. Pain mechanisms: a new theory. Science 1965;150(699):971–9.
24. Latremoliere A, Woolf CJ. Central sensitization: a generator of pain hypersensitivity by central neural plasticity. J Pain 2009;10(9):895–926.
25. Woolf CJ. Central sensitization: implications for the diagnosis and treatment of pain. Pain 2011;152(3 Suppl.):S2–15.
26. Price DD, Staud R. Neurobiology of fibromyalgia syndrome. J Rheumatol Suppl 2005;75:22–8.
27. Van Oosterwijck J, et al. Evidence for central sensitization in chronic whiplash: a systematic literature review. Eur J Pain 2013;17(3):299–312.
28. Staud R. Evidence for shared pain mechanisms in osteoarthritis, low back pain, and fibromyalgia. Curr Rheumatol Rep 2011;13(6):513–20.
29. Torres-Cueco R. Chronic low back pain: Biopsychosocial approach and physical therapy, in 6th Interdisciplinary World Congress on Low Back & Pelvic Pain Diagnosis and Treatment. The Balance between Research and Clinic. Barcelona 2007.
30. Roussel NA, et al. Central sensitization and altered central pain processing in chronic low back pain: fact or myth? Clin J Pain 2013;29(7):625–38.

31. Cagnie B, et al. Central sensitization in fibromyalgia? A systematic review on structural and functional brain MRI. Semin Arthritis Rheum 2014;44(1):68–75.

32. Graven-Nielsen T, Arendt-Nielsen L. Assessment of mechanisms in localized and widespread musculoskeletal pain. Nat Rev Rheumatol 2010;6(10):599–606.

33. Jull G, et al. Does the presence of sensory hypersensitivity influence outcomes of physical rehabilitation for chronic whiplash?–A preliminary RCT. Pain 2007;129(1–2):28–34.

34. Daenen L, et al. Dysfunctional pain inhibition in patients with chronic whiplash-associated disorders: an experimental study. Clin Rheumatol 2013;32(1):23–31.

35. Sterling M, et al. Pressure pain thresholds in chronic whiplash associated disorder: further evidence of altered central pain processing. J Musculoskelet Pain 2002;10:69–81.

36. Sterling M, et al. Sensory hypersensitivity occurs soon after whiplash injury and is associated with poor recovery. Pain 2003;104(3):509–17.

37. Herren-Gerber R, et al. Modulation of central hypersensitivity by nociceptive input in chronic pain after whiplash injury. Pain Med 2004;5(4):366–76.

38. Bruehl S. An update on the pathophysiology of complex regional pain syndrome. Anesthesiology 2010;113(3):713–25.

39. Kaya S, et al. Central sensitization in urogynecological chronic pelvic pain: a systematic literature review. Pain Physician 2013;16(4):291–308.

40. Ferreira Gurian MB, et al. Reduction of Pain Sensitivity is Associated with the Response to Treatment in Women with Chronic Pelvic Pain. Pain Med 2014.

41. Yang CC, et al. Pain sensitization in male chronic pelvic pain syndrome: why are symptoms so difficult to treat? J Urol 2003;170(3):823–6, discussion 826-7.

42. Brawn J, et al. Central changes associated with chronic pelvic pain and endometriosis. Hum Reprod Update 2014;20(5):737–47.

43. Sadownik LA. Etiology, diagnosis, and clinical management of vulvodynia. Int J Womens Health 2014;6:437–49.

44. Desmeules J, et al. Central pain sensitization, COMT Val-158Met polymorphism, and emotional factors in fibromyalgia. J Pain 2014;15(2):129–35.

45. Staud R, Spaeth M. Psychophysical and neurochemical abnormalities of pain processing in fibromyalgia. CNS Spectr 2008;13(3 Suppl. 5):12–17.

46. Staud R. Evidence of involvement of central neural mechanisms in generating fibromyalgia pain. Curr Rheumatol Rep 2002;4(4):299–305.

47. Arendt-Nielsen L, Graven-Nielsen T. Central sensitization in fibromyalgia and other musculoskeletal disorders. Curr Pain Headache Rep 2003;7(5):355–61.

48. Staud R, et al. Enhanced central pain processing of fibromyalgia patients is maintained by muscle afferent input: a randomized, double-blind, placebo-controlled study. Pain 2009;145(1–2):96–104.

49. Meeus M, Nijs J. Central sensitization: a biopsychosocial explanation for chronic widespread pain in patients with fibromyalgia and chronic fatigue syndrome. Clin Rheumatol 2007;26(4):465–73.

50. Fernandez-Carnero J, et al. Widespread mechanical pain hypersensitivity as sign of central sensitization in unilateral epicondylalgia: a blinded, controlled study. Clin J Pain 2009;25(7):555–61.

51. Lluch E, et al. Evidence for central sensitization in patients with osteoarthritis pain: A systematic literature review. Eur J Pain 2014.

52. Van de Ven TJ, John Hsia HL. Causes and prevention of chronic postsurgical pain. Curr Opin Crit Care 2012;18(4):366–71.

53. Hubscher M, et al. Relationship between quantitative sensory testing and pain or disability in people with spinal pain-a systematic review and meta-analysis. Pain 2013;154(9):1497–504.

54. McLean SA, et al. The development of persistent pain and psychological morbidity after motor vehicle collision: integrating the potential role of stress response systems into a biopsychosocial model. Psychosom Med 2005;67(5):783–90.

55. Chapman CR. The psychophysiology of pain. In: Fishman S, Ballantyne J, Rathmell J, editors. Bonica's Management of Pain. Philadelphia.: Wolters Kluwer Lippincott Williams & Wilkins; 2010. p. 375–88.

56. Chapman CR, Nakamura Y. A passion of the soul: an introduction to pain for consciousness researchers. Conscious Cogn 1999;8(4):391–422.

57. Donaldson GW, et al. Pain and the defense response: structural equation modeling reveals a coordinated psychophysiological response to increasing painful stimulation. Pain 2003;102(1–2):97–108.

58. Chapman CR, Gavrin J. Suffering: the contributions of persistent pain. Lancet 1999;353(9171):2233–7.

59. Torpy DJ, Chrousos GP. The three-way interactions between the hypothalamic-pituitary-adrenal and gonadal axes and the immune system. Baillieres Clin Rheumatol 1996;10(2): 181–98.

60. O'Connor KA, et al. Peripheral and central proinflammatory cytokine response to a severe acute stressor. Brain Res 2003;991(1–2):123–32.

61. Chrousos GP. The stress response and immune function: clinical implications. The 1999 Novera H. Spector Lecture. Ann N Y Acad Sci 2000;917:38–67.

62. Watkins LR, Maier SF. The pain of being sick: implications of immune-to-brain communication for understanding pain. Annu Rev Psychol 2000;51:29–57.

63. Maier SF. Bi-directional immune-brain communication: Implications for understanding stress, pain, and cognition. Brain Behav Immun 2003;17(2):69–85.

64. Maier SF, Watkins LR. Cytokines for psychologists: implications of bidirectional immune-to-brain communication for understanding behavior, mood, and cognition. Psychol Rev 1998;105(1):83–107.

65. Watkins LR, Maier SF. Immune regulation of central nervous system functions: from sickness responses to pathological pain. J Intern Med 2005;257(2):139–55.

66. Johnson EO, et al. Mechanisms of stress: a dynamic overview of hormonal and behavioral homeostasis. Neurosci Biobehav Rev 1992;16(2):115–30.

67. Melzack R, et al. Central neuroplasticity and pathological pain. Ann N Y Acad Sci 2001;933:157–74.

68. Koelbaek Johansen M, et al. Generalised muscular hyper-algesia in chronic whiplash syndrome. Pain 1999;83(2):229–34.

69. Lidbeck J. Central hyperexcitability in chronic musculoskeletal pain: a conceptual breakthrough with multiple clinical implications. Pain Res Manag 2002;7(2):81–92.

70. Banic B, et al. Evidence for spinal cord hypersensitivity in chronic pain after whiplash injury and in fibromyalgia. Pain 2004;107(1–2):7–15.

71. Apkarian AV, et al. Imaging the pain of low back pain: functional magnetic resonance imaging in combination with monitoring subjective pain perception allows the study of clinical pain states. Neurosci Lett 2001;299(1–2):57–60.

72. Gracely RH, et al. Functional magnetic resonance imaging evidence of augmented pain processing in fibromyalgia. Arthritis Rheum 2002;46(5):1333–43.

73. Giesecke T, et al. Evidence of augmented central pain processing in idiopathic chronic low back pain. Arthritis Rheum 2004;50(2):613–23.

74. Jensen KB, et al. Evidence of dysfunctional pain inhibition in Fibromyalgia reflected in rACC during provoked pain. Pain 2009;144(1–2):95–100.

75. Kong J, et al. Exploring the brain in pain: activations, deactivations and their relation. Pain 2010;148(2):257–67.

76. Gracely RH, Ambrose KR. Neuroimaging of fibromyalgia. Best Pract Res Clin Rheumatol 2011;25(2):271–84.

77. Davis KD, Moayedi M. Central mechanisms of pain revealed through functional and structural MRI. J Neuroimmune Pharmacol 2013;8(3):518–34.

78. Engel GL. The need for a new medical model: a challenge for biomedicine. Science 1977;196(4286):129–36.

79. Main CJ, Richards HL, Fortune DG. Why put new wine in old bottles: the need for a biopsychosocial approach to the assessment, treatment, and understanding of unexplained and explained symptoms in medicine. J Psychosom Res 2000;48(6):511–14.

80. Melzack R, Wall P. The Challenge of Pain. Penguin Books Ltd; 1996.

81. Waddell G. 1987 Volvo award in clinical sciences. A new clinical model for the treatment of low-back pain. Spine 1987;12(7):632–44.

82. Torres-Cueco R. Aproximación biopsicosocial del dolor crónico y de la fibromialgia. In: Salvat IS, editor. Fisioterapia del Dolor Miofascial y de la Fibromialgia. Sevilla: Universidad Internacional de Andalucía; 2009. p. 78–110.

83. Merskey H, Bogduk N. Classification of chronic pain: descriptions of chronic pain syndromes anda definitions of pain terms. 2nd ed. Seattle, WA: IASP Press; 1994.

84. Butler D. The Sensitive Nervous System. Adelaide: Noigroup Publications; 2000.

85. Watt-Watson J, Siddall PJ, Carr E. Interprofessional pain education: the road to successful pain management outcomes. Pain Manag 2012;2(5):417–20.

86. Legrain V, et al. Cognitive aspects of nociception and pain: bridging neurophysiology with cognitive psychology. Neurophysiol Clin 2012;42(5):325–36.

87. Flor H, Turk D. Basic concepts of pain. In: Flor H, Turk D, editors. Chronic Pain. A integrated biobehavioral approach. Seattle.: IASP press; 2011. p. 3–23.

88. Nijs J, Van Houdenhove B. From acute musculoskeletal pain to chronic widespread pain and fibromyalgia: application of pain neurophysiology in manual therapy practice. Man Ther 2009;14(1):3–12.

89. Lee MC, Mouraux A, Iannetti GD. Characterizing the cortical activity through which pain emerges from nociception. J Neurosci 2009;29(24):7909–16.

90. Osborn J, Derbyshire SW. Pain sensation evoked by observing injury in others. Pain 2010;148(2):268–74.

91. Derbyshire SW, et al. Cerebral activation during hypnotically induced and imagined pain. Neuroimage 2004;23(1):392–401.

92. Raij TT, et al. Brain correlates of subjective reality of physically and psychologically induced pain. Proc Natl Acad Sci USA 2005;102(6):2147–51.

93. Lumley MA, et al. Pain and emotion: a biopsychosocial review of recent research. J Clin Psychol 2011;67(9):942–68.

94. Linton SJ, Shaw WS. Impact of psychological factors in the experience of pain. Phys Ther 2011;91(5):700–11.

95. Ramachandran V, Blakeslee S. Phantoms in the Brain. Probing the mysteries of the human mind. New York: HarperCollins Publishers; 1999.

96. Arntz A, Claassens L. The meaning of pain influences its experienced intensity. Pain 2004;109(1–2):20–5.

97. Moseley GL, Arntz A. The context of a noxious stimulus affects the pain it evokes. Pain 2007.

98. Turk DC. Understanding pain sufferers: the role of cognitive processes. Spine J 2004;4(1):1–7.

99. Wiech K, Ploner M, Tracey I. Neurocognitive aspects of pain perception. Trends Cogn Sci 2008;12(8):306–13.

100. Jensen MP, et al. Patient beliefs predict patient functioning: further support for a cognitive-behavioural model of chronic pain. Pain 1999;81(1–2):95–104.

101. Stroud MW, et al. The relation between pain beliefs, negative thoughts, and psychosocial functioning in chronic pain patients. Pain 2000;84(2–3):347–52.

102. Ramirez-Maestre C, Esteve R, Lopez AE. Cognitive appraisal and coping in chronic pain patients. Eur J Pain 2008;12(6):749–56.

103. Van Damme S, et al. Is distraction less effective when pain is threatening? An experimental investigation with the cold pressor task. Eur J Pain 2008;12(1):60–7.

104. Butler D, Moseley G. Explain Pain. Adelaide: Noigroup Publications; 2003.

105. Moseley GL, Butler DS. 15 Years of Explaining Pain - The Past, Present and Future. J Pain 2015.

106. Van Damme S, et al. Keeping pain in mind: a motivational account of attention to pain. Neurosci Biobehav Rev 2010;34(2):204–13.

107. Hofbauer RK, et al. Cortical representation of the sensory dimension of pain. J Neurophysiol 2001;86(1):402–11.

108. Bushnell MC, et al. Imaging pain in the brain: The role of the cerebral cortex in pain perception and modulation. J Musculoskelet Pain 2002;10(1–2):59–72.

109. Valet M, et al. Distraction modulates connectivity of the cingulo-frontal cortex and the midbrain during pain–an fMRI analysis. Pain 2004;109(3):399–408.

110. Fecteau JH, Munoz DP. Salience, relevance, and firing: a priority map for target selection. Trends Cogn Sci 2006;10(8):382–90.

111. Wall PD. Pain and the placebo response. Ciba Found Symp 1993;174:187–211, discussion 212-6.

112. Tracey I, Mantyh PW. The cerebral signature for pain perception and its modulation. Neuron 2007;55(3):377–91.

113. Eccleston C, Crombez G. Pain demands attention: a cognitive-affective model of the interruptive function of pain. Psychol Bull 1999;125(3):356–66.

114. Sanders SH. Chronic pain: conceptualization and epidemiology. Ann Behav Med 1985;7:3–5.

115. Price DD. Psychological and neural mechanisms of the affective dimension of pain. Science 2000;288(5472):1769–72.

116. Moseley GL. A pain neuromatrix approach to patients with chronic pain. Man Ther 2003;8(3):130–40.

117. Favril L, et al. Shifting attention between the space of the body and external space: electrophysiological correlates of visual-nociceptive crossmodal spatial attention. Psychophysiology 2014;51(5):464–77.

118. Legrain V, et al. The pain matrix reloaded: a salience detection system for the body. Prog Neurobiol 2011;93(1):111–24.

119. Moseley GL, Gallace A, Spence C. Bodily illusions in health and disease: physiological and clinical perspectives and the concept of a cortical 'body matrix. Neurosci Biobehav Rev 2012;36(1):34–46.

120. Neugebauer V, et al. Forebrain pain mechanisms. Brain Res Rev 2009;60(1):226–42.

121. Lotze M, Moseley GL. Role of distorted body image in pain. Curr Rheumatol Rep 2007;9(6):488–96.

122. Pleger B, et al. Patterns of cortical reorganization parallel impaired tactile discrimination and pain intensity in complex regional pain syndrome. Neuroimage 2006;32(2):503–10.

123. Lewis JS, et al. Body perception disturbance: a contribution to pain in complex regional pain syndrome (CRPS). Pain 2007;133(1–3):111–19.

124. Wand BM, et al. Cortical changes in chronic low back pain: current state of the art and implications for clinical practice. Man Ther 2011;16(1):15–20.

125. Moseley GL, Zalucki NM, Wiech K. Tactile discrimination, but not tactile stimulation alone, reduces chronic limb pain. Pain 2008;137(3):600–8.

126. Moriarty O, McGuire BE, Finn DP. The effect of pain on cognitive function: a review of clinical and preclinical research. Prog Neurobiol 2011;93(3):385–404.

127. Berryman C, et al. Evidence for working memory deficits in chronic pain: a systematic review and meta-analysis. Pain 2013;154(8):1181–96.

128. Berryman C, et al. Do people with chronic pain have impaired executive function? A meta-analytical review. Clin Psychol Rev 2014;34(7):563–79.

129. Kirby ED, et al. Basolateral amygdala regulation of adult hippocampal neurogenesis and fear-related activation of newborn neurons. Mol Psychiatry 2011.

130. Fordyce W. Behavioral Methods for Chronic Pain and Illness. San Luis: Mosby; 1976.

131. Fordyce W. Dolor aprendido: dolor como función conductual. In: Loeser JD, editor. Bonica Terapéutica del Dolor. Mexico: McGraw-Hill Interamericana; 2003. p. 575–81.

132. Flor H. The functional organization of the brain in chronic pain. Prog Brain Res 2000;129:313–22.

133. Flor H. Painful memories. Can we train chronic pain patients to 'forget' their pain? EMBO Rep 2002;3(4):288–91.

134. Apkarian AV. Pain perception in relation to emotional learning. Curr Opin Neurobiol 2008;18(4):464–8.

135. Apkarian AV, Baliki MN, Geha PY. Towards a theory of chronic pain. Prog Neurobiol 2009;87(2):81–97.

136. Flor H. New developments in the understanding and management of persistent pain. Curr Opin Psychiatry 2012;25(2):109–13.

137. Zaman J, et al. Associative fear learning and perceptual discrimination: A perceptual pathway in the development of chronic pain. Neurosci Biobehav Rev 2015;51:118–25.

138. Vlaeyen JW, Linton SJ. Fear-avoidance and its consequences in chronic musculoskeletal pain: a state of the art. Pain 2000;85(3):317–32.

139. Meulders A, Vansteenwegen D, Vlaeyen JW. The acquisition of fear of movement-related pain and associative learning: a novel pain-relevant human fear conditioning paradigm. Pain 2011;152(11):2460–9.

140. Lorenz J, Tracey I. Brain correlates of psychological amplification of pain. In: Mayer E, Bushnell M, editors. Functional pain syndromes: presentation and pathophysiology. Seattle: IASP PRESS; 2009. p. 385–401.

141. Schaible HG. Peripheral and central mechanisms of pain generation. Handb Exp Pharmacol 2007;177:3–28.

142. Apkarian AV, et al. Human brain mechanisms of pain perception and regulation in health and disease. Eur J Pain 2005;9(4):463–84.

143. Kandel ER, Schwartz J, Jesell T, editors. Principios de Neurociencia. 4ª ed. Madrid: McGraw-Hill Interamericana; 2000.

144. Woolf C, Salter M. Plasticity and pain: role of the dorsal horn. In: McMahon S, Koltzenburg M, editors. Wall and Melzack's Textbook of Pain. Philadelphia: Elsevier Churchill Livingstone; 2006. p. 91–105.

145. Woolf CJ, Salter MW. Neuronal plasticity: increasing the gain in pain. Science 2000;288(5472):1765–9.

146. Mannion RJ, Woolf CJ. Pain mechanisms and management: a central perspective. Clin J Pain 2000;16(3 Suppl.):S144–56.

147. Arendt-Nielsen L, Fernandez-de-Las-Penas C, Graven-Nielsen T. Basic aspects of musculoskeletal pain: from acute to chronic pain. J Man Manip Ther 2011;19(4):186–93.

148. Mifflin KA, Kerr BJ. The transition from acute to chronic pain: understanding how different biological systems interact. Can J Anaesth 2014;61(2):112–22.

149. Coombes BK, Bisset L, Vicenzino B. Thermal hyperalgesia distinguishes those with severe pain and disability in unilateral lateral epicondylalgia. Clin J Pain 2012;28(7):595–601.

150. Staud R, et al. Abnormal sensitization and temporal summation of second pain (wind-up) in patients with fibromyalgia syndrome. Pain 2001;91(1–2):165–75.

151. Vikman KS, Kristensson K, Hill RH. Sensitization of dorsal horn neurons in a two-compartment cell culture model: wind-up and long-term potentiation-like responses. J Neurosci 2001;21(19):RC169.

152. Li J, Simone DA, Larson AA. Windup leads to characteristics of central sensitization. Pain 1999;79(1):75–82.

153. Eide PK. Wind-up and the NMDA receptor complex from a clinical perspective. Eur J Pain 2000;4(1):5–15.

154. Bennett GJ. Update on the neurophysiology of pain transmission and modulation: focus on the NMDA-receptor. J Pain Symptom Manage 2000;19(1 Suppl.):S2–6.

155. Graven-Nielsen T, Arendt-Nielsen L. Peripheral and central sensitization in musculoskeletal pain disorders: an experimental approach. Curr Rheumatol Rep 2002;4(4):313–21.

156. Wall PD, Woolf CJ. Muscle but not cutaneous C-afferent input produces prolonged increases in the excitability of the flexion reflex in the rat. J Physiol 1984;356:443–58.

157. Mense S. The pathogenesis of muscle pain. Curr Pain Headache Rep 2003;7(6):419–25.

158. Neugebauer V, Li W. Differential sensitization of amygdala neurons to afferent inputs in a model of arthritic pain. J Neurophysiol 2003;89(2):716–27.

159. Wei F, Zhuo M. Potentiation of sensory responses in the anterior cingulate cortex following digit amputation in the anaesthetised rat. J Physiol 2001;532(Pt 3):823–33.

160. Yezierski RP, et al. Excitotoxic spinal cord injury: behavioral and morphological characteristics of a central pain model. Pain 1998;75(1):141–55.

161. Woolf CJ. Central sensitization: uncovering the relation between pain and plasticity. Anesthesiology 2007;106(4):864–7.

162. Watkins LR, et al. "Listening" and "talking" to neurons: implications of immune activation for pain control and increasing the efficacy of opioids. Brain Res Rev 2007;56(1):148–69.

163. Ji RR, et al. Possible role of spinal astrocytes in maintaining chronic pain sensitization: review of current evidence with focus on bFGF/JNK pathway. Neuron Glia Biol 2006;2(4):259–69.

164. Ji RR, Berta T, Nedergaard M. Glia and pain: is chronic pain a gliopathy? Pain 2013;154(Suppl. 1):S10–28.

165. Ji RR, Suter MR. p38 MAPK, microglial signaling, and neuropathic pain. Mol Pain 2007;3:33.

166. Kawasaki Y, et al. Cytokine mechanisms of central sensitization: distinct and overlapping role of interleukin-1beta, interleukin-6, and tumor necrosis factor-alpha in regulating synaptic and neuronal activity in the superficial spinal cord. J Neurosci 2008;28(20):5189–94.

167. Watkins LR, Milligan ED, Maier SF. Glial activation: a driving force for pathological pain. Trends Neurosci 2001;24(8):450–5.

168. Watkins LR, Milligan ED, Maier SF. Glial proinflammatory cytokines mediate exaggerated pain states: implications for clinical pain. Adv Exp Med Biol 2003;521:1–21.

169. Wieseler-Frank J, Maier SF, Watkins LR. Glial activation and pathological pain. Neurochem Int 2004;45(2–3):389–95.

170. Hansson E. Could chronic pain and spread of pain sensation be induced and maintained by glial activation? Acta Physiol (Oxf) 2006;187(1–2):321–7.

171. Uceyler N, Sommer C. Cytokine-related and histological biomarkers for neuropathic pain assessment. Pain Manag 2012;2(4):391–8.

172. Milligan ED, et al. Spinal glia and proinflammatory cytokines mediate mirror-image neuropathic pain in rats. J Neurosci 2003;23(3):1026–40.

173. Loggia ML, et al. Evidence for brain glial activation in chronic pain patients. Brain 2015.

174. Newman HM, Stevens RT, Apkarian AV. Direct spinal projections to limbic and striatal areas: anterograde transport studies from the upper cervical spinal cord and the cervical enlargement in squirrel monkey and rat. J Comp Neurol 1996;365(4):640–58.

175. Gauriau C, Bernard JF. A comparative reappraisal of projections from the superficial laminae of the dorsal horn in the rat: the forebrain. J Comp Neurol 2004;468(1):24–56.

176. Braz JM, et al. Parallel "pain" pathways arise from subpopulations of primary afferent nociceptor. Neuron 2005;47(6):787–93.

177. Willis WD, Westlund KN. Neuroanatomy of the pain system and of the pathways that modulate pain. J Clin Neurophysiol 1997;14(1):2–31.

178. Fields H, Basbaum A, Heinricher M. Central nervous system mechanisms of pain modulation. In: McMahon S, Koltzenburg M, editors. Wall and Melzack's Textbook of Pain. Philadelphia.: Elsevier Churchill Livingstone; 2006. p. 125–42.

179. Salter MW. The neurobiology of central sensitization. J Musculoskelet Pain 2002;10(1–2):23–33.

180. Millan MJ. Descending control of pain. Prog Neurobiol 2002;66(6):355–474.

181. Suzuki R, Rygh LJ, Dickenson AH. Bad news from the brain: descending 5-HT pathways that control spinal pain processing. Trends Pharmacol Sci 2004;25(12):613–17.

182. Zambreanu L, et al. A role for the brainstem in central sensitisation in humans. Evidence from functional magnetic resonance imaging. Pain 2005;114(3):397–407.

183. Porreca F, Ossipov MH, Gebhart GF. Chronic pain and medullary descending facilitation. Trends Neurosci 2002;25(6):319–25.

184. Yarnitsky D. Role of endogenous pain modulation in chronic pain mechanisms and treatment. Pain 2015;156(Suppl. 1):S24–31.

185. Le Bars D, Dickenson AH, Besson JM. Diffuse noxious inhibitory controls (DNIC). I. Effects on dorsal horn convergent neurones in the rat. Pain 1979;6(3):283–304.

186. Bouhassira D, et al. Involvement of the subnucleus reticularis dorsalis in diffuse noxious inhibitory controls in the rat. Brain Res 1992;595(2):353–7.

187. Lima D, Almeida A. The medullary dorsal reticular nucleus as a pronociceptive centre of the pain control system. Prog Neurobiol 2002;66(2):81–108.

188. Yarnitsky D, et al. Recommendations on terminology and practice of psychophysical DNIC testing. Eur J Pain 2010;14(4):339.

188a. Katon W, Egan K, Miller D. Chronic pain: lifetime psychiatric diagnoses and family history. Am J Psychiatry 1985; 142(10):1156–60.

189. Daenen L, et al. Changes in Pain Modulation Occur Soon After Whiplash Trauma but are not Related to Altered Perception of Distorted Visual Feedback. Pain Pract 2013.

190. Yarnitsky D, et al. Prediction of chronic post-operative pain: pre-operative DNIC testing identifies patients at risk. Pain 2008;138(1):22–8.

191. Wilder-Smith OH, et al. Patients with chronic pain after abdominal surgery show less preoperative endogenous pain inhibition and more postoperative hyperalgesia: a pilot study. J Pain Palliat Care Pharmacother 2010;24(2):119–28.

192. Yarnitsky D. Conditioned pain modulation (the diffuse noxious inhibitory control-like effect): its relevance for acute and chronic pain states. Curr Opin Anaesthesiol 2010;23(5): 611–15.

193. Nir RR, et al. Cognitive manipulation targeted at decreasing the conditioning pain perception reduces the efficacy of conditioned pain modulation. Pain 2012;153(1):170–6.

194. Cormier S, Piche M, Rainville P. Expectations modulate heterotopic noxious counter-stimulation analgesia. J Pain 2013; 14(2):114–25.

195. Goodin BR, et al. The association of greater dispositional optimism with less endogenous pain facilitation is indirectly transmitted through lower levels of pain catastrophizing. J Pain 2013;14(2):126–35.

196. Goodin BR, et al. Testing the relation between dispositional optimism and conditioned pain modulation: does ethnicity matter? J Behav Med 2013;36(2):165–74.

197. Millan MJ. The induction of pain: an integrative review. Prog Neurobiol 1999;57(1):1–164.

198. Lumb BM. Hypothalamic and midbrain circuitry that distinguishes between escapable and inescapable pain. News Physiol Sci 2004;19:22–6.

199. Bingel U, et al. Somatotopic organization of human somatosensory cortices for pain: a single trial fMRI study. Neuroimage 2004;23(1):224–32.

200. Mouraux A, et al. A multisensory investigation of the functional significance of the "pain matrix. Neuroimage 2011; 54(3):2237–49.

201. Lorenz J, Hauck M. Supraspinal mechanisms of pain and nociception. In: Fishman S, Ballantyne J, Rathmell J, editors. Bonica's Management of Pain. Philadelphia.: Wolters Kluwer Lippincott Williams & Wilkins; 2010. p. 61–73.

202. Nagai M, Kishi K, Kato S. Insular cortex and neuropsychiatric disorders: a review of recent literature. Eur Psychiatry 2007;22(6):387–94.

203. Brooks JC, Tracey I. The insula: a multidimensional integration site for pain. Pain 2007;128(1–2):1–2.

204. Craig AD. How do you feel–now? The anterior insula and human awareness. Nat Rev Neurosci 2009;10(1):59–70.

205. Craig AD. How do you feel? Interoception: the sense of the physiological condition of the body. Nat Rev Neurosci 2002; 3(8):655–66.

206. Vogt BA. Pain and emotion interactions in subregions of the cingulate gyrus. Nat Rev Neurosci 2005;6(7):533–44.

207. Lorenz J, Tracey I. Brain correlates of psychological amplification of pain. In: Mayer EA, Bushnell MC, editors. Functional Pain Syndromes: presentation and pathophysiology. Seattle: IASP Press; 2009.

208. Bush G, Luu P, Posner MI. Cognitive and emotional influences in anterior cingulate cortex. Trends Cogn Sci 2000;4(6):215–22.

209. Neugebauer V, et al. The amygdala and persistent pain. Neuroscientist 2004;10(3):221–34.

210. Simons LE, et al. The human amygdala and pain: evidence from neuroimaging. Hum Brain Mapp 2014;35(2):527–38.

211. O'Doherty JP, et al. Neural responses during anticipation of a primary taste reward. Neuron 2002;33(5):815–26.

212. Bechara A, et al. Double dissociation of conditioning and declarative knowledge relative to the amygdala and hippocampus in humans. Science 1995;269(5227):1115–18.

213. Bingel U, et al. Subcortical structures involved in pain processing: evidence from single-trial fMRI. Pain 2002;99(1–2):313–21.

214. Zola SM, et al. Impaired recognition memory in monkeys after damage limited to the hippocampal region. J Neurosci 2000;20(1):451–63.

215. Miller EK, Cohen JD. An integrative theory of prefrontal cortex function. Annu Rev Neurosci 2001;24:167–202.

216. Lorenz J, Minoshima S, Casey KL. Keeping pain out of mind: the role of the dorsolateral prefrontal cortex in pain modulation. Brain 2003;126(Pt 5):1079–91.

217. Lorenz J, et al. A unique representation of heat allodynia in the human brain. Neuron 2002;35(2):383–93.

218. Wiech K, et al. Anterolateral prefrontal cortex mediates the analgesic effect of expected and perceived control over pain. J Neurosci 2006;26(44):11501–9.

219. Burgmer M, et al. Cerebral mechanisms of experimental hyperalgesia in fibromyalgia. Eur J Pain 2012;16(5): 636–47.

220. Iannetti GD, et al. Determinants of laser-evoked EEG responses: pain perception or stimulus saliency? J Neurophysiol 2008;100(2):815–28.

221. Mouraux A, Iannetti GD. Nociceptive laser-evoked brain potentials do not reflect nociceptive-specific neural activity. J Neurophysiol 2009;101(6):3258–69.

222. Shackman AJ, et al. The integration of negative affect, pain and cognitive control in the cingulate cortex. Nat Rev Neurosci 2011;12(3):154–67.

223. Downar J, et al. A cortical network sensitive to stimulus salience in a neutral behavioral context across multiple sensory modalities. J Neurophysiol 2002;87(1):615–20.

224. Downar J, Mikulis DJ, Davis KD. Neural correlates of the prolonged salience of painful stimulation. Neuroimage 2003;20(3):1540–51.

225. Moayedi M. All roads lead to the insula. Pain 2014; 155(10):1920–1.

226. Davis KD, et al. Human anterior cingulate cortex neurons encode cognitive and emotional demands. J Neurosci 2005;25(37):8402–6.

227. Uddin LQ. Salience processing and insular cortical function and dysfunction. Nat Rev Neurosci 2015;16(1):55–61.

228. Apkarian AV. The brain in chronic pain: clinical implications. Pain Manag 2011;1(6):577–86.

229. Baliki MN, et al. Chronic pain and the emotional brain: specific brain activity associated with spontaneous fluctuations of intensity of chronic back pain. J Neurosci 2006;26(47): 12165–73.

230. Sawamoto N, et al. Expectation of pain enhances responses to nonpainful somatosensory stimulation in the anterior cingulate cortex and parietal operculum/posterior insula: an event-related functional magnetic resonance imaging study. J Neurosci 2000;20(19):7438–45.

231. Deus J, et al. Resonancia magnética funcional de la respuesta cerebral al dolor en pacientes con diagnóstico de fibromialgia. Psiq Biol 2006;13(2):39–46.

232. Pujol J, et al. Mapping brain response to pain in fibromyalgia patients using temporal analysis of FMRI. PLoS ONE 2009;4(4):e5224.

233. Burgmer M, et al. Altered brain activity during pain processing in fibromyalgia. Neuroimage 2009;44(2):502–8.

234. Burgmer M, et al. Fibromyalgia unique temporal brain activation during experimental pain: a controlled fMRI Study. J Neural Transm 2010;117(1):123–31.

235. Parks EL, et al. Brain activity for chronic knee osteoarthritis: dissociating evoked pain from spontaneous pain. Eur J Pain 2011;15(8):843 e1–14.

236. Hashmi JA, et al. Shape shifting pain: chronification of back pain shifts brain representation from nociceptive to emotional circuits. Brain 2013;136(Pt 9):2751–68.

237. Schweinhardt P, et al. An fMRI study of cerebral processing of brush-evoked allodynia in neuropathic pain patients. Neuroimage 2006;32(1):256–65.

238. Schweinhardt P, et al. Investigation into the neural correlates of emotional augmentation of clinical pain. Neuroimage 2008;40(2):759–66.

239. Castren E. Is mood chemistry? Nat Rev Neurosci 2005;6(3):241–6.

240. Chen R, Cohen LG, Hallett M. Nervous system reorganization following injury. Neuroscience 2002;111(4):761–73.

241. Flor H, Birbaumer N. Phantom limb pain: cortical plasticity and novel therapeutic approaches. Curr Opin Anaesthesiol 2000;13(5):561–4.

242. Wall JT, Xu J, Wang X. Human brain plasticity: an emerging view of the multiple substrates and mechanisms that cause cortical changes and related sensory dysfunctions after injuries of sensory inputs from the body. Brain Res Brain Res Rev 2002;39(2–3):181–215.

243. Flor H. Cortical reorganisation and chronic pain: implications for rehabilitation. J Rehabil Med 2003;41(Suppl.):66–72.

244. Moseley L. Gifford L, editor. Making sense of "S1 mania" - Are things really that simple?,. Falmouth: CNS Press; 2006.

245. Juottonen K, et al. Altered central sensorimotor processing in patients with complex regional pain syndrome. Pain 2002;98(3):315–23.

246. Maihofner C, et al. Patterns of cortical reorganization in complex regional pain syndrome. Neurology 2003;61(12): 1707–15.

247. Schwenkreis P, Maier C, Tegenthoff M. Functional imaging of central nervous system involvement in complex regional pain syndrome. AJNR Am J Neuroradiol 2009;30(7):1279–84.

248. Flor H, et al. Phantom-limb pain as a perceptual correlate of cortical reorganization following arm amputation. Nature 1995;375(6531):482–4.

249. Flor H, et al. Cortical reorganization and phantom phenomena in congenital and traumatic upper-extremity amputees. Exp Brain Res 1998;119(2):205–12.

250. Knecht S, et al. Plasticity of plasticity? Changes in the pattern of perceptual correlates of reorganization after amputation. Brain 1998;121(Pt 4):717–24.

251. Grusser SM, et al. The relationship of perceptual phenomena and cortical reorganization in upper extremity amputees. Neuroscience 2001;102(2):263–72.

252. Karl A, et al. Reorganization of motor and somatosensory cortex in upper extremity amputees with phantom limb pain. J Neurosci 2001;21(10):3609–18.

253. Flor H, Nikolajsen L, Staehelin Jensen T. Phantom limb pain: a case of maladaptive CNS plasticity? Nat Rev Neurosci 2006;7(11):873–81.

254. Flor H, et al. Extensive reorganization of primary somatosensory cortex in chronic back pain patients. Neurosci Lett 1997;224(1):5–8.

255. Janig W, Baron R. Complex regional pain syndrome is a disease of the central nervous system. Clin Auton Res 2002;12(3):150–64.

256. Swart CM, Stins JF, Beek PJ. Cortical changes in complex regional pain syndrome (CRPS). Eur J Pain 2009;13(9): 902–7.

257. Maihofner C, Seifert F, Markovic K. Complex regional pain syndromes: new pathophysiological concepts and therapies. Eur J Neurol 2010;17(5):649–60.

258. Pleger B, et al. Mean sustained pain levels are linked to hemispherical side-to-side differences of primary somatosensory cortex in the complex regional pain syndrome I. Exp Brain Res 2004;155(1):115–19.

259. Yang TT, et al. Sensory maps in the human brain. Nature 1994;368(6472):592–3.

260. Maihofner C, et al. Mislocalization of tactile stimulation in patients with complex regional pain syndrome. J Neurol 2006;253(6):772–9.

261. McCabe CS, et al. Referred sensations in patients with complex regional pain syndrome type 1. Rheumatology (Oxford) 2003;42(9):1067–73.

262. Moseley GL. Distorted body image in complex regional pain syndrome. Neurology 2005;65(5):773.

263. Soler MD, et al. Referred sensations and neuropathic pain following spinal cord injury. Pain 2010;150(1):192–8.

264. Schwenkreis P, et al. Bilateral motor cortex disinhibition in complex regional pain syndrome (CRPS) type I of the hand. Neurology 2003;61(4):515–19.

265. Krause P, Forderreuther S, Straube A. TMS motor cortical brain mapping in patients with complex regional pain syndrome type I. Clin Neurophysiol 2006;117(1):169–76.

266. Maihofner C, et al. The motor system shows adaptive changes in complex regional pain syndrome. Brain 2007;130(Pt 10):2671–87.

267. Gieteling EW, et al. Cerebral activation during motor imagery in complex regional pain syndrome type 1 with dystonia. Pain 2008;134(3):302–9.

268. Flor H, Diers M, Andoh J. The neural basis of phantom limb pain. Trends Cogn Sci 2013;17(7):307–8.

269. Moseley GL. Widespread brain activity during an abdominal task markedly reduced after pain physiology education: fMRI evaluation of a single patient with chronic low back pain. Aust J Physiother 2005;51(1):49–52.

270. Moseley GL, Gandevia SC. Sensory-motor incongruence and reports of 'pain. Rheumatology (Oxford) 2005;44(9):1083–5.

271. McCabe CS, et al. Simulating sensory-motor incongruence in healthy volunteers: implications for a cortical model of pain. Rheumatology (Oxford) 2005;44(4):509–16.

272. Frettloh J, Huppe M, Maier C. Severity and specificity of neglect-like symptoms in patients with complex regional pain syndrome (CRPS) compared to chronic limb pain of other origins. Pain 2006;124(1–2):184–9.

273. Kerkhoff G. Spatial hemineglect in humans. Prog Neurobiol 2001;63(1):1–27.

274. Galer BS, Jensen M. Neglect-like symptoms in complex regional pain syndrome: results of a self-administered survey. J Pain Symptom Manage 1999;18(3):213–17.

275. Moseley GL. Why do people with complex regional pain syndrome take longer to recognize their affected hand? Neurology 2004;62(12):2182–6.

276. Moseley GL, Gallagher L, Gallace A. Neglect-like tactile dysfunction in chronic back pain. Neurology 2012;79(4):327–32.

277. Moseley GL, Parsons TJ, Spence C. Visual distortion of a limb modulates the pain and swelling evoked by movement. Curr Biol 2008;18(22):R1047–8.

278. Maihofner C, et al. Cortical reorganization during recovery from complex regional pain syndrome. Neurology 2004;63(4):693–701.

279. Pleger B, et al. Sensorimotor retuning [corrected] in complex regional pain syndrome parallels pain reduction. Ann Neurol 2005;57(3):425–9.

280. Mercier C, Sirigu A. Training with virtual visual feedback to alleviate phantom limb pain. Neurorehabil Neural Repair 2009;23(6):587–94.

281. Moseley GL, Flor H. Targeting cortical representations in the treatment of chronic pain: a review. Neurorehabil Neural Repair 2012;26(6):646–52.

282. Simons LE, Elman I, Borsook D. Psychological processing in chronic pain: a neural systems approach. Neurosci Biobehav Rev 2014;39:61–78.

283. Ji RR, et al. Central sensitization and LTP: do pain and memory share similar mechanisms? Trends Neurosci 2003;26(12):696–705.

284. Kim JJ, Jung MW. Neural circuits and mechanisms involved in Pavlovian fear conditioning: a critical review. Neurosci Biobehav Rev 2006;30(2):188–202.

285. Price TJ, Inyang KE. Commonalities between pain and memory mechanisms and their meaning for understanding chronic pain. Prog Mol Biol Transl Sci 2015;131:409–34.

286. Mansour AR, et al. Chronic pain: the role of learning and brain plasticity. Restor Neurol Neurosci 2014;32(1):129–39.

287. Acerra NE, Moseley GL. Dysynchiria: watching the mirror image of the unaffected limb elicits pain on the affected side. Neurology 2005;65(5):751–3.

288. Moseley GL. Imagined movements cause pain and swelling in a patient with complex regional pain syndrome. Neurology 2004;62(9):1644.

289. Castellanos FX, Cortese S, Proal E. Connectivity. Curr Top Behav Neurosci 2014;16:49–77.

290. Melzack R. Pain–an overview. Acta Anaesthesiol Scand 1999;43(9):880–4.

291. Deco G, et al. Key role of coupling, delay, and noise in resting brain fluctuations. Proc Natl Acad Sci USA 2009;106(25):10302–7.

292. Raichle ME, Mintun MA. Brain work and brain imaging. Annu Rev Neurosci 2006;29:449–76.

293. Zhang D, Raichle ME. Disease and the brain's dark energy. Nat Rev Neurol 2010;6(1):15–28.

294. Biswal B, et al. Functional connectivity in the motor cortex of resting human brain using echo-planar MRI. Magn Reson Med 1995;34(4):537–41.

295. Raichle ME, et al. A default mode of brain function. Proc Natl Acad Sci USA 2001;98(2):676–82.

296. Gusnard DA, Raichle ME. Searching for a baseline: functional imaging and the resting human brain. Nat Rev Neurosci 2001;2(10):685–94.

297. Buckner RL, Andrews-Hanna JR, Schacter DL. The brain's default network: anatomy, function, and relevance to disease. Ann N Y Acad Sci 2008;1124:1–38.

298. Greicius MD, et al. Functional connectivity in the resting brain: a network analysis of the default mode hypothesis. Proc Natl Acad Sci USA 2003;100(1):253–8.

299. Baliki MN, et al. Beyond feeling: chronic pain hurts the brain, disrupting the default-mode network dynamics. J Neurosci 2008;28(6):1398–403.

300. Weissman-Fogel I, et al. Abnormal cortical activity in patients with temporomandibular disorder evoked by cognitive and emotional tasks. Pain 2011;152(2):384–96.

301. Kucyi A, Salomons TV, Davis KD. Mind wandering away from pain dynamically engages antinociceptive and default mode brain networks. Proc Natl Acad Sci USA 2013;110(46):18692–7.

302. Behrens TE, Sporns O. Human connectomics. Curr Opin Neurobiol 2012;22(1):144–53.

303. Van Essen DC, et al. The Human Connectome Project: a data acquisition perspective. Neuroimage 2012;62(4):2222–31.

304. Craddock RC, et al. Imaging human connectomes at the macroscale. Nat Methods 2013;10(6):524–39.

305. Legrain V, et al. A neurocognitive model of attention to pain: behavioral and neuroimaging evidence. Pain 2009;144(3):230–2.

306. Menon V. Salience Network. In: Toga A, editor. Brain Mapping: An Encyclopedic Reference. Academic Press: Elsevier.; 2015. p. 597–611.

307. Wager TD, et al. Placebo-induced changes in FMRI in the anticipation and experience of pain. Science 2004;303(5661): 1162–7.

308. Smith SM, et al. Tract-based spatial statistics: voxel-wise analysis of multi-subject diffusion data. Neuroimage 2006;31(4):1487–505.

309. Hutton C, et al. A comparison between voxel-based cortical thickness and voxel-based morphometry in normal aging. Neuroimage 2009;48(2):371–80.

310. Apkarian AV, et al. Chronic back pain is associated with decreased prefrontal and thalamic gray matter density. J Neurosci 2004;24(46):10410–15.

311. Apkarian AV, et al. Chronic pain patients are impaired on an emotional decision-making task. Pain 2004;108(1–2): 129–36.

312. Dick BD, et al. Disruption of cognitive function in fibromyalgia syndrome. Pain 2008;139(3):610–16.

313. Schmidt-Wilcke T, et al. Affective components and intensity of pain correlate with structural differences in gray matter in chronic back pain patients. Pain 2006;125(1–2):89–97.

314. Kuchinad A, et al. Accelerated brain gray matter loss in fibromyalgia patients: premature aging of the brain? J Neurosci 2007;27(15):4004–7.

315. Lutz J, et al. White and gray matter abnormalities in the brain of patients with fibromyalgia: a diffusion-tensor and volumetric imaging study. Arthritis Rheum 2008;58(12): 3960–9.

316. Burgmer M, et al. Decreased gray matter volumes in the cingulo-frontal cortex and the amygdala in patients with fibromyalgia. Psychosom Med 2009;71(5):566–73.

317. Wood PB, et al. Changes in gray matter density in fibromyalgia: correlation with dopamine metabolism. J Pain 2009;10(6):609–18.

318. Robinson ME, et al. Gray matter volumes of pain-related brain areas are decreased in fibromyalgia syndrome. J Pain 2011;12(4):436–43.

319. McCrae CS, et al. Fibromyalgia patients have reduced hippocampal volume compared with healthy controls. J Pain Res 2015;8:47–52.

320. Geha PY, et al. The brain in chronic CRPS pain: abnormal gray-white matter interactions in emotional and autonomic regions. Neuron 2008;60(4):570–81.

321. Davis KD, et al. Cortical thinning in IBS: implications for homeostatic, attention, and pain processing. Neurology 2008;70(2):153–4.

322. Seminowicz DA, et al. Regional gray matter density changes in brains of patients with irritable bowel syndrome. Gastroenterology 2010;139(1):48–57 e2.

323. As-Sanie S, et al. Changes in regional gray matter volume in women with chronic pelvic pain: a voxel-based morphometry study. Pain 2012;153(5):1006–14.

324. Rocca MA, et al. Brain gray matter changes in migraine patients with T2-visible lesions: a 3-T MRI study. Stroke 2006;37(7):1765–70.

325. Valfre W, et al. Voxel-based morphometry reveals gray matter abnormalities in migraine. Headache 2008;48(1): 109–17.

326. Kim JH, et al. Regional grey matter changes in patients with migraine: a voxel-based morphometry study. Cephalalgia 2008;28(6):598–604.

327. Schmidt-Wilcke T, et al. Subtle grey matter changes between migraine patients and healthy controls. Cephalalgia 2008;28(1):1–4.

328. Schmitz N, et al. Frontal lobe structure and executive function in migraine patients. Neurosci Lett 2008;440(2):92–6.

329. Schmitz N, et al. Attack frequency and disease duration as indicators for brain damage in migraine. Headache 2008;48(7):1044–55.

330. Schmidt-Wilcke T, et al. Gray matter decrease in patients with chronic tension type headache. Neurology 2005;65(9):1483–6.

331. Schmidt-Wilcke T, Hierlmeier S, Leinisch E. Altered regional brain morphology in patients with chronic facial pain. Headache 2010;50(8):1278–85.

332. Younger JW, et al. Chronic myofascial temporomandibular pain is associated with neural abnormalities in the trigeminal and limbic systems. Pain 2010;149(2):222–8.

333. Gerstner G, et al. Changes in regional gray and white matter volume in patients with myofascial-type temporomandibular disorders: a voxel-based morphometry study. J Orofac Pain 2011;25(2):99–106.

334. de Lange FP, et al. Gray matter volume reduction in the chronic fatigue syndrome. Neuroimage 2005;26(3):777–81.

335. Villarreal G, et al. Reduced hippocampal volume and total white matter volume in posttraumatic stress disorder. Biol Psychiatry 2002;52(2):119–25.

336. Schweinhardt P, Bushnell MC. Pain imaging in health and disease how far have we come? J Clin Invest 2010;120(11):3788–97.

337. Park DC, et al. Cognitive function in fibromyalgia patients. Arthritis Rheum 2001;44(9):2125–33.

338. Obermann M, et al. Gray matter changes related to chronic posttraumatic headache. Neurology 2009;73(12):978–83.

339. Valet M, et al. Patients with pain disorder show gray-matter loss in pain-processing structures: a voxel-based morphometric study. Psychosom Med 2009;71(1):49–56.

340. Jensen KB, et al. Overlapping structural and functional brain changes in patients with long-term exposure to fibromyalgia pain. Arthritis Rheum 2013;65(12):3293–303.

341. Rodriguez-Raecke R, et al. Brain gray matter decrease in chronic pain is the consequence and not the cause of pain. J Neurosci 2009;29(44):13746–50.

342. Gwilym SE, et al. Thalamic atrophy associated with painful osteoarthritis of the hip is reversible after arthroplasty: a longitudinal voxel-based morphometric study. Arthritis Rheum 2010;62(10):2930–40.

343. Luerding R, et al. Working memory performance is correlated with local brain morphology in the medial frontal and anterior

cingulate cortex in fibromyalgia patients: structural correlates of pain-cognition interaction. Brain 2008;131(Pt 12):3222–31.

344. Matharu MS, et al. No change in the structure of the brain in migraine: a voxel-based morphometric study. Eur J Neurol 2003;10(1):53–7.

345. Hsu MC, et al. No consistent difference in gray matter volume between individuals with fibromyalgia and age-matched healthy subjects when controlling for affective disorder. Pain 2009;143(3):262–7.

346. Tracey I. Nociceptive processing in the human brain. Curr Opin Neurobiol 2005;15(4):478–87.

347. McEwen BS, Gianaros PJ. Central role of the brain in stress and adaptation: links to socioeconomic status, health, and disease. Ann N Y Acad Sci 2010;1186:190–222.

348. Wood PB. Variations in brain gray matter associated with chronic pain. Curr Rheumatol Rep 2010;12(6):462–9.

349. Gianaros PJ, et al. Prospective reports of chronic life stress predict decreased grey matter volume in the hippocampus. Neuroimage 2007;35(2):795–803.

350. Schweinhardt P, et al. Increased gray matter density in young women with chronic vulvar pain. Pain 2008;140(3):411–19.

351. Blankstein U, et al. Altered brain structure in irritable bowel syndrome: potential contributions of pre-existing and disease-driven factors. Gastroenterology 2010;138(5):1783–9.

352. Moayedi M, et al. Contribution of chronic pain and neuroticism to abnormal forebrain gray matter in patients with temporomandibular disorder. Neuroimage 2011;55(1):277–86.

353. Walther K, et al. Anti-inflammatory drugs reduce age-related decreases in brain volume in cognitively normal older adults. Neurobiol Aging 2011;32(3):497–505.

354. Younger JW, et al. Prescription opioid analgesics rapidly change the human brain. Pain 2011;152(8):1803–10.

355. Rodriguez-Raecke R, et al. Structural brain changes in chronic pain reflect probably neither damage nor atrophy. PLoS ONE 2013;8(2):e54475.

356. Dolman AJ, et al. Phenotype matters: the absence of a positive association between cortical thinning and chronic low back pain when controlling for salient clinical variables. Clin J Pain 2014;30(10):839–45.

357. Munoz M, Esteve R. Reports of memory functioning by patients with chronic pain. Clin J Pain 2005;21(4):287–91.

358. Oosterman JM, et al. Memory functions in chronic pain: examining contributions of attention and age to test performance. Clin J Pain 2011;27(1):70–5.

359. Etherton JL, et al. Pain, malingering, and performance on the WAIS-III Processing Speed Index. J Clin Exp Neuropsychol 2006;28(7):1218–37.

360. Dick BD, Rashiq S. Disruption of attention and working memory traces in individuals with chronic pain. Anesth Analg 2007;104(5):1223–9, tables of contents.

361. Glass JM. Review of cognitive dysfunction in fibromyalgia: a convergence on working memory and attentional control impairments. Rheum Dis Clin North Am 2009;35(2):299–311.

362. Verdejo-Garcia A, Perez-Garcia M. Profile of executive deficits in cocaine and heroin polysubstance users: common and differential effects on separate executive components. Psychopharmacology (Berl) 2007;190(4):517–30.

363. Schiltenwolf M, et al. Evidence of specific cognitive deficits in patients with chronic low back pain under long-term substitution treatment of opioids. Pain Physician 2014;17(1):9–20.

364. Apkarian AV, Hashmi JA, Baliki MN. Pain and the brain: specificity and plasticity of the brain in clinical chronic pain. Pain 2011;152(3 Suppl.):S49–64.

365. Farmer MA, Baliki MN, Apkarian AV. A dynamic network perspective of chronic pain. Neurosci Lett 2012;520(2):197–203.

366. Bushnell MC, et al. Effect of environment on the long-term consequences of chronic pain. Pain 2015;156(Suppl. 1):S42–9.

367. Baliki MN, Baria AT, Apkarian AV. The cortical rhythms of chronic back pain. J Neurosci 2011;31(39):13981–90.

368. Coderre TJ, et al. Contribution of central neuroplasticity to pathological pain: review of clinical and experimental evidence. Pain 1993;52(3):259–85.

369. Melzack R. Recent concepts of pain. J Med 1982;13(3):147–60.

370. Melzack R. From the gate to the neuromatrix. Pain 1999;Suppl 6:S121–6.

371. Melzack R. Gate Control Theory. On the evolution of pain concepts. Pain Forum 1996;5(1):128–38.

372. Melzack R, Casey K. Sensory, motivational and central control determinants of pain. In: Kenshalo D, editor. The skin senses. Springfield.: Charles C Thomas; 1968. p. 423–39.

373. Melzack R. Phantom limbs and the concept of a neuromatrix. Trends Neurosci 1990;13(3):88–92.

374. Melzack R. Evolution of the neuromatrix theory of pain. The prithvi raj lecture: presented at the third world congress of world institute of pain, barcelona 2004. Pain Pract 2005;5(2):85–94.

375. Melzack R. Pain and the neuromatrix in the brain. J Dent Educ 2001;65(12):1378–82.

376. Melzack R. Pain: past, present and future. Can J Exp Psychol 1993;47(4):615–29.

377. Eisenberger NI, Lieberman MD, Williams KD. Does rejection hurt? An FMRI study of social exclusion. Science 2003;302(5643):290–2.

378. Singer T, et al. Empathy for pain involves the affective but not sensory components of pain. Science 2004;303(5661):1157–62.

379. Raij TT, et al. Strength of prefrontal activation predicts intensity of suggestion-induced pain. Hum Brain Mapp 2009;30(9):2890–7.

380. Chapman CR. Neuromatrix theory Do we need it? Pain Forum 1996;5(2):139–42.

381. Tracey I. Imaging pain. Br J Anaesth 2008;101(1):32–9.

382. Tracey I, Johns E. The pain matrix: reloaded or reborn as we image tonic pain using arterial spin labelling. Pain 2010;148(3):359–60.

383. Derbyshire SW. Exploring the pain "neuromatrix". Curr Rev Pain 2000;4(6):467–77.

384. Melzack R. The future of pain. Nat Rev Drug Discov 2008;7(8):629.

385. Chapman CR, Nakamura Y. Consciousness, Complexity, and Causality. Concerns and Conundrums. Pain Forum 1999;8(3):136–8.

386. Gifford L. The mature organism model. In: Gifford L, editor. Topical issues in pain 1. Falmouth: CNS Press; 1998. p. 45–56.

387. Jones M, Rivett D. Introduction to clinical reasoning. In: Jones M, Rivett D, editors. Clinical reasoning for manual therapist. Philadelphia.: Elsevier Butterworth-Heinemann; 2004. p. 3–24.

388. Gifford L, Thacker M, Jones M. Physiotherapy and pain. In: McMahon S, Koltzenburg M, editors. Wall and Melzack's Textbook of Pain. Philadelphia: Philadelphia; 2006. p. 603–17.

389. Gifford L. Tissue and input related mechanisms. In: Gifford L, editor. Topical issues in pain 1. Falmouth: CNS Press; 1998. p. 57–65.

390. Chapman CR. Aspectos psicofisiológicos del dolor. In: Loeser JD, editor. Bonica Terapútica del Dolor. Mexico: McGraw-Hill Interamericana; 2003. p. 555–74.

391. Stratakis CA, Chrousos GP. Neuroendocrinology and pathophysiology of the stress system. Ann N Y Acad Sci 1995;771:1–18.

392. Feldman S, Conforti N, Weidenfeld J. Limbic pathways and hypothalamic neurotransmitters mediating adrenocortical responses to neural stimuli. Neurosci Biobehav Rev 1995;19(2):235–40.

393. McLean SA, et al. Cerebrospinal Fluid Corticotropin-Releasing Factor Concentration is Associated with Pain but not Fatigue Symptoms in Patients with Fibromyalgia. Neuropsychopharmacology 2006.

394. Charmandari E, Tsigos C, Chrousos G. Endocrinology of the stress response. Annu Rev Physiol 2005;67:259–84.

395. Chrousos GP. Stressors, stress, and neuroendocrine integration of the adaptive response. The 1997 Hans Selye Memorial Lecture. Ann N Y Acad Sci 1998;851:311–35.

396. Habib KE, Gold PW, Chrousos GP. Neuroendocrinology of stress. Endocrinol Metab Clin North Am 2001;30(3):695–728, vii-viii.

397. Pitman RK. Post-traumatic stress disorder, hormones, and memory. Biol Psychiatry 1989;26(3):221–3.

398. McGaugh JL, et al. Involvement of the amygdaloid complex in neuromodulatory influences on memory storage. Neurosci Biobehav Rev 1990;14(4):425–31.

399. McGaugh JL, Roozendaal B. Role of adrenal stress hormones in forming lasting memories in the brain. Curr Opin Neurobiol 2002;12(2):205–10.

400. Roozendaal B. Stress and memory: opposing effects of glucocorticoids on memory consolidation and memory retrieval. Neurobiol Learn Mem 2002;78(3):578–95.

401. Delahanty DL, et al. Initial urinary epinephrine and cortisol levels predict acute PTSD symptoms in child trauma victims. Psychoneuroendocrinology 2005;30(2):121–8.

402. Nugent NR, Christopher NC, Delahanty DL. Initial physiological responses and perceived hyperarousal predict subsequent emotional numbing in pediatric injury patients. J Trauma Stress 2006;19(3):349–59.

403. Shalev AY, et al. Prospective study of posttraumatic stress disorder and depression following trauma. Am J Psychiatry 1998;155(5):630–7.

404. Shalev AY, et al. A prospective study of heart rate response following trauma and the subsequent development of posttraumatic stress disorder. Arch Gen Psychiatry 1998;55(6):553–9.

405. Cohen H, et al. Prevalence of post-traumatic stress disorder in fibromyalgia patients: overlapping syndromes or posttraumatic fibromyalgia syndrome? Semin Arthritis Rheum 2002;32(1):38–50.

406. Zatzick DF, et al. Reevaluating the association between emergency department heart rate and the development of posttraumatic stress disorder: A public health approach. Biol Psychiatry 2005;57(1):91–5.

407. Schubert R, et al. Now you feel it–now you don't: ERP correlates of somatosensory awareness. Psychophysiology 2006;43(1):31–40.

408. Azanon E, et al. The posterior parietal cortex remaps touch into external space. Curr Biol 2010;20(14):1304–9.

409. Macaluso E, Maravita A. The representation of space near the body through touch and vision. Neuropsychologia 2010;48(3):782–95.

410. Keefe FJ, et al. Psychological aspects of persistent pain: current state of the science. J Pain 2004;5(4):195–211.

411. Gauthier N, et al. Investigating risk factors for chronicity: the importance of distinguishing between return-to-work status and self-report measures of disability. J Occup Environ Med 2006;48(3):312–18.

412. Young Casey C, et al. Transition from acute to chronic pain and disability: a model including cognitive, affective, and trauma factors. Pain 2008;134(1–2):69–79.

413. Nicholas MK, et al. Early identification and management of psychological risk factors ("yellow flags") in patients with low back pain: a reappraisal. Phys Ther 2011;91(5):737–53.

414. Flor H, Turk D. Psychobiological mechanisms in chronic pain. In: Flor H, Turk D, editors. Chronic Pain. A integrated biobehavioral approach. Seattle.: IASP press; 2011. p. 89–136.

415. Kim H, Clark D, Dionne RA. Genetic contributions to clinical pain and analgesia: avoiding pitfalls in genetic research. J Pain 2009;10(7):663–93.

416. Lacroix-Fralish ML, Ledoux JB, Mogil JS. The Pain Genes Database: An interactive web browser of pain-related transgenic knockout studies. Pain 2007;131(1–2):3 e1–4.

417. Schur EA, et al. Feeling bad in more ways than one: comorbidity patterns of medically unexplained and psychiatric conditions. J Gen Intern Med 2007;22(6):818–21.

418. Levy RL, et al. Irritable bowel syndrome in twins: heredity and social learning both contribute to etiology. Gastroenterology 2001;121(4):799–804.

419. Van Houdenhove B. Listening to CFS: why we should pay more attention to the story of the patient. J Psychosom Res 2002;52(6):495–9.

420. Paras ML, et al. Sexual abuse and lifetime diagnosis of somatic disorders: a systematic review and meta-analysis. JAMA 2009;302(5):550–61.

421. Tietjen GE, et al. Childhood maltreatment and migraine (part I). Prevalence and adult revictimization: a multicenter headache clinic survey. Headache 2010;50(1):20–31.

422. Saariaho TH, et al. Early maladaptive schemas in Finnish adult chronic pain patients and a control sample. Scand J Psychol 2011;52(2):146–53.

423. Hart-Johnson T, Green CR. The impact of sexual or physical abuse history on pain-related outcomes among blacks and whites with chronic pain: gender influence. Pain Med 2012;13(2):229–42.

424. Symes L, et al. The association of pain severity and pain interference levels with abuse experiences and mental health symptoms among 300 mothers: baseline data analysis for a 7-year prospective study. Issues Ment Health Nurs 2013;34(1):2–16.

425. Lampe A, et al. Chronic pelvic pain and previous sexual abuse. Obstet Gynecol 2000;96(6):929–33.

426. Harlow BL, Stewart EG. Adult-onset vulvodynia in relation to childhood violence victimization. Am J Epidemiol 2005;161(9):871–80.

427. Raphael KG, Widom CS, Lange G. Childhood victimization and pain in adulthood: a prospective investigation. Pain 2001;92(1–2):283–93.

428. Raphael KG, Widom CS. Post-traumatic stress disorder moderates the relation between documented childhood victimization and pain 30 years later. Pain 2011;152(1):163–9.

429. Von Korff M, et al. Childhood psychosocial stressors and adult onset arthritis: broad spectrum risk factors and allostatic load. Pain 2009;143(1–2):76–83.

430. Nicolson NA, et al. Childhood maltreatment and diurnal cortisol patterns in women with chronic pain. Psychosom Med 2010;72(5):471–80.

431. Miller-Graff LE, et al. Victimization in childhood: General and specific associations with physical health problems in young adulthood. J Psychosom Res 2015;79(4):265–71.

432. Van Houdenhove B. Psychosocial stress and chronic pain. Eur J Pain 2000;4(3):225–8.

433. Van Houdenhove B, et al. Victimization in chronic fatigue syndrome and fibromyalgia in tertiary care: a controlled study on prevalence and characteristics. Psychosomatics 2001;42(1):21–8.

434. Van Houdenhove B, Egle UT. Comment on Raphael, K.G., Widom, C.S., Lange, G., Childhood victimization and pain in adulthood: a prospective investigation, PAIN 92 (2001) 283-293. Pain 2002;96(1–2):215–16, author reply 216-7.

435. Poleshuck EL, et al. Contributions of physical and sexual abuse to women's experiences with chronic pelvic pain. J Reprod Med 2005;50(2):91–100.

436. Sullivan MJ, et al. Integrating psychosocial and behavioral interventions to achieve optimal rehabilitation outcomes. J Occup Rehabil 2005;15(4):475–89.

437. Van Houdenhove B, Egle U, Luyten P. The role of life stress in fibromyalgia. Curr Rheumatol Rep 2005;7(5):365–70.

438. Afari N, et al. Psychological trauma and functional somatic syndromes: a systematic review and meta-analysis. Psychosom Med 2014;76(1):2–11.

439. Williams AC, Eccleston C, Morley S. Psychological therapies for the management of chronic pain (excluding headache) in adults. Cochrane Database Syst Rev 2012;(11):CD007407.

440. Liedl A, Knaevelsrud C. Chronic pain and PTSD: the Perpetual Avoidance Model and its treatment implications. Torture 2008;18(2):69–76.

441. Hinton DE, et al. The 'multiplex model' of somatic symptoms: application to tinnitus among traumatized Cambodian refugees. Transcult Psychiatry 2008;45(2):287–317.

442. Shipherd JC, et al. Veterans seeking treatment for posttraumatic stress disorder: what about comorbid chronic pain? J Rehabil Res Dev 2007;44(2):153–66.

443. Diagnostic and Statistical Manual of Mental Disorders. 5th ed. American Psychiatric Association; 2013.

444. Liedl A, et al. Support for the mutual maintenance of pain and post-traumatic stress disorder symptoms. Psychol Med 2010;40(7):1215–23.

445. Latthe P, et al. Factors predisposing women to chronic pelvic pain: systematic review. BMJ 2006;332(7544):749–55.

446. Greco LA, Freeman KE, Dufton L. Overt and relational victimization among children with frequent abdominal pain: links to social skills, academic functioning, and health service use. J Pediatr Psychol 2007;32(3):319–29.

447. Weaver TL. Impact of rape on female sexuality: review of selected literature. Clin Obstet Gynecol 2009;52(4):702–11.

448. Wuest J, et al. Abuse-related injury and symptoms of posttraumatic stress disorder as mechanisms of chronic pain in survivors of intimate partner violence. Pain Med 2009;10(4):739–47.

449. Tietjen GE, et al. Childhood maltreatment and migraine (part III). Association with comorbid pain conditions. Headache 2010;50(1):42–51.

450. Taft C, Schwartz S, Liebschutz JM. Intimate partner aggression perpetration in primary care chronic pain patients. Violence Vict 2010;25(5):649–61.

451. Luce H, Schrager S, Gilchrist V. Sexual assault of women. Am Fam Physician 2010;81(4):489–95.

452. Ulirsch JC, et al. Pain and somatic symptoms are sequelae of sexual assault: results of a prospective longitudinal study. Eur J Pain 2014;18(4):559–66.

453. Johnston NE, Atlas LY, Wager TD. Opposing effects of expectancy and somatic focus on pain. PLoS ONE 2012;7(6): e38854.

454. Atlas LY, Wager TD. How expectations shape pain. Neurosci Lett 2012;520(2):140–8.

455. Legrain V, et al. Attentional modulation of the nociceptive processing into the human brain: selective spatial attention, probability of stimulus occurrence, and target detection effects on laser evoked potentials. Pain 2002;99(1–2):21–39.

456. Villemure C, Bushnell MC. Cognitive modulation of pain: how do attention and emotion influence pain processing? Pain 2002;95(3):195–9.

457. Zampini M, et al. 'Prior entry' for pain: attention speeds the perceptual processing of painful stimuli. Neurosci Lett 2007;414(1):75–9.

458. Spence C, Parise C. Prior-entry: a review. Conscious Cogn 2010;19(1):364–79.

459. Leeuw M, et al. The Fear-Avoidance Model of Musculoskeletal Pain: Current State of Scientific Evidence. J Behav Med 2006.

460. McCracken LM, Turk DC. Behavioral and cognitive-behavioral treatment for chronic pain: outcome, predictors of outcome, and treatment process. Spine 2002;27(22):2564–73.

461. Wiech K, et al. Modulation of pain processing in hyperalgesia by cognitive demand. Neuroimage 2005;27(1):59–69.

462. Schrooten MG, et al. Nonpain goal pursuit inhibits attentional bias to pain. Pain 2012;153(6):1180–6.

463. Bushnell MC, et al. Pain perception: is there a role for primary somatosensory cortex? Proc Natl Acad Sci USA 1999;96(14):7705–9.

464. Spence C, et al. Selective attention to pain: a psychophysical investigation. Exp Brain Res 2002;145(3):395–402.

465. Lorenz J, Garcia-Larrea L. Contribution of attentional and cognitive factors to laser evoked brain potentials. Neurophysiol Clin 2003;33(6):293–301.

466. Tracey I, et al. Imaging attentional modulation of pain in the periaqueductal gray in humans. J Neurosci 2002;22(7):2748–52.

467. Petrovic P, et al. Pain-related cerebral activation is altered by a distracting cognitive task. Pain 2000;85(1–2):19–30.

468. Bantick SJ, et al. Imaging how attention modulates pain in humans using functional MRI. Brain 2002;125(Pt 2):310–19.

469. Crombez G, Van Damme S, Eccleston C. Hypervigilance to pain: an experimental and clinical analysis. Pain 2005;116(1–2):4–7.

470. Herbert MS, et al. Pain hypervigilance is associated with greater clinical pain severity and enhanced experimental pain sensitivity among adults with symptomatic knee osteoarthritis. Ann Behav Med 2014;48(1):50–60.

471. Song GH, et al. Cortical effects of anticipation and endogenous modulation of visceral pain assessed by functional brain MRI in irritable bowel syndrome patients and healthy controls. Pain 2006;126(1–3):79–90.

472. Porro CA, et al. Does anticipation of pain affect cortical nociceptive systems? J Neurosci 2002;22(8):3206–14.

473. Flor H, Turk DC. Chronic back pain and rheumatoid arthritis: predicting pain and disability from cognitive variables. J Behav Med 1988;11(3):251–65.

474. Asmundson GJ, Hadjistavropoulos HD. Is high fear of pain associated with attentional biases for pain-related or general threat? A categorical reanalysis. J Pain 2007;8(1):11–18.

475. DeGood DE, Kiernan B. Perception of fault in patients with chronic pain. Pain 1996;64(1):153–9.

476. DeGood D, Tait R. Assessment of pain beliefs and coping. In: Turk D, Melzack R, editors. Handbook of Pain Assessment. New York.: Guilford Press; 2001. p. 320–45.

477. Main CJ, Watson PJ. Psychological aspects of pain. Man Ther 1999;4(4):203–15.

478. Main CJ, Foster N, Buchbinder R. How important are back pain beliefs and expectations for satisfactory recovery from back pain? Best Pract Res Clin Rheumatol 2010;24(2):205–17.

479. Darlow B, et al. Easy to Harm, Hard to Heal: Patient Views About the Back. Spine 2015;40(11):842–50.

480. Petrie KJ, Jago LA, Devcich DA. The role of illness perceptions in patients with medical conditions. Curr Opin Psychiatry 2007;20(2):163–7.

481. van Wilgen P, et al. Physical therapists should integrate illness perceptions in their assessment in patients with chronic musculoskeletal pain; a qualitative analysis. Man Ther 2014;19(3):229–34.

482. Gehrt TB, et al. The Role of Illness Perceptions in Predicting Outcome After Acute Whiplash Trauma: A Multicenter 12-month Follow-up Study. Clin J Pain 2015;31(1):14–20.

483. Jensen MP, et al. Relationship of pain-specific beliefs to chronic pain adjustment. Pain 1994;57(3):301–9.

484. Peters ML, Vlaeyen JW, Weber WE. The joint contribution of physical pathology, pain-related fear and catastrophizing to chronic back pain disability. Pain 2005;113(1–2):45–50.

485. Swinkels-Meewisse EJ, et al. Psychometric properties of the Tampa Scale for kinesiophobia and the fear-avoidance beliefs questionnaire in acute low back pain. Man Ther 2003;8(1):29–36.

486. Turner JA, Mancl L, Aaron LA. Pain-related catastrophizing: a daily process study. Pain 2004;110(1–2):103–11.

487. Sullivan MJ, Lynch ME, Clark AJ. Dimensions of catastrophic thinking associated with pain experience and disability in patients with neuropathic pain conditions. Pain 2005;113(3):310–15.

488. Gheldof EL, et al. Pain and pain-related fear are associated with functional and social disability in an occupational setting: evidence of mediation by pain-related fear. Eur J Pain 2006;10(6):513–25.

489. Swinkels-Meewisse IE, et al. Acute low back pain: pain-related fear and pain catastrophizing influence physical performance and perceived disability. Pain 2006;120(1–2):36–43.

490. Vervoort T, et al. Catastrophic thinking about pain is independently associated with pain severity, disability, and somatic complaints in school children and children with chronic pain. J Pediatr Psychol 2006;31(7):674–83.

491. Lame IE, et al. Quality of life in chronic pain is more associated with beliefs about pain, than with pain intensity. Eur J Pain 2005;9(1):15–24.

492. Kleinman A, et al. Pain as Human Experience: An Introduction. In: Good MD, et al., editors. Pain as Human Experience An Anthropological perspective. Oxford: University of California Press; 1992.

493. Sullivan MJ, et al. Catastrophizing, pain, and disability in patients with soft-tissue injuries. Pain 1998;77(3):253–60.

494. Sullivan MJ, et al. Theoretical perspectives on the relation between catastrophizing and pain. Clin J Pain 2001;17(1):52–64.

495. Edwards RR, et al. Catastrophizing as a mediator of sex differences in pain: differential effects for daily pain versus laboratory-induced pain. Pain 2004;111(3):335–41.

496. Crombez G, et al. The effects of catastrophic thinking about pain on attentional interference by pain: no mediation of negative affectivity in healthy volunteers and in patients with low back pain. Pain Res Manag 2002;7(1):31–9.

497. Roelofs J, et al. The role of fear of movement and injury in selective attentional processing in patients with chronic low back pain: a dot-probe evaluation. J Pain 2005;6(5):294–300.

498. Edwards RR, et al. Catastrophizing and pain in arthritis, fibromyalgia, and other rheumatic diseases. Arthritis Rheum 2006;55(2):325–32.

499. Sullivan MJ, et al. Path model of psychological antecedents to pain experience: experimental and clinical findings. Clin J Pain 2004;20(3):164–73.

500. Gracely RH, et al. Pain catastrophizing and neural responses to pain among persons with fibromyalgia. Brain 2004;127(Pt 4):835–43.

501. Eccleston C, et al. Worry and chronic pain patients: a description and analysis of individual differences. Eur J Pain 2001;5(3):309–18.

502. Severeijns R, et al. Pain catastrophizing predicts pain intensity, disability, and psychological distress independent of the level of physical impairment. Clin J Pain 2001;17(2):165–72.

503. Lee H, et al. How does pain lead to disability? A systematic review and meta-analysis of mediation studies in people with back and neck pain. Pain 2015;156(6):988–97.

504. Picavet HS, Vlaeyen JW, Schouten JS. Pain catastrophizing and kinesiophobia: predictors of chronic low back pain. Am J Epidemiol 2002;156(11):1028–34.

505. Linton SJ, et al. The role of depression and catastrophizing in musculoskeletal pain. Eur J Pain 2011;15(4):416–22.

506. Wertli MM, et al. Catastrophizing-a prognostic factor for outcome in patients with low back pain: a systematic review. Spine J 2014;14(11):2639–57.

507. Goubert L, Crombez G, Van Damme S. The role of neuroticism, pain catastrophizing and pain-related fear in vigilance to pain: a structural equations approach. Pain 2004;107(3):234–41.

508. Bostick GP, et al. Predictive capacity of pain beliefs and catastrophizing in Whiplash Associated Disorder. Injury 2013;44(11):1465–71.

509. Schanberg LE, et al. The relationship of daily mood and stressful events to symptoms in juvenile rheumatic disease. Arthritis Care Res 2000;13(1):33–41.

510. Yang JC, et al. Preoperative Multidimensional Affect and Pain Survey (MAPS) scores predict postcolectomy analgesia requirement. Clin J Pain 2000;16(4):314–20.

511. Beck AT. Cognitive Therapy and the Emotional Disorders. New York: International University Press; 1979.

512. McWilliams LA, Cox BJ, Enns MW. Mood and anxiety disorders associated with chronic pain: an examination in a nationally representative sample. Pain 2003;106(1–2):127–33.

513. Bair MJ, et al. Depression and pain comorbidity: a literature review. Arch Intern Med 2003;163(20):2433–45.

514. Tunks ER, Crook J, Weir R. Epidemiology of chronic pain with psychological comorbidity: prevalence, risk, course, and prognosis. Can J Psychiatry 2008;53(4):224–34.

515. Sullivan MJ, et al. Initial depression severity and the trajectory of recovery following cognitive-behavioral intervention for work disability. J Occup Rehabil 2006;16(1):63–74.

516. Main C, Sullivan M, Watson P. Pain Management. Practical applications of the biopsychosocial perspective in clinical and occupational settings. 2nd ed. Philadelphia Churchill Livingstone: ELSEVIER; 2008.

517. Lethem J, et al. Outline of a Fear-Avoidance Model of exaggerated pain perception–I. Behav Res Ther 1983;21(4):401–8.

518. Vlaeyen JW, et al. Fear of movement/(re)injury in chronic low back pain and its relation to behavioral performance. Pain 1995;62(3):363–72.

519. Waddell G, et al. A Fear-Avoidance Beliefs Questionnaire (FABQ) and the role of fear-avoidance beliefs in chronic low back pain and disability. Pain 1993;52(2):157–68.

520. Asmundson GJ, Taylor S. Role of anxiety sensitivity in pain-related fear and avoidance. J Behav Med 1996;19(6):577–86.

521. Kori S, Miller R, Todd D. Kinisiophobia: a new view of chronic pain behavior. Pain Manag 1990;3:35–43.

522. George SZ, Beneciuk JM. Psychological predictors of recovery from low back pain: a prospective study. BMC Musculoskelet Disord 2015;16:49.

523. Soderlund A, Asenlof P. The mediating role of self-efficacy expectations and fear of movement and (re)injury beliefs in two samples of acute pain. Disabil Rehabil 2010;32(25):2118–26.

524. Turk DC, Robinson JP, Burwinkle T. Prevalence of fear of pain and activity in patients with fibromyalgia syndrome. J Pain 2004;5(9):483–90.

525. Bortz WM 2nd. The disuse syndrome. West J Med 1984;141(5):691–4.

526. Philips HC. Avoidance behaviour and its role in sustaining chronic pain. Behav Res Ther 1987;25(4):273–9.

527. Council JR, et al. Expectancies and functional impairment in chronic low back pain. Pain 1988;33(3):323–31.

528. Bennett RM, Jacobsen S. Muscle function and origin of pain in fibromyalgia. Baillieres Clin Rheumatol 1994;8(4):721–46.

529. Burton AK, et al. Psychosocial predictors of outcome in acute and subchronic low back trouble. Spine 1995;20(6):722–8.

530. Klenerman L, et al. The prediction of chronicity in patients with an acute attack of low back pain in a general practice setting. Spine 1995;20(4):478–84.

531. Buer N, Linton SJ. Fear-avoidance beliefs and catastrophizing: occurrence and risk factor in back pain and ADL in the general population. Pain 2002;99(3):485–91.

532. Grotle M, et al. Fear-avoidance beliefs and distress in relation to disability in acute and chronic low back pain. Pain 2004;112(3):343–52.

533. Gheldof EL, et al. The differential role of pain, work characteristics and pain-related fear in explaining back pain and sick leave in occupational settings. Pain 2005;113(1–2):71–81.

534. Nederhand MJ, et al. Predictive value of fear avoidance in developing chronic neck pain disability: consequences for clinical decision making. Arch Phys Med Rehabil 2004;85(3):496–501.

535. Wertli MM, et al. The role of fear avoidance beliefs as a prognostic factor for outcome in patients with nonspecific low back pain: a systematic review. Spine J 2014;14(5):816–36 e4.

536. Zale EL, et al. The relation between pain-related fear and disability: a meta-analysis. J Pain 2013;14(10):1019–30.

537. Main C, Watson P. The distressed and angry low back pain patient. In: Gifford L, editor. Topical issues in pain 3. Falmouth: CNS Press; 2002. p. 175–92.

538. Nisenzon AN, et al. The role of anger in psychosocial subgrouping for patients with low back pain. Clin J Pain 2014;30(6):501–9.

539. Bandura A. Self-efficacy: toward a unifying theory of behavioral change. Psychol Rev 1977;84(2):191–215.

540. Flor H, Birbaumer N, Turk D. The psichobiology of chronic pain. Advances en Behaviour Research and Therapy 1990;12:47–84.

541. Jensen MP, et al. Coping with chronic pain: a critical review of the literature. Pain 1991;47(3):249–83.

542. Asghari A, Nicholas MK. Pain self-efficacy beliefs and pain behaviour. A prospective study. Pain 2001;94(1):85–100.

543. Arnstein P. The mediation of disability by self efficacy in different samples of chronic pain patients. Disabil Rehabil 2000;22(17):794–801.

544. Asenlof P, Soderlund A. A further investigation of the importance of pain cognition and behaviour in pain rehabilitation: longitudinal data suggest disability and fear of movement are most important. Clin Rehabil 2010;24(5):422–30.

545. Woby SR, et al. The relation between cognitive factors and levels of pain and disability in chronic low back pain patients presenting for physiotherapy. Eur J Pain 2007;11(8):869–77.

546. Costa Lda C, et al. Self-efficacy is more important than fear of movement in mediating the relationship between pain and disability in chronic low back pain. Eur J Pain 2011;15(2):213–19.

547. Salomons TV, et al. Perceived controllability modulates the neural response to pain. J Neurosci 2004;24(32):7199–203.

548. Linton SJ. A review of psychological risk factors in back and neck pain. Spine 2000;25(9):1148–56.

549. Flor H, Turk D. Chronic Pain. A integrated biobehavioral approach. Seattle: IASP press; 2011.

550. Weiten W, et al. Psychology Applied to Modern Life: Adjustment in the 21st Century. 9th ed. Cengage Learning; 2008.

551. Waddell G, et al. Chronic low-back pain, psychologic distress, and illness behavior. Spine 1984;9(2):209–13.

552. George SZ, Bialosky JE, Donald DA. The centralization phenomenon and fear-avoidance beliefs as prognostic factors for acute low back pain: a preliminary investigation involving patients classified for specific exercise. J Orthop Sports Phys Ther 2005;35(9):580–8.

553. Swinkels-Meewisse IE, et al. Fear of movement/(re)injury predicting chronic disabling low back pain: a prospective inception cohort study. Spine 2006;31(6):658–64.

554. Swinkels-Meewisse IE, et al. Fear-avoidance beliefs, disability, and participation in workers and non-workers with acute low back pain. Clin J Pain 2006;22(1):45–54.

555. Richards JS, et al. Assessing pain behavior: the UAB Pain Behavior Scale. Pain 1982;14(4):393–8.

556. Waddell G, et al. Nonorganic physical signs in low-back pain. Spine 1980;5(2):117–25.

557. Main CJ, Waddell G. Behavioral responses to examination. A reappraisal of the interpretation of "nonorganic signs. Spine 1998;23(21):2367–71.

558. Sobel JB, et al. Cervical nonorganic signs: a new clinical tool to assess abnormal illness behavior in neck pain patients: a pilot study. Arch Phys Med Rehabil 2000;81(2):170–5.

559. Waddell G, Main CJ. Assessment of severity of low back disorders. Acta Orthop Belg 1987;53(2):269–71.

560. Ahern DK, et al. Correlation of chronic low-back pain behavior and muscle function examination of the flexion-relaxation response. Spine 1990;15(2):92–5.

561. Waddell G, Burton AK. Concepts of rehabilitation for the management of low back pain. Best Pract Res Clin Rheumatol 2005;19(4):655–70.

562. de Waal MW, et al. Somatoform disorders in general practice: prevalence, functional impairment and comorbidity with anxiety and depressive disorders. Br J Psychiatry 2004;184:470–6.

563. Watson P, Kendall N. Assessing psychosocial yellow flags. In: Gifford L, editor. Topical issues in pain 2. Falmouth: CNS Press; 1998. p. 111–29.

564. Kendall N, Linton S, Main C. Guide to assessing psychosocial yellow flags in acute low back pain: Risk factors for long-term disabilty and work loss. Wellington: Accident Rehabilitation & Compensation Insurance Corporation of New Zealand and the National Health Committee; 1997.

565. Gonzalez-Anleo J. Sociología del Dolor. In: Dou A, editor. El Dolor. Madrid: UPCO; 1992. p. 338.

566. OMS, Clasificación Internacional del Funcionamiento, de la Discapacidad y de la Salud. 2001: Ministerio de Trabajo y Asuntos Sociales. Secretaría General de Asuntos Sociales. Instituto de Migraciones y Servicios Sociales (IMSERSO).

567. Hoftun GB, Romundstad PR, Rygg M. Association of parental chronic pain with chronic pain in the adolescent and young adult: family linkage data from the HUNT Study. JAMA Pediatr 2013;167(1):61–9.

568. Turk DC, Flor H, Rudy TE. Pain and families. I. Etiology, maintenance, and psychosocial impact. Pain 1987;30(1):3–27.

569. Rickard K. The occurrence of maladaptive health-related behaviors and teacher-rated conduct problems in children of chronic low back pain patients. J Behav Med 1988;11(2):107–16.

570. Goubert L, et al. Learning about pain from others: an observational learning account. J Pain 2011;12(2):167–74.

571. Helsen K, et al. Observational learning and pain-related fear: an experimental study with colored cold pressor tasks. J Pain 2011;12(12):1230–9.

572. Goubert L, et al. Parental emotional responses to their child's pain: the role of dispositional empathy and catastrophizing about their child's pain. J Pain 2008;9(3):272–9.

573. Caes L, et al. Parental catastrophizing about child's pain and its relationship with activity restriction: the mediating role of parental distress. Pain 2011;152(1):212–22.

574. Goubert L, et al. The impact of parental gender, catastrophizing and situational threat upon parental behaviour to child pain: a vignette study. Eur J Pain 2012;16(8):1176–84.

575. Sieberg CB, Williams S, Simons LE. Do parent protective responses mediate the relation between parent distress and child functional disability among children with chronic pain? J Pediatr Psychol 2011;36(9):1043–51.

576. Logan DE, Simons LE, Carpino EA. Too sick for school? Parent influences on school functioning among children with chronic pain. Pain 2012;153(2):437–43.

577. Schanberg LE, et al. Family pain history predicts child health status in children with chronic rheumatic disease. Pediatrics 2001;108(3):E47.

578. Ottman R, Hong S, Lipton RB. Validity of family history data on severe headache and migraine. Neurology 1993;43(10): 1954–60.

579. Fillingim RB, Edwards RR, Powell T. Sex-dependent effects of reported familial pain history on recent pain complaints and experimental pain responses. Pain 2000;86(1–2):87–94.

580. Christensen MF, Mortensen O. Long-term prognosis in children with recurrent abdominal pain. Arch Dis Child 1975;50(2):110–14.

581. Lier R, Nilsen TI, Mork PJ. Parental chronic pain in relation to chronic pain in their adult offspring: family-linkage within the HUNT Study, Norway. BMC Public Health 2014;14:797.

582. Leonard MT, Cano A. Pain affects spouses too: personal experience with pain and catastrophizing as correlates of spouse distress. Pain 2006;126(1–3):139–46.

583. Flor H, Kerns RD, Turk DC. The role of spouse reinforcement, perceived pain, and activity levels of chronic pain patients. J Psychosom Res 1987;31(2):251–9.

584. Romano JM, et al. Chronic pain patient-spouse behavioral interactions predict patient disability. Pain 1995;63(3):353–60.

585. Kerns RD, et al. The role of marital interaction in chronic pain and depressive symptom severity. J Psychosom Res 1990;34(4):401–8.

586. Flor H, Turk DC, Rudy TE. Relationship of pain impact and significant other reinforcement of pain behaviors: the mediating role of gender, marital status and marital satisfaction. Pain 1989;38(1):45–50.

587. Romano JM, Jensen MP, Turner JA. The Chronic Pain Coping Inventory-42: reliability and validity. Pain 2003;104(1–2):65–73.

588. Romano JM, et al. Sequential analysis of chronic pain behaviors and spouse responses. J Consult Clin Psychol 1992;60(5):777–82.

589. Schwartz L, Jensen MP, Romano JM. The development and psychometric evaluation of an instrument to assess spouse responses to pain and well behavior in patients with chronic pain: the Spouse Response Inventory. J Pain 2005;6(4): 243–52.

590. Raichle KA, Romano JM, Jensen MP. Partner responses to patient pain and well behaviors and their relationship to patient pain behavior, functioning, and depression. Pain 2011;152(1):82–8.

591. Cunningham JL, et al. Associations between spousal or significant other solicitous responses and opioid dose in patients with chronic pain. Pain Med 2012;13(8):1034–9.

592. Newton-John T. When helping does not help: responding to pain behaviours. In: Gifford L, editor. Topical issues in Pain 2. Falmouth: CNS Press; 2000.

593. Attention and social responsiveness. In: Main CJ, et al., editors. Fordyce's Behavioral Methods for Chronic Pain and Illness. IASP Press.; 2015. p. 367–403.

594. Swift CM, Reed K, Hocking C. A new perspective on family involvement in chronic pain management programmes. Musculoskeletal Care 2014;12(1):47–55.

595. Keefe FJ, et al. Effects of spouse-assisted coping skills training and exercise training in patients with osteoarthritic knee pain: a randomized controlled study. Pain 2004;110(3):539–49.

596. Cano A, Leonard M. Integrative behavioral couple therapy for chronic pain: promoting behavior change and emotional acceptance. J Clin Psychol 2006;62(11):1409–18.

597. Waddell G, Burton A. Concepts of Rehabilitation for the Management of Common Health Problems. London: The Stationery Office; 2004.

598. Steenstra IA, et al. Prognostic factors for duration of sick leave in patients sick listed with acute low back pain: a systematic review of the literature. Occup Environ Med 2005;62(12):851–60.

599. Marhold C, Linton SJ, Melin L. Identification of obstacles for chronic pain patients to return to work: evaluation of a questionnaire. J Occup Rehabil 2002;12(2):65–75.

600. Anema JR, et al. Ineffective disability management by doctors is an obstacle for return-to-work: a cohort study on low back pain patients sicklisted for 3-4 months. Occup Environ Med 2002;59(11):729–33.

601. Waddell G, Aylward M. Models of sickness and disability. Applied to common health problems. London: Royal Society of Medicine Press; 2010.

602. Wynn PA, et al. Undergraduate occupational health teaching in medical schools–not enough of a good thing? Occup Med (Lond) 2003;53(6):347–8.

603. Beaumont D. Rehabilitation and retention in the workplace– the interaction between general practitioners and occupational health professionals: a consensus statement. Occup Med (Lond) 2003;53(4):254–5.

604. Frank JW, et al. Disability resulting from occupational low back pain. Part II: What do we know about secondary prevention? A review of the scientific evidence on prevention after disability begins. Spine 1996;21(24):2918–29.

605. Main CJ, Williams AC. Musculoskeletal pain. BMJ 2002;325(7363):534–7.

606. Main CJ, Burton AK. Economic and occupational influences on pain and disability. In: Main C, Spanswick C, editors. Pain Management: An Interdisciplinary Approach. Edinburgh.: Churchill Livingstone; 2000. p. 63–87.

607. Kendall B. Main, & Watson Tackling Musculoskeletal Problems: A Guide for Clinic and Workplace - Identifying Obstacles Using the Psychosocial Flags Framework. Norwich: TSO; 2009.

608. Shaw WS, et al. Early patient screening and intervention to address individual-level occupational factors ("blue flags") in back disability. J Occup Rehabil 2009;19(1): 64–80.

609. Ferrari R, Russell AS. Development of persistent neurologic symptoms in patients with simple neck sprain. Arthritis Care Res 1999;12(1):70–6.

610. Cassidy JD, et al. Effect of eliminating compensation for pain and suffering on the outcome of insurance claims for whiplash injury. N Engl J Med 2000;342(16):1179–86.

611. Houben RM, et al. Health care providers' attitudes and beliefs towards common low back pain: factor structure and psychometric properties of the HC-PAIRS. Clin J Pain 2004;20(1):37–44.

612. Houben RM, et al. Health care providers' orientations towards common low back pain predict perceived harmfulness of physical activities and recommendations regarding return to normal activity. Eur J Pain 2005;9(2):173–83.

613. Houben RM, et al. Do health care providers' attitudes towards back pain predict their treatment recommendations? Differential predictive validity of implicit and explicit attitude measures. Pain 2005;114(3):491–8.

614. Coudeyre E, et al. General practitioners' fear-avoidance beliefs influence their management of patients with low back pain. Pain 2006;124(3):330–7.

615. Poiraudeau S, et al. Outcome of subacute low back pain: influence of patients' and rheumatologists' characteristics. Rheumatology (Oxford) 2006;45(6):718–23.

616. Bonathan C, Hearn L, Williams AC. Socioeconomic status and the course and consequences of chronic pain. Pain Manag 2013;3(3):159–62.

617. Kristenson M, et al. Psychobiological mechanisms of socioeconomic differences in health. Soc Sci Med 2004;58(8):1511–22.

618. Steptoe A, Feldman PJ. Neighborhood problems as sources of chronic stress: development of a measure of neighborhood problems, and associations with socioeconomic status and health. Ann Behav Med 2001;23(3):177–85.

619. Roth RS, Geisser ME. Educational achievement and chronic pain disability: mediating role of pain-related cognitions. Clin J Pain 2002;18(5):286–96.

620. Geertz G. The Interpretation of Cultures. New York: Basic Books Inc; 1973.

621. Kleinman A. Patients and healers in the context of culture: an exploration of the borderland between anthropology, medicine, and psychiatry. Berkeley. University of California Press; 1980.

622. Zborowski M. Cultural Components in Responses to Pain. J Soc Issues 1952;8(4):16–30.

623. Gooberman-Hill R. Ethnographies of pain: culture, context and complexity. Br J Pain 2015;9(1):32–5.

624. Stanaway FF, et al. Back pain in older male Italian-born immigrants in Australia: the importance of socioeconomic factors. Eur J Pain 2011;15(1):70–6.

625. Bates MS, Rankin-Hill L. Control, culture and chronic pain. Soc Sci Med 1994;39(5):629–45.

626. Honeyman PT, Jacobs EA. Effects of culture on back pain in Australian aboriginals. Spine 1996;21(7):841–3.

627. Rahim-Williams B, et al. A quantitative review of ethnic group differences in experimental pain response: do biology, psychology, and culture matter? Pain Med 2012;13(4):522–40.

628. Otegui R. Factores socioculturales del dolor y el sufrimiento. In: Perdiguero E, Comelles J, editors. Medicina y Cultura. Estudios entre la antropología y la medicina. Barcelona: Bellaterra; 2000.

629. Le Breton D. Antropología del Dolor. Ed Seix Barral; 1999.

630. Barsky AJ. The paradox of health. N Engl J Med 1988;318(7):414–18.

631. DALYs, G.B.D., et al. Global, regional, and national disability-adjusted life years (DALYs) for 306 diseases and injuries and healthy life expectancy (HALE) for 188 countries, 1990-2013: quantifying the epidemiological transition. Lancet 2015.

632. Barsky AJ, Borus JF. Somatization and medicalization in the era of managed care. JAMA 1995;274(24):1931–4.

633. Chodoff P. The medicalization of the human condition. Psychiatr Serv 2002;53(5):627–8.

634. Wildes KW. Medicalization and social ills. America (NY) 1999;180(11):16–18.

635. Hadler NM. "Fibromyalgia" and the medicalization of misery. J Rheumatol 2003;30(8):1668–70.

636. Nye RA. The evolution of the concept of medicalization in the late twentieth century. J Hist Behav Sci 2003;39(2):115–29.

637. Conrad P, Leiter V. Medicalization, markets and consumers. J Health Soc Behav 2004;45(Suppl.):158–76.

638. Kalanithi P. The medicalization of personality: mind-body relations in scientific culture. Princet J Bioeth 2001;4:46–63.

639. Conrad P. The shifting engines of medicalization. J Health Soc Behav 2005;46(1):3–14.

640. Filc D. The medical text: between biomedicine and hegemony. Soc Sci Med 2004;59(6):1275–85.

641. Thomas-MacLean R, Stoppard JM. Physicians' constructions of depression: inside/outside the boundaries of medicalization. Health (London) 2004;8(3):275–93.

642. Orueta R, et al. Medicalización de la vida (I). Rev Clin Med Fam 2003;4:150–61.

643. Moynihan R, Smith R. Too much medicine? BMJ 2002;324(7342):859–60.

644. Maturo A. Medicalization: current concept and future directions in a bionic society. Mens Sana Monogr 2012;10(1):122–33.

645. Hadler NM, Greenhalgh S. Labeling woefulness: the social construction of fibromyalgia. Spine 2005;30(1):1–4.

646. Illich I, Némesis médica: la expropiación de la salud. 1975, Barcelona Barral Editores.

647. Page L, Wessely S. Medically unexplained symtoms: exacerbating factors in the doctor-patient encounter. J R Soc Med 2003;96:223–7.

648. Hadler NM, Ehrlich GE. Fibromyalgia and the conundrum of disability determination. J Occup Environ Med 2003;45(10):1030–3.

649. Hazemeijer I, Rasker JJ. Fibromyalgia and the therapeutic domain. A philosophical study on the origins of fibromyalgia in a specific social setting. Rheumatology (Oxford) 2003;42(4):507–15.

650. Ehrlich GE. Pain is real; fibromyalgia isn't. J Rheumatol 2003;30(8):1666–7.

651. Hadler NM, Greenhalgh S. Labeling woefulness: the social construction of fibromyalgia. Spine 2005;30(1):1–4.

652. Ferrari R, Schrader H. The late whiplash syndrome: a biopsychosocial approach. J Neurol Neurosurg Psychiatry 2001;70(6):722–6.

653. Smythe HA, Moldofsky H. Two contributions to understanding of the "fibrositis" syndrome. Bull Rheum Dis 1977;28(1):928–31.

654. Wolfe F, et al. The American College of Rheumatology 1990 Criteria for the Classification of Fibromyalgia. Report of the Multicenter Criteria Committee. Arthritis Rheum 1990;33(2):160–72.

655. Bentall RP, et al. Predictors of response to treatment for chronic fatigue syndrome. Br J Psychiatry 2002;181:248–52.

656. Friedberg F, Leung DW, Quick J. Do support groups help people with chronic fatigue syndrome and fibromyalgia? A comparison of active and inactive members. J Rheumatol 2005;32(12):2416–20.

657. Moynihan R, Heath I, Henry D. Selling sickness: the pharmaceutical industry and disease mongering. BMJ 2002;324(7342):886–91.

658. Moynihan R. Scientists find new disease: motivational deficiency disorder. BMJ 2006;332(7544):745.

659. Loeser JD, Black RG. A taxonomy of pain. Pain 1975;1(1):81–4.

660. Nolan M. Pain: the experience and its expression. Clin Manage 1990;10(22).

661. Main C, Spanswick C. Pain management: An interdisciplinary approach. Edinburgh: Churchill Livingstone; 2000.

662. Loeser J. Perspectives on pain. In: Turner P, editor. Clinical Pharmacy and therapeutics. London.: Macmillan; 1980. p. 313–16.

663. Bausbaum AI, Jessell TM. La percepción del dolor. In: Kandel ER, Schwartz JH, Jessell TM, editors. Principios de Neurociencia. Mc Graw-Hill Interamericana; 2001.

664. Gatzounis R, et al. Operant learning theory in pain and chronic pain rehabilitation. Curr Pain Headache Rep 2012;16(2):117–26.

665. Waddell G. The Back Pain Revolution. 2 ed. London: Churchill Livingstone; 2004.

666. Vlaeyen JW, Linton SJ. Fear-avoidance model of chronic musculoskeletal pain: 12 years on. Pain 2012;153(6):1144–7.

667. Vlaeyen J, et al. Pain-Related Fear. Exposure treatment of chronic pain. Seattle: IASP press; 2012.

668. Weiner BK. Spine update: the biopsychosocial model and spine care. Spine 2008;33(2):219–23.

669. Pransky G, Buchbinder R, Hayden J. Contemporary low back pain research - and implications for practice. Best Pract Res Clin Rheumatol 2010;24(2):291–8.

670. Jull G, Moore A. Hands on, hands off? The swings in musculoskeletal physiotherapy practice. Man Ther 2012;17(3):199–200.

671. Ford JJ, Hahne AJ. Pathoanatomy and classification of low back disorders. Man Ther 2013;18(2):165–8.

672. Hancock M, et al. MRI findings are more common in selected patients with acute low back pain than controls? Eur Spine J 2012;21(2):240–6.

673. Merskey H, Bogduk N. Part III: Pain Terms, A Current List with Definitions and Notes on Usage. In: Classification of Chronic Pain: Descriptions of chronic pain syndromes and definitions of pain terms. Seattle: IASP Press; 1994.

674. Turk DC, Okifuji A. Pain terms and taxonomies of pain. In: Fishman SM, Ballantyne J, Rathmell J, editors. Bonica's Management of Pain. Wolters Kluwer Lippincott Willams & Wilkins; 2010. p. 13–23.

675. Dickinson BD, et al. Maldynia: pathophysiology and management of neuropathic and maladaptive pain–a report of the AMA Council on Science and Public Health. Pain Med 2010;11(11):1635–53.

676. Dubois MY, Gallagher RM, Lippe PM. Pain medicine position paper. Pain Med 2009;10(6):972–1000.

677. Gallagher RM, Fraifeld EM. Vision and purpose: AAPM members lead national initiative to improve pain care, education, and training. Pain Med 2010;11(2):154–7.

678. Gallagher RM. Chronification to maldynia: biopsychosocial failure of pain homeostasis. Pain Med 2011;12(7):993–5.

679. Crook J, Tunks E. Defining the "chronic pain syndrome": An epidemiological method. Pain 1984;18:S121.

680. Diatchenko L, et al. Idiopathic pain disorders–pathways of vulnerability. Pain 2006;123(3):226–30.

681. Addison RG. Chronic pain syndrome. Am J Med 1984;77(3A):54–8.

682. Yunus MB. Central sensitivity syndromes: a new paradigm and group nosology for fibromyalgia and overlapping conditions, and the related issue of disease versus illness. Semin Arthritis Rheum 2008;37(6):339–52.

683. Doege T, Houston T. Guides to the evaluation of permanent impairment. 4 ed. Chicago: American Medical Association; 1993.

684. Huijnen IP, et al. Subgrouping of low back pain patients for targeting treatments: evidence from genetic, psychological, and activity-related behavioral approaches. Clin J Pain 2015;31(2):123–32.

685. Phillips K, Clauw DJ. Central pain mechanisms in chronic pain states–maybe it is all in their head. Best Pract Res Clin Rheumatol 2011;25(2):141–54.

686. Borsook D, Sava S, Becerra L. The pain imaging revolution: advancing pain into the 21st century. Neuroscientist 2010;16(2):171–85.

687. May A. Chronic pain may change the structure of the brain. Pain 2008;137(1):7–15.

688. Tracey I, Bushnell MC. How neuroimaging studies have challenged us to rethink: is chronic pain a disease? J Pain 2009;10(11):1113–20.

689. Sullivan MD, et al. What does it mean to call chronic pain a brain disease? J Pain 2013;14(4):317–22.

690. Sullivan MD. Finding pain between minds and bodies. Clin J Pain 2001;17(2):146–56.

691. Cohen M, Quintner J, Buchanan D. Is chronic pain a disease? Pain Med 2013;14(9):1284–8.

692. American, Psychiatric, and Association. Diagnostic and Statistical Manual of Mental Disorders DSM-5. Arlington; 2013.

693. Merskey H. Pain disorder, hysteria or somatization? Pain Res Manag 2004;9(2):67–71.

694. Treede RD, et al. A classification of chronic pain for ICD-11. Pain 2015.

695. Woolf CJ, et al. Towards a mechanism-based classification of pain? Pain 1998;77(3):227–9.

696. Backonja MM. Defining neuropathic pain. Anesth Analg 2003;97(3):785–90.

697. Bennett MI, et al. Can pain can be more or less neuropathic? Comparison of symptom assessment tools with ratings of certainty by clinicians. Pain 2006;122(3):289–94.

698. Bennett MI, et al. Using screening tools to identify neuropathic pain. Pain 2007;127(3):199–203.

699. Treede RD, et al. Neuropathic pain: redefinition and a grading system for clinical and research purposes. Neurology 2008;70(18):1630–5.

700. Merskey H, Bogduk N. Classification of Chronic Pain: Descriptions of chronic pain syndromes and definitions of pain terms. 2nd ed. Seattle: IASP Press; 1994.

701. Smart KM, et al. The reliability of clinical judgments and criteria associated with mechanisms-based classifications of pain in patients with low back pain disorders: a preliminary reliability study. J Man Manip Ther 2010;18(2):102–10.

702. Smart KM, et al. The Discriminative validity of "nociceptive," "peripheral neuropathic," and "central sensitization" as mechanisms-based classifications of musculoskeletal pain. Clin J Pain 2011;27(8):655–63.

703. Nijs J, Van Houdenhove B, Oostendorp RA. Recognition of central sensitization in patients with musculoskeletal pain: Application of pain neurophysiology in manual therapy practice. Man Ther 2010;15(2):135–41.

704. Smart KM, et al. Self-reported pain severity, quality of life, disability, anxiety and depression in patients classified with 'nociceptive', 'peripheral neuropathic' and 'central sensitisation' pain. The discriminant validity of mechanisms-based classifications of low back (+/-leg) pain. Man Ther 2012;17(2):119–25.

705. Nijs J, et al. Low back pain: guidelines for the clinical classification of predominant neuropathic, nociceptive, or central sensitization pain. Pain Physician 2015;18(3):E333–46.

706. Nijs J, et al. Applying modern pain neuroscience in clinical practice: criteria for the classification of central sensitization pain. Pain Physician 2014;17(5):447–57.

707. Desmeules JA, et al. Neurophysiologic evidence for a central sensitization in patients with fibromyalgia. Arthritis Rheum 2003;48(5):1420–9.

708. Meeus M, et al. Evidence for generalized hyperalgesia in chronic fatigue syndrome: a case control study. Clin Rheumatol 2010;29(4):393–8.

709. Kasch H, et al. Reduced cold pressor pain tolerance in non-recovered whiplash patients: a 1-year prospective study. Eur J Pain 2005;9(5):561–9.

710. Martenson ME, Cetas JS, Heinricher MM. A possible neural basis for stress-induced hyperalgesia. Pain 2009;142(3):236–44.

711. Nielsen LA, Henriksson KG. Pathophysiological mechanisms in chronic musculoskeletal pain (fibromyalgia): the role of central and peripheral sensitization and pain disinhibition. Best Pract Res Clin Rheumatol 2007;21(3):465–80.

712. Staud R, Rodriguez ME. Mechanisms of disease: pain in fibromyalgia syndrome. Nat Clin Pract Rheumatol 2006;2(2):90–8.

713. Kamper SJ, et al. Relationship between pressure pain thresholds and pain ratings in patients with whiplash-associated disorders. Clin J Pain 2011;27(6):495–501.

714. Sterling M. Testing for sensory hypersensitivity or central hyperexcitability associated with cervical spine pain. J Manipulative Physiol Ther 2008;31(7):534–9.

715. Scott D, Jull G, Sterling M. Widespread sensory hypersensitivity is a feature of chronic whiplash-associated disorder but not chronic idiopathic neck pain. Clin J Pain 2005;21(2):175–81.

716. Kosek E, et al. Evidence of different mediators of central inflammation in dysfunctional and inflammatory pain - Interleukin-8 in fibromyalgia and interleukin-1 beta in rheumatoid arthritis. J Neuroimmunol 2015;280:49–55.

717. O'Neill S, et al. Generalized deep-tissue hyperalgesia in patients with chronic low-back pain. Eur J Pain 2006.

718. Staud R, Robinson ME, Price DD. Temporal summation of second pain and its maintenance are useful for characterizing widespread central sensitization of fibromyalgia patients. J Pain 2007;8(11):893–901.

719. Imamura M, et al. Changes in pressure pain threshold in patients with chronic nonspecific low back pain. Spine 2013;38(24):2098–107.

720. Pavlakovic G, Petzke F. The role of quantitative sensory testing in the evaluation of musculoskeletal pain conditions. Curr Rheumatol Rep 2010;12(6):455–61.

721. Blumenstiel K, et al. Quantitative sensory testing profiles in chronic back pain are distinct from those in fibromyalgia. Clin J Pain 2011;27(8):682–90.

722. Sjors A, et al. An increased response to experimental muscle pain is related to psychological status in women with chronic non-traumatic neck-shoulder pain. BMC Musculoskelet Disord 2011;12:230.

723. Edwards RR, et al. Pain, catastrophizing, and depression in the rheumatic diseases. Nat Rev Rheumatol 2011;7(4):216–24.

724. Kosek E, Ordeberg G. Lack of pressure pain modulation by heterotopic noxious conditioning stimulation in patients with painful osteoarthritis before, but not following, surgical pain relief. Pain 2000;88(1):69–78.

725. Kosek E, Ordeberg G. Abnormalities of somatosensory perception in patients with painful osteoarthritis normalize following successful treatment. Eur J Pain 2000;4(3):229–38.

726. Gwilym SE, et al. Psychophysical and functional imaging evidence supporting the presence of central sensitization in a cohort of osteoarthritis patients. Arthritis Rheum 2009;61(9):1226–34.

727. Arendt-Nielsen L, et al. Sensitization in patients with painful knee osteoarthritis. Pain 2010;149(3):573–81.

728. Leffler AS, et al. Somatosensory perception and function of diffuse noxious inhibitory controls (DNIC) in patients suffering from rheumatoid arthritis. Eur J Pain 2002;6(2):161–76.

729. Vladimirova N, et al. Pain Sensitisation in Women with Active Rheumatoid Arthritis: A Comparative Cross-Sectional Study. Arthritis 2015;2015:434109.

730. Hochman JR, et al. Neuropathic pain symptoms on the modified painDETECT correlate with signs of central sensitization in knee osteoarthritis. Osteoarthritis Cartilage 2013;21(9):1236–42.

731. Malfliet A, et al. Lack of evidence for central sensitization in idiopathic, non-traumatic neck pain: a systematic review. Pain Physician 2015;18(3):223–36.

732. Woolf CJ. What is this thing called pain? J Clin Invest 2010;120(11):3742–4.

733. Costigan M, Scholz J, Woolf CJ. Neuropathic pain: a maladaptive response of the nervous system to damage. Annu Rev Neurosci 2009;32:1–32.

734. Salomons TV, et al. Pain flashbacks in posttraumatic stress disorder. Clin J Pain 2004;20(2):83–7.

735. Small DM, Apkarian AV. Increased taste intensity perception exhibited by patients with chronic back pain. Pain 2006;120(1–2):124–30.

736. Smart KM, et al. Clinical indicators of 'nociceptive', 'peripheral neuropathic' and 'central' mechanisms of musculoskeletal pain. A Delphi survey of expert clinicians. Man Ther 2010;15(1):80–7.

737. Smart K, Doody C. The clinical reasoning of pain by experienced musculoskeletal physiotherapists. Man Ther 2007;12(1):40–9.

738. Fuentes J, et al. Enhanced therapeutic alliance modulates pain intensity and muscle pain sensitivity in patients with chronic low back pain: an experimental controlled study. Phys Ther 2014;94(4):477–89.

739. Di Blasi Z, et al. Influence of context effects on health outcomes: a systematic review. Lancet 2001;357(9258):757–62.

740. Huibers MJ, Wessely S. The act of diagnosis: pros and cons of labelling chronic fatigue syndrome. Psychol Med 2006;36(7):895–900.

741. Kraemer HC, et al. Mediators and moderators of treatment effects in randomized clinical trials. Arch Gen Psychiatry 2002;59(10):877–83.

742. Carroll LJ, et al. Recovery in whiplash-associated disorders: do you get what you expect? J Rheumatol 2009;36(5):1063–70.

743. Ozegovic D, Carroll LJ, David Cassidy J. Does expecting mean achieving? The association between expecting to return to work and recovery in whiplash associated disorders: a population-based prospective cohort study. Eur Spine J 2009;18(6):893–9.

744. Kongsted A, et al. Expectation of recovery from low back pain: a longitudinal cohort study investigating patient characteristics related to expectations and the association between expectations and 3-month outcome. Spine 2014;39(1):81–90.

745. Daykin AR, Richardson B. Physiotherapists' pain beliefs and their influence on the management of patients with chronic low back pain. Spine 2004;29(7):783–95.

746. Turner JA, Holtzman S, Mancl L. Mediators, moderators, and predictors of therapeutic change in cognitive-behavioral therapy for chronic pain. Pain 2007;127(3):276–86.

747. Higgs J, Burn A, Jones M. Integrating clinical reasoning and evidence-based practice. AACN Clin Issues 2001;12(4):482–90.

748. Dworkin RH, et al. Interpreting the clinical importance of treatment outcomes in chronic pain clinical trials: IMMPACT recommendations. J Pain 2008;9(2):105–21.

749. Cleeland CS, Ryan KM. Pain assessment: global use of the Brief Pain Inventory. Ann Acad Med Singapore 1994;23(2):129–38.

750. Mendoza T, et al. Reliability and validity of a modified Brief Pain Inventory short form in patients with osteoarthritis. Eur J Pain 2006;10(4):353–61.

751. Von Korff M, et al. Grading the severity of chronic pain. Pain 1992;50(2):133–49.

752. Turk DC, Rudy TE. Toward an empirically derived taxonomy of chronic pain patients: integration of psychological assessment data. J Consult Clin Psychol 1988;56(2):233–8.

753. Kerns RD, Turk DC, Rudy TE. The West Haven-Yale Multidimensional Pain Inventory (WHYMPI). Pain 1985;23(4):345–56.

754. Westaway MD, Stratford PW, Binkley JM. The patient-specific functional scale: validation of its use in persons with neck dysfunction. J Orthop Sports Phys Ther 1998;27(5):331–8.

755. Ware JE Jr, Sherbourne CD. The MOS 36-item short-form health survey (SF-36). I. Conceptual framework and item selection. Med Care 1992;30(6):473–83.

756. Ware J Jr, Kosinski M, Keller SD. A 12-Item Short-Form Health Survey: construction of scales and preliminary tests of reliability and validity. Med Care 1996;34(3):220–33.

757. Roland M, Fairbank J. The Roland-Morris Disability Questionnaire and the Oswestry Disability Questionnaire. Spine 2000;25(24):3115–24.

758. Roland M, Morris R. A study of the natural history of back pain. Part I: development of a reliable and sensitive measure of disability in low-back pain. Spine 1983;8(2):141–4.

759. Vernon H, Mior S. The Neck Disability Index: a study of reliability and validity. J Manipulative Physiol Ther 1991;14(7):409–15.

760. Leak AM, et al. The Northwick Park Neck Pain Questionnaire, devised to measure neck pain and disability. Br J Rheumatol 1994;33(5):469–74.

761. Beck AT, Steer RA, Brown GK. Manual for Beck Depression Inventory-II. San Antonio: TX: Psychological Corporation; 1996.

762. Zigmond AS, Snaith RP. The hospital anxiety and depression scale. Acta Psychiatr Scand 1983;67(6):361–70.

763. McNair D, Lorr M, Droppleman L. Profile of Mood States. San Diego: CA: Educational and Industrial Testing Service; 1971.

764. McNeil DW, Rainwater AJ 3rd. Development of the Fear of Pain Questionnaire–III. J Behav Med 1998;21(4):389–410.

765. McCracken LM, Zayfert C, Gross RT. The Pain Anxiety Symptoms Scale: development and validation of a scale to measure fear of pain. Pain 1992;50(1):67–73.

766. Crowley D, Kendall A. Development and initial validation of a questionnaire for measuring fear-avoidance associated with pain: the fear-avoidance of pain scale. J Musculoskelet Pain 1999;7(3):3–19.

767. Miller R, Kori S, Todd D. The Tampa Scale. USA: Tampa, Fla; 1991.

768. Woby SR, et al. Psychometric properties of the TSK-11: a shortened version of the Tampa Scale for Kinesiophobia. Pain 2005;117(1–2):137–44.

769. Kugler K, Wijn J, Geilen M. The Photograph Series of Daily Activities (PHODA). The Netherlands, Amsterdam: Heerlen; 1999.

770. Sandborgh M, Lindberg P, Denison E. Pain belief screening instrument: Development and preliminary validation of a screening instrument for disabling persistent pain. J Rehabil Med 2007;39(6):461–6.

771. Linton SJ, Hallden K. Can we screen for problematic back pain? A screening questionnaire for predicting outcome in acute and subacute back pain. Clin J Pain 1998;14(3):209–15.

772. Riley JF, Ahern DK, Follick MJ. Chronic pain and functional impairment: assessing beliefs about their relationship. Arch Phys Med Rehabil 1988;69(8):579–82.

773. Hill JC, et al. Comparison of stratified primary care management for low back pain with current best practice (STarT Back): a randomised controlled trial. Lancet 2011;378(9802):1560–71.

774. Sullivan M, Bishop S, Pivik J. The Pain Catastrophizing Scale: development and validation. Psychol Assess 1995;7(4):524–32.

775. Tang NK, Salkovskis PM, Hanna M. Mental defeat in chronic pain: initial exploration of the concept. Clin J Pain 2007;23(3):222–32.

776. Brown GK, Nicassio PM. Development of a questionnaire for the assessment of active and passive coping strategies in chronic pain patients. Pain 1987;31(1):53–64.

777. Nicholas MK. The pain self-efficacy questionnaire: Taking pain into account. Eur J Pain 2007;11(2):153–63.

778. McCracken LM, Vowles KE, Eccleston C. Acceptance of chronic pain: component analysis and a revised assessment method. Pain 2004;107(1–2):159–66.

779. Guy W. ECDEU assessment manual for psychopharmacology (DHEW Publication No. ADM 76–338). Washington, DC: US Government Printing Office; 1976.

780. Kamper SJ, Maher CG, Mackay G. Global rating of change scales: a review of strengths and weaknesses and considerations for design. J Man Manip Ther 2009;17(3):163–70.

781. Linton SJ, Kamwendo K. Low back schools. A critical review. Phys Ther 1987;67(9):1375–83.

782. Cohen JE, et al. Group education interventions for people with low back pain. An overview of the literature. Spine 1994;19(11):1214–22.

783. Koes BW, et al. The efficacy of back schools: a review of randomized clinical trials. J Clin Epidemiol 1994;47(8):851–62.

784. Gross AR, et al. Patient education for mechanical neck disorders. Cochrane Database Syst Rev 2000;(2):CD000962.

785. Roland M, et al. The Back Book. 2nd ed. TSO The Stationery Office; 2002.

786. Waddell G. The Neck Book. TSO The Stationery Office; 2004.

787. Burton K, McClune T, Waddell G. The Whiplash Book. 2002.

788. Jull G. The Whiplash Injury Recovery. The University of Queensland; 2005.

789. McClune T, Burton AK, Waddell G. Evaluation of an evidence based patient educational booklet for management of whiplash associated disorders. Emerg Med J 2003;20(6):514–17.

790. Moseley GL, Nicholas MK, Hodges PW. A randomized controlled trial of intensive neurophysiology education in chronic low back pain. Clin J Pain 2004;20(5):324–30.

791. Ellis A. Rational Emotive Behavior Therapy: It Works for Me - It Can Work for You. New York: Prometheus Books; 2009.

792. Van Damme S, Crombez G, Eccleston C. Disengagement from pain: the role of catastrophic thinking about pain. Pain 2004;107(1–2):70–6.

793. Woby SR, Roach NK, Watson PJ. Outcome following a physiotherapist-led intervention for chronic low back pain: the important role of cognitive processes. Physiotherapy 2008;94:115–24.

794. Crombez G, et al. Pain-related fear is more disabling than pain itself: evidence on the role of pain-related fear in chronic back pain disability. Pain 1999;80(1–2):329–39.

795. Malenbaum S, et al. Pain in its environmental context: implications for designing environments to enhance pain control. Pain 2008;134(3):241–4.

796. Moseley G. Motor control in chronic pain: new ideas for effective intervention. In: Vleeming A, Mooney V, Stoeckart R, editors. Movement, Stability & Lumbopelvic Pain. Edinburgh.: Churchill Livingstone ELSEVIER; 2007. p. 513–25.

797. Acerra NE, Souvlis T, Moseley GL. Stroke, complex regional pain syndrome and phantom limb pain: can commonalities direct future management? J Rehabil Med 2007;39(2):109–14.

798. Moseley GL. Graded motor imagery is effective for long-standing complex regional pain syndrome: a randomised controlled trial. Pain 2004;108(1–2):192–8.

799. Moseley GL. Is successful rehabilitation of complex regional pain syndrome due to sustained attention to the affected limb? A randomised clinical trial. Pain 2005;114(1–2):54–61.

800. Ramachandran VS, Rogers-Ramachandran D. Synaesthesia in phantom limbs induced with mirrors. Proc Biol Sci 1996;263(1369):377–86.

801. Murray CD, et al. Immersive virtual reality as a rehabilitative technology for phantom limb experience: a protocol. Cyberpsychol Behav 2006;9(2):167–70.

802. Murray CD, et al. Can immersive virtual reality reduce phantom limb pain? Stud Health Technol Inform 2006;119:407–12.

803. Gallese V, et al. Action recognition in the premotor cortex. Brain 1996;119(Pt 2):593–609.

804. Rizzolatti G, Sinigaglia C. Mirror neurons and motor intentionality. Funct Neurol 2007;22(4):205–10.

805. Harris JC. Social neuroscience, empathy, brain integration, and neurodevelopmental disorders. Physiol Behav 2003;79(3):525–31.

806. McCabe CS, et al. A controlled pilot study of the utility of mirror visual feedback in the treatment of complex regional pain syndrome (type 1). Rheumatology (Oxford) 2003;42(1):97–101.

807. Liepert J, et al. Treatment-induced cortical reorganization after stroke in humans. Stroke 2000;31(6):1210–16.

808. Garry MI, Loftus A, Summers JJ. Mirror, mirror on the wall: viewing a mirror reflection of unilateral hand movements facilitates ipsilateral M1 excitability. Exp Brain Res 2005;163(1):118–22.

809. Funase K, et al. Increased corticospinal excitability during direct observation of self-movement and indirect observation with a mirror box. Neurosci Lett 2007;419(2):108–12.

810. McCabe CS, Haigh RC, Blake DR. Mirror visual feedback for the treatment of complex regional pain syndrome (type 1). Curr Pain Headache Rep 2008;12(2):103–7.

811. Karmarkar A, Lieberman I. Mirror box therapy for complex regional pain syndrome. Anaesthesia 2006;61(4):412–13.

812. Vladimir Tichelaar YI, et al. Mirror box therapy added to cognitive behavioural therapy in three chronic complex regional pain syndrome type I patients: a pilot study. Int J Rehabil Res 2007;30(2):181–8.

813. Selles RW, Schreuders TA, Stam HJ. Mirror therapy in patients with causalgia (complex regional pain syndrome type II) following peripheral nerve injury: two cases. J Rehabil Med 2008;40(4):312–14.

814. Chan BL, et al. Mirror therapy for phantom limb pain. N Engl J Med 2007;357(21):2206–7.

815. Graziano MS. Where is my arm? The relative role of vision and proprioception in the neuronal representation of limb position. Proc Natl Acad Sci USA 1999;96(18):10418–21.

816. Ro T, et al. Visual enhancing of tactile perception in the posterior parietal cortex. J Cogn Neurosci 2004;16(1):24–30.

817. Moseley GL, Gallace A, Spence C. Is mirror therapy all it is cracked up to be? Current evidence and future directions. Pain 2008;138(1):7–10.

818. Lundborg G, Rosen B. Hand function after nerve repair. Acta Physiol (Oxf) 2007;189(2):207–17.

819. Moseley GL. Graded motor imagery for pathologic pain: a randomized controlled trial. Neurology 2006;67(12):2129–34.

820. Priganc VW, Stralka SW. Graded motor imagery. J Hand Ther 2011;24(2):164–8, quiz 169.

821. Daly AE, Bialocerkowski AE. Does evidence support physiotherapy management of adult Complex Regional Pain Syndrome Type One? A systematic review. Eur J Pain 2009;13(4):339–53.

822. Moseley GL. I can't find it! Distorted body image and tactile dysfunction in patients with chronic back pain. Pain 2008;140(1):239–43.

823. Flor H, et al. Effect of sensory discrimination training on cortical reorganisation and phantom limb pain. Lancet 2001;357(9270):1763–4.

824. Dolce JJ, et al. Exercise quotas, anticipatory concern and self-efficacy expectancies in chronic pain: a preliminary report. Pain 1986;24(3):365–72.

825. Vlaeyen JW, et al. The treatment of fear of movement/(re)injury in chronic low back pain: further evidence on the effectiveness of exposure in vivo. Clin J Pain 2002;18(4):251–61.

826. Fordyce W, et al. Pain complaint–exercise performance relationship in chronic pain. Pain 1981;10(3):311–21.

INDEX